ATI

Management of Fractures in Severely Osteoporotic Bone

Springer
London
Berlin
Heidelberg
New York
Barcelona
Hong Kong
Milan
Paris
Singapore
Tokyo

Karl Obrant (Ed)

Management of Fractures in Severely Osteoporotic Bone

Orthopedic and Pharmacologic Strategies

Springer

Karl Obrant, Professor of Orthopaedics
Head of the Department of Medicine, Surgery and Orthopaedics
Malmö University Hospital
S-205 02 Malmö
Sweden

ISBN 1-85233-220-4 Springer-Verlag London Berlin Heidelberg

British Library Cataloguing in Publication Data
Management of fractures in severely osteoporotic bone:
orthopaedic and pharmacologic strategies
1. Osteoporosis 2. Fractures – Treatment
I. Obrant, Karl
616.7'16
ISBN 1852332204

Library of Congress Cataloging-in-Publication Data
Management of fractures in severely osteoporotic bone: orthopaedic and pharmacologic strategies/Karl Obrant (ed).
p. ; cm.
Includes bibliographical references and index.
ISBN 1-85233-220-4 (alk. paper)
1. Fractures. 2. Osteoporosis – Complications. I. Obrant, Karl, 1948– .
[DNLM: 1. Fractures – surgery. 2. Fractures – etiology. 3. Fractures – prevention & control. 4. Osteoporosis – complications. 5. Osteoporosis – drug therapy. WE 175 M266 2000
RD101.M28 2000
617.1'5 – dc21 99-053907

Printed in Great Britain

Typeset by Florence Production Ltd, Stoodleigh, Devon
Printed and bound at The Cromwell Press, Trowbridge, Wiltshire, England
28/3830-543210 Printed on acid-free paper SPIN 10745424

Foreword

Over the past decade, major advances have taken place in the management of osteoporosis. New classes of pharmaceutical agents have been developed, tested, and used to treat millions of patients; education and early detection programs have been instituted around the world; and bone densitometry has received widespread recognition by healthcare agencies as being central to the preventive health strategy necessary to care for an aging population. With all these advances, scientists continue to explore new methods to understand and treat this disease. The field of orthopaedic surgery has a great opportunity to bring this new information to its clinics and operating rooms. It is critically important that the practicing surgeon be armed with this knowledge.

Fractures are clearly the most common orthopaedic problem associated with osteoporosis. The goals of treatment are rapid restoration of mobility and function and return of patients to a level of activity that supports their general health. The ability to control the metabolic condition or to treat the underlying cause of the osteoporosis with pharmacological intervention will improve surgical results. Moreover, the special techniques required to succeed in the operative treatment of bone, which is already weakened by osteoporosis, must be carefully developed, tested, and understood. This book provides the first attempt to bring this body of information to the orthopaedic surgeon in a clearly organized and comprehensive way.

Historically, few orthopaedic surgery or trauma training programs have offered much in the way of education in the science of bone metabolism. Moreover, few such programs have the expertise to teach the newer concepts of this evolving field in a way which adequately addresses the different aspects of management of osteoporotic patients and the latest methods of diagnosis. The development of pharmacological agents and how they should be used in conjunction with surgical or operative strategies is just now beginning to evolve as a new subdiscipline of orthopaedics. The involvement of orthopaedists and trauma surgeons in osteoporosis prevention programs and public awareness efforts is a necessary step towards the ultimate goal of reducing the prevalence of this problem in the future.

The reader of this text will have a unique opportunity to acquire an understanding of this field that differs from that obtained from existing books on osteoporosis or articles on new technologies in assessing bone quality or quantity. As the basic information on advances in detection and diagnosis, and on medical and surgical management, weave their way through each chapter, a higher order of knowledge will be achieved and this is precisely the type of knowledge required in order to bring the best care to our patients. The editor and contributors are deserving of both our praise and thanks. It is a privilege to introduce this book to you.

Thomas A. Einhorn, M.D.
Boston University School of Medicine

Preface

A substantial number, not to say the majority, of patients seeking medical advice or treatment from an orthopaedic surgeon, have osteoporosis. As late as in 1992, at an international conference, in a discussion with a world-famous professor of orthopaedic surgery, he asked me why I was interested in osteoporosis research. His opinion, and probably the prevailing opinion among orthopaedic surgeons at that time and, unfortunately, still today, was that osteoporosis "was an inevitable disease with an increased prevalence with age just like having grey hair. There is nothing that can be done about it." Also, in a recent volume (1998) of one of the highest-ranked orthopaedic journals it was stated that "osteoporosis can be definitely diagnosed only on the basis of histologic examination but it is suggested by dual energy x-ray absorptiometry (DEXA) values 2 standard deviations from the norm". Such profoundly erroneous information, given in highly reputed scientific journals on orthopaedics, alone is sufficient motivation to produce this book.

A further intention of the book is to combine into one volume our present body of knowledge concerning all aspects of the treatment of osteoporosis and osteoporotic fracture. Thus there are chapters on diagnosis and prevention as well as on the treatment of patients who have already sustained fractures due to osteoporosis. I believe that this book, with its 41 chapters, each written by international experts in their fields, will contribute to a better understanding of the disease and to a profound insight into different orthopaedic treatment options in fractures of severely osteoporotic bone. It is also my hope that the physician who is not an orthopaedic surgeon but who treats these patients, either in order to prevent fractures or in rehabilitation practice, will be enlightened by the information given in this book.

Karl Obrant

Contents

III: Orthopaedic Management Options

Hip Fracture

IV: Nonpharmacological Prevention of Osteoporotic Fractures

V: Pharmacological Prevention of Osteoporotic Fractures

VI: Identification and Management of Secondary or Localized Bone Loss

Contributors

R. Barkmann
Osteoporosediagnostik Kiel, Klinik für Diagnostiche Radiologie, Christian-Albrechts-Universität du Kiel, Michaelisstrasse 9, D-24105 Kiel, Germany

M. R. Baumgaertner
Department of Orthopaedics, Yale School of Medicine, P.O. Box 208071, New Haven, CT 06520-8071, USA

U. Berlemann
Department of Orthopaedic Surgery, Inselspital Bern, Freiburgstrasse, CH-3010 Bern, Switzerland

S. Brandsson
Department of Orthopaedics, Östra Hospital, SE-41685 Göteborg, Sweden

S. Boonen
Division of Geriatric Medicine, UZ Gasthuisberg, B-3000 Leuven, Belgium

P. L. O. Broos
Department of Traumatology, University Hospital Gasthuisberg, Herestraat 49, B-3000 Leuven, Belgium

Å. Carlsson
Department of Orthopaedics, Malmö University Hospital, S-20502 Malmö, Sweden

M. Chigira
Department of Orthopaedic Surgery, Faculty of Medicine, Gunma University, 3-39-22 Showa, Maebashi, Gunma, Japan

J. E. Compston
Department of Medicine Box 157, University of Cambridge, School of Medicine, Addenbrooke's Hospital, Cambridge CB2 2QQ, UK

J. Dequeker
Department of Rheumatology, Weligerveld 1, B-3212 Pellenberg, Belgium

P. U. Dijkstra
Pain Centre, University Hospital Groningen, Groningen, The Netherlands

E. F. Eriksen
University Department of Endocrinology, Aarhus Amtssygehus, DK-8000 Aarhus C, Denmark

H. Fleisch
Avenue Déscartes 5, CH-1009 Pully, Switzerland

J. H. B. Geertzen
Department of Rehabilitation, University Hospital Groningen, Groningen, The Netherlands

C. Gerber
Department of Orthopaedics, University of Zurich, Balgrist, Forchstrasse 340, CH-8008 Zurich, Switzerland

P. Geusens
Clinical Research Unit for Bone and Joint Diseases, Biomedical Research Institute, Limburgs Universitaire Centrum, B-3590 Diepenbeek, Belgium

L. Willems Instituut, Limburgs Universitair Centrum, B-3590 Diepenbeek, Belgium

H. Glerup
University Department of Endocrinology, Aarhus Amtssygehus, DK-8000 Aarhus C, Denmark

C.-C. Glüer
Osteoporosediagnostik Kiel, Klinik für Diagnostiche Radiologie, Christian-Albrechts-Universität du Kiel, Michaelisstrasse 9, D-24105 Kiel, Germany

V. Halkin
Bone and Cartilage Research Unit, University of Liège, CHU Centre-Ville, 45 Quai Godefroid Kurth (+9), B-4020 Liège, Belgium

H. Hastings II
The Indiana Hand Center, 8501 Harcourt Road, Indianapolis, IN 46250, USA

W. C. Hayes
Oregon State University, 312 Kerr Administration Building, Corvallis, OR 97331-2140, USA

P. F. Heini
Department of Orthopaedic Surgery, Inselspital Bern, Freiburgstrasse, CH-3010 Bern, Switzerland

M. H. Hessmann
Department of Traumatology, University Hospitals of the Johannes Gutenberg University of Mainz, Lagenbeckenstrasse 1, D-55131 Mainz, Germany

R. Hoffmann
Städtische Kliniken Offenbach, Unfallchirurgische Klinik, Starkenburgring 66, Postfach 101964, D-63019 Offenbach, Germany

R. Honkanen
Research Institute of Public Health, University of Kuopio, Kuopio, Finland

R. Huiskes
Orthopaedic Research Laboratory, University of Nijmegen, PO Box 9101, 6500 HB Nijmegen, The Netherlands

J. Z Ilich
School of Allied Health, University of Connecticut, 358 Mansfield Road, Box U-101, Storrs, CT 06269-2101, USA

Manabu Ito
Department of Orthopaedic Surgery, Hokkaido University School of Medicine, Kita-15, Nishi-7, Kitaku 060-8638, Sapporo, Japan

J.-E. B. Jensen
The Osteoporosis Centre, Copenhagen Municipal Hospital, Øster Farimagsgade 5, DK-1399 Copenhagen, Denmark

T. R Johnson
Hospital for Special Surgery, 535 East 70th Street, New York NY 10021, USA

T. S Kaastad
Orthopaedic Research Laboratory, University of Nijmegen, PO Box 9101, 6500 HB Nijmegen, The Netherlands

K. Kaneda
Department of Orthopaedic Surgery, Hokkaido University School of Medicine, Kita-15, Nishi-7, Kitaku 060-8638, Sapporo, Japan

P. Kannus
Accident and Trauma Research Center, UKK Institute for Health Promotion Research, P.O. Box 30, FIN-33501 Tampere, Finland

J. Karlsson
Department of Orthopaedics, Östra Hospital, SE-41685 Göteborg, Sweden

J. E. Kerstetter
School of Allied Health, University of Connecticut, 358 Mansfield Road, Box U-101, Storrs, CT 06269-2101, USA

S Kolbeck
Charité, Humboldt-Universität zu Berlin, Campus Virchow Klinikum, Unfall- und Wiederherstellungschirurgie, Augustenburger Platz 1, D-13353 Berlin, Germany

H. Kröger
Department of Surgery, Kuopio University Hospital, FIN-70211 Kuopio, Finland

J. M. Lane
Hospital for Special Surgery, 535 East 70th Street, New York, NY 10021, USA

E. M. C. Lau
The Chinese University of Hong Kong, Department of Community and Family Medicine, 4/F Lek Yuen Health Centre, Shatin, N.T., Hong Kong

K.-H. W. Lau
Musculoskeletal Disease Center (151), Jerry L. Pettis Memorial V.A. Medical Center, 11201 Benton Street, Loma Linda, CA 92357, USA

J. B. Lauritzen
Department of Orthopaedic Surgery 333, Hvidovre Hospital, University of Copenhagen, Kettegaard Alle 30, DK-2650 Copenhagen, Denmark

P. C. Leung
The Chinese University of Hong Kong, Department of Community and Family Medicine, 4/F Lek Yuen Health Centre, Shatin, N.T., Hong Kong

J. E. Madsen
Orthopaedic Department, Ullevål Hospital, N-0407 Oslo, Norway

J. Magaziner
Division of Gerontology, Department of Epidemiology and Preventive Medicine, School of Medicine, 660 W Redwood St, Suite 200, Baltimore, MD 21201, USA

J. L. Marsh
Department of Orthopaedics, University of Iowa Hospitals and Clinics, Iowa City, IA 52242, USA

M. McClung
Oregon Osteoporosis Center, 5050 N.E. Hoyt, Suite 651, Portland, OR 97213, USA

M. Möller
Department of Orthopaedics, Östra Hospital, SE-41685 Göteborg, Sweden

L. Nordsletten
Orthopaedic Department, Ullevål Hospital, N-0407 Oslo, Norway

K. Obrant
Department of Orthopaedics, Malmö University Hospital, S-205 02 Malmö, Sweden

A. Oladipo
Endocrinology and Metabolic Medicine, Imperial College School of Medicine, London W2 1PG, UK

S. L. Olmsted
Department of Orthopaedic Surgery, University of California, Davis, School of Medicine, 4860 Y Street, Suite 3800, Sacramento, CA 95817, USA

S. Ortolani
Centro Malattie Metaboliche Dell'Osso, Istituto Auxologico Italiano IRCCS, Via Ariosto 13, I-20145 Milan, Italy

R. L. Prince
Department of Medicine, University of Western Australia, Nedlands, WA 6907, Australia

G. A. Pryor
Edith Cavell Hospital, Bretton Gate, Peterborough PE3 9GZ, UK

M. D. Putnam
Department of Orthopaedic Surgery, University of Minnesota, 420 Delaware Street SE, Box 992, Minneapolis, MN 55455, USA

I. Ravelingien
Department of Rheumatology, Weligerveld 1, B-3212 Pellenberg, Belgium

J.-Y. Reginster
Bone and Cartilage Research Unit, University of Liège, CHU Centre-Ville, 45 Quai Godefroid Kurth (+9), B-4020 Liège, Belgium

M. R Robichaux
The Indiana Hand Center, 8501 Harcourt Road, Indianapolis, IN 46250, USA

F. M. A. Robijns
Department of Traumatology, University Hospital Gasthuisberg, Herestraat 49, B-3000 Leuven, Belgium

P. M. Rommens
Department of Traumatology, University Hospitals of the Johannes Gutenberg University of Mainz, Lagenbeckenstrasse 1, D-55131 Mainz, Germany

H. E Rubash
GRJ 1125 Biomaterials Research, Massachusetts General Hospital, 55 Fruit Street, Boston, MA 02114, USA

L. Sanzén
Department of Orthopaedics, Malmö University Hospital, S-20502 Malmö, Sweden

A. S. Shanbhag
GRJ 1125 Biomaterials Research, Massachusetts General Hospital, 55 Fruit Street, Boston, Massachusetts MA 02114, USA

H. Sievänen
Accident and Trauma Research Center, UKK Institute for Health Promotion Research, PO Box 30, FIN-33501 Tampere, Finland

H. A. Sørensen
The Osteoporosis Centre, Copenhagen Municipal Hospital, Øster Farimagsgade 5, DK-1399 Copenhagen, Denmark

O. H. Sørensen
The Osteoporosis Centre, Copenhagen Municipal Hospital, Øster Farimagsgade 5, DK-1399 Copenhagen, Denmark

J. C. Stevenson
Endocrinology and Metabolic Medicine, Imperial College School of Medicine, London W2 1PG, UK

R. M. Szabo
Department of Orthopaedic Surgery, University of California, Davis, School of Medicine, 4860 Y Street, Suite 3800, Sacramento, CA 95817, USA

E. Tomin
Hospital for Special Surgery, 535 East 70th Street, New York NY 10021, USA

C. Trevisan
Clinica Ortopedica, Ospedale San Gerardo, Via Donizzetti 106, I-20052 Monza (MI), Italy

Dirk Vanderschueren
Department of Endocrinology, UZ Gasthuisberg, B-3000 Leuven, Belgium

Patrick Vienne
Department of Orthopaedics, University of Zurich, Balgrist, Forchstrasse 340, CH-8008 Zurich, Switzerland

C. Wahl
Department of Orthopaedics, Yale School of Medicine, PO Box 208071, New Haven, CT 06520-8071, USA

L. Wehren
Division of Gerontology, Department of Epidemiology and Preventive Medicine, School of Medicine, 660 W Redwood Street, Suite 200, Baltimore, MD 21201, USA

R. Westhovens
Department of Rheumatology, Weligerveld 1, B-3212 Pellenberg, Belgium

C. Wüster
University of Heidelberg, Department of Internal Medicine I, Endocrinology and Metabolism, Im Neuenheimer Feld 400, D-69120 Heidelberg, Germany

Part I

General Aspects of Osteoporosis and Fracture

1 The Size of the Problem

E. M. C. Lau and P. C. Leung

Introduction

Osteoporosis has been present in human populations for thousands of years. This condition was described in ancient Egypt as early as 1990 BC [1]. As the world population ages, osteoporosis is presenting itself as a "silent epidemic". Although osteoporosis is largely asymptomatic, it is associated with significant mortality and morbidity. The health care cost for this condition is also very high. It is predicted that the burden of illness due to osteoporosis will continue to increase exponentially.

The Size of the Problem

The size of the problem of osteoporosis can be considered from two perspectives: the incidence of fractures and the prevalence of "low bone mass". Both will be reviewed here.

Fracture Epidemiology

Fractures of the hip, vertebra and forearm are known to be due to osteoporosis. They share common epidemiological features: the incidence is higher in women than in men, incidence increases exponentially with age, and the fractures occur at sites with a large proportion of trabecular bone [2].

It is increasingly being recognized, however, that osteoporosis can lead to fracture at other sites. For instance, fractures of the proximal humerus [3] and pelvis [4] are considered to be osteoporosis related. This implies that the size of the problem of osteoporotic fractures is probably much larger than has been realized in the past.

Hip Fracture

World Pattern. There is pronounced geographical variation in the incidence of hip fracture, with rates being highest in Caucasians living in North Europe, followed

Table 1.1. Age-adjusted rate[a] of hip fracture per 100 000 population for women and men, by ethnic group and year of study

Ethnic group	Site	Female to Year of study	Women	Men	Male ratio
Black	Maryland, USA	1979–1988	345	191	1.8
	California, USA	1983–1984	241	153	1.6
	Johannesburg, South Africa	1950–1964	26	29	1.3
Hispanic	California, USA	1983–1984	219	97	2.3
	Texas, USA	1980	305	128	2.4
Asian	Hong Kong	1985	389	196	2.0
	Hong Kong	1965–1967	179	113	1.6
	Tottori, Japan	1986–1987	227	79	2.9
	Okinawa, Japan	1984–1985	325	86	3.8
	California, USA	1983–1984	383	116	3.3
	Hawaii, USA	1979–1981	224	66	3.4
	New Zealand	1973–1976	212	121	1.8
	Singapore	1955–1962	83	111	0.7
Caucasian	Sweden	1972–1981	730	581	1.3
	Kuopio, Finland	1968	280	107	2.6
	Malmö, Sweden	1950–1960	468	153	3.1
	Norway	1983–1984	737	298	2.5
	Edinburgh, UK	1978–1979	529	174	3.0
	Oxford,UK	1983	603	114	5.3
	California, USA	1983–1984	617	215	2.9
	Hawaii, USA	1979–1981	645	205	3.1
	New Zealand	1973–1976	466	139	3.4

Reproduced with permission from Villa and Nelson [5].

[a]Rates were age- and gender-adjusted to the 1990 US non-Hispanic Caucasian population.

by rates in Caucasians living in North America. The rates are intermediate in Orientals and lowest in black populations (Table 1.1) [5]. Moreover, the female to male ratio for hip fracture is 3:1 in Caucasians but 1:1 in Chinese and the Bantu.

There is some evidence that the incidence of hip fracture is rising rapidly in developing Asian countries. For instance, in Hong Kong, a highly urbanized city in China, the incidence of hip fracture has increased by 200% in the past three decades [6]. Such an increase draws the Asian rates much closer to Caucasian rates. Indeed, Cooper et al. [7] have projected that, by the year 2050, more than half of all hip fractures in the world will occur in Asia (Fig.1.1). The projected number of fractures will be 6.3 million, with 3.2 million occurring in Asia.

Secular Trends. Recent research suggests that the incidence of hip fracture has experienced either a levelling off or a slight downturn in North America and Europe. In Malmö, Sweden, Gulberg et al. [8] describe a levelling off of hip fracture incidence during the mid-1980s. Nungu et al. [9] reported that the age-adjusted incidence of hip fracture remained at around 6 per 1000 population in Uppsala county, Sweden in the same period. In the canton of Vaud, Switzerland, Jéquier et al. [10] found a slight increase in hip fracture incidence in Swiss men, but not in women, from 1986 to 1991. In Siena, Italy, the incidence of hip fracture increased slightly in men, but not in women from 1980 to 1991 [11].

The time trends for hip fracture in the UK from 1968 to 1986 were studied by Spector et al. [12], using data from the Hospital Inpatient Enquiry. The standard-

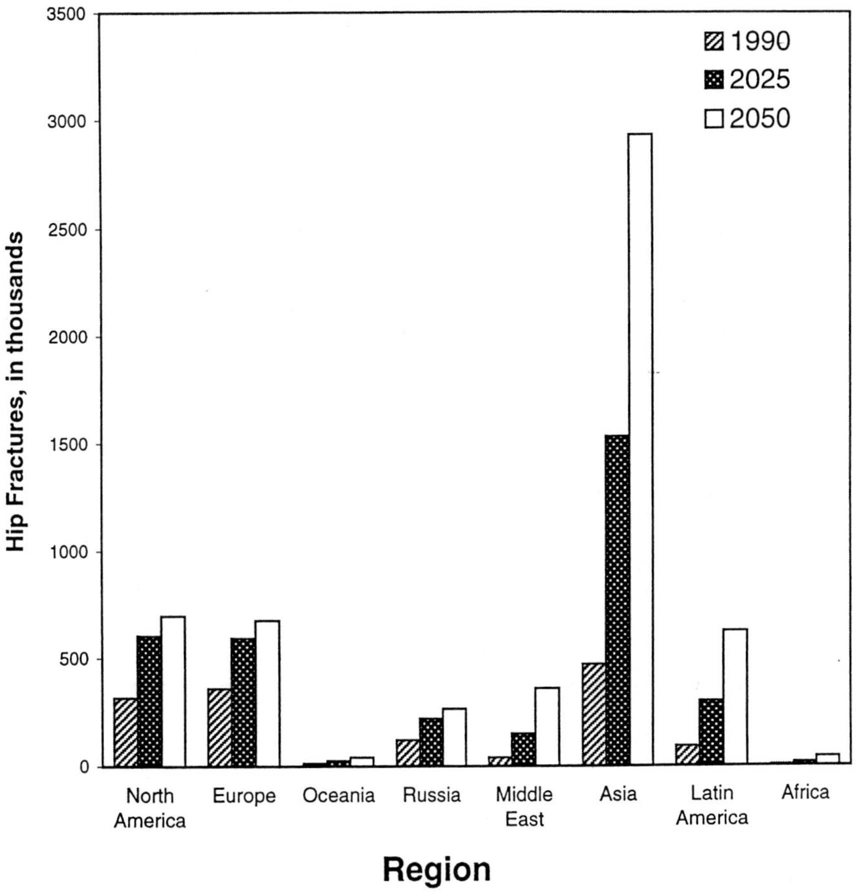

Figure 1.1. Estimated numbers of hip fractures in eight geographic regions in 1990, 2025 and 2050. Reproduced with permission from Cooper et al. [7].

ized admission rates for hip fracture increased tremendously from 1968 to 1980 in both sexes, after which the rates levelled off. A more recent study by Evans et al. [13] confirmed these results.

Similar trends have been observed in North America. Melton et al. [14] reported a downturn in hip fracture incidence in Rochester, Minnesota, between 1984 and 1987. It is not known whether such changes are due to health education, lifestyle changes or cohort effects. Assuming no increase in hip fracture incidence, the number of hip fracture patients will continue to rise in all continents, as a result of population aging (Fig. 1.1) [7].

Incidence by Sex and Age. The incidence of hip fracture by age in men and women in Rochester, Minnesota, was described by Cooper and Melton [15] (Fig. 1.2). The incidence in Rochester rose from 2 per 100 000 person-years among women less than 35 years old to 3032 per 100 000 for women 85 years old and over [15]. Although the annual incidence among young men was similar to that in young women, the

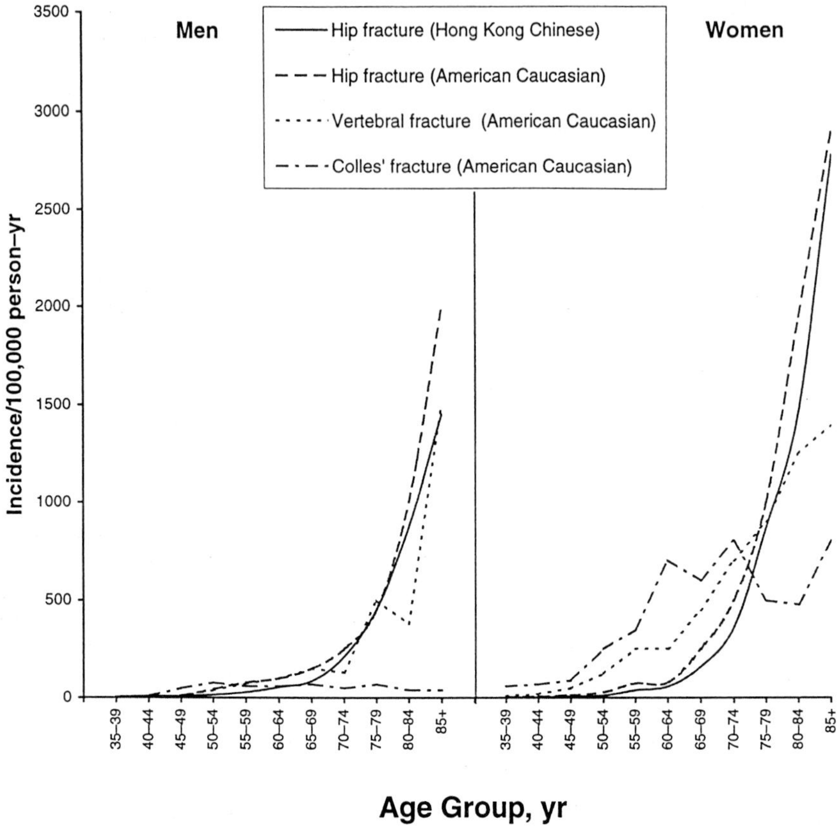

Figure 1.2. Age-specific incidence rates of hip, vertebral and Colles" fracture in Caucasian and Chinese men and women. Data for American Caucasians are reproduced with permission from Cooper and Melton [15]; data for Hong Kong Chinese are fromLau (unpublished data).

rates in elderly men were only half those in elderly women [15]. These patterns were representative of those in Caucasian populations.

The age-specific rates of hip fracture in Hong Kong Chinese in 1995 are also presented in Fig. 1.2 [Lau, unpublished data]. The changes in the incidence of hip fracture with age are similar to those observed in Rochester. While the incidence was similar in young men and women, an exponential rise was seen in women from 65 years of age onwards and in men from 70 years onwards. The rates in elderly women remained twice as high as those in elderly men. In general, the incidence rates for hip fracture in elderly Chinese men were 75% of those observed in Rochester, while the rates in elderly women approached 90% of those observed in Rochester.

The large increase in hip fracture incidence with age can be attributed both to a decrease in bone mass and an increase in falls with age. Results from the Study of Osteoporotic Fractures showed that women with bone density in the lowest quartile had an 8.5-fold greater risk of hip fracture than those in the highest quartile [16]. This concurred with a previous observation by Riggs and Melton [17] that bone mineral density was a consistent and strong predictor of osteoporotic fractures. As bone density declines rapidly after 60 years of age, the incidence of hip fracture rises rapidly. The incidence of falls also rises rapidly with age, more so in women than in men. The probability of experiencing at least one fall in a year rises from 25% in women 60–64 years old to 35% in women 80–84 years old [18].

Vertebral Fracture

In early epidemiological studies of vertebral fracture, a diagnosis of wedge, crush and biconcave deformities was made by subjective reading of X-ray films. Such procedures were poorly reproducible and made comparative epidemiological studies difficult. Standardization of methods for defining vertebral fracture was carried out by researchers in the last decade. In recent studies, radiographs have been taken under standard conditions, allowing vertebral height ratios to be calculated for defining vertebral fracture by fixed cutoff values. Standardization of methods has enhanced international comparison of vertebral fracture prevalence.

International Pattern. The results of the European Vertebral Osteoporosis Study (EVOS) [19] are presented with data from American Caucasians [20–22] and Hong Kong Chinese [23] in Fig. 1.3. In all these studies a diagnosis of vertebral fracture was made from lateral spine radiographs, defining a fracture as a reduction in vertebral height ratio by 3 standard deviations or more below the mean. The results of EVOS showed that the prevalence of vertebral fracture was highest in Scandinavia and lowest in Eastern Europe. The prevalence rates of vertebral fracture in American Caucasian women and Hong Kong Chinese women were as high as in Northern Europeans, while the rates in Hong Kong Chinese men and American Caucasian men were lower than in European men.

The Incidence of Vertebral Fracture. The incidence of vertebral fracture in Rochester has been precisely described (Fig. 1.2) [19]. In this study, the incidence of vertebral fracture rose from less than 0.2 per 1000 per year in men and women under 45 years of age, to 12 per 1000 in men and women aged 85 years and over.

Temporal Trends. The temporal trends for vertebral fracture are not as well studied as for hip fracture, and the results are mixed. According to Bengnèr et al. [25], the prevalence of vertebral fracture increased in Sweden between the periods 1950–1952 and 1982–1983. Nevertheless, the temporal trend was found to be stable in Denmark from 1979 to 1989 [26]; and in Rochester, Minnesota, from 1950 to 1989 [27].

Distal Forearm Fracture

The change in incidence with age for distal forearm fracture is different from that for fractures of the hip and vertebra. Study results from the Mayo Clinic found that incidence rates increased linearly from age 40 to 65 years and then stabilized [15]. However, in men the incidence remained relatively constant between 20 and 80 years of age. The female to male ratio for forearm fracture was 4 to 1. This ratio was much larger than that of 2 to 1 for vertebral and hip fracture.

The reasons why the incidence of forearm fracture plateaus with age are unknown. Nevitt and Cummings [28] proposed that elderly women have a slower gait and impaired neuromuscular coordination, and are hence more likely to fall backwards to land on their hip. On the other hand, younger women tended to fall on their

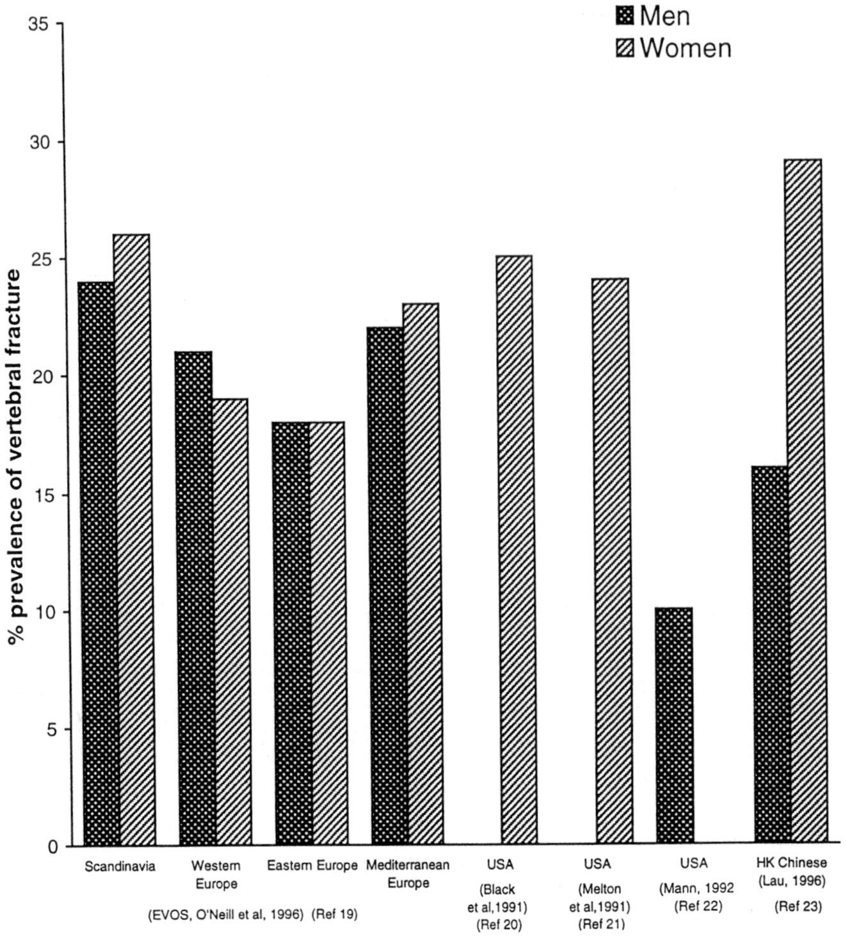

Figure 1.3. The prevalence of vertebral deformity in men and women from various countries.

outstretched arms. The changes in the incidence of forearm fracture with age concur with the pattern of age-related bone loss [29].

The international pattern for forearm fracture is not well described. There is some evidence to suggest that forearm fracture is much less frequent in Asian [30] and black [31] populations than in Caucasians.

Other Fractures

Besides fractures of the hip, vertebra and forearm, several other fractures may be related to osteoporosis. These include fracture of the proximal humerus, pelvis, proximal tibia and distal femur. The epidemiology of these fractures is similar to that of other osteoporotis-related fractures. Firstly, these fractures are more common in elderly women than in men, with 75% of proximal humerus fractures [3] and 70% of pelvic fractures occurring in women [4]. Such fractures also occur with minimal trauma: with 75% of proximal humerus fractures [3,32], 80% of pelvic

Table 1.2. The prevalence (%) of osteoporosis in American Caucasians and Hong Kong Chinese

Age (years)	At the spine		At the hip	
	American Caucasians	Hong Kong Chinese	American Caucasians	Hong Kong Chinese
50–59	15%	9%	1.2%	0%
60–69	32%	46%	22%	23%
70–79	44%	54%	37%	55%
⩾80	48%	56%	68%	71%
Total	24%	36%	23%	28%

Data for American Caucasians are reproduced with permission from Melton [34]. Data for Hong Kong Chinese are reproduced with permission from Ho SC et al. [35].

fractures [4], 60% of tibia fractures and 50% of distal forearm fractures [33] result from mild trauma. Exclusion of such fractures will result in underestimation of the magnitude of the problem due to osteoporosis.

The Prevalence of Osteoporosis

The prevalence of osteoporosis can be defined as the percentage of the population with a bone mineral density of 2.5 standard deviations or more below the young normal mean. Such data for American Caucasian and Hong Kong Chinese are presented in Table 1.2 [34,35]. The prevalence of osteoporosis was extremely high in both populations, with a quarter of postmenopausal women designated as being osteoporotic. It has been estimated that 26 million white women in America are afflicted with osteoporosis [34].

Consequences of Osteoporotic Fractures

Mortality

The mortality attributable to osteoporosis results largely from hip fractures. Hip fracture causes a 12–20% reduction in expected survival [36]. Hospital-based studies have shown that mortality rates are higher in men [37], older patients [38] and in non-white populations [38,39]. Such observations can be explained by the difference in the prevalence of chronic and degenerative disease in population subgroups [40]. Most of the excess mortality occurs in the 6 months after a hip fracture [41].

Morbidity and Quality of Life

Many hip fracture patients become permanently disabled. The percentage who cannot walk rises from 20% to 50% after a hip fracture [42]. Up to a third become totally dependent, necessitating institutionalization [43].

Although vertebral fracture causes many fewer deaths than hip fracture, it affects morbidity and quality of life considerably. Ettinger et al. demonstrated in two separate studies [44,45] that vertebral fracture caused significant back pain, disability and height loss in Americans. Two other studies showed that vertebral fracture caused a reduction in quality of life by pain, functional limitations and low mood [46,47]. The effects of vertebral fracture on back pain and low morale were consistently demonstrated in Chinese men and women [48].

Costs of Osteoporosis

Hip fracture is a major cause of hospital admission in the elderly. The acute care cost associated with hip fracture is tremendous in all developed countries. In the USA, the direct cost of hip fractures was around US$7035 million per year recently [49]. In the UK, the direct cost for hip fracture was £750 million per year in 1994 [50]. In Hong Kong, the acute hospital care cost of hip fracture per annum amounted to 1% of the total hospital budget, or US$17 million, for a population of 6 million [Lau, unpublished data].

In the USA, nursing home care cost for hip fracture was as much as US$1565 million in 1992 [49]. This approximated 22% of the total direct cost for hip fracture. As death due to hip fracture occurs mainly in the elderly, the indirect cost due to reduced productivity is much lower than for other chronic disorders such as ischemic heart disease, stroke or breast cancer.

Conclusion

Osteoporosis is a major public health problem. As the world population ages, the magnitude of the problem will continue to rise on an exponential scale. Prevention will be the only cost-effective means to deal with this problem.

References

1. Dequeker J, Ortner DJ, Stix AI. Hip fracture and osteoporosis in a XIIth Dynasty female skeleton from Lisht, Upper Egypt. J Bone Miner Res 1997;12:881–888.
2. Melton LJ III. Epidemiology of fractures. In: Riggs BL, Melton LJ III, editors. Osteoporosis: etiology, diagnosis and management. New York: Raven Press, 1995:225–248.
3. Rose SH, Melton LJ III, Morrey BF, Ilstrup DM, Riggs BL. Epidemiologic features of humeral fractures. Clin Orthop 1982;168:24–30.
4. Melton LJ III, Sampson JM, Morrey BF, Ilstrup DM. Epidemiologic features of pelvic fractures. Clin Orthop 1981;155:43–47.
5. Villa ML, Nelson L. Race, ethnicity, and osteoporosis. In: Marcus R, Feldman D, Kelsey J, editors. Osteoporosis. San Diego: Academic Press, 1996:435–447.
6. Lau EMC, Cooper C, Wickham C, Donnan S, Barker DJB. Hip fracture in Hong Kong and Britain. Int J Epidemiol. 1990;19:1119–1121.
7. Cooper C, Campion G, Melton LJ III. Hip fractures in the elderly: a world-wide projection. Osteoporos Int 1992;2:285–289.
8. Gulberg B, Duppe H, Nilsson B, et al. Incidence of hip fractures in Malmö, Sweden. Bone 1993;14:S23–S29.
9. Nungu S, Olerud C, Rehnberg L. The incidence of hip fracture in Uppsala Country. Acta Orthop Scand 1993;64:75–78.
10. Jéquier V, Burnand B, Vader J-P, Paccaud F. Hip fracture incidence in the Canton of

Vaud, Switzerland, 1986–1991. Osteoporos Int 1995;5:191–195.
11. Agnusdei D, Camporeale A, Gerardi D, Rossi S, Bocchi L, Gennari C. Trends in the incidence of hip fracture in Siena, Italy, from 1980 to 1991. Bone 1993;14:S31–34.
12. Spector TD, Cooper C, Fenton Lewis A. Trends in admission for hip fracture in England and Wales, 1968–85. BMJ 1990;300:1173–1174.
13. Evans JG, Seagroatt V, Goldacre MJ. Secular trends in proximal femur fracture, Oxford record linkage study area and England 1968–86. J Epidmiol Community Health 1997;51:424–429.
14. Melton LJ III, Atkinson EJ, Madhok R. Downturn in hip fracture incidence. Public Health Rep 1996;111:146–150.
15. Cooper C, Melton LJ III. Epidemiology of osteoporosis. Trends Endocrinol Metab 1992;314:224–229.
16. Cummings SR, Blash DM, Nevitt MC, et al. Bone density at various sites for the prediction of hip fractures. Lancet 1993;341:72–5.
17. Riggs BL, Melton LJ III. Medical progress: involutional osteoporosis. N Engl J Med 1986;314:1676–1686.
18. Melton LJ III, Chao EYS, Lane J. Biochemical aspects of fractures. In: Riggs AL, Melton LJ III, editors. Osteoporosis: etiology, diagnosis, and management. New York: Raven Press, 1988:111–131.
19. O'Neill TW, Felsenberg D, Varlow J, Cooper C, Kanis JA, Silman AJ and the European Vertebral Osteoporosis Study Group. The prevalence of vertebral deformity in European men and women: the European Vertebral Osteoporosis Study. J Bone Miner Res 1996;11:1010–1018.
20. Black DM, Cummings SR, Stone K, Hudes E, Palermo L, Steiger P. A new approach to defining normal vertebral dimensions. J Bone Miner Res 1991;6:883–892.
21. Melton LJ III, Lane AW, Cooper C, Eastell R, O'Fallon WM, Riggs BL. Prevalence and incidence of vertebral deformities. Osteoporos Int 1993;3:113–119.
22. Mann T, Oviatt SK, Wilson D, Nelson D, Orwoll ES. Vertebral deformity in men. J Bone Miner Res 1992;11:1259–1265.
23. Lau EMC, Chan HHL, Woo J, Lin F, Black D, Nevitt M, Leung PC. Normal ranges for vertebral height ratios and prevalence of vertebral fracture in Hong Kong Chinese: a comparison with American Caucasians. J Bone Miner Res 1996;11:1364–1368.
24. Cooper C, Atkinson EJ, O'Fallon WM, Melton LJ III. Incidence of clinically diagnosed vertebral fractures: a population-based study in Rochester, Minnesota, 1985–1989. J Bone Miner Res 1992;7:221–227.
25. Bengnér U, Johndl O, Redlund-Johnell. Changes in the incidence and prevalence of vertebral fractures during 30 years. Calcif Tissue Int 1988;42:293–296.
26. Hansen MA, Overgaard K, Gotfriedson A, Christiansen C. Does the prevalence of vertebral fractures increase? In: Christiansen C, Overgaard K, editors. Osteoporosis 1990. Copenhagen: Osteopress, 1990:95.
27. Cooper C, Atkinson EJ, Kotowicz M, O'Fallon WM, Melton LJ. Secular trends in the incidence of postmenopausal vertebral fractures. Calcif Tissue Int 1992;51:100–104.
28. Nevitt MC, Cummings SR and the Study of Osteoporotic Fractures Research Group. Type of fall and risk of hip and wrist fractures: the Study of Osteoporotic Fractures. J Am Geriatr Soc 1993;41:1226–1234.
29. Horsman A, Burkinshaw L. Stochastic models of bone loss and fracture risk. In: Ring EFJ, Evan WD, Dixon AS, editors. Osteoporosis and bone mineral measurement. York, UK: Institute of Physical Sciences in Medicine, 1989:15–30.
30. Hagino H, Yamamoto K, Teshima R, Kishimoto H, Kuranobu K, Nakamura T. The incidence of fractures of the proximal femur and the distal radius in Tottori prefecture, Japan. Arch Orthop Trauma Surg 1989;109:43–44.
31. Griffin MR, Ray WA, Fought RL, Melton LJ III. Black–white difference in fracture rates. Am J Epidemiol 1992;136: 1378–1385.
32. Kristiansen B, Barfod G, Bredesen J, Erin-Madsen J, Grum B, Horsnaes MW, et al.

Epidemiology of proximal humeral fractures. Acta Orthop Scand 1987;58:75–77.
33. Arneson TJ, Melton LJ III, Lewallen DG, O'Fallon WM. Epidemiology of diaphyseal and distal femoral fractures in Rochester, Minnesota, 1965–1984. Clin Orthop 1988;234: 188–194.
34. Melton LJ III. How many women have osteoporosis now? J Bone Miner Res 1995;10: 175–177.
35. Ho SC, Lau EMC, Woo J, Leung PC. The prevalence of osteoporosis in Hong Kong Chinese female population. Maturitas, Eur Menopause J 1999; 32: 171–178.
36. Cummings SR, Kelsey JL, Nevitt MC, O'Down KJ. Epidemiology of osteoporosis and osterporotic fractures. Epidemiol Rev 1985;7:178–208.
37. Sexson SB, Lehner JT. Factors affecting hip fracture mortality. J Orthop Trauma 1988;1:298–305.
38. Kellie SE, Brody JA. Sex-specific and race-specific hip fracture rates. Am J Public Health 1990;80:326–328.
39. Myers AH, Robinson EG, Van Natta ML, Michelson JD, Collins K, Baker SP. Hip fractures among the elderly: factors associated with in-hospital mortality. Am J Epidemiol 1991;14:1128–1137.
40. Magaziner J, Simonsick EM, Kashner TM, Hebel JR, Kenzora JE. Survival experience of aged hip fracture patients. Am J Public Health 1989;79:274–278.
41. Weiss NS, Liff JM, Ure CL, Ballard JH, Abbott GH, Daling JR. Mortality in women following hip fracture. J Chron Dis 1983;36:879–882.
42. Holbrook TL, Grazier K, Kelsey JL, Stauffer RN. The frequency of occurrence, impact and cost of selected musculoskeletal conditions in the United States. Chicago: American Academy of Orthopedic Surgeons, 1984.
43. Bonar SK, Tinetti ME, Speechley M, Cooney LM. Factors associated with short- versus long-term skilled nursing facility placement among community-living hip fracture patients. J Am Geriatr Soc 1990;38:1139–1144.
44. Ettinger B, Block JE, Smith R, Cummings SR, Harris ST, Genant HK. An examination of the association among vertebral deformities, physical disabilities and psychosocial problems. Maturitas 1988;10:283–296.
45. Ettinger B, Black DM, Nevitt MC, Cauley JA, Cummings SR and the Study of Osteoporosis Fractures Research Group. Contribution of vertebral deformity, chronic back pain and disability. J Bone Miner Res 1992;7:449–456.
46. Leidig G, Helmut WM, Sauer P, Wuster C, Wuster J, Lojen M, et al. A study of complaints and their relation to vertebral destruction in patients with osteoporosis. Bone Miner 1990;8:217–229.
47. Lyles KW, Gold DT, Shipp KM, Pieper CF, Martinez S, Mulhausen PL. Association of osteoporotic vertebral compression fractures with impaired functional status. Am J Med 1993;94:595–601.
48. Lau EMC, Woo J, Chan H, et al. The Health Consequences of vertebral deformity in elderly Chinese men and women. Calcif Tissue Int 1998;63:1–4.
49. Praemer A, Furner S, Rice DP. Musculoskeletal Condition in the United States. Park Ridge, IL: American Academy of Orthopaedic Surgeons, 1992.
50. Department of Health. Department of Health, Advisory Group on Osteoporosis. London: Department of Health, 1994.

2 Pathogenesis of Osteoporosis

E. F. Eriksen and H. Glerup

Introduction

Osteoporosis is defined pathologically as "a systemic disease causing an absolute decrease in the amount of bone and microstructural changes, leading to skeletal fragility and consequent fractures after minimal trauma (low energy fractures)". The classical osteoporotic fractures affect primarily bones with large amounts of cancellous bone, i.e. spine, hip and forearm. Cancellous bone is metabolically much more active than cortical bone; therefore this phenomenon suggests that perturbations in bone remodelling play a pivotal role in the development of osteoporosis. In this chapter we will re-examine the different factors that may lead to perturbations of bone remodelling.

Secondary Osteoporosis

When a patient over the age of 50 years presents with a fracture the first task is to assess whether the fracture was caused by low- or high energy trauma. If the circumstances point toward low-energy fracture the next step is to rule out other disease that may cause reduced skeletal mass (osteopenia). Twenty percent of women are found to have secondary osteoporosis, i.e., osteoporosis due to underlying specific diseases; the remaining 80% are diagnosed with idiopathic osteoporosis. In males the distribution between idiopathic and secondary osteoporosis is about 50/50. Potential diseases to look for are listed in Table 2.1, and include hormonal, nutritional, gastrointestinal, rheumatological, renal and hematological disorders as well as certain hereditary diseases.

Hormonal Causes

Hypogonadism in men and women increases the rate of bone loss (see below). Cushing's syndrome is a rare variant of corticosteroid-induced osteoporosis. The mechanisms underlying osteoporosis associated with Addison's disease are still unknown.

Hyperthyroidism leads to high turnover and a negative bone balance in turn leading to accelerated bone loss, but in the vast majority of cases the disease is

Table 2.1. Diseases causing secondary osteoporosis (parentheses indicate that data on bone loss and fractures are equivocal)

Hormonal	*Rheumatological*
Hypogonadism	Rheumatoid arthritis and related diseases
Cushing's syndrome	(Ankylosing spondylitis)
Addison's disease	
(Hyperthyroidism)	*Hematological*
(Hyperparathyroidism)	Multiple myeloma and related diseases
(Acromegaly)	Hemochromatosis
	Hemophilia
Nutritional	Mastocytosis
Severe malnutrition (e.g., anorexia nervosa)	Thalassemia
Malabsorption (e.g., postgastrectomy)	Leukemia and lymphoma
Severe liver disease	
	Other
Hereditary	Paralysis or total immobilization
Osteogenesis imperfecta	Chronic obstructive lung disease
Ehlers-Danlos syndrome	Diffuse metastatic carcinoma
Homocystinuria	Hypercalcemia of malignancy
Congenital porphyria	
(Hypophosphatasia)	

detected very early, and has very little impact on skeletal integrity. Epidemiological studies have demonstrated previous hyperthyroidism to be a risk factor for osteoporotic fractures, so even short-term disease may have adverse effects on bone structure.

Traditionally, primary hyperparathyroidism is listed as a risk factor for osteoporosis. Recent data suggest that mild primary hyperparathyroidism has no long-term adverse effects on bone mass. Individuals with severe primary hyperparathyroidism (serum calcium > 3.00 mmol/l) should still be considered at increased risk, due to the effects of high turnover on skeletal homeostasis.

The effects of acromegaly on bone mass are controversial, with some studies showing increased bone mass and others showing reduced bone mass [5]. The latter findings may reflect accompanying hypogonadism, a frequent finding in acromegaly.

The data on bone mass and fractures in diabetic subjects and endometriosis are conflicting.

Nutritional Causes

Nutritional deficiencies affect the skeleton via impaired supply of calcium and vitamin D, leading to secondary hyperparathyroidism and osteomalacia. This is the case after gastric resections and short bowel syndromes. In anorexia nervosa the nutritional deficiency is exacerbated by amenorrhea.

Hereditary Causes

The common denominator behind osteoporosis associated with hereditary disorders of bone (e.g., osteogenesis imperfecta and Ehlers–Danlos syndrome) is impaired quality of bone matrix due to disturbances in collagen synthesis. Hypophosphatasia is characterized by very low levels of alkaline phosphatase. In severely affected individuals this will lead to impaired matrix mineralization.

Rheumatological Disease

Rheumatological diseases are characterized by general inflammatory processes liberating proinflammatory cytokines such as interleukins and tumor necrosis factors. These peptides also stimulate osteoclastic activity, which leads to increased bone resorption and bone loss.

Hematological Disease

Most hematological malignancies are associated with increased liberation of proinflammatory cytokines, leading to stimulation of osteoclasts. Systemic mastocytosis is a more benign variant, which may be very difficult to demonstrate without bone biopsy.

Other Causes

Immobilization and multiple sclerosis cause bone loss due to reduced mechanosensation. Diffuse metastatic disease causes increased bone resorption due to liberation of proinflammatory cytokines, while hypercalcemia of malignancy increases bone loss due to increased osteoclastic stimulation mediated by parathyroid hormone related peptide (PTHrp) liberated from the tumors (primarily breast and lung cancers).

Drugs and Lifestyle Factors Causing Osteoporosis

Drugs and lifestyle factors increasing the risk for osteoporotic fractures are listed in Table 2.2. Glucocorticoid-induced osteoporosis is a clinically very important problem. In cross-sectional studies 50% of patients on long-term corticosteroids will exhibit spinal fractures.

Glucocorticoids

Bone cells contain large numbers of nuclear receptors for corticosteroids. The main effect of corticosteroids in vitro is an inhibition of protein synthesis. Therefore, chronic corticosteroid administration (usually defined as doses > 7.5 mg/day for more than 6 months) leads to reduced bone matrix synthesis and, in the long term, bone loss. Analysis of bone biopsies from patients undergoing long term treatment with cortiocsteroids have demonstrated a reduced thickness of bone structural units reflecting impaired osteoblast function, corroborating reduced bone matrix synthesis.

It has also been claimed that corticosteroid excess decreases intestinal calcium absorption and increases renal excretion of calcium, resulting in secondary hyper-

Table 2.2. Drugs and lifestyle factors causing osteoporosis (parentheses indicate that data on bone loss and fractures are equivocal)

Glucocorticoids
Cytotoxic drugs
Gonadotropin-releasing hormone agonists
Heparin
Lithium
(Anticonvulsants)
(Aluminum)
Excessive alcohol
(Cigarette smoking)

parathyroidism. This theory is mainly based on studies performed in rodents, and in recent human studies employing new specific PTH assays no hyperparathyroidism was demonstrable.

Glucocorticoids also interfere with bone metabolism in other ways. They bind to sex hormone receptors and inhibit sex hormone action at the cellular level. They also increase the degree of programmed cell death (apoptosis) of osteoblasts, thus reducing the number of osteoblasts participating in bone formation. The reduction in osteocyte numbers may also have deleterious effects on bone by interfering with mechanosensation. Cytotoxic drugs seem to impair osteoblast function by much the same mechanisms.

Other Drugs

Gonadotropin-releasing hormone agonists reduce circulating estrogen levels and thereby cause excessive bone loss. Tamoxifen used in premenopausal women will interfere with binding of estradiol to nuclear receptors and thereby impair the cellular action of the hormone.

Long-term treatment with heparin also causes osteoporosis. In vitro the drug reduces osteoblastic acitivty and decreases osteoblast adhesion to matrix proteins.

Aluminum impairs osteoblast function and causes osteomalacia. Like aluminum, lithium also interferes with intracellular signalling. Antiepileptic drugs, especially phenytoin, have been shown to increase the risk for osteoporotic fractures. They interfere with vitamin D metabolism, and interference with intracellular singalling has also been invoked as a possible mechanism.

Lifestyle Factors (Tobacco and Alcohol)

As already demonstrated by Daniell smoking is a risk factor for osteoporosis. The following factors are generally considered to be the most important: (a) smokers enter menopause earlier than nonsmokers; (b) smokers are slimmer than nonsmokers, which reduces extraglandular production of estrogens; (c) smokers may have an increased metabolic clearance rate of estrogens; (d) smoke may directly inhibit osteoblast function.

Several-large scale epidemiological studies and a recent meta-analysis reported a significant impact of smoking on osteoporosis. Two large-scale European studies were, however, unable to show any significant effect of smoking on osteoporotic fractures.

Previous or present alcoholism is a risk factor for the development of osteoporosis. Alcohol exerts a direct toxic effect on bone cells. It affects osteoblastic proliferation in vitro and reduces matrix protein synthesis in vivo, and of course current alcohol abuse increases the risk for falls. Thus, excessive alcohol consumption is a risk factor for osteoporotic fracture. Two large European studies have, however, been unable to show any significant effect of moderate alcohol consumption on the risk for osteoporotic fracture in women.

Osteoporosis in Men

Contrary to women, only 20% of whom exhibit signs of secondary osteoporosis, 50% of men have secondary osteoporosis. Alcoholism, malignant disease and long-term corticosteroid use are the three first causes to look for. More rarely (< 5%) male osteoporosis is caused by hypogonadism (Table 2.3).

In the remaining men classified as having idiopathic osteoporosis, new data point towards estrogen deficiency as a main contributor to bone loss. Men with aromatase deficiency causing reduced conversion from testosterone to estrogen develop osteopenia. Total absence of estrogen receptors also results in severe osteopenia. Riggs et al. demonstrated that the bone loss rate in older men is correlated to circulating levels of estrogen and not testosterone. Finally, several papers have demonstrated that estrogens and not testosterone determine skeletal homeostasis in males (Fig. 2.1).

Table 2.3. Causes of osteoporosis in 110 males admitted consecutively to our clinic

Primary osteoporosis	61%
Secondary osteoporosis	39%
Steroid induced	13%
Alcoholism	10%
Hypogonadism	5%
Immobilization	2%
Rachitis	2%
Hypogonadism + alcohol/steroid	2%
Other causes	5%

Rare Forms of Osteoporosis

In rare cases severe osteopenia may develop in adolescents and younger individuals (juvenile osteoporosis). These individuals present mainly vertebral fractures and the causes are less well understood. High turnover in relation to growth processes may play a role. Another rare form is postpartum osteoporosis, where multiple spinal fractures develop in young women around or after childbirth. This disease has been linked to changes in bone remodelling caused by lactation. In particular, excessive secretion of PTHrp has been invoked as a possible eliciting factor.

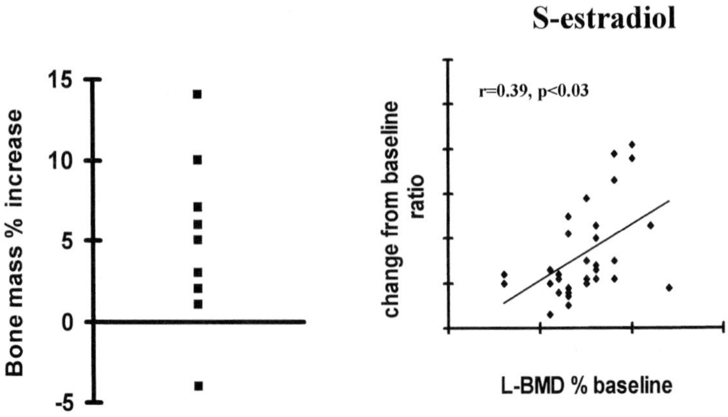

Figure 2.1. *Left*: Effects on bone mass of testosterone supplementation in old eugonadal men. *Right*: Regression of estrogen and androgen levels on changes in lumbar bone mineral density (L-BMD). Note the significant regression on estrogen levels. (From Andersson et al. J Bone Miner Res 1997;12:472–478 with permission.)

Causes of Ideopathic Osteoporosis

In the remaining 80% of women without demonstrable underlying medical causes, a diagnosis of ideopathic osteoporosis can be made. Riggs and Melton proposed further subdivision of this group into type I and type II osteoporosis. Type I osteoporosis was directly linked to the loss of ovarian function after menopause, while type II osteoporosis was considered a mere exaggeration of the physiological aging processes in the skeleton. Recently, with new results re-emphasizing the importance of estrogen for the late phase of bone loss in both men and women, a unitary concept linking type I and type II osteoporosis has been proposed. This model considers both the early postmenopausal bone loss of women and the later age-dependent bone loss in both sexes a result of estrogen deficiency. In the early phases estrogen deficiency causes osteoclastic hyperactivity. Changes in calcium metabolism with reduced vitamin D levels and resulting secondary hyperparathyrodism caused by low estrogen levels are considered responsible for the age-dependent bone loss.

The natural history of the skeleton can be illustrated schematically as consisting of four phases (Fig. 2.2): (a) growth phase resulting in peak bone mass, (b) a plateau phase where bone mass is relatively stable, (c) menopausal bone loss and (d) age-dependent bone loss. Perturbations in bone formation or resorption leading to aberrations in bone accretion or loss during these phases may all eventually lead to low-energy fracture. Apart from the acknowledged crucial role of sex hormone deficiency in the pathogenesis of ideopathic osteoporosis, the causes of ideopathic osteoporosis are multifactorial, and the roles of many factors are still poorly characterized. The listing below is meant as a summary of current knowledge, but the relative importance of the different factors remains to be established.

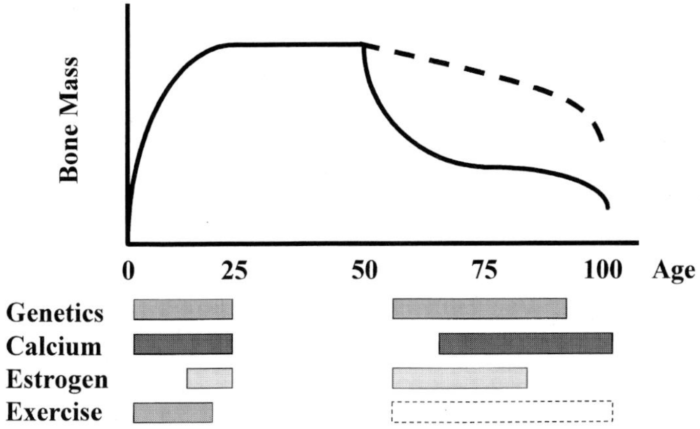

Figure 2.2. The most important factors affecting changes in bone mass at different ages. The changes in skeletal mass in women (*continuous line*) and males (*broken line*) throughout life are shown schematically. The *bars* below show the periods of life where the four factors listed exert their main action. The *broken bar* denoting the effects of exercise after menopause signifies that the data pertaining to these effects are controversial.

Genetic Determinants of Bone Mass

Twin studies have demonstrated that 80% of bone mass is determined by genetic factors. Daughters of mothers with osteoporosis also exhibit lower bone mass than age-matched daughters of mothers without osteoporosis.

Kelly et al. were the first to demonstrate a relation between a genetic polymorphism and bone mass. Later the results in the first paper were withdrawn, and many subsequent studies could not demonstrate the highly significant association between polymorphisms in the vitamin D receptor and bone mass. The study by Kelly et al., however, sparked a tremendous interest in genetic determinants of bone mass. Later studies have shown that polymorphisms in the type I collagen, transforming growth factor β and the estrogen receptor all increase the risk for osteoporotic fracture. So far the most promising marker seems to be the polymorphisms in the binding site for the sp1 transcription factor in the type I collagen gene (COLIA1). Individuals who are homozygous for the ss polymorphism in the COLIA1 gene carry a 10-fold higher risk for osteoporotic fracture.

Osteoporosis is a polygenic disease. Therefore no single gene will provide sufficient information in relation to prediction of future fracture risk. A combination of 5 to 10 genes may, though, yield additional information in combination with bone mass measurements.

Peak Bone Mass

The bone mass achieved at the age of 30 years is called the "peak bone mass", and the factors determining this entity are still poorly delineated. As mentioned above, genetics may play a role in peak bone mass. Blacks achieve higher peak bone mass than Caucasians or Asians. Twin studies indicate that 80% of bone mass in determined by genes; thus only 20% is subject to modulation by environmental factors.

Twin studies have shown that calcium intake determines the increase in bone mass during the growth spurt. Exercise also stimulates bone mass accretion during the growth spurt. Finally, some studies suggest that the circulating levels of testosterone and estrogen during early puberty may play a role.

Menopause

The menopause begins with the last episode of menstrual bleeding induced by cyclic endogenous secretion of steroids. It normally occurs at the age of 51–52 years (range 42–60 years). Estradiol and estrone drop to around 25% and 75% of their premenospausal values, respectively. Most of the estriol still present in the circulation after menopause represents extraglandular conversion of androgen precursors (mainly androstenedione) by aromatases in muscles and adipose tissues to estrone and then to estriol. This is one of the reasons why obesity protects against osteoporosis.

It is generally accepted that an early menopause is associated with osteoporotic fractures and oophorectomized women are subject to accelerated bone loss in the first few years after the operation, with biochemical evidence of an increased bone turnover and bone mineral mobilization. After 4–6 years, however, the rate of bone loss may show great individual variation. This indicates that early oophorectomy may be of clinical significance for the development of later osteoporosis. Amenorrhea also predisposes to osteoporosis. Women with early menopause usually have experienced prolonged periods with oligomenorrhea. Thus, their skeleton has experienced low estrogen levels for an extendedtime, resulting in increased bone loss and low bone mass.

Several different studies have demonstrated an increase in bone turnover after menopause and oopohorectomy. This increase in the number of sites undergoing active remodelling (i.e. increased activation frequency) leads to an increased probability for trabecular perforation, and thus accelerated, irreversible bone loss. The increase in bone turnover in postmenopausal women has also been demonstrated using bone histomorphometry in a group of women with a mean age of 65 years. In the same study estrogen treatment was shown to reduce bone turnover by 50%. In a more recent study on women within 5 years of menopause estrogen deficiency was shown to increase osteoclastic activity and erosion depth. Women treated with a combined cyclic etrogen/progestogen regimen did not exhibit the increase in osteoclastic activity and preserved bone balance. (Fig. 2.3). The basic mechanisms underlying the induction of high bone turnover after menopause are the still subject of debate, but several stand out. Although direct action of estradiol on osteoclasts has only been shown for avian osteoclasts, this mechanism remains a clear possibility. Estrogen deficiency causes increased secretion of proinflammatory, osteoclast stimulating cytokines, mainly interleukins 1 and 6 and tumor necrosis factor alpha, all known osteoclast stimulators. Recently, estrogen has been shown to regulate secretion of osteoprotegerin, an inhibitor of osteoclast differentiation, which may turn out to be the most important mechanism. Other cellular mechanisms (estrogen-deficiency-mediated changes in cellular responsivity of hormones and growth factors) as well as indirect mechanisms (e.g., estrogen–PTH interactions) may also play a role. A recent study has also demonstrated increased cellular sensitivity to PTH in osteoporotics.

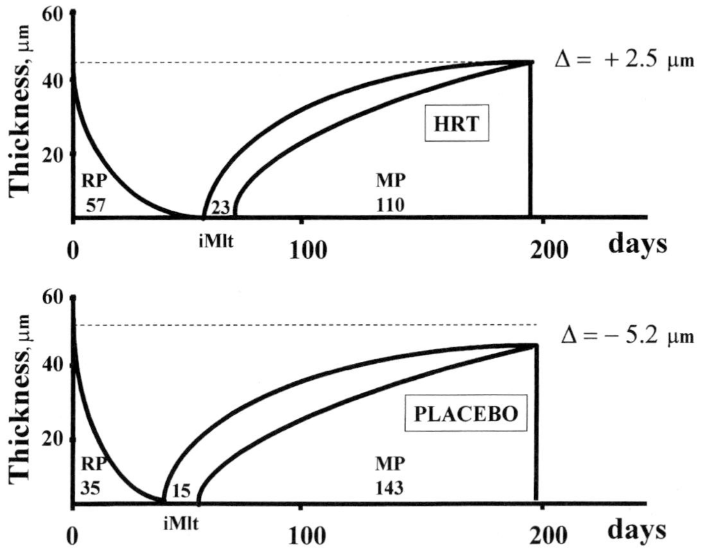

Figure 2.3. Bone remodelling sequences in women going through menopause untreated, and in women treated with hormone replacement therapy (*HRT*). The *curves* are a schematic representation of the bone remodelling sequence of cancellous bone based on histomorphometric analysis. To the *left* is the resorptive phase, to the *right* the formative phase. The *x*-axis shows time in days, the *y*-axis denotes the thickness of bone either removed during bone resorption or formed during subsequent bone formation. The *numbers* above denote the duration of individual phases: resorptive phase (*RP*), initial mineralization lag time (*iMlt*, i.e., the time taken for matrix to mineralize) and the mineralization phase (*MP*). Imlt + MP constitute the formative phase (*FP*). The *broken line* above the curves denotes the thickness of bone removed, i.e., erosion depth, and can be compared with the thickness of bone formed (the *vertical line* on the right), i.e., mean wall thickness. In women on HRT (*upper panel*) no free space is visible below the broken line on the right; thus bone balance is preserved, and is slightly positive (+2.5 μm). In women going through the early phase of menopause without HRT (*lower panel*) a free space is visible below the *broken line* on the right, i.e., mean wall thickness is lower than erosion depth, indicating a negative bone balance of −5.2 μm. (From Erikson et al. J Bone Miner Res 1999:14:1217–1221 with permission.)

Early and late estrogen deficiency probably affect bone mass by different mechanisms. Early estrogen deficiency, developed before peak bone mass is achieved around the age of 25 years (e.g., Turner's syndrome, most cases of hyperprolactinemic amenorrhea and amenorrhea among athletes), probably affect bone maturation and formation during bone modelling, leading to a thinner and more slender skeleton. On the other hand late estrogen deficiency (e.g., oophorectomy, normal menopause) could induce a state of accelerated bone loss due to increased activation frequency as previously discussed. This mechanism would mainly affect cancellous bone due to increased incidence of trabecular perforations.

Other Factors Affecting Age-Dependent Bone Loss

The aging processes leads to loss of bone after the age of 35 yearsas described above, and the crucial role for estrogen deficiency in this process has been emphasized

Table 2.4. Pathophysiologic mechanisms of age-related bone loss

Increased bone resorption	
Estrogens	↓
Androgens	↓
1,25-dihydroxyvitamin D3	↓
Serum parathyroid hormone	↑
Impaired bone formation	
age-dependent decreases in osteoblastic activity	
Insulin-like growth factors	↓
Other growth factors	↓
Responsivity to anabolic effects of hormones and growth factors	↓

above. The other mechanisms underlying the age-dependent bone loss are poorly defined, but several factors have been implicated as shown in Table 2.4.

Like fibroblasts, osteoblasts undergo cellular aging. In long-term culture the cells undergo up to the limiting 50 population doublings, but with increasing age collagen synthesis and secretion of other osteotropic factors goes down. Furthermore, cells cultured from osteoporotic individuals seem to undergo fewer populations doublings. This reduction in osteoblast function may explain the osteoblastic insufficiency that has been demonstrated in osteoporotics and with increasing age (see below).

With increasing age the calcium intake goes down. Calcium absorption is also reduced. Age-dependent reductions in calcium absorption and reduced production of active vitamin D due to thinning of the skin and reduced sun exposure play a role in this respect. As mentioned above, reduced calcium absorption may lead to secondary hyperparathyroidism and accelerated bone loss. This process seems to be amplified by estrogen deficiency.

Defective Osteoblastic Function in Osteoporosis

At the cellular level osteoporotics reveal certain abnormalities especially in relation to osteoblastic function. Compared with age-matched women without osteoporotic fractures, osteoporotic women exhibit reduced bone formation, reflected in decreased thickness of newly formed bone (Fig. 2.4). Resorption depth in the two groups is about the same. Thus, the main difference between osteoporotic women and their non-osteoporotic peers seems to be related mainly to defective bone formation. The lacunae eroded by osteoclasts are not completely refilled, which leads to bone loss. If this defect is already present around menopause, when bone turnover is increased, it would lead to accelerated bone loss. Bone turnover in osteoporotics may be elevated, normal or reduced, but the imbalance between resorption and formation seems to be present at all turnover states and becomes even more pronounced with increased turnover (Fig. 2.5). As already mentioned, aging phenomena play a role in the development of osteoblastic insufficiency that impairs the ability of bone formation to match bone resorption, but genetic factors such as polymorphisms in the sp1 binding site of the type I collagen molecule also play a role.

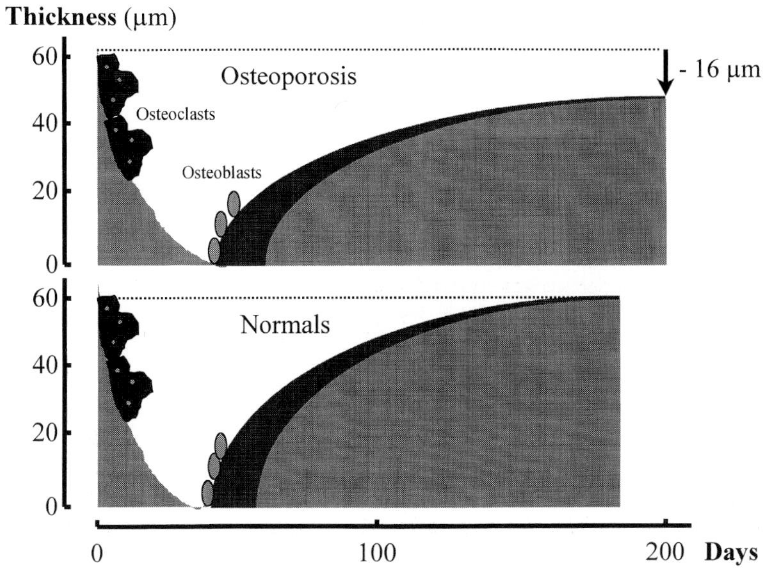

Figure 2.4. Schematic representation of cancellous bone remodelling sequences in osteoporotic women with low-energy spine fractures and age-matched women without osteoporotic fractures. The general outline is similar to that of Figure 2.3. Note the pronounced negative bone balance in osteoporotic women and the preservation of bone balance in age-matched normal women. (From Erikson et al. J Bone Miner Res 1990:5:311–319 with permission.)

Environmental Factors

Nutrition (Calcium Intake)

The calcium ion is crucial for several important functions in the body (nerve function, muscle function, mineralization of bone, control of intracellular processes, etc.). Therefore the serum level of calcium has to be kept within narrow limits, and several hormonal systems participate in calcium control as mentioned above.

Calcium is absorbed in the gut through the action of vitamin D on the gut epithelium, leading to the synthesis of a calcium-transporting protein. Calcium is then transported via the blood stream to bone, where it is incorporated in the bone matrix during calcification. In case of calcium depletion or decreased calcium absorption bone may act as a buffer securing a steady level of calcium in blood. Calcium can be removed from bone either by transport over the osteocyte-lining cell system, which is resposible for the rapid regulation of serum calcium, or by liberation from bone matrix through osteoclastic resorption. Calcium is further excreted through gut (fecal loss), urine (renal loss) and skin. The kidney also plays an important role in calcium homeostasis; it is able to retain calcium or increase calcium excretion mainly via changes in PTH.

The individual daily calcium intake in Denmark is 800 mg. In the USA the average intake is 50% lower. The minimal sufficient intake of calcium is difficult to define, but if calcium intake is very low, compensatory mechanisms (mainly increased secretion of PTH) will start to operate and lead to a high turnover state and possible negative effects on bone mass. Recent studies from the USA have shown that a diet

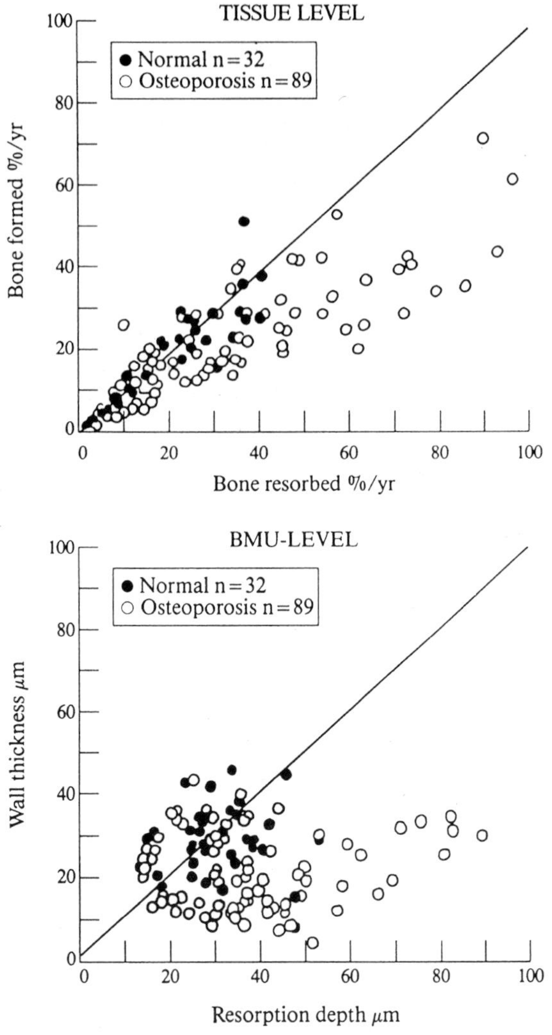

Figure 2.5. Balance between volume referent bone resorption and volume referent bone formation as calculated from histomorphometric analysis of bone in in osteoporotic women with low-energy spine fractures and age-matched women without osteoporotic fractures. The x-axis denotes the volume of bone removed during bone resoprtion, and is given as the percentage of cancellous bone volume present in the bone biopsy. The *y*-axis represents the amount of bone formed, also given as the percentage of cancellous bone volume present in the bone biopsy. If a point is situated below the line of identity, bone resorption is exceeding bone formation, i.e. cancellous bone balance is negative. If a point is situated above the line of identity, bone formation is exceeding bone resorption, i.e., cancellous bone balance is positive. Points situated on the line of the line of identity denote that cancellous bone balance is preserved. The higher the turnover in osteoporotic women, the more pronounced the negative balance. Note furthermore the preservation of balance across different turnover states in normal women. Antiresorptive therapies lower bone turnover, and will move a given point down and to the left. Based on the results shown in this figure, this should result in a less negative balance. (From Erikson et al. J Bone Miner Res 1990;5:311–319 with permission.)

rich in phosphate and low in calcium (e.g., burger diet with soft drinks) may lead to a permanent state of secondary hyperparathyroidism even in the young.

Nutrition may affect peak bone mass. In a study by Matkovic et al. in the former Yugoslavia, two valleys with a low degree of exchange and pronounced differences in calcium content of the drinking water were compared with respect to the incidence of femoral neck fractures. A reduced incidence of femoral neck fractures was demonstrable in the valley with the higher calcium intake. The difference is probably attributable to differences in peak bone mass.

Physical Activity

Osteoblasts are sensitive to mechanical stress. In vitro experiments have demonstrated increased osteoblastic activity after stretching or torsion of the cells. Changes in bone structure due to physical stress are also seen in vivo. In vertebrae the preferential loss of horizontal trabeculae leads to compensatory thickening of vertical trabeculae, and correction of teeth exploits physical stress in order to create changes in bone remodelling in the jaw. Experiments using repetitive physical stress on bone have demonstrated profound increases in bone formation in the stimulated areas.

The skeleton seems to need continuous physical stimulation, otherwise bone loss ensues. This is seen after immobilization or during space flight – in both cases pronounced bone losses have been recorded. Women with a reasonable level of physical activity have a higher bone mineral content than less active women and some studies have demonstrated a direct correlation between maximal oxygen uptake and bone density. Activities involving antigravity exercises (e.g., dancing or running) seem to be more effective than swimming.

The steady decrease in general physical activity in the population is probably one of the main factors responsible for the increased prevalence of osteoporosis seen over the last 10 years. In perimenopausal women several studies have shown increases in bone mass of 5–7% over a 3-year period associated with physical exercise. Therefore a reasonable amount of physical activity throughout life protects against bone loss. Whether physical activity alone will be able to offset the 30–40% loss of bone occurring after menopause is, however, questionable. Most studies in postmenopausal women have been able to show increases in bone mass of only 1–2%. A meta-analysis on all controlled clinical trials was unable to show significant effects on bone mass. No long-term clinical trials have been able to show the antifracture efficacy of exercise. It is neceassary to stress the term "moderate physical activity" because excessive physical activity in young women may produce hypothalamic amenorrhea with estrogen deficiency.

Body Weight

Several studies have reported an inverse relation between body weight and hip fracture rate. In the Framingham study the relative risk of fracture was found to be 0.63 in individuals 114–123% overweight and 0.33 in individuals more than 138% overweight. Obesity may protect the skeleton in several ways: (a) by increased extraglandular production of estrone in fatty tissue; (b) improved vitamin D status due to storage of vitamin D in fatty tissues; (c) by providing a cushioning effect in association with falls; and (d) by creating a larger skeleton due to increased weight bearing.

Recent data suggest that increased weight loss over a short period greatly increases the risk for osteoporotic frailty fractures (defined as fractures of the proximal femur, pelvis, and proximal humerus).

Table 2.5. Historical risk factors for osteoporosis (From NOF Physician's guide to the treatment of osteoporosis with permission)

Personal history of fracture as an adult
History of fracture in first degree relative
Caucasian race
Advanced age
Female sex
Dementia
Poor health or frailty
Current cigarette smoking
Low body weight (< 58 kg)
Estrogen deficiency (early menopause, bilateral ovariectomy, prolonged premenopausal amenorrhea)
Low calcium intake (lifelong)
Alcoholism
Impaired eyesight despite adequate correction
Recurrent falls
Inadequate physical activity

Evaluation of Risk Factors

The historical risk factors are summarized in Table 2.5. They are important when counselling women as to whether they should take estrogen or not, and today they constitute the best guidelines for counseling. Other variables such as the thickness of skin or hair and/or joint hypermobility have been used as indicators of poor collagen synthesis, but their discriminative power still needs to be investigated on a large scale.

Hormones

Parathyroid hormone

Circulating PTH levels increase with increasing age. Several factors have been invoked as being causative. The primary cause seems to be reduced calcium absorption leading to secondary hyperparathyroidism.

Heaney put forward the hypothesis that estrogens might act as antiresorptive agents through inhibition of PTH-mediated effects at the cellular level. Recently two in vitro studies have shown 17ß-estradiol-mediated inhibition of PTH-related increases in cAMP and prostaglandin E_2 production in bone cells. Riggs et al. hypothesized, that the main factor regulating the changes in calcium metabolism was estrogen deficiency in both males and females.

Calcitonin

Several investigators have reported considerably lower plasma calcitonin levels and secretory reserve in women. These findings, together with the demonstration of increased immunoreactive calcitonin levels after estrogen treatment, led to the hypothesis that the antiresorptive action of estrogen is mediated by the increase in calcitonin levels. The whole concept of estrogen exerting any action via alterations in calcitonin levels is, however, losing impact.

Vitamin D

Estrogen treatment increases serum levels of hydroxyvitamin D_3. As osteoporotic women have decreased calcium absorption that increases with calcitriol supplementation, this effect has been taken as one of the indirect effects of estradiol, which might explain its beneficial role in the prophylaxis against postmenopausal osteoporosis.

Vitamin D may also affect the risk for osteoporotic fractures by exerting positive effects on muscle function. It seems that vitamin D deficiency may cause longstanding myopathy, before skeletal involvement with osteomalacia ensues. The myopathy affects primarily the antigravity muscles, and affects balance leading to an increased risk for falls. Vitamin D treatment improves muscle function and balance.

Growth Hormone

Perturbations of the growth hormone (GH)/insulin-like growth factor (IGF) axis have been implicated in the pathogenesis of osteoporosis. The 24-h integrated GH concentration is greater in women than in men, and greater in young women than in postmenopausal women, and the differences are highly significantly correlated with endogenous concentrations of estradiol. Moreover, after correcting for effects of estradiol no significant effects of age or sex were demonstrable. This would suggest estrogen-mediated amplification of the pulsatile GH release. How the reduction in GH amplitude affects bone loss in perimenopausal women remains unknown. Several studies have also reported reduced circulating IGF levels in osteoporotic women. Wüster et al. examined large groups of women with crush fracture osteoporosis, osteoarthritis and healthy age-matched controls. They found that osteoporotic patients exhibited reduced circulating levels of IGF-I and -II and IGF binding protein 3 (IGFBP-3), while patients with osteoarthritis had increased levels of IGFBP-3. They also reported a positive correlation between IGFBP-3 levels and bone mass in control women on hormone replacement therapy. Ljunghall et al. have described a subgroup of osteoporotic men with low IGF-I levels. In this subgroup of male osteoporotics bone mineral density was correlated both with serum IGF-I levels and with peak GH levels at night or after GH-releasing hormone stimulation. Further analysis demonstrated that these men were characterized by reduced IGFBP-3 levels and histomorphometric analysis demonstrated the mean thickness of new bone structural units to be reduced. The latter finding corroborates the significant role of IGFs in the coupling between resorption and formation during bone remodelling.

Kassem et al. compared the response to stimulation with GH (0.2 IU/kg per day for 3 days) in osteoporotic women and age-matched controls without fractures and bone mass in the upper 50% of the normal distribution. Both groups displayed stimulation of both resorption and formation as assessed by biochemical markers. Resorption markers such as cross-linked carboxyterminal telopeptide of collagen type I (ICTP) and hydroxyproline increased by a factor 2–3, but no difference was demonstrable between the two groups (Fig. 2.6). Formative markers such as alkaline phosphatase, osteocalcin and carboxyterminal propeptide of procollagen type I (PICP) also increased upon GH stimulation, but no differences were demonstrable for these markers either. Serum levels of IGF-I, IGF-II and IGFBP-3 were also assessed, but here also no difference was demonstrable between osteoporotic and control subjects. The authors also cultured osteoblasts from marrow aspirates

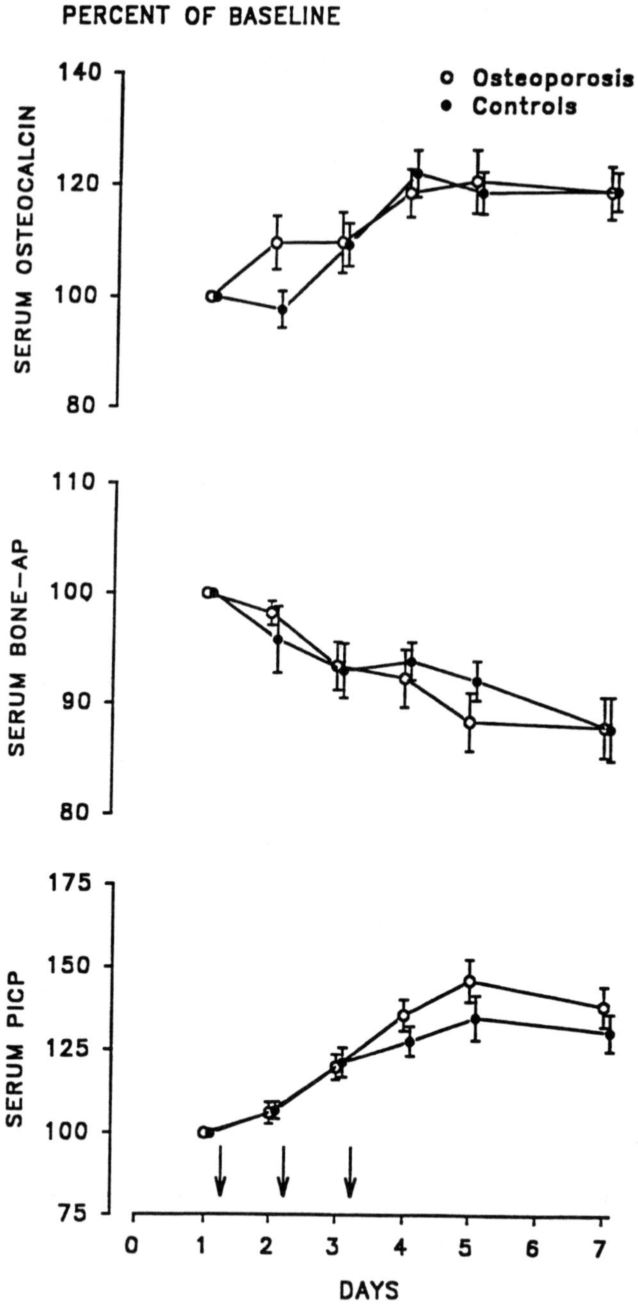

Figure 2.6. Changes in biochemical markers of formation and resorption in osteoporotics and normal age- and sex-matched controls after 1 week of stimulation with human growth hormone (hGH). The responses do not differ. *AP*, alkaline phosphatase; *PICP*, carboxyterminal propeptide of procollagen type I. (From Kassem et al. Eur J Endocrinol 1994;131:150–155 with permission.)

obtained from subjects undergoing in vivo stimulation with GH. Similar to the in vivo experiments, no difference with respect to the proliferative or differentiation response to GH of these cells was demonstrable between osteoporotic and control subjects.

Thus, it seems that certain subgroups of osteoporotics may be characterized by reduced circulating IGF levels, but a general defect in GH secretion or perturbations in the GH–IGF axis in osteoporosis cannot be demonstrated.

Summary and Conclusions

Osteoporosis is a multifactorial disease. Different phases of life each participate in the development of low bone mass and low-energy fractures late in life. One common denominator is impaired osteoblast function. It may be caused by genetic, hormonal or environmental factors. Recent data suggest that estrogen deficiency plays a pivotal role in age-dependent bone loss in men and women. Furthermore, aging phenomena play a pivotal role. It seems that osteoblasts are more sensitive to aging than osteoclasts, which causes the progressive bone loss after attainmaint of peak bone mass at the age of 30 years. Aging phenomena and estrogen deficiency also cause perturbations in calcium metabolism leading, to impaired calcium absorption and increased bone turnover due to secondary hyperparathyroidism. This increase in bone turnover further exaggerates the negative balance caused by other factors. Antiresorptive drugs, which constitute the dominant treatment regimens for osteoporosis today, both reverse the negative bone balance and decrease bone turnover.

References

1. Eriksen EF, Mosekilde L, Melsen F. Trabecular bone remodelling and bone balance in hyperthyroidism. Bone 1985;6:421–428.
2. Langdahl BL, Loft AG, Eriksen EF, Mosekilde L, Charles P. Bone mass, bone turnover, body composition, and calcium homeostasis in former hyperthyroid patients treated by combined medical therapy. Thyroid. 1996;6:161–168.
3. Masiukiewicz US, Insogna KL. The role of parathyroid hormone in the pathogenesis, prevention and treatment of postmenopausal osteoporosis [in process citation]. Aging (Milano) 1998;10:232–239.
4. Halse J, Melsen F, Mosekilde L. Iliac crest bone mass and remodelling in acromegaly. Acta Endocrinol (Copenh) 1981;97:18–22.
5. Longobardi S, Di Somma C, Di Rella F, Angelillo N, Ferone D, Colag A, et al. Bone mineral density and circulating cytokines in patients with acromegaly. J Endocrinol Invest 1998;21:688–693.
6. Bisballe S, Eriksen EF, Melsen F, Mosekilde L, Sorensen OH, Hessov I. Osteopenia and osteomalacia after gastrectomy: interrelations between biochemical markers of bone remodelling, vitamin D metabolites, and bone histomorphometry [see comments]. Gut 1991;32:1303–1307.
7. Hergenroeder AC. Bone mineralization, hypothalamic amenorrhea, and sex steroid therapy in female adolescents and young adults. J Pediatr 1995;126:683–689.
8. Mundy GR. Inflammatory mediators and the destruction of bone. J Periodontal Res 1991;26:213–217.
9. Mundy GR. Local control of osteoclast function. Osteoporos Int 1993;3(Suppl 1):126–127.
10. Chines A, Pacifici R, Avioli LV, Teitelbaum SL, Korenblat PE. Systemic mastocytosis

presenting as osteoporosis: a clinical and histomorphometric study. J Clin Endocrinol Metab 1991;72:140–144.
11. Dempster DW. Bone histomorphometry in glucocorticoid-induced osteoporosis. J Bone Miner Res 1989;4:137–141.
12. Weinstein RS, Jilka RL, Parfitt AM, Manolagas SC. Inhibition of osteoblastogenesis and promotion of apoptosis of osteoblasts and osteocytes by glucocorticoids: potential mechanisms of their deleterious effects on bone. J Clin Invest 1998;102:274–282.
13. Hurley MM, Kessler M, Gronowicz G, Raisz LG. The interaction of heparin and basic fibroblast growth factor on collagen synthesis in 21-day fetal rat calvariae. Endocrinology 1992;130:2675–2682.
14. Puleo DA, Bizios R. Mechanisms of fibronectin-mediated attachment of osteoblasts to substrates in vitro. Bone Miner 1992;18:215–226.
15. Goodman WG. Short-term aluminum administration in the rat: reductions in bone formation without osteomalacia. J Lab Clin Med 1984;103:749–757.
16. May LG, Gay CV. Multiple G-protein involvement in parathyroid hormone regulation of acid production by osteoclasts. J Cell Biochem 1997;64:161–170.
17. Daniell HW. Osteoporosis of the slender smoker: vertebral compression fractures and loss of metacarpal cortex in relation to postmenopausal cigarette smoking and lack of obesity. Arch Intern Med. 1976;136:298–304.
18. Bauer DC, Browner WS, Cauley JA, et al. Factors associated with appendicular bone mass in older women: the Study of Osteoporotic Fractures Research Group [see comments]. Ann Intern Med 1993;118:657–665.
19. Ensrud KE, Nevitt MC, Yunis C, et al. Correlates of impaired function in older women. J Am Geriatr Soc 1994;42:481–489.
20. Naves DM, O'Neill TW, Silman AJ. The influence of alcohol consumption on the risk of vertebral deformity. European Vertebral Osteoporosis Study Group. Osteoporos Int 1997;7:65–71.
21. Johnell O, Gullberg B, Kanis JA, et al. Risk factors for hip fracture in European women: the MEDOS Study. J Bone Miner Res 1995;10:1802–1815.
22. Nielsen HK, Lundby L, Rasmussen K, Charles P, Hansen C. Alcohol decreases serum osteocalcin in a dose-dependent way in normal subjects. Calcif Tissue Int 1990;46:173–178.
23. Toussirot E, Royet O, Wendling D. [Aetiologic features of osteoporosis in male patients aged less than 50 years: study of 28 cases with a comparative series of 30 patients over the age of 50]. Rev Med Intern 1998;19:479–485.
24. Vanderschueren D, Van HE, De CR, Bouillon R. Aromatization of androgens is important for skeletal maintenance of aged male rats. Calcif Tissue Int 1996;59:179–183.
25. Riggs BL, Khosla S, Melton LJ. A unitary model for involutional osteoporosis: estrogen deficiency causes both type I and type II osteoporosis in postmenopausal women and contributes to bone loss in aging men. J Bone Miner Res 1998;13:763–773.
26. Anderson FH, Francis RM, Peaston RT, Wastell HJ. Androgen supplementation in eugonadal men with osteoporosis: effects of six months' treatment on markers of bone formation and resorption. J Bone Miner Res 1997;12:472–478.
27. Sowers M. Pregnancy and lactation as risk factors for subsequent bone loss and osteoporosis. J Bone Miner Res 1996;11:1052–1060.
28. Riggs BL, Melton LJ III. Clinical review 8. Clinical heterogeneity of involutional osteoporosis: implications for preventive therapy. J Clin Endocrinol Metab 1990;70: 1229–1232.
29. Seeman E, Tsalamandris C, Formica C, Hopper JL, McKay J. Reduced femoral neck bone density in the daughters of women with hip fractures: the role of low peak bone density in the pathogenesis of osteoporosis. J Bone Miner Res 1994;9:739–743.
30. Kelly PJ, Morrison N, Sambrook PN, Eisman JA. Genetics and osteoporosis: role of the vitamin D receptor gene. Agents Actions 1994;42:i–ii.
31. Grant SFA, Reid DM, Blake G, Herd R, Fogelman I, Ralston SH. Reduced bone density and osteoporosis associated with a polymorphic SP1 binding site in the collagen type I alpha 1 gene. Nature Genet 1996;14:203–205.

32. Langdahl BL, Knudsen JY, Jensen HK, Gregersen N, Eriksen EF. A sequence variation: 713-8delC in the transforming growth factor-beta 1 gene has higher prevalence in osteoporotic women than in normal women and is associated with very low bone mass in osteoporotic women and increased bone turnover in both osteoporotic and normal women. Bone 1997;20:289–294.
33. Kobayashi S, Inoue S, Hosoi T, Ouchi Y, Shiraki M, Orimo H. Association of bone mineral density with polymorphism of the estrogen receptor gene. J Bone Miner Res 1996;11:306–311.
34. Uitterlinden AG, Burger H, Huang Q, et al. Relation of alleles of the collagen type I alpha 1 gene to bone density and the risk of osteoporotic fractures in postmenopausal women [see comments]. N Engl J Med 1998;338:1016–1021.
35. Langdahl BL, Ralston SH, Grant SF, Eriksen EF. An Sp1 binding site polymorphism in the COLIA1 gene predicts osteoporotic fractures in both men and women. J Bone Miner Res 1998;13:1384–1389.
36. Johnston CC Jr, Miller JZ, Slemenda CW, et al. Calcium supplementation and increases in bone mineral density in children. N Engl J Med 1992;327:82–87.
37. Bass S, Pearce G, Bradney M, Hendrich E, Delmas PD, Harding A, et al. Exercise before puberty may confer residual benefits in bone density in adulthood: studies in active prepubertal and retired female gymnasts.J Bone Miner Res 1998;13:500–507.
38. Ryan KJ. Estrogen use and postmenopausal women: a National Institutes of Health Consensus Development Conference. Ann Intern Med 1979;91:921–922.
39. Lindsay R, Hart DM, Forest C, Baird C. Prevention of spinal osteoporosis in oophorectomized women. Lancet 1980;II:1151–1154.
40. Katz E, McClamrock HD, Adashi EY. Ovarian failure including menopause, premature menopause, and resistant ovarian syndrome, and hormonal replacement. Curr Opin Obstet Gynecol 1990;2:392–397.
41. Eastell R, Delmas PD, Hodgson SF, Eriksen EF, Mann KG, Riggs BL. Bone formation rate in older normal women: concurrent assessment with bone histomorphometry, calcium kinetics, and biochemical markers. J Clin Endocrinol Metab 1988;67:741–748.
42. Parfitt AM. Age-related structural changes in trabecular and cortical bone: cellular mechanisms and biomechanical consequences. Calcif Tissue Int 1984;36(Suppl 1): S123–S128.
43. Eriksen EF. Normal and pathological remodelling of human trabecular bone: three dimensional reconstruction of the remodelling sequence in normals and in metabolic bone disease. Endocr Rev 1986;7:379–408.
44. Steiniche T, Hasling C, Charles P, Eriksen EF, Mosekilde L, Melsen F. A randomized study on the effects of estrogen/gestagen or high dose oral calcium on trabecular bone remodelling in postmenopausal osteoporosis. Bone 1989;10:313–320.
45. Eriksen EF, Langdahl B, Vesterby A, Rungby J, Kassem M. Hormone replacement therapy prevents osteoclastic hyperactivity: a histomorphometric study in early postmenopausal women. J Bone Miner Res 1999;14:1217–1221.
46. Pacifici R, Rifas L, Teitelbaum S, et al. Spontaneous release of interleukin 1 from human blood monocytes reflects bone formation in idiopathic osteoporosis. Proc Natl Acad Sci USA 1987;84:4616–4620.
47. Hofbauer LC, Khosla S, Dunstan CR, Lacey DL, Spelsberg TC, Riggs BL. Estrogenstimulates gene expression and protein production of osteoprotergerin in human osteoblastic cells. Endocrinology 1999;140:4367–4370.
48. Kotowicz MA, Klee GG, Kao PC, et al. Relationship between serum intact parathyroid hormone concentrations and bone remodelling in type I osteoporosis: evidence that skeletal sensitivity is increased. Osteoporos Int 1990;1:14–22.
49. Kassem M, Ankersen L, Eriksen E, Clark B, Rattan S. Demonstration of cellular aging and senescence in serially passaged long-term cultures of human trabecular osteoblasts. Osteoporos Int 1997;7:514–524.
50. Eriksen EF, Hodgson SF, Eastell R, Cedel SL, O'Fallon WM, Riggs BL. Cancellous bone remodelling in type I (postmenopausal) osteoporosis: quantitative assessment of rates

of formation, resorption, and bone loss at tissue and cellular levels. J Bone Miner Res 1990;5:311–319.
51. Matkovic V, Kostial K, Simonovici L, Buzina R, Broadarec A, Nordin BEC. Bone status and fracture rates in two regions of Yugoslavia. Am J Clin Nutr 1979;32:540–544.
52. Lanyon LE. Functional strain as a determinant for bone remodelling. Calcif Tissue Int 1984;36(Suppl 1):S56–S61.
53. Pocock NA, Eisman JA, Yeates MG, Sambrook PN, Eberl S. Physical fitness is a major determinant of femoral neck and lumbar spine bone mineral density. J Clin Invest 1986;78:618–621.
54. Berard A, Bravo G, Gauthier P. Meta-analysis of the effectiveness of physical activity for the prevention of bone loss in postmenopausal women. Osteoporos Int 1997;7:331–337.
55. Glazener CM, Sargood AJ, Jackson PC, et al. Osteoporosis and amenorrhea in young women. Gynecol Endocrinol 1987;1:255–261.
56. Kiel DF, Felson DT, Anderson JJ, Wilson FWF, Moskowitz MA. Hip fracture and the use of estrogens in postmenopausal women: The Framingham Study. N Engl J Med 1987;317:1169–1174.
57. Ensrud KE, Cauley J, Lipschutz R, Cummings SR. Weight change and fractures in older women. Study of Osteoporotic Fractures Research Group. Arch Intern Med 1997;157:857–863.
58. Dawson-Hughes B, Harris S, Dallal GE. Serum ionized calcium, as well as phosphorus and parathyroid hormone, is associated with the plasma 1,25-dihydroxyvitamin D_3 concentration in normal postmenopausal women. J Bone Miner Res 1991;6:461–468.
59. Eastell R, Yergey AL, Vieira NE, Cedel SL, Kumar R, Riggs BL. Interrelationship among vitamin D metabolism, true calcium absorption, parathyroid function, and age in women: evidence of an age-related intestinal resistance to 1,25-dihydroxyvitamin D action. J Bone Miner Res 1991;6:125–132.
60. Chapuy MC, Arlot ME, Duboeuf F, et al. Vitamin D_3 and calcium to prevent hip fractures in the elderly women. N Engl J Med 1992;327:1637–1642.
61. Heaney RP. Estrogen-calcium interactions in the postmenopause: a quantitative description. Bone Miner 1990;11:67–84.
62. Raisz LG, Pilbeam CC, Fall PM. Prostaglandins: mechanisms of action and regulation of production in bone. Osteoporos Int 1993;3(Suppl 1):136–140.
63. Fukayama S, Tashjian AH Jr. Direct modulation by estradiol of the response of human bone cells (SaOS-2) to human parathyroid hormone (PTH) and PTH-related protein. Endocrinology 1989;124:397–401.
64. Stevenson JC. Pathogenesis, prevention, and treatment of osteoporosis. Obstet Gynecol 1990;75:36S–41S.
65. Sorensen OH, Lund B, Andersen RB, et al. Effects of 1-alpha vitamin D on bone and muscle in senile osteopenia. Mol Endocrinol 1979;oo:309–318.
66. Prince RL, Smith M, Dick IM, et al. Prevention of postmenopausal osteoporosis. A comparative study of exercise, calcium supplementation, and hormone-replacement therapy. N Engl J Med 1991;325:1189–1195
67. Ho KKY, Evans WS, Blizzard RM. Effects of sex and age on the 24-hour profile of growth hormone secretion in man: importance of endogenous estradiol concentrations. J Clin Endocrinol Metab 1987;64:51–58.
68. Wuster C, Blum WF, Schlemilch S, Ranke MB, Ziegler R. Decreased serum levels of insulin-like growth factors and IGF binding protein 3 in osteoporosis. J Intern Med 1993;234:249–55
69. Ljunghall S, Johansson AG, Burman P, Kampe O, Lindh E, Karlsson FA. Low plasma levels of insulin-like growth factor 1 (IGF-1) in male patients with idiopathic osteoporosis. J Intern Med 1992;232:59–64
70. Kassem M, Brixen K, Blum W, Mosekilde L, Eriksen EF. No evidence for reduced spontaneous or growth-hormone-stimulated serum levels of insulin-like growth factor (IGF)-I, IGF-II or IGF binding protein 3 in women with spinal osteoporosis. Eur J Endocrinol 1994;131:150–155.

3 Assessing Bone Mass by X-ray Absorptiometry: The WHO Definition of Osteoporosis

M. McClung

Introduction

The ability to measure bone mass in both peripheral and central skeletal sites with accuracy and precision has been one of the most significant advances in the field of osteoporosis. Bone density is related to bone strength in both animals and in vitro. The original measurements obtained by photon absorption techniques have evolved into today's technology using dual-energy X-ray absorptiometry (DXA). DXA is now the most widely used and accepted technique for the assessment of bone mineral density (BMD). DXA and its predecessors have been used in large, prospective epidemiological studies to define the relationship between bone density and fracture risk and a major end-point in clinical trials evaluating new drug therapies to prevent bone loss. These techniques are now used clinically to predict fracture risk, establish or confirm the diagnosis of osteoporosis, select patients for therapy and monitor the effectiveness of therapy [1]. Quantitative computed tomography and quantitative ultrasound (see Ch. 4) are other techniques for measuring bone mass that are based on different technical principles also useful in clinical practice.

DXA Technology

The technique of photon absorptiometry relies upon the relationship between bone mineral content and the ease with which photons pass through skeletal tissue. The denser the skeleton, the more photons are "absorbed" by the bone. Fewer photons pass through the bone and are thus capable of being detected and counted. The original absorptiometric techniques for measuring BMD used single-energy radionuclides (usually ^{125}I). This technique, called single photon absorptiometry (or SPA), was limited to use in areas where the soft tissue thickness could be standardized by immersing the body part in water or wrapping it in a bag of tissue-equivalent material. The radius and calcaneus were the sites measured with SPA. To measure BMD in sites where soft tissue is variable (spine, hip or total body), dual photon absorptiometry (DPA) was developed using isotopes such as ^{153}Gd with two different photon energies. Bone mass of these central skeletal sites could then be measured by factoring out the soft tissue contribution to photon absorption. Several DPA devices were developed for research and clinical use. They required long scan times (20–40 min for spine and hip scans) and constant adjustment for isotope decay. Because of its relatively high precision error relative to the rate of bone density changes, DPA was not suitable for monitoring longitudinal changes.

A major advance in bone density assessment occurred in 1987 when the first DXA system was introduced that used X-rays as the dual-energy photon source [2]. The use of X-rays avoided the problem of isotope source decay and replacement. The increased photon flux with DXA reduced scan times to 5–7 min and markedly improved scan image quality and resolution. Most importantly, the percent coefficient of variation (%CV) of measurements in the spine (1–1.5%) and hip (1.8–2.5%) was adequate for longitudinal monitoring of bone density, especially in response to pharmacological intervention. It is no coincidence that the large clinical trials evaluating the efficacy of estrogen, bisphosphonates and calcitonin were all begun after the availability of DXA machines to measure spine and hip density.

Single energy X-ray based units (SXA) for the heel and forearm have also been developed, supplanting SPA. These units share the advantage of using X-ray tubes instead of radionuclides as the photon generator, but they still require the use of a water bath or tissue-equivalent bags to standardize soft tissue thickness. More recently, DXA devices specifically designed to quantify bone mass in the forearm, calcaneus and phalanx have been developed and introduced into clinical practice. These devices do not require a water bath or bags, provide scan times as short as 5 s, excellent image quality (helpful for quality control) and outstanding precision (%CV = 0.5–2%).

Bone density is not directly measured by DXA or SXA devices. All absorptiometric devices measure the bone mineral content (BMC) of a specified skeletal region (in grams of mineral) and the area (in square centimeters) of that region. The resultant BMD value is an areal density, expressed in grams per square centimeter. True volumetric BMD is not measured since the third dimension (depth of the bone) is not assessed. Only quantitative computed tomography provides a true volumetric bone density measurement. This is not a significant limitation of DXA since the depth of the bone in most individuals is proportional to other dimensions. Furthermore, areal BMD by DXA and volumetric BMD by quantitative computed tomography of the same site are highly correlated [3].

Since BMD is the quotient of BMC divided by area, artifactual changes in BMD can occur if the area of the region of interest is artifactually distorted or is not correctly measured by the scanner and technologist. Examples of such artifacts include vertebral fractures or the failure of the edge detection algorithm, especially in the proximal femur in patients with very low bone density. Proper quality control requires review of the BMC and area results to validate the BMD value.

Pencil Beam Versus Fan Beam Systems

Bone density is determined pixel by pixel over the skeletal region scanned. The original DXA scanners (Hologic QDR-1000, Lunar DPX) acquire BMD data by performing a rectilinear scan over the spine, hip or other skeletal region with a pinhole collimator and a single photon detector. The next generation of scanners (Hologic QDR-2000) acquires data from many pixels simultaneously by using a fan beam of X-rays coupled to an array of multiple detectors in the scanning arm. In a single pass, data from the entire lumbar spine or hip region can be acquired. The most recent fan beam systems (Hologic QDR-4500, Lunar Prodigy, Norland Eclipse) acquire hip and spine scans in 1–2 min and total-body scans in less than 5 min. Fan beam systems use high-voltage X-ray tubes, that provide better image resolution but at the expense of increased radiation dose to patients and staff, although the effective absorbed dose per scan with the newest scanners remains very low (between 2 and 10 μSv) [3]. The advantages of fan beam systems are their acquisition speed, image quality and their ability to perform special tasks such as lateral spine scanning and vertebral morphometry. Fan beam systems do not improve precision of measurements [4]. One potential limitation in the fan beam system is a magnification error related to differences in height between the scanned part and the X-ray tube [5]. This is not an issue with pencil beam systems. In clinical practice, however, this is rarely a significant problem.

Recently, new DXA systems have been introduced by the major manufacturers that use pencil beam technology coupled with higher-voltage X-ray units (Norland Eclipse, Lunar IQ, Hologic QDR-4000). These systems are less expensive than the fan beam systems but still provide enhanced image quality and faster scan times compared with the original pencil beam systems.

Both pencil beam and fan beam systems provide excellent bone density data. Either is suitable for clinical practice or clinical research studies. Making the choice between system types is dependent upon the specific application desired in a particular laboratory.

DXA Scanning Sites

The common sites of bone density measurement and the technologies available to measure them are listed in Table 3.1.

Table 3.1. Bone mineral density measurement sites

Site	Technology	% trabecular bone
Lumbar spine - PA	DXA	67
Lumbar spine - PA	QCT	100
Lumbar spine - lateral	DXA	75 (?)
Proximal femur		
Femoral neck	DXA	25
Trochanter	DXA	50
Total hip	DXA	10–20
Radius		
Proximal (1/3)	DXA/SXA	1
Distal	DXA/SXA	20–40
Trabecular	pQCT	100
Phalanx	DXA/QUS	40
Calcaneus	DXA/SXA/QUS	95
Total body	DXA	20

DXA,dual-energy X-ray absorptiometry; QCT, quantitative computed tomography; SXA, single photon absorptiometry; pQCT, peripheral quantitative computed tomography; QUS, quantitative ultrasound.

PA Lumbar Spine

BMD measurement of the spine by DXA is limited to the L1–L4 region; the thoracic spine cannot be measured because of overlying ribs and sternum. Lumbar spine BMD is usually acquired in the posterior/anterior (PA) projection with the patient in a supine position with legs elevated to minimize the lumbar lordosis. Proper positioning and alignment are essential components of appropriate DXA technique. The L1–L4 or L2–L4 region is typically measured. Vertebral bodies with significant artifact (e.g., fracture) should be excluded from the analysis. Accuracy and precision of individual vertebral body measurements are limited because of the small region of interest, and major clinical decisions should not be based on values from single vertebral bodies alone.

DXA measurements in the PA projection include both the vertebral body and the posterior elements of the spine. Artifacts including scoliosis, facet joint and end-plate sclerosis, osteophytes and fractures often limit the use of spine DXA measurements in older individuals [6]. In some patients, degenerative changes in the spine result in such artifact that measurement of bone density in the spine is not possible. PA spine results are most useful in younger postmenopausal women (age less than 65 years). Loss of bone mass occurs more rapidly in the spine in early menopause than in other skeletal sites. In addition, BMD response to antiresorptive therapy is usually greater in the spine than other skeletal sites because of the high trabecular bone content of the spine.

Lumbar spine BMD measurements can also be acquired in a lateral projection of a supine subject by rotating the C-arm of specially equipped fan beam scanners. This measurement includes only the vertebral bodies and excludes the posterior elements of the spine. Thus, some artifacts that interfere with PA measurements can be minimized with lateral scanning. By excluding these artifacts and the posterior elements, the rate of bone loss (1.1%/year) is greater with lateral versus PA (0.4%/year) measurements in older women [7]. Despite the attractiveness of lateral spine measurements, however, this technique has apparently limited clinical utility. Other artifacts such as scoliosis, fractures and end-plate deformity or sclerosis still affect lateral spine BMD values. In younger menopausal women, the rate of bone loss without therapy and the skeletal response to antiresorptive treatment are similar in lateral and PA spine measurements [8]. Because the precision of lateral spine measurements is reduced compared with PA measurements, the PA spine value is actually a more sensitive method of monitoring spinal BMD response in these younger patients. Furthermore, there are minimal data relating lateral spine BMD values with fracture risk in older adults.

Proximal Femur Scans

BMD measurement in the proximal femur is more complex than in the spine because the geometry of the hip makes consistent positioning at that site more difficult. The scan is performed in the supine position with both legs extended. The leg is first abducted so that the femoral neck is well separated from the pelvis and is then internally rotated to bring the femoral neck into the most favorable alignment for scanning. When the femur is appropriately positioned, the lesser trochanter is barely visible on the inner margin of the femoral shaft.

Hip measurements are made in four distinct subregions as well as the total hip region of interest. These regions are defined somewhat differently by the various bone densitometer manufacturers. The femoral neck and trochanteric regions have usually been used in clinical trials and clinical practice. The trochanter is primarily trabecular bone and usually responds to therapy in a manner similar to the spine. The femoral neck measurement is compromised by its somewhat higher precision error. This is attributable to its small area and its sensitivity to small changes in the rotation of the femur and to small differences in the placement of the region of interest box. Ward's region does not have specific anatomical boundaries. It is located by the computer software as the area of lowest density in the proximal femur. The intertrochanteric region is used only to complete the total hip area, which consists of the femoral neck, trochanteric and intertrochanteric areas. Because of its larger area, the precision of total hip measurement is slightly better (%CV about 1.7%) than that of the subregions. The response of total hip BMD to treatment and its use in predicting hip fractures in older women is similar to the femoral neck BMD. The International Committee on Standardization in Bone Measurement has recommended that the total hip region be the preferred site in the proximal femur [9].

Forearm

Traditionally, two sites in the forearm have been studied. The mid-shaft or 1/3 site is at the junction of the middle two-thirds and distal one-third of the forearm. This site is predominantly cortical bone. The distal and ultradistal sites are regions in the distal portion of the forearm which are predominantly trabecular bone.

BMD either of the radius or of both the radius and ulna can be determined. The mid-radial site has proven the more useful forearm measurement. Precision error is small, and the mid-radial site is somewhat more predictive of fracture risk in longitudinal studies than are distal sites. Recently, a new region in the ultradistal radius was defined for use in Osteometer DXA forearm machines. Preliminary studies suggest that this may be a useful site for monitoring response to estrogen therapy, but these observations require confirmation.

Calcaneus

In gross terms, the calcaneus resembles a vertebra in that it is a highly trabecular bone with a thin cortical shell. BMD in the calcaneus is measured in the lateral projection. Regions in the mid-portion of this bone are defined by Lunar, Osteometer and Norland for use with their DXA heel scanners. Images of the heel are provided with some scanners, and this may improve scan reproducibility by allowing operators to assure consistent placement of the region of interest.

Total-Body Calcium

Specific DXA scanners from each of the manufacturers are capable of whole-body scanning and the quantification of total-body calcium. This measurement can be made very precisely (%CV $<$ 1%) and can be analyzed by subregions (arm, thorax, pelvis, legs, etc.). Total-body calcium is predominantly cortical bone (about 80%).

Values in adults change slowly with time and only modestly in response to therapy. As a consequence, total-body BMD measurements are less useful than regional scanning sites in adults. Total-body BMC or BMD is very useful, however, in assessing and monitoring skeletal changes in children and adolescents whose skeletons are still growing.

Specialized Uses of DXA Scanners

Body Composition

Using total-body scans, body composition (fat mass and lean body mass) can be determined by DXA [10]. The values obtained by DXA are highly correlated with traditional methods of assessing body composition in young people [11]. In older subjects, DXA has proven to be the most accurate measure for assessing lean and fat mass. DXA avoids both the logistic problems associated with hydrostatic weighing and the inaccuracies induced by age-related bone loss which are not taken into account by most techniques. This capability of DXA has been exploited in many clinical studies on the effects of various wasting diseases, nutritional deficiencies and therapeutic interventions with agents such as growth hormone.

Vertebral Morphometry

Specialized software is available on Lunar Expert and Hologic QDR 4500 scanners to obtain spine images from T4 to L4 in the lateral projection [12]. Morphometric measurements on the individual vertebral bodies can then be performed, and vertebral deformities can be identified and classified. To date, this capability has been useful in screening potential research candidates for the presence of fractures, but standardized techniques using actual radiographs are still the most appropriate methods for the assessment of fractures.

Quantitative Computed Tomography

Computed tomography is a powerful tool that measures the density of tissue and uses this information to generate diagnostic images [13]. Standard CT scanners can be adapted to provide quantitative density measurements. Bone mineral density by quantitative computed tomography (QCT) is obtained by comparing the density measurements obtained in a skeletal part with a set of calibrated mineral-equivalent standards contained in a phantom that is scanned with the patient. QCT is the only bone density test that measures actual volumetric bone density, and the results are expressed in grams per cubic centimeter. The standard lumbar spine QCT measurement selects a region of interest in the central portion of the vertebral body and thus measures the true density of trabecular bone. Other regions of interest can be selected which specifically measure the vertebral body shell (predominantly cortical bone) or the integral bone density of the vertebral body with or without the posterior elements of the spine. In this way, QCT can actually measure density of the same region measured by DXA machines. Dedicated smaller peripheral QCT units have been manufactured that are capable of measuring bone density in the forearm and the leg. These instruments, too, define regions of interest which measure trabecular, cortical or combined skeletal compartments. The early QCT units had much higher radiation exposure and poorer reproducibility than did DXA. Both of these drawbacks have been minimized with the new versions of QCT software.

Spinal QCT may be the most sensitive site for monitoring BMD changes in early menopause or in response to glucocorticoid therapy – clinical conditions in which trabecular bone loss predominates. The rate of measured loss is greater with spinal QCT than with PA spinal DXA. Similarly, larger changes are observed in the trabecular compartment of the radius measured by peripheral QCT than with DXA or SXA. Whether these changes reflect changes in fracture risk is not yet clear.

Evaluating and Comparing Bone Density Results

Absolute BMD values obtained at the same site by scanners of different manufacturers may differ because of different definitions of the regions of interest (especially in the hip, forearm and calcaneus) and variations in edge-detection software and calibration. Despite differences in absolute values, BMD measurements obtained at the same skeletal site by different types of DXA equipment are very highly correlated [14]. Equations and methods for standardizing measurements at the given skeletal site across DXA manufacturers are available [15]. The IBDSC recommends using such standardized BMD values in the spine. This aids comparison of values obtained in the same person on scanners of different manufacturers. However, differences in scanner calibration exist, even among scanners of the same manufacturer, limiting the ability to use different scanners to monitor interval change in an individual even if standardized BMD values are used.

BMD values obtained by DXA are expressed as grams per square centimeter and vary substantially across different skeletal sites. The average values in young women in the spine and mid-radius, measured by Hologic DXA instruments, are 1.05 and 0.70 gm/cm^2, respectively. In an attempt to compare bone density values at different skeletal sites, results have traditionally been expressed as standardized scores in comparison with young-normal or age-matched values. The *Z*-score refers to the number of standard deviations above (a positive number) or below (a negative number) the average values obtained in individuals of the same age and gender. The *T*-score (sometimes referred to as the "age-adjusted *Z*-score") is the number of standard deviations above or below the average bone density values in young adults. This reporting method has proven useful in comparing and discussing bone density values at different skeletal sites.

BMD Diagnostic Criteria for Osteoporosis

Traditionally, the diagnosis of osteoporosis was made clinically when a patient presented with a fragility fracture. Because of the strong relationship between BMD values and fracture risk, the diagnosis of osteoporosis can now be made on the basis of BMD values according to the World Health Organization definitions [16] (Table 3.2). These definitions are only applicable to Caucasian women, are based on the relationship between BMD and fracture risk in postmenopausal women and were not originally designed to be used as criteria for therapeutic intervention.

Table 3.2. World Health Organization diagnostic criteria for osteoporosis

Diagnostic category	Definition	BMD T-score
Normal bone mass	BMD more than 1 standard deviation below the average young adult value	> -1
Osteopenia (low bone mass)	BMD between 1 and 2.5 standard deviations below the average young adult value	< -1 to > -2.5
Osteoporosis	BMD more than 2.5 standard deviations below the average young adult value	< -2.5
Severe osteoporosis	BMD more than 2.5 standard deviations below the average young adult value and one or more osteoporotic fractures	< -2.5

Using these criteria, osteoporosis in postmenopausal women is defined as a BMD *T*-score of < -2.5. Any specific level of a continuous variable used to define a clinical entity or disease must be arbitrary. The *T*-score threshold for osteoporosis was selected to identify the appropriate proportion of the population at increased risk for fracture. This proportion is estimated to be about 30% of the postmenopausal female population. In a subsequent large population survey of femoral neck BMD values in American postmenopausal women, 30% were categorized as having osteoporosis by the WHO criteria [17]. The definition of osteopenia or low bone mass is meant to describe a group of individuals at increased risk of developing osteoporosis in the future but who are not now at high risk for fracture. The classification of severe or established osteoporosis recognizes the additional risk for fracture associated with having had a previous fracture [18].

T- and *Z*-scores are very dependent upon the nature and quality of the normative databases from which the values are derived. Despite attempts to "standardize" the result of bone density tests, significant disparities do exist in diagnostic categorization among bone density measurements at different skeletal sites even when they are expressed as *T*-scores [6,19]. These disparities arise because of differences, in a given individual, in peak bone mass values at different skeletal sites, and different rates of age-related bone loss at different skeletal sites, as well as differences in the databases. Part of the problem could be eliminated if normative databases were derived from the same set of patients. Improved concordance of BMD values in a large group of older women exists when comparisons are made with the group averages of BMD at different skeletal sites, in contrast to their comparison with manufacturers' databases [20]. Having a single set of individuals to serve as the reference population for all bone density technologies, however, is impractical. Furthermore, true differences in BMD values exist among different racial or geographic populations. Discussion continues about whether bone density interpretations should be based on local or regional normative databases or a single database to be used for all populations. Bone density, expressed in absolute units, appears to be similarly predictive of fracture risk in different populations and in both men and women [21,22]. This suggests that, for the purpose of diagnosing osteoporosis and predicting fracture risk, a single database, carefully matched to fracture risk, would be most appropriate for all older adults.

Predicting Fracture Risk

Several large population studies, usually involving older women, have evaluated the association of BMD values and fracture risk. The relationship is usually described as the relative risk (RR) of fractures associated with a 1 standard deviation (SD) decrease in BMD compared with the age-adjusted BMD mean of the population study. DXA measurements of the hip, spine, forearm and calcaneus predict the risk of any fragility fracture in older women similarly, each with a relative risk for any fracture of 1.5 per age-adjusted standard deviation decrease. However, the risk of specific types of fractures, especially hip fractures, is more strongly predicted by measuring bone density at that site. The RR for hip fracture per SD of age-adjusted BMD in the femoral neck is 2.6, while in the mid-radius the RR is 1.5 [23]. For an older woman with a BMD value 2 SD below her age-adjusted mean, her relative risk for hip fracture is about 7 (2.6×2.6), compared with a women with "average" bone density. A similar BMD (Z-score $= -2$) in the radius is associated with a 2.25-fold (1.5×1.5) increase in fracture risk compared with age-matched controls.

Combining BMD and Other Risk Factors for Fracture

Although BMD is a strong and important risk factor for fracture, other risk factors exist which are independent of BMD. These include age, a history of previous fractures, biochemical markers of bone turnover, differences in skeletal geometry, and a variety of clinical risk factors identified in prospective studies. The most important clinical risk factors are body weight (small body mass increases fracture risk), smoking, maternal history of hip fracture, the risk of falls and indices of fragility. Any of these risk factors can be used to identify individuals within a cohort of older patients who are at relatively high risk for fracture. Clearly, postmenopausal women with a previous history of fragility fractures are at high risk for subsequent fracture, irrespective of their BMD values [18]. In the Study of Osteoporotic Fractures, Caucasian women over 65 years of age were classified both into tertiles of calcaneal BMD and by the number of their clinical risk factors for hip fracture [24]. The relationship between BMD and fracture risk was minimally apparent in the women with few clinical risk factors. Women in the highest BMD tertile and with more than four risk factors were at greater risk for hip fracture than were women in the lowest BMD tertile with few risk factors. However, clinical risk factors and biochemical markers are most effectively used to predict fracture risk when combined with bone density results. The subset of women in the Study of Osteoporotic Fractures in the lowest BMD tertile who also had more than four clinical risk factors were at much higher risk for hip fracture than were any other group. Thus, fracture risk and indications for pharmacological intervention should be based on the combination of bone density testing and clinical evaluation.

Summary

Bone density measured by DXA and QCT in multiple skeletal sites provides the clinician, as well as the clinical investigator, with a set of powerful tools to assess skeletal health, predict fracture risk and monitor response to therapeutic interventions. The availability of DXA opened the door for the evaluation of new treatments for osteoporosis, and the subsequent availability of these new therapies now provides the basis for the appropriate application of bone density testing in routine clinical practice.

References

1. Miller PD, Bonnick SL, Rosen CJ. Consensus of an international panel on the clinical utility of bone mass measurements in the detection of low bone mass in the adult population. Calcif Tissue Int 1996;58:207–214.
2. Kelly T, Slovick D, Schoenfield D, et al. Quantitative digital radiography versus dual photon absorptiometry of the lumbar spine. J Clin Endocrinol Metab 1987;67:839–844.
3. Yu W, Gluer CC, Grampp S, et al. Spinal bone mineral assessment in postmenopausal women: a comparison between dual X-ray absorptiometry and quantitative computed tomography. Osteoporos Int 1995;5:433–439.
4. Blake GM, Parker JC, Buxton FMA, Fogelman I. Dual X-ray absorptiometry: a comparison between fan beam and pencil beam scans. Br J Radiol 1993;66:902–906.
5. Patel R, Blake GM, Batchelor S, et al. Occupational dose to the radiographer in dual X-ray absorptiometry: a comparison of pencil-beam and fan-beam systems. Br J Radiol 1996;69:539–542.
6. von der Recke P, Hansen MA, Overgaard K, Christiansen C. The impact of degenerative conditions in the spine on bone mineral density and fracture risk prediction. Osteoporos Int 1996;6:43–49.
7. Yu W, Gluer CC, Fuerst T, Grampp S, Li J, Lu Y, Genant HK. Influence of degenerative joint disease on spinal bone mineral measurements in postmenopausal women. Calcif Tissue Int 1995;57:169–174.
8. Faulkner KG, McClung MR, Ravn P, et al. Monitoring skeletal response to therapy in early postmenopausal women: which bone to measure? J Bone Miner Res 1996;11(suppl 1):S96.
9. Hanson J. Standardization of femur bone mineral density [letter]. J Bone Miner Res 1997;12(8):1316–1317.
10. Mazess RB, Barden HS, Bisek JP, et al. Dual–energy X-ray absorptiometry for total-body and regional bone-mineral and soft-tissue composition. Am J Clin Nutr 1990;51:1106–1112.
11. Brodowicz GR, Mansfield RA, McClung MR, Althoff SA. Measurement of body composition in the elderly: dual energy X-ray absorptiometry, underwater weighing, bioelectrical impedance analysis, and anthropometry. Gerontology 1994;40:332–339.
12. Steiger P, Cummings SR, Genant HK, et al. Morphometric X-ray absorptiometry of the spine: Correlation in vivo with morphometric radiography. Osteoporos Int 1994;4:238–244.
13. Genant HK, Cann CE, Ettinger B, Gordan GS. Quantitative computed tomography of vertebral spongiosa: a sensitive method for detecting early bone loss after oophorectomy. Ann Intern Med 1982;97:699–705.
14. Lai KC, Goodsitt MM, Murano R, et al. A comparison of two dual-energy X-ray absorptiometry systems for spinal bone mineral measurement. Calcif Tissue Int 1992;50: 203–208.
15. Genant HK, Grampp S, Gluer CC, Faulkner KG, et al. Universal standardization for dual X-ray absorptiometry: patient and phantom cross-calibration results. J Bone Miner Res 1994;9:1503–1514.
16. WHO Study Group. Assessment of fracture risk and its application to screening for postmenopausal osteoporosis. WHO Technical Report Series no. 843. Geneva: World Health Organization, 1994:1–129.

17. Looker AC, Wahner HW, Dunn WL, et al. Proximal femur bone mineral levels of US adults. Osteoporos Int 1995;5:389–409.
18. Ross PD, Davis JW, Epstein RS, et al. Pre-existing fractures and bone mass predict vertebral fracture incidence in women. Ann Intern Med 1991;114:914–923.
19. Grampp S, Genant HK, Mathur A, et al. Comparisons of noninvasive bone mineral measurements in assessing age-related loss, fracture discrimination, and diagnostic classification. J Bone Miner Res 1997;12:697–711.
20. Genant HK, Lu Y, Mathur AK, Fuerst TP, Cummings SR. Classification based on DXA measurement for assessing the risk of hip fractures. J Bone Miner Res 1996;11(Suppl 1):S120.
21. DeLaet CEDH, van Hout Ben A, Burger H, Hofman A, Pols HAP. Bone density and risk of hip fracture in men and women: cross-sectional analysis. BMJ 1997;315:221–225.
22. Ross PD, Kim S, Wasnich RD.. Bone density predicts vertebral fracture risk in both men and women: a prospective study. J Bone Miner Res 1996;1(Suppl 1): S127.
23. Cummings SR, Black DM, Nevitt MC, et al. Bone density at various sites is predictive of hip fractures. Lancet 1993;341:72–75.
24. Cummings SR, Nevitt MC, Browner WS, et al. Risk factors for hip fracture in white women. N Engl J Med 1995;332:767–773.

4 Assessment of Bone Status by Quantitative Ultrasound

C.-C. Glüer and R. Barkmann

Introduction

Although early studies using ultrasound to assess bone status had shown some potential [1,2] the development of quantitative ultrasound (QUS) approaches as they are used today started in 1984 with the introduction of a new quantitative measuring parameter, broadband ultrasound attenuation (BUA) by Langton et al. [3]. After results of an early prospective study with 1000 elderly women were reported which showed that a low BUA is an indicator for an increased hip fracture risk [4], it became obvious that there was sense in further investigating this method. Many studies in the 1990s confirmed this result [5,6]. Prospective fracture studies [7–12] as well as some experimental studies taking into consideration biomechanical [13–16] and micromorphological aspects [16–18] were carried out. Today, there is broad consensus that QUS techniques can provide relevant information about bone status, specifically for but not limited to osteoporosis [19].

Technology of QUS Approaches

From the technological point of view those ultrasound approaches that are used in the field of osteoporosis diagnosis differ fundamentally from sonographic approaches which are commonly used in a clinical setting. To transmit signals through the bone, much lower frequencies, typically in the range of 100 kHz up to 2 MHz, have to be applied. QUS approaches are parametrical, normally non-imaging investigation procedures, analyzing the interaction of ultrasound when penetrating the bone. In this context "parametrical" means that instead of obtaining (visual) information which is used for subjective interpretation a quantitative measuring result is gained, which provides information on bone features such as mass, structure or quality. Even QUS imaging approaches [20,21] do not use the image as a source of diagnostic information but only as an aid for the anatomically correct positioning of the region of interest to be evaluated.

The interaction between ultrasound waves and bone tissue leads to a change in the sound velocity and to a reduction in the transmitted power of sound. In the context of QUS approaches, sound velocity is usually called "speed of sound" (SOS) and is specified in units of meters per second (m/s). Analyses of SOS play an important role in materials testing and are also of importance for other applications of ultrasound. For osteoporosis diagnosis, however, an additional special measuring parameter, characterizing sound attenuation proved successful: the so-called broadband ultrasound attenuation (BUA) [3]. The attenuation is primarily caused by scattering, and to a lesser extent, also by absorption. Consequently bone structure, which determines the scattering process to a greater extent than the bone mass, is of decisive importance for the generation and thus also for interpretation of the ultrasonic signal. This distinguishes QUS approaches from other osteodensitometric methods. The adjective "broadband" indicates that broadband signals, i.e. sound waves with a broad spectrum of frequencies (typically 200–600 kHz) are analyzed. A high BUA value indicates a strong linear increase in the attenuation with increased frequencies. It can be supposed that the lower increase found in subjects suffering from osteoporosis is caused by bones with fewer structures of high spatial density. Consequently, scattering of sound waves with high frequencies, i.e., shorter wavelength, is lower. While this appears to be in agreement with theories [22] one has to recognize that this is only a simplified model. Bone architecture is very complex and a conclusive model needs to be developed.

Differences Among QUS Approaches

The evaluation of QUS methodology has become more difficult as different ultrasound approaches and yet more commercial devices are offered on the market. It is necessary to differentiate. QUS is not always equal to QUS, although there are many similarities between the different approaches and devices.

Different devices measure sonic speed in different ways. Very rarely, the real mean bone velocity is determined; in some cases instead, SOS reflects the mean sound velocity through bones and of the soft tissue in the transmission path of the sound waves; and in other cases the sound velocity in the coupling medium water is also included [23]. This is not necessarily a disadvantage but it should be taken into consideration that different definitions might lead to different sensitivity regarding metabolic changes. Another version of the sonic speed is the "amplitude-dependent speed of sound" (AD-SOS) which is obtained when measuring at the finger phalanges; it reflects the influence of sound attenuation and SOS due to measurement at an increased trigger threshold. Even more important than the question of different definitions of SOS are the differences in the approaches with regard to measuring site, bone type measured and the method of signal transmission. Due to different metabolic sensitivity QUS approaches that measure cortical versus cancellous or weight-bearing versus non-weight-bearing bones cannot all be treated alike without proving diagnostic equivalence. Furthermore, different aspects are measured if the bone is irradiated with ultrasonic waves in transverse transmission, in which case the inner structure of the bone influences the signal, as opposed to when it is measured in axial transmission, in which case only the outer millimeters of the cortex contribute to generating the signal. Therefore, study results can only be inferred from one SOS category to another in a limited way.

Even if the definitions of BUA are not as different as those for SOS parameters, BUA values are calculated differently using different devices. Similar to SOS it would be necessary to categorize BUA according to the measurement site but so far BUA has commercially been determined only at a weight-bearing, cancellous bone: the calcaneus.

When looking in more detail at the QUS technology further differences have to be considered: Coupling by an ultrasound gel as it is offered for all measuring sites might be easier with regard to handling than coupling by means of a water bath as is usually done at the calcaneus. As in this case the water temperature is not of any influence, an important error source, especially for measuring SOS is eliminated. On the other hand, coupling of the ultrasound transmitter and receiver has to be done with great care. Due to movements of the transducer during the scanning process image creation is easier in a water bath than with coupling by gel; however, a first ultrasound device with a scanning mechanism working with gel coupling was introduced recently.

In addition to the basic parameters, further combination parameters are calculated. The most commonly used parameter is the ultrasound "stiffness" value, a weighted average of BUA and SOS. Further combination parameters, defined in similar ways, are called the quantitative ultrasound index (QUI), "soundness", etc. These neither reflect the implied biomechanical parameters (ultrasound stiffness is not identical to biomechanical stiffness) nor do they supply other information than that provided by the basic parameters SOS and BUA. They are, however, of practical value as they summarize the two parameters and have a lower precision error, i.e., they are better suited for monitoring (e.g., due to lower sensitivity to temperature [24]). This, however, only applies if SOS and BUA reflect the same trend over time. For age-related processes this is true, but in the case of drug therapy discrepant changes were reported for BUA and SOS in some cases [25]. Therefore, it still has to be checked which parameters are best suited to therapy monitoring and whether combination parameters can always be used without problems. With regard to fracture risk evaluation, combination parameters – taking into consideration all known results – do not offer major advantages or disadvantages. As a mean value they should not give better results than the better of the two single parameters; on the other hand they are somewhat more stable. Apart from combination values derived from BUA and SOS there are, especially for the finger phalanges, more complex measuring parameters that seem to be promising. Their diagnostic value, however, has not been finally clarified.

To facilitate the overview, we suggest grouping QUS approaches into categories. The devices presently commercially available fall into five categories of QUS parameters: four SOS and one BUA parameter (Table 4.1). Figures 4.1 to 4.3 show their measuring procedures in a schematic manner.

Assessing Fracture Risk by QUS Approaches

Similar to bone densitometry approaches, QUS techniques could be used for the (initial) diagnosis, fracture risk evaluation, and monitoring. We currently have limited data regarding the utility of QUS approaches for diagnosis and monitoring, but for assessment of fracture risk numerous studies, including those with a prospective design, have been carried out. Results published in the peer-reviewed literature document that QUS approaches are well suited to the assessment of fracture risk. Still, the abovementioned differences between the five categories need to be considered. We will summarize the results obtained in prospective fracture studies. For further information on cross-sectional studies and a discussion of the applications for diagnosis and monitoring we recommend some recent review articles [5,6,19,26,27] and a book on QUS approaches [28].

Table 4.1. Overview of five main QUS measurement categories currently implemented in commercial devices

Parameter	Site	Weight-bearing	Cortical	Cancellous	Transmission	Amplitude-dependent	Prospective fracture studies	Figure
BUA	Calcaneus	Yes	Minimal	Yes	Transverse	Yes	Several	1
SOS	Calcaneus	Yes	Minimal	Yes	Transverse	No	Several	1
AD-SOS	Phalanges	No	Yes	Variable	Transverse	Yes	One	2
SOS	Phalanges							
	Radius	No	Yes	No	Axial	No	None	3
SOS	Tibia	Yes	Yes	No	Axial	No	None	3

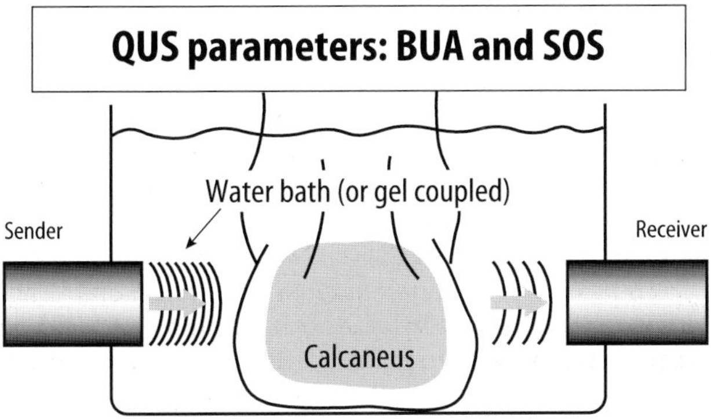

Figure 4.1. Schematic drawing of QUS measurement at the calcaneus (transverse transmission, coupling can alternatively be performed by ultrasound gels).

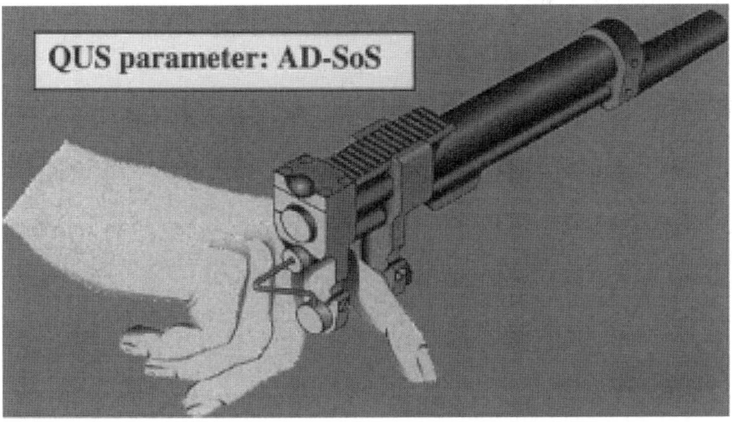

Figure 4.2. Schematic drawing of QUS measurement at the finger phalanges (transverse transmission).

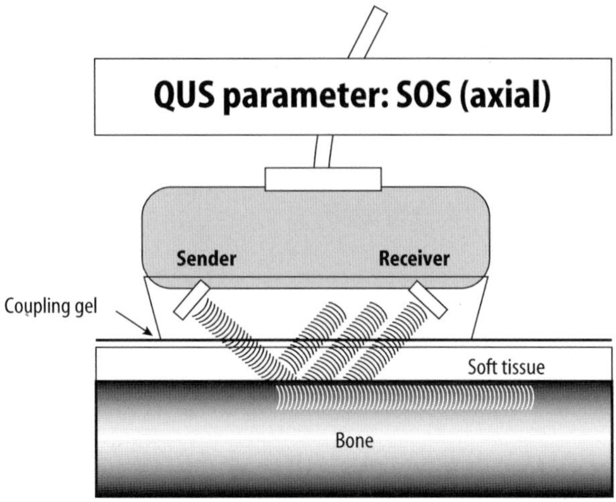

Figure 4.3. Schematic drawing of QUS measurement along the cortex of long bones (axial transmission; e.g., tibia, phalanges, radius).

Review of Prospective Fracture Studies

To date, prospective studies of QUS have been published for devices that measure the weight-bearing cancellous bone of the calcaneus and the non-weight-bearing bone of the finger phalanges, which are comprised of mostly cortical bone at the site investigated. Another study used a device measuring non-weight-bearing trabecular bone of the patella, but this is no longer commercially available. The two largest prospective studies, with sample sizes of 6500 to 10 000 women, showed that QUS results (as measured at the calcaneus) can be used to predict future hip fracture risk in older women [7,9]. Both SOS and BUA were shown to perform equally well [9]. The gradients of risk reported for QUS were similar to those for DXA. A significant but weaker relationship between BUA and non-spine fractures (a 40% increase in risk per standard deviation [7]) was also observed, confirming results of an earlier study in perimenopausal women women [12]. Combinations of BUA and SOS as reflected in the "stiffness" parameter did not improve fracture risk prediction [9]. Smaller prospective studies have documented a relationship between calcaneal BUA and incident vertebral fractures [29], patellar ultrasound velocity and incident vertebral fractures [10], and phalangeal AD-SOS and non-spine fractures [30]. There are no prospective studies of SOS assessed in axial transmission (feasible at, for example, the tibia, radius and phalanges) and fracture risk.

Validation of QUS Devices for Risk Assessment

A device's suitability for fracture risk evaluation should ideally have been documented in prospective fracture studies in comparable populations. Such studies take several years and necessitate more than 1000 participants. Within limits a proof can also be furnished if (a) the device shows results for the study population which closely correlate with those of an already-established device belonging to the same device category and (b) several independently run cross-sectional studies for fracture discrimination are available which unambiguously support the suitability of the device. However, at present there is no consensus about the details of such requirements.

Interpretation of QUS Results

Provided that adequate reference data are available for a given device and that its performance can be monitored by appropriate quality assurance measures, the results of the fracture studies reviewed above can be used to evaluate the magnitude of the fracture risk in individual patients. Typically, the fracture risk increases by approximately a factor of 1.5–2 if a QUS value is reduced by 1 standard deviation, but this can vary between devices and QUS parameters and also for different types of fractures. To estimate fracture risk it is necessary to know (a) the QUS parameter for the patient, (b) the age-correlated or premenopausal peak value of the same QUS parameter (mean value of the population), (c) the population variance, i.e., the mean variation of the values around the mean value given as standard deviation, and (d) the percentage of risk increase per standard deviation (so-called standardized relative risk) as derived from prospective studies. These figures can be used for calculating the extent of fracture risk increase. For example, for a BUA value of the patient of 70 dB/MHz, a population variance of 10 dB/MHz and a standardized relative risk for hip fractures for the device in question of 1.8, the patient would have a 5.4-fold increased risk of hip fracture [$(100 - 70)/10 \times 1.8$] compared with a young healthy woman and a 1.8-fold increased risk of hip fracture [$(80 - 70)/10 \times 1.8$) compared with a healthy woman of the same age.

For any examination it is necessary that the results are evaluated by an experienced and qualified physician. Does the result fall into the age-matched normal range and, if not, by how much is the fracture risk increased? Which other risk factors are to be considered additionally? These and other aspects are required to evaluate the extent of the bone strength impairment and to determine therapy options. If, for example, a patient has suffered a fracture after minimal trauma, a QUS investigation could be performed to establish the extent of skeletal impairment. While it is obvious that no simple recipe such as "if BUA or SOS is smaller than X, then prescribe Y" can be given, the example illustrates how QUS-based fracture risk information can be used clinically.

QUS Versus Bone Densitometry: What Is the Difference?

The utility of QUS for assessment of bone status has been clearly established but a number of questions remain regarding the respective advantages and disadvantages of QUS versus bone densitometry approaches. Both QUS and bone densitometry techniques such as dual-energy X-ray absorptiometry (DXA) and quantitative computed tomography (QCT) can be used to assess characteristics of bone status that are relevant for the estimation of bone strength and along with that of fracture risk. The classical bone densitometry techniques measure the attenuation of X-rays when passing through bone. This is largely governed by the amount of calcium in the path of the X-rays and, therefore, aside from sources of error such as soft tissue and extraskeletal calcifications, the results closely reflect bone mass. Sound waves, on the other hand, are *mechanical* waves and, therefore, are affected by all the characteristics of bone that determine its mechanical properties. From an orthopaedic point of view one would be more interested in the overall mechanical state of bone than in the specific question of how much calcium there is. Therefore, from this point of view QUS approaches have the potential to provide a more direct and thus potentially more comprehensive insight into skeletal status as it relates to mechanical strength. For example, bone strength is known to depend both on bone mass and on bone structure. Bone densitometry approaches, however, unlike QUS methods, reflect only to a very low degree the structural influence on bone strength [19].

This difference between densitometric and ultrasound approaches has led to some confusion regarding the interpretation of results. Since QUS parameters are affected by characteristics of bone other than density the correlation of bone mineral density (BMD) and QUS parameters is imperfect. While it may reach levels exceeding $r = 0.7$ for carefully site-matched measurements [31,32], it is typically much lower when comparing QUS results obtained at the calcaneus and BMD of the main fracture sites such as spine and proximal femur, with correlations ranging around $r = 0.3$–0.5 [33,35]. This, however, does not imply that QUS techniques are inferior to densitometry approaches in the assessment of bone strength and fracture risk. QUS approaches may probe relevant characteristics of bone not measurable by bone densitometry and, on the other hand, they may be affected by error sources not relevant for densitometric techniques. Both techniques have advantages and disadvantages and in clinical fracture studies have generally been shown to yield comparable results [7,9]. Bone densitometry thus cannot be regarded as the gold standard and, therefore, it is methodologically incorrect to gauge QUS performance by comparing the technique with bone densitometry approaches [19]. Moreover, familiar concepts such as accuracy errors (i.e., the deviation of the measured and the true result) are more difficult to apply. QUS parameters do not measure a single simple-to-determine property of bone (such as bone mass) and, therefore, should be judged on their ability to reflect the overall mechanical competence. A direct assessment of fracture risk predictive power or the ability to determine bone strength in vitro is required for a proper evaluation of the performance of QUS versus densitometric techniques.

From a practical point of view QUS approaches offer additional advantages. During ultrasound assessments the patient is not exposed to ionizing radiation. This enhances the patient's acceptance of the test. Moreover, ultrasound technology is less expensive than X-ray technology and devices can be designed to be portable. Nevertheless, one has to recognize that a number of low-cost X-ray techniques for the assessment of the peripheral skeleton have recently successfully been introduced to the market. They also measure BMD at peripheral skeletal sites such as the calcaneus, the radius and the hand. It remains to be seen how such devices perform in direct comparison with QUS approaches. The lack of ionizing radiation facilitates placement, licencing and operation of equipment because of less demanding regulations for personnel and space. Therefore, ultrasound has a potential for wider applicability compared with X-ray based methods. Nevertheless, appropriate training of personnel and sufficient quality assurance measures need to be ensured.

Prospects

The description given above shows that at least the better-validated QUS devices – if operated carefully and the results are interpreted correctly – are suitable for fracture risk evaluation. The open questions with regard to diagnosis and technological improvements regarding reproducibility will probably be solved in the future. The potential of QUS approaches to provide a measurement parameter that not only depends on bone mass but also reflects influences on bone microstructure and bone material properties shows a perspective for future ultrasound developments: It might be possible to overcome the limitations of traditional bone densitometry, i.e., the restriction of measuring bone mass only, by QUS approaches. If structural features can be differentiated from mass features, then different quality aspects of the bone status can be distinguished and a more sophisticated diagnosis would become feasible. Differential diagnosis of osteoporosis and osteomalacia as well as distinguishing different types of renal osteodystrophy are a possibility. As yet, however, it is too early to talk about a breakthrough, and further investigations will be necessary.

The other, very different future prospect is based on the potential of a widespread use of QUS approaches. QUS devices are inexpensive, the examination does not expose either patient or doctor or MTRA to ionizing rays (an advantage, although radiation exposure is already very low – about 1–5 μSv – with common X-ray based osteodensitometry) and it is very well accepted by patients. Commercial incentives resulting from this, more widespread indications for use of QUS, the assumed easier interpretation of results – all these factors may lead to an improper use if operators are not sufficiently instructed or motivated. To avoid this it is absolutely necessary to train operators thoroughly, to regularly perform quality assurance measures, to formulate and distribute appropriate guidelines and to develop rules about who may use QUS approaches under what circumstances. Uncontrolled use of this powerful approach may easily lead to misuse. Experiences with bone densitometry show that prevention of such misuse is extremely important. Certification courses as they are presently prepared by the International Osteoporosis Foundation, the parent association of European osteoporosis organisations, show a promising way forward. It should be possible to introduce detailed quality assurance measures as they are already common in laboratory medicine. Misuse must be avoided, QUS approaches in particular offer the possibility of reducing the diagnosis gap currently present in osteoporosis. Early diagnosis plays an important role in a disorder such as osteoporosis that is characterized by a slow and gradual progress. For finalizing a concrete strategy for clinical use – no one is going to advocate unrestricted screening – population-based QUS studies that are presently carried out will provide the required data bases. If QUS is used in a responsible fashion it will be of decisive importance for the assessment of bone status, specifically for but not limited to osteoporosis.

References

1. Abendschein W, Hyatt GW. Ultrasonics and selected physical properties of bone. Clin Orthop 1970;69:294–301.
2. Lang SB. Elastic coefficients of animal bone. Science 1969;165:287–288.
3. Langton CM, Palmer SB, Porter RW. The measurement of broadband ultrasound attenuation in cancellous bone. Eng Med 1984;13:89–91.

4. Porter R, Miller C, Grainger D, Palmer S. Prediction of hip fracture in elderly women: a prospective study. BMJ 1990;301:638–641.
5. Gregg EW, Kriska AM, Salamone LM, et al. The epidemiology of quantitative ultrasound: a review of the relationships with bone mass, osteoporosis and fracture risk. Osteoporos Int 1997;7:89–99.
6. Njeh CF, Boivin CM, Langton CM. The role of ultrasound in the assessment of osteoporosis: a review. Osteoporos Int 1997;7:7–22.
7. Bauer DC, Glüer CC, Cauley JA, et al. Bone ultrasound predicts fractures strongly and independently of densitometry in older women: a prospective study. Arch Intern Med 1997;157:629–634.
8. Cadossi R, Mele R, Masci G, Ventura V, de Aloysio D, Bicocchi M. Fracture risk assessment by quantitative ultrasound at the hand phalanx: three year longitudinal study. J Bone Miner Res. 1997;12(Suppl.1):S383.
9. Hans D, Dargent-Molina P, Schott AM, et al. Ultrasonographic heel measurements to predict hip fracture in elderly women: the EPIDOS prospective study. Lancet 1996;348:511–514.
10. Heaney RP, Avioli LV, Chesnut CH III, Lappe J, Recker RR, Brandenburger GH. Ultrasound velocity through bone predicts incident vertebral deformity. J Bone Miner Res 1995;10:341–345.
11. Pluijm SMF, Graafmans WC, Bouter LM, Lips P. Ultrasound measurements for the prediction of osteoporotic fractures in elderly people. J Bone Miner Res 1997;12 (Suppl.1):S362.
12. Stewart A, Torgerson DJ, Reid DM. Prediction of fractures in perimenopausal women: a comparison of dual energy x-ray absorptiometry and broadband ultrasound attenuation. Ann Rheum Dis 1996;55:140–142.
13. Bouxsein ML, Courtney AC, Hayes WC. Ultrasound and densitometry of the calcaneus correlate with the failure loads of cadaveric femurs. Calcif Tissue Int 1995;56: 99–103.
14. Grimm MJ, Williams JL. Prediction of Young's modulus in trabecular bone with a combination of ultrasound velocity and attenuation measurements. In: Langrana NA, Friedman MH, Grood ES, editors. Bioengineering conference, Breckenridge, CO: The American Society of Mechanical Engineers, 1993: 608–609.
15. Langton CM, Njeh CF, Hodgskinson R, Currey JD. Prediction of mechanical properties of the human calcaneus by broadband ultrasonic attentuation. Bone 1996;18: 495–503.
16. Turner CH, Eich M. Ultrasonic velocity as a predictor of strength in bovine cancellous bone. Calcif Tissue Int 1991;49:116–119.
17. Glüer CC, Wu CY, Genant HK. Broadband Ultrasound Attenuation signals depend on trabecular orientation: an in vitro study. Osteoporosis Int 1993;3(4):185–191.
18. Takano Y, Turner CH, Burr DB. Mineral anisotropy in mineralized tissues is similar among species and mineral growth occurs independently of collagen orientation in rats: results from acoustic velocity measurements. J Bone Miner Res 1996;11:1292–1301.
19. Glüer CC, The International Quantitative Ultrasound Consensus Group. Quantitative ultrasound techniques for the assessment of osteoporosis: expert agreement on current status. J Bone Mineral Res 1997;12:1280–1288.
20. Laugier P, Giat P, Berger G. Broadband ultrasonic attenuation imaging: a new imaging technique of the os calcis. Calcif Tissue Int 1994;54:83–86.
21. Roux C, Fournier B, Laugier P, et al. Broadband ultrasound attenuation imaging: a new imaging method in osteoporosis. J Bone Miner Res 1996;11:1112–1118.
22. Biot MA. Generalized theory of acoustic propagation in porous dissipative media. J Acoust Soc Am 1962;34:1254–1264.
23. Miller CG, Herd RJM, Ramalingam T, Fogelman I, Blake GM. Ultrasonic velocity measurements through the calcaneus: which velocity should be measured? Osteoporos Int 1993;3:31–35.

24. Morris R, Mazess R, Trempe J, Hanson J. Stiffness compensates for temperature variation in ultrasound densitometry. J Bone Miner Res 1997;12(Suppl.1):S388.
25. Rosenthall L, Caminis J, Tenenhouse A. Calcaneal ultrasonometry: response to treatment compared to DXA of the lumbar spine and femur. J Bone Miner Res 1997;12 (Suppl.1):S120.
26. Hans D, Fuerst T, Duboeuf F. Quantitative ultrasound bone measurement. Eur Radiol 1997;7(Suppl 2):S43–S50.
27. Prins SH, Jørgensen HL, Jørgensen LV, Hassager C. The role of quantitative ultrasound in the assessment of bone: a review. Clin Physiol 1998;18:3–17.
28. Njeh CF, Hans D, Fuerst T, Glüer CC, Genant HK. Quantitative ultrasound; assessment of osteoporosis and bone status. London: Martin Dunitz, 1999.
29. Huang C, Ross PD, Yates AJ, et al. Prediction of fracture risk by radiographic absorptiometry and quantitative ultrasound: a prospective study. Calcif Tissue Int 1998;63: 380–384.
30. Mele R, Masci G, Ventura V, de Aloysio D, Bicocchi M, Cadossi R. Three-year longitudinal study with quantitative ultrasound at the hand phalanx in a femal population. Osteoporos Int 1997;7:550–557.
31. Glüer CC, Vahlensieck M, Faulkner KG, Engelke K, Black D, Genant HK. Site-matched calcaneal measurements of broadband ultrasound attenuation and single x-ray absorptiometry: do they measure different skeletal properties? J Bone Miner Res 1992;7: 1071–1079.
32. Waud C, Lew R, DT. B. The relationship between ultrasound and densitometric measurements of bone mass at the calcaneus in women. Calcif Tissue Int 1992;51: 415–418.
33. Faulkner KG, McClung MR, Coleman LJ, Kingston-Sandahl E. Quantitative ultrasound of the heel: correlation with densitometric measurements at different skeletal sites. Osteoporos Int 1994;4:42–47.
34. Massie A, Reid DM, Porter RW. Screening for osteoporosis: comparison between dual energy x-ray absorptiometry and broadband ultrasound attenuation in 1000 perimenopausal women. Osteoporos Int 1993;3:107–110.
35. van Daele PLA, Burger H, Algra D, et al. Age-associated changes in ultrasound measurements of the calcaneus in men and women: the Rotterdam study. J Bone Miner Res 1994;9:1751–1757.

5 Biomechanics, Bone Quality and Strength

R. Huiskes and T. S. Kaastad

Introduction

Osteoporosis is a biomechanical problem. It is not a problem by itself – on the contrary, osteoporosis gives you less weight to carry around. But osteoporotic bone is less strong than normal bone, and it is only the prospect of a fracture that gives it an undesirable aspect. Fracture is a matter of stress versus strength; hence, it is a biomechanical problem. A fracture will only occur if the force on a bone is higher than its strength, or when its strength is lower than the force it is subjected to. In the case of a hip or a wrist fracture, a super-normal, traumatic impact force is usually involved, and one may wonder whether the bone would not have broken equally well if it was not osteoporotic. But in the case of a vertebral fracture the forces are usually not much higher than normal; the fracture is often spontaneous. Whatever the difference, the principle remains the same: fracture risk is found in the balance of force versus resistance to force; stress versus strength (Fig. 5.1).

There are four main areas in which biomechanical research and technology are of particular importance to osteoporosis. The first is the evaluation of bone strength. This is important for the diagnosis of osteoporosis, evaluation of fracture risk, prevention of fractures and management of fracture fixation. The second area concerns the prevention of falls and the attenuation of impact loading. The third relates to Wolff's law and the effects of forces on bone mass maintenance and adaptation. The revelation of remodelling mechanisms, which enhance bone mass and strength through mechanical stimuli, could give us the opportunity to determine those activities and exercises that might prevent osteoporosis, or could maybe even reverse it. The fourth area relates to treatment of osteoporosis as well, as it concerns preclinical testing of drugs. The preclinical assessment of the efficacy of drugs in the prevention of fractures requires evaluation of bone strength in experimental animals. As these animals tend to be small – rats, usually – the design of suitable post-mortem strength tests of bone with adequate precision is not trivial.

Most osteoporotic fractures occur in cancellous bone, and we have limited ourselves to cancellous bone in this chapter for a discussion of mechanical bone quality, as it relates to bone strength and fracture risk. *Quality* is meant here in the sense of "degree of excellence" [*Webster's Dictionary*, 1996], as a property

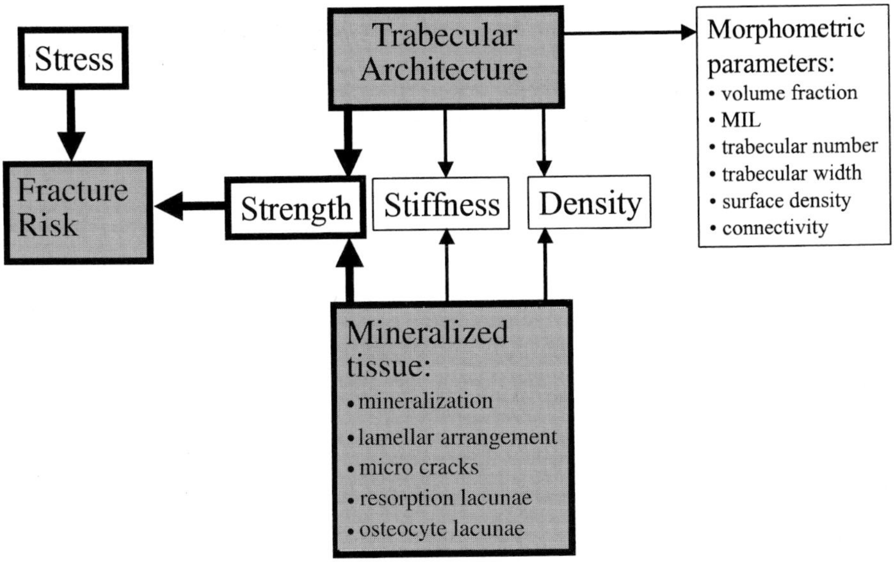

Figure 5.1. Fracture risk depends on the balance between stress on bone, as an effect of normal or traumatic forces, and its strength, as it depends on the mechanical quality of the architecture and the mineralized tissue. The same properties that determine bone strength also determine its stiffness and its density. Architectural quality can be expressed in several morphometric parameters, which can be given values, as discussed in the text.

complementary to *quantity*, as it is used most often in bone biology. It is common to differentiate the properties of bone that determine bone strength into quantity, expressed as bone mass, or density, and quality, as represented by its trabecular architecture and the characteristics of the mineralized matrix [1]. One should be aware, however, that these terms are ambiguous. Sometimes the meaning of *bone quality* is restricted to that of the mineralized matrix only [2], while in orthopaedic biomechanics *quality* is used in the sense of a property, to summarize a "particular character or part; capacity; function" [*Webster's Dictionary*, 1996]. Thus the *mechanical quality of bone* refers to its capacity to withstand mechanical load, while morphological qualities such as bone mass and architecture, and the mechanical quality of the mineralized tissue, are the factors on which this capacity depends. To complicate things even further, *architecture* is often used as a quality combining both the spatial arrangement of trabeculae and the amount of bone mass, but other times as spatial arrangement only [2]. We did not select a particular convention for this chapter, but just ask the reader to be aware of these alternatives. We have tried to be as explicit as possible about the meaning of terms used.

Another source of confusion is the matter of material versus structural mechanical quality of bone. The former refers to (cancellous or cortical) bone as a *material*, the latter to bones themselves, as *structures* made out of bone material, for which also anatomical dimensions play a role. Here we discuss only material qualities, expressed per unit of volume. We will see that this also introduces ambiguity, as cancellous bone can be seen as either a porous material or as a trabecular structure.

Bone Fracture

If a bone fractures, for whatever reason, its strength is less than the stress it is subjected to. This phenomenon, fracture, is a process rather than an event. Although it seems to occur instantly, in slow motion it is the effect of a cascade of phenomena. The strength of the bone material and the stresses it is subjected to due to external loads are not normally distributed uniformly. Thus a fracture is initiated locally, at a particular spot, as a *crack*. If the stress in that spot is only slightly higher than the strength, and lasts only momentarily, it is possible that such a crack (or micro-crack) is the only effect. But when it is not, the crack will propagate through the bone material, causing a gross fracture of the bone as a whole. Due to high impact loading, as during a fall on the hip, this *crack propagation process* occurs very rapidly. But it can also occur very slowly, for instance as a few micrometers per step taken, and then result in what is called a *stress fracture* in orthopaedics but a *fatigue fracture* in mechanics. All solid materials are known to be subject to fatigue, which is nothing else other than the accumulation of micro-cracks during repetitive loading. Bone, as an essentially composite material at all morphological levels, is particularly prone to fatigue, and we all have a certain percentage of micro-cracks in our bones at any moment in time [3]. As opposed to other solids, however, bone removes the micro-cracks by repair and remodelling. Thus normally, although micro-cracks develop as an effect of our typical daily loading patterns, this process does not result in a fatigue fracture, owing to the counteracting remodelling process. But we must realize that at any particular time the strength of our bones can be less than at other times – as, for instance, after long, strenuous exercise. The strength of bone is, in short, not constant, but time dependent.

The time dependency of bone strength is not just caused by the fatigue process described above, but is also an effect of the remodelling process, or of defects in the remodelling process. In the course of life, generally after the age of 30 years, bone mass and strength gradually reduce in both men and women. This is probably caused by reductions in mechanical usage [2], and its effects in the sense of Wolff's law. Women, in addition, undergo a disturbance in the strain-adaptive remodelling process due to estrogen loss after the menopause.

An entirely different mechanical failure modality for bone is *buckling*. Buckling relates to stiffness, rather than strength. Take a plastic stirring rod, such as is often supplied with coffee or tea in a cafeteria, between the thumb and forefinger and compress it. It will bend outwards and then break. That is buckling. Resistance against buckling is fully dependent on the resistance to bending outwards, and that, in turn, depends on the stiffness of the material and the slenderness of the rod. If the rod is made out of a flexible material, relatively long and thin, it is sensitive to buckling failure. This phenomenon is thought to occur in spontaneous failure of trabeculae in vertebral bodies, particularly due to the resorption of horizontal trabeculae normally supporting the vertical ones [4]. As the resistance to buckling is dependent on bone remodelling and resorption, it is time dependent as well, just like the resistance against fracture.

Thus when we discuss the balance between the strength of bone and the stress it is subjected to, it must be realized that this should be placed in a dynamic context of both spatial and temporal variations. Stress is non-uniformly distributed in the bone material, while at any given location it varies in time as well, due to variations in both the magnitude and direction of external forces. The time scales of stress and strength variations differ. Stress is variable on the order of seconds, the strength effects of the fatigue process on the order of hours, and those of the remodelling process on the order of weeks.

At any particular moment, however, bone strength depends only on morphology, at several microscopic levels, and the quality of its constituent materials. In Fig. 5.1 these factors are specified for cancellous bone and grouped into two levels: quality of architecture and quality of the mineralized matrix. Note that in this scheme the *quantity* of bone is included in the architectural factor. The reason is that although quantity can be defined and measured, there is no practical definition or measure for *spatial trabecular arrangement* independent of quantity. The factors that determine cancellous bone strength, as listed in Fig. 5.1, are exactly the same as those that determine its *stiffness*.

Mechanical Bone Quality: Stiffness and Strength

Bone stiffness (resistance against deformation) and strength (resistance against fracture) are the mechanical qualities of bone that matter. Both can be defined and evaluated by the same test. In a compression test (Fig. 5.2) a bone sample is gradually compressed, which produces a reduction in height by a displacement of the test machine's cross-head, and requires a force (F). The reduction in height is normalized to the original height of the sample, as a displacement per unit length, called *strain* (ε), which is dimensionless. The force is normalized to the area of the surface on which it is applied (the upper face of the bone cube), as *stress* (σ), expressed in N/mm^2 or MPa. While the test runs, increasing stress and strain are monitored in the form of a *stress–strain curve* (Fig. 5.2).

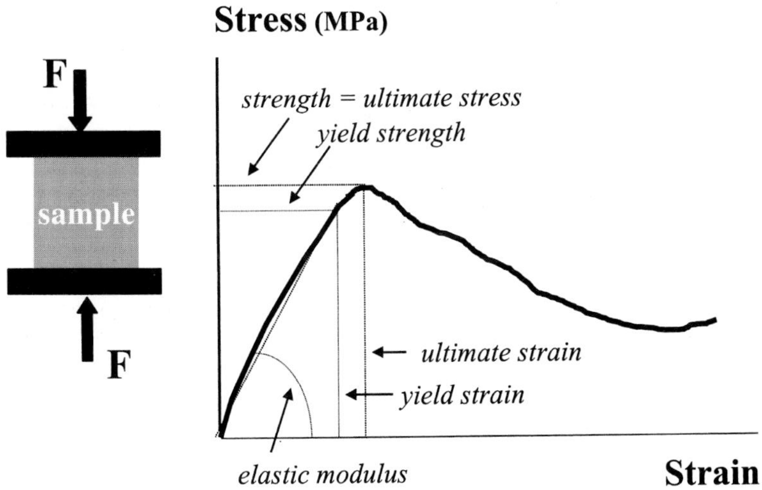

Figure 5.2. A material sample is tested to failure in compression. Its properties are characterized in a stress–strain curve. In the first phase bone behaves in a linear elastic manner by approximation, and the angle of the stress–strain curve determines its elastic modulus. At higher loads cracks start to form when the stress reaches the yield strength of the material, associated with its yield strain. Eventually, total fracture occurs when the stress level reaches the strength (or ultimate stress), associated with the ultimate strain.

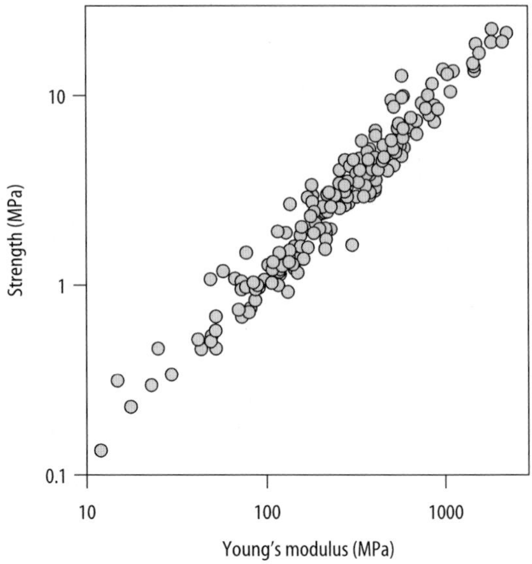

Figure 5.3. Strength versus stiffness in cancellous bone from several species, in a wide variety of densities, shown on a log-log scale. Note that although strength and stiffness are highly correlated statistically, prediction of strength from stiffness in individual cases is still subject to large standard deviations. Courtesy of Professor John D. Currey, PhD, York, UK [5].

In the first part of the curve (Fig. 5.2) we see an approximately linear relationship between stress and strain. This is an expression of the *linear elastic* quality of bone. Later the curve deviates from linearity, meaning that the region of irreversible *plastic* deformation was reached, in which micro-cracks start to form. The stress value at which this occurs is called the *yield strength* of the material. The stress at which fracture eventually occurs is called the *strength* or *ultimate stress* of the material (sometimes also called *failure stress*). In the example of Fig. 5.2 the yield strength is close to the ultimate stress, which is usually so for bone in compression. The linear relationship between stress and strain in the initial loading phase, implying linear elastic behavior of bone, allows us to express strain as a function of stress according to $\varepsilon = \sigma/E$, where E (MPa) is a material constant called the *elastic* (*or Young's*) *modulus*. Thus, if we know the strain in an arbitrary region of the material, we can calculate the stress, and vice versa. The elastic modulus thus measures the *stiffness* of the material. Generally, there tends to be a correlation between strength and stiffness of a material; stiff materials are usually strong, while flexible materials are weak, as shown for bone in Fig. 5.3 [5].

In the above example it was assumed that the material tested is continuous (without pores), homogeneous (the same constitution in the entire volume) and isotropic (similar mechanical properties in all loading directions). But even cortical bone has pores; and although reasonably homogeneous when considered over a macroscopic volume, it is certainly not isotropic. Along the *grain* of its structure, the axial direction in the cortex, both strength and elastic moduli are considerably higher than in both the radial and tangential directions, up to some 50%. For cancellous bone the deviations are even worse, as at the level where it matters, that of the trabecular architecture, it is a structure, rather than a material. The consequences

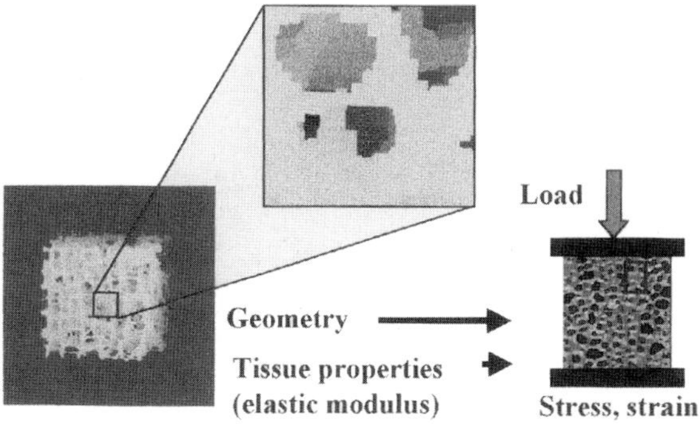

Figure 5.4. The trabecular architecture of bone can now be measured with microcomputed tomography (μCT) scanners, and reconstructed in graphics computer programs, in which the mineralized matrix is imaged in small cubes, called voxels, typically 20 μm in size [11,12]. The voxel mesh can be transformed into a finite-element mesh which, given the elastic tissue properties, can be used for micro-finite element analysis (μFEA) computer simulation of a bone sample test. In this way, the elastic modulus of the bone sample can be estimated, and stress transfer through the trabecular architecture can also be evaluated [6].

of this are visualized in Fig. 5.4, which stems from a finite element analysis (FEA) computer simulation of a compression test, similar to the one above (Fig. 5.2). Evidently, the stress distribution in the bone sample is not homogeneous, as was presumed in the evaluation above. The force applied on the upper face of the cube is transferred through the sample as water flows from a hill through its gullies after rainfall: some trabeculae carry much of the load, some carry nothing, and some only a little. Although the sample as a whole is loaded in compression, some individual trabeculae are loaded in tension, and many in bending [6]. To what extent can we treat cancellous bone as a *material*, and apply the associated principles of mechanics? The answer is that we can, with reasonable approximation, if a sample contains more than five trabeculae, measured along any direction [7]. In that case we may treat the sample as though it were a continuous material. The qualities we measure, in that case, we call *apparent* qualities. For example, the *apparent density* of the cube is its total bone mass, divided by its volume. So it is treated as a sort of average, depending on *actual density* of the mineralized matrix and the *bone volume fraction* of the trabecular architecture (volume of mineralized matrix per volume cancellous bone). Likewise, the *apparent elastic modulus* and the *apparent strength* are defined and determined according to the same test as described above (Fig. 5.2).

Strength and Stiffness as Related to Bone Quantity and Quality

Quantity

Osteoporosis is defined and commonly assessed in terms of bone mass or density; hence in terms of quantity. Well-controlled studies showed that radiographic data,

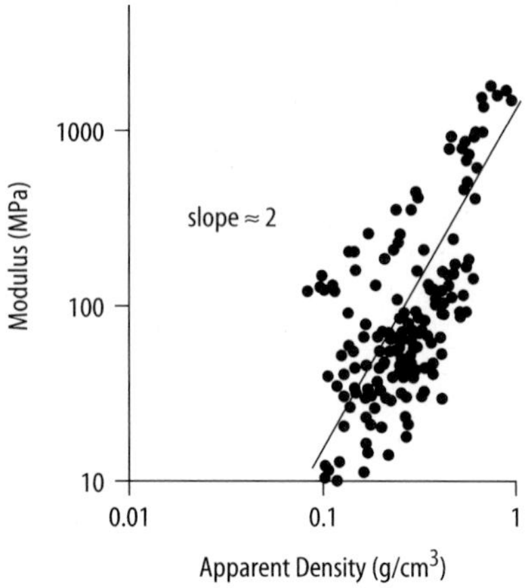

Figure 5.5. Correlation between apparent density and elastic modulus of cancellous bone, as measured in compressive tests of samples from various sites in various species. Typically, 60–80% of modulus values are explained by density. Reproduced from Bouxsein et al. [9], with permission.

as from quantitative computed tomography (QCT) measurements of bone mass, could account for 48–90% of the variability in structural bone strength [8]; therefore the unexplained 10–52% relied on other modalities of the bone. Hence, cancellous bone strength does not depend on quantity alone, as the quality of trabecular morphology, the architecture, plays a role as well, as does the quality of the mineralized tissue. It has been found in post-mortem tests with bone samples like the one described above, that bone strength and stiffness are both proportional, by approximation, to the apparent density squared, as illustrated in Fig. 5.5 [9]. This implies that when, for example, bone mass has reduced by 20%, strength has reduced by about 36%. But this relationship is indicative only, as the statistical correlation between density and stiffness is not very strong (Fig. 5.5). Depending on the homogeneity of specimens tested in well-controlled laboratory experiments, it was found that some 60–70% of the strength values could be explained by density [10]. Thus 30–40% of cancellous bone strength depends not on the quantity of bone, but on the quality of the trabecular architecture and that of the mineralized tissue. For stiffness, this is about 20–40% [9].

Architectural Quality

The properties of cancellous bone seen as a material depend on its characteristics as a structure. At the microscopic level we see trabecular architecture and the material it is made of, the mineralized tissue. Looking again at the stress transfer in the bone sample of Fig. 5.4, it is evident how these two morphological qualities, microscopic architecture and mineralized tissue, play separate roles. The trabecular architecture decides where the stresses are spread; it is up to the tissue, locally, to deal with it in terms of stiffness and strength. Stiffness and strength of cancellous bone therefore depend on trabecular architecture and tissue matrix properties as separate entities, as depicted in Fig. 5.1. The tissue matrix properties, in their turn, depend on the degree of mineralization, the submicroscopic texture, the properties of the collagen matrix and on defects such as osteocyte and resorption lacunae, and micro-cracks (Fig. 5.1).

In the results of mechanical tests the effects of architectural and mineralized tissue qualities on specimen stiffness can not be discriminated. But owing to recent technological developments, this can now be done in computer simulations of tests with micro-finite element analysis (μFEA) illustrated in Fig. 5.4. The trabecular architecture of specimens can be graphically reconstructed with serial sectioning or microcomputed tomography (μCT) scanning, which provide a resolution high enough to represent trabecular refinement [11–13]. From the voxel-density mesh thus obtained, a μFEA mesh can be constructed, for which suitable computer algorithms have been developed to simulate mechanical tests [6]. In this case an arbitrary "effective" isotropic elastic modulus is assigned to the mineralized tissue, hence only the architecture plays a role in such analyses.

To date, only the stiffness of a cancellous bone specimen can be evaluated with this method, not its strength. Cancellous bone is anisotropic. Hence, the elastic modulus values found in a test depend on the test direction. However, according to the theory of elasticity, the elastic constants of anisotropic materials can also be quantified. What helps us here is that the anisotropy of cancellous bone is not arbitrary but *orthotropic* [14,15]. This means it has a particular symmetry which allows us to express its elastic properties as measured along three perpendicular orientations, called the principal material directions. So in practice, the elastic moduli of a sample can be determined by repeating a test as shown in Fig. 5.2 for other directions, which must also include shear tests. In total, an orthotropic material requires nine elastic constants to be fully characterized in its elastic properties; six of these can be determined experimentally, but all can be determined in a μFEA simulation [6].

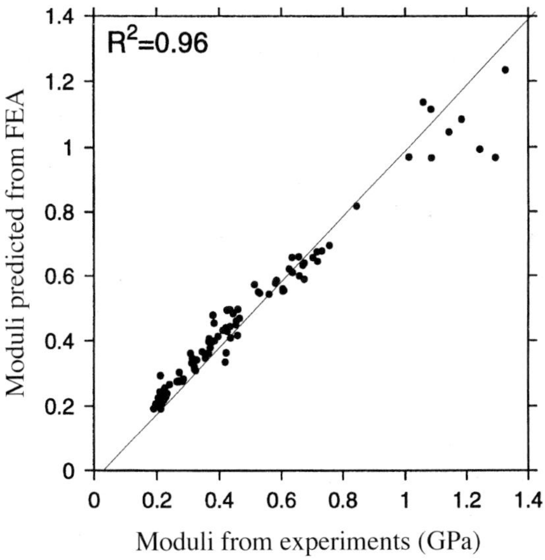

Figure 5.6. Correlation between elastic moduli measured in compressive tests and as predicted with μFEA simulation for (relatively homogeneous) vertebral whale bone. Assuming a uniform modulus value for the mineralized tissue, a correlation of 92% was obtained. By scaling the tissue modulus to the apparent density of each sample, the correlation was improved to 96% . Courtesy of Jesper Kabel, MD, PhD, Aarhus, Denmark [16].

By comparing the results of the simulations (which do not include information about mineralized tissue qualities) with those of actual tests on the same specimens (which include both architectural and mineralized tissue qualities) up to 96% correlation was found between experimental and analytical elastic moduli [16,17], as illustrated in Fig. 5.6. This implies that the stiffness of (normal) cancellous bone is determined predominantly by variations in architecture, while the mineralized tissue stiffness is rather constant at an effective elastic modulus value of an average 5.6 GPa (SD 0.2) [16].

Morphometric Measures of Architectural Quality

Above it was shown that the stiffness properties of cancellous bone are highly correlated with trabecular architecture alone (implicitly including both quantity and spatial trabecular arrangement). This begs the question whether a similar correlation can be found with morphometric parameters which capture the quality of the architecture in some way (Fig. 5.1). Examples of these are scalar quantities such as *specific trabecular surface, trabecular number, trabecular width* and *trabecular separation*, popular in histomorphometry. None of these discriminates architectural quality from quantity, and none produces improved correlation with strength as compared with *trabecular volume fraction* or *apparent density* (hence quantity) alone [18]. Parameters independent of quantity are *connectivity* and *fractal number*. Little can be said about the latter, but connectivity was shown not to improve upon the correlation between bone mass and strength or stiffness either [10,18,19], at least not in normal bone.

As shown in mechanical testing, the most serious disturbance of the relationship between strength (or stiffness) and density is produced by variations in the test direction of the specimens. In vertebral specimens the strength anisotropy (ratio between axial and transverse yield-strength values) was found to be 2 in young and 3.5 in old subjects [20]. The stiffness of a specimen tested in the principal material direction can be up to 8 times as high as when tested in either transverse direction [21,22]. Directionality of trabecular architecture can be quantified by a parameter called *mean intercept length* (MIL) [18,21,22], as illustrated in Fig. 5.7. Like most of the other morphometric parameters, MIL is not independent of volume fraction, so its inclusion in statistical analyses does not always improve upon correlation with bone quantity alone. It was shown in sophisticated analyses of compressive experiments on bone specimens that 72–94% of variation in the three-dimensional elastic (stiffness) constants could be explained by apparent density and MIL combined [21]. This suggests that 6–28% of stiffness variations would depend on variations in the mechanical quality of the mineralized tissue, but that is not entirely true. First, MIL is a parameter for directionality only by approximation, and secondly, experimental assessment of cancellous bone elastic constants is notoriously imprecise [23,24]. A better evaluation of the significance of MIL for the prediction of stiffness can be obtained from μFEA simulations, as in that case neither experimental errors nor variations in mineralized matrix properties are included. It was found in this way that volume fraction and MIL together explain the variance in the individual elastic constants of (relatively homogeneous) vertebral whale bone for 92–98% [22], as illustrated in Fig. 5.8. For more variable human bone specimens a typical correlation of 93% was found, using the same methods [25]. This shows that MIL can be a powerful predictor for architectural mechanical

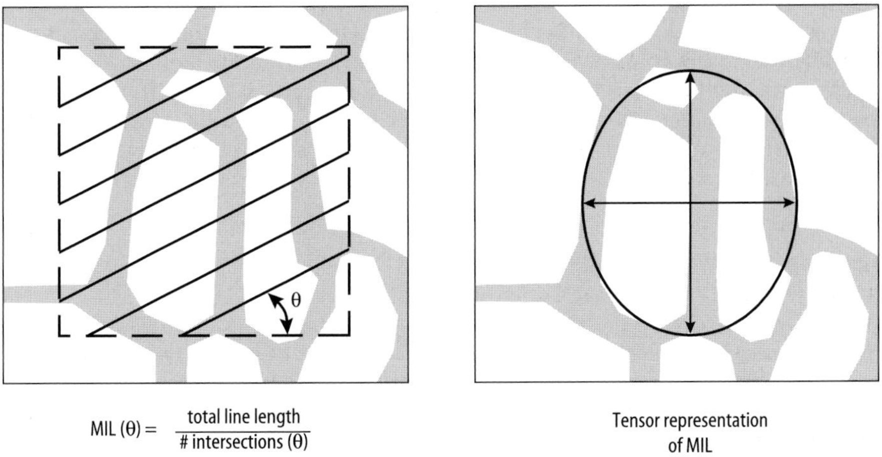

Figure 5.7. Mean intercept length (MIL) in a trabecular surface is determined by projecting a grid of lines over that surface and counting the total number of intersections between bone and marrow. This is repeated for stepwise increasing values of θ; hence MIL is determined as a function of orientation. When plotted in a polar graph, this function yields an ellipse, with the longest axis indicating the principal material direction. If the material is isotropic, the ellipse is circular. Such measurement procedures are now computer-automated, and can also be performed three-dimensionally, if a computer reconstruction of the architecture is available. In that case a spatial ellipsoid is obtained. The orientation of the longest MIL axis coincides with the one of maximal stiffness. Courtesy of Harry van Lenthe, MS, Nijmegen, The Netherlands [26].

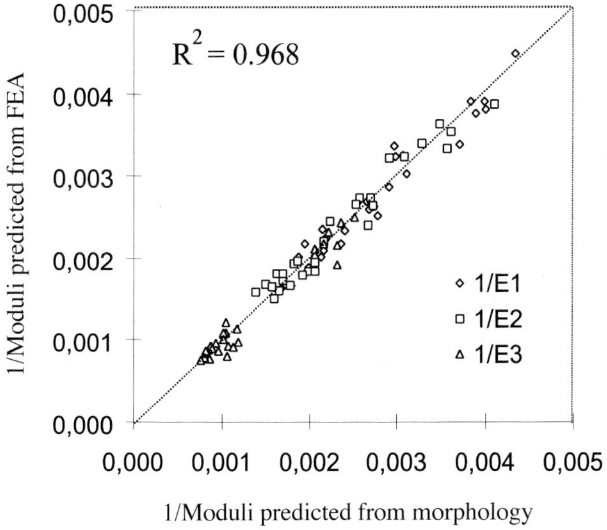

Figure 5.8. Correlation of elastic properties in whale vertebral cancellous bone, as predicted from volume fraction and MIL combined (using an analytical model [21]) and as predicted from μFEA analyses. Shown are the principal compliances, which are the inverse elastic moduli in the three principal material directions. Adapted from van Rietbergen et al. [22].

quality of cancellous bone. However, this is due to the particular morphological features of bone, which it owes to its maintenance, based on mechanical usage (remodelling homeostasis according to Wolff's law); porous structures are not well characterized by MIL as a rule [26]. Hence, it is not certain that MIL would characterize the mechanical quality of osteoporotic bone equally well. There are alternative measures for MIL [18], but these have not been shown to give better predictions for bone [22,25,26].

Quality of the Mineralized Matrix

The factors that determine the mechanical quality (stiffness and strength) of the mineralized matrix were shown in Fig. 5.1. The degree of mineralization is known to determine the stiffness of the material to a large extent. Currey [27] found the elastic modulus to be proportional to the third power of the calcium content in cortical bone. Kabel et al. [16] found a linear correlation of 75% between average tissue density in trabecular bone specimens (varying between about 1.3 and 1.6 g/cm^3) and the effective tissue modulus (between 4.5 and 7.5 GPa). Trabecular tissue is some 20% less strong than cortical tissue (Fig. 5.9), although mineral density is some 6% less in cortical tissue; hence the submicroscopic bone structure in trabeculae is probably less effective in withstanding load [28]; but strength is likely to vary with trabecular mineral density in a similar way to stiffness. To what extent osteocyte and resorption lacunae play independent roles in these relationships is

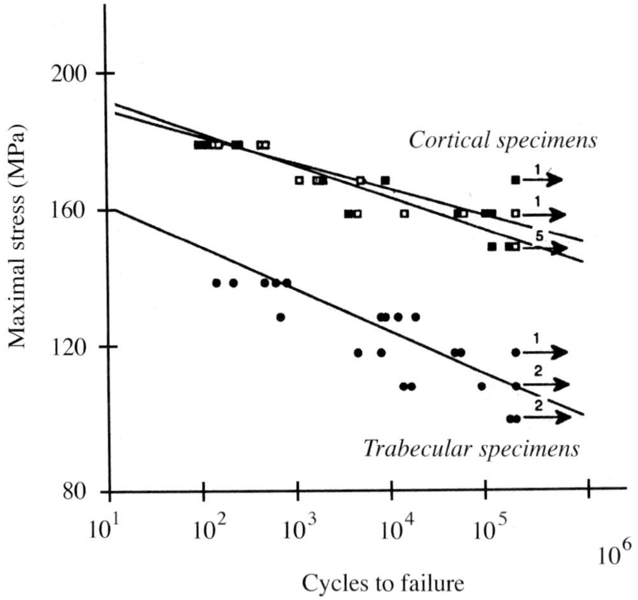

Figure 5.9. Results of fatigue tests on cortical and trabecular tissue (micro)specimens. In such tests the specimens are divided in groups, and each group is cycled at another stress level. Depending on the stress level (S), the number of cycles to failure (N) varies. The so-called SN curves this provides nicely illustrate that bone tissue will crack even at low stresses if cycled for a long time. Trabecular tissue is significantly weaker than cortical tissue. Adapted from Choi and Goldstein [28].

not known. An osteoclast resorption lacuna can be 40–60 μm deep [2], which is on the order of 30% of average trabecular thickness [29], so it may have a significant effect on the mechanical quality of an individual trabecula. Since such a lacuna has a local effect, the reduction of strength due to increased resorption (e.g., after menopause) may be more prominent than suggested by the overall reduction of bone density.

Bone tissue is prone to fatigue failure, as illustrated in Fig. 5.9. When micro-cracks develop due to repetitive loading, both strength and stiffness reduce. The relationship between crack density and loss of stiffness is hyperbolic [30]. A similar relationship exists between age and crack density [31]; hence the effects of crack density on bone stiffness are bound to be quite progressive. However, it is difficult to measure crack density accurately in histological specimens. It was found that, next to mineral density, crack density is a main determining factor for bone strength [31].

Quality of Osteoporotic Bone

Not much is known about the mechanical quality of osteoporotic bone. Although much experimental work has been done to study relationships between mechanical properties and architectural quality, as discussed above, virtually all studies concerned normal bone, or older bone in general at the most. Two effects of bone loss on architectural quality can be discriminated: the reduction in trabecular thickness, which is not homogeneous as a rule, and may be different in postmenopausal as compared with senile osteoporosis; and trabecular interruption and a general reduction of trabecular number and connectivity [4]. It stands to reason that while bone mass reduces and these phenomena proceed, the relationships between architectural properties and mechanical quality will deviate increasingly from the normal. For example, although connectivity, assessed three-dimensionally, has shown not to improve upon the correlation between architectural quality parameters (such as MIL and density [19]), it might become a significant indicator of bone fragility in the case that a large number of trabeculae are severed.

How osteoporosis affects the mechanical quality of the mineralized matrix is not entirely certain, either [32]. As discussed above, strength and stiffness are determined foremost by degree of mineralization, which was found to decrease with age [33]. Crack density is another important variable, which increases with age. A dramatic increase in trabecular crack density in women was found after the age of about 70 years [34]. This increase coincided with a similar reduction in osteocyte lacunae, suggesting that micro-cracks are no longer adequately repaired in the elderly, as the osteocytic network is assumed to play an important role in remodelling [34]. A third possible factor, also increasing with age, is fluoride accumulation. Fluoride treatment increases bone mass but reduces the strength of the mineralized matrix [35]. There are findings, however, suggesting that normal fluoride accumulation does not play a significant role in the reduction of bone strength with age [36]. In any case, all this suggests that the reduction in cancellous bone strength in the elderly – including osteoporotics – is more progressive than the reduction of bone mass suggests. In density-matched specimens it was found that cancellous bone strength of subjects older than 60 years was an average 40% less than in those younger than 40 years [37]. In this sense, it is probably not realistic that the WHO definition of osteoporosis uses linear scales to discriminate normal, osteopenic and osteoporotic bone. More thorough investigations of osteoporotic bone are needed to clarify mechanical bone quality effects. New tools in biomechanics, discussed above, will be shown proficient for this purpose.

Biomechanical Strategies to Enhance Bone Quality

In the context of methods to enhance bone strength, biomechanical strategies must be discussed as well. In Ch. 27 the effects of exercise on bone mass are treated, for example. With the prominence of biomechanics as a basic science in orthopaedics in mind, one could even call these *orthopaedic treatment strategies* for osteoporosis. The question is here whether exercise can have a beneficial effect, not just on bone quantity but on quality as well. The evidence for a dependence of bone mass on mechanical usage (Wolff's law) is overwhelming [38–40]. It is widely assumed that osteocytes, or at least the osteocytic network at large, provide a mechanosensitive system, governing osteoclastic resorption and osteoblastic formation of bone, based on the maximal or typical bone loading rates experienced daily [41,42], as illustrated in Fig. 5.10. Such a biological control process was shown to be able in principle to regulate both bone mass and its spatial distribution realistically [42]. According to these paradigms, senile osteoporosis could potentially be explained as an effect of reduced mechanical usage, hence a reduction of the stimulus for the process, and postmenopausal osteoporosis as a result of defects in the biochemical process machinery itself. Hence, in principle, physical exercise should suffice for prevention, or maybe even a treatment, for at least senile osteoporosis.

There are limitations to its efficacy for this purpose, however. First, exercise has produced only slight increases in bone mass in representative, older populations – up to a few percent only [43]. Dramatic effects on bone mass can only be expected from high-impact exercises (running rather than hiking). But these are not the types of exercise for an older population. Secondly, the strain-adaptive bone remodelling

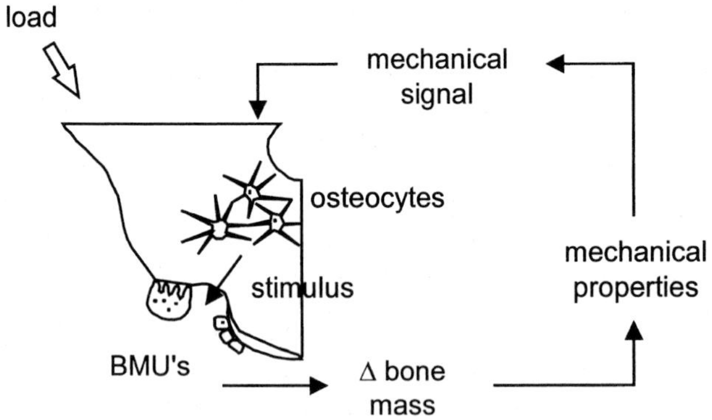

Figure 5.10. A regulatory scheme for mechanical bone adaptation. Loads produce a mechanical signal (e.g., stress, strain, strain energy) in the mineralized tissue, which is sensed by the osteocytes, and compared with a *mechanostat* set point. Based on a disuse or overload deviation, stimuli for bone mass adaptations are provided to the *basic modelling units* (osteoclasts and osteoblasts) at the local bone surface. The changes in bone mass affect the mechanical signal, and thus a self-limiting feedback loop is obtained. This scheme, actualized in a computer simulation program, produced realistic explanations for trabecular morphogenesis and adaptation. Adapted from Mullender and Huiskes [42].

regulatory process will not bring back trabeculae which were severed and resorbed [4,44]. And thirdly, those exercises which are most effective in producing new bone are also the ones likely to enhance crack density, thereby reducing the mechanical quality of the mineralized matrix. Exercise is definitely effective for increasing peak bone mass in the young, but – and this is the fourth limitation – as soon as one stops training, bone mass will adapt to the new, actual loading history [45]. Hence, those who reach high peak bone mass through excessive sports activities at a young age, but then stop exercising, will lose bone faster than others.

Enhancement of architectural quality can be obtained in *error-rich* exercises [L.E. Lanyon, personal communication], by which is meant that the character of the loads, in terms of the stress distributions they provoke in the trabecular structure, must deviate considerably from the normal [46]. High-bar gymnastics, for example, is a very effective exercise for enhancement of bone-mass and architectural quality.

Future Prospects: Clinical Assessment of Bone Quality

Strength of bone can only be measured directly with autopsies, in a test as discussed above (Fig. 5.2). However, apart from the inconvenience for the person concerned, bone autopsies are usually too small to obtain dependable results [7]. Thus the reality is that for clinical, diagnostic purposes, strength will have to be inferred from other qualities, the best candidate for which is stiffness. The only method which measures bone stiffness directly is ultrasound (see Ch. 4). Cancellous bone stiffness correlates closely with quantitative ultrasound measurements as speed of sound (SOS) and broadband ultrasound attenuation (BUA). Both SOS and BUA predict risk of fracture as well as bone mineral density, and ultrasound could develop into a practical method to estimate bone strength in vivo. In the laboratory, excellent (89%) correlation was found between the elastic properties of bovine bone specimens, in three perpendicular directions, determined by SOS and with μFEA simulation [47], as illustrated in Fig. 5.11. It will not be easy to obtain similar accuracy in vivo, though, as bone marrow and soft tissues grossly disturb the attenuation of sound.

Alternatively, stiffness can be estimated using μFEA to simulate mechanical testing, based on computer reconstructions of the three-dimensional architecture. For this purpose an architectural computer reconstruction is required, however, which remains a technical barrier. μCT scans can only be made from autopsies, and the resolution of peripheral quantitative CT (pQCT) and whole-body CT scanners is inadequate for this purpose. Much has been done to develop magnetic resonance imaging methods to evaluate bone architecture for clinical purposes, but presently this method also is limited to applications for small samples. Nevertheless, refined bone imaging methods are bound to become available for clinical use in the future. When they do, the question is still whether the elaborate μFEA approach is fortuitous. Only architectural mechanical quality is assessed with this method; the quality of the mineralized matrix remains unknown. However, it might be possible to infer tissue mineralization from μFEA data combined with bone density measurements [16]; or even estimate tissue stiffness from a combination of μFEA with ultrasound data [47].

Alternative prospects are to estimate architectural quality directly from morphometric parameters (e.g., apparent density, MIL), using relationships with stiffness (or even strength) as determined in laboratory experiments [22,25]. But these

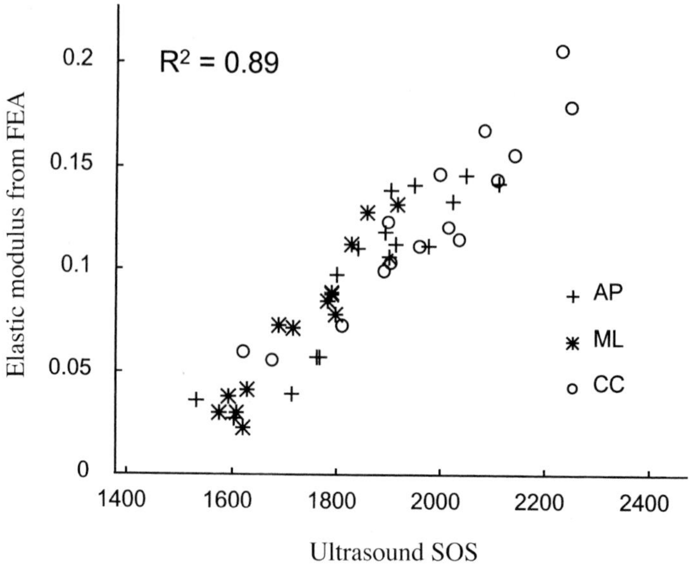

Figure 5.11. A correlation of ultrasound speed of sound (SOS) values and elastic moduli predicted by micro-finite element analysis (μFEA), measured in bovine cancellous bone specimens in three directions. The results suggest that 11% of the variability is due to the quality of the mineralized tissue. Courtesy of Joop van de Bergh, MD and Harry van Lenthe, MS, Nijmegen, The Netherlands [47].

methods require refined clinical imaging tools for computer reconstructions of architecture as well. In addition, the relationships between morphometric parameters and mechanical quality were invariably established from testing normal bone, not osteoporotic bone. Information about tissue quality (e.g., crack density) is not provided in this way. It must be added that μCT scans are already useful for evaluating the three-dimensional morphometric parameters of cancellous bone quality in biopsies [48]

The methods mentioned above are all being considered or developed, and their applicability and precision remain to be determined. But there may be an alternative route to assessing bone fragility with more precision in the future. Although elastic modulus values of cancellous bone determined experimentally could not be explained by density alone with a high precision (60–80% correlation), excellent correlation of 94–97% was found between density and *average* elastic moduli [19,49]. It may be possible to relate average moduli to strength, possibly in a site-dependent way. Also, it was recently discovered that the architectural quality of cancellous bone (stiffness) can be estimated from bone mineral density measurements alone, by using data on local architectural directionality in addition [50]. As principal material orientations per anatomical site are fairly constant in humans and other vertebrates, and well known, the three-dimensional elastic constants could be directly correlated with apparent density, using empirical statistical relationships, with remarkable precision (88–92% correlation for the main elastic constants in a series of 141 human specimens from several sites and individuals). Again, these relationships were established for normal bone, not osteoporotic bone, and only architectural quality is assessed in this way, no information being obtained about tissue quality. Thus the practical applicability of this finding is still uncertain. But the point is rather in its scientific significance. Architecture, in terms of both quantity and spatial arrangement of mineralized tissue, is formed and maintained by mechanical stimuli. This new information can be used to better understand these processes, and how they are disturbed by osteoporosis. It may be that the new tools for measurements and analysis – such as ultrasound, μCT and μFEA – will show their values not so much in direct clinical applications, but rather in research of normal and osteoporotic bone. It is very possible that the solution to problems of in vivo mechanical bone quality assessment is not to be found in better measurement tools, but rather in knowing when and where to assess bone density, and how to judge its significance.

References

1. Chavassieux P, Arlot M, Meunier PJ. Clinical use of bone biopsy. In: Marcus M, Feldman D, Kelsey J editors. Osteoporosis. San Diego: Academic Press, 1996;1113–1121.
2. Kanis JA. Osteoporosis. London: Blackwell Healthcare Communications, 1997.
3. Schaffler MB, Choi K, Milgrom C. Aging and bone matrix microdamage accumulation in human compact bone. Bone 1995;17:521–525.
4. Mosekilde Li, Mosekilde Le, Danielsen CC. Biomechanical competence of vertebral trabecular bone in relation to ash density and age in normal individuals. Bone 1987;8:79–85.
5. Hodgskinson R, Currey JD. Separate effects of osteoporosis and density on the strength and stiffness of human cancellous bone. Clin Biomech 1993;8:262–268.
6. van Rietbergen B, Weinans H, Huiskes R, Odgaard A. A new method to determine trabecular bone elastic properties and loading using micromechanical finite-element models. J Biomech 1995;28:69–81.
7. Harrigan TP, Jasty M, Mann RW, Harris WH. Limitations of the continuum assumption in cancellous bone. J Biomech 1988;21:269–275.
8. Martin RB. Determinants of the mechanical properties of bone. J Biomech 1991;24 (Suppl):S79–88.
9. Bouxsein ML, Myers ER, Hayes WC. Biomechanics of age-related fractures. In: Marcus M, Feldman D, Kelsey J editors. Osteoporosis. San Diego: Academic Press, 1996: 373–393.
10. Goulet RW, Goldstein SA, Ciarelli ME, Kuhn JL, Brown MB, Feldkamp LA. The relationship between the structural and orthogonal compressive properties of trabecular bone. J Biomech 1994;27:375–389.
11. Odgaard A, Andersen K, Melsen F, Gundersen HJG. A direct method for fast three-dimensional serial reconstruction. J Microsc 1990;159:335–342
12. Feldkamp LA, Goldstein SA, Parfitt AM, Jesion G, Kleerekoper M. The direct examination of three-dimensional bone architecture in vitro by computed tomography, J Bone Miner Res 1989;4:3–11.
13. Ruegsegger P, Koller B, Muller R. A microtomographic system for the nondestructive evaluation of bone architecture. Calcif Tissue Int 1996;58:24–29.
14. Cowin SC, Mehrabadi M. Identification of the elastic symmetry of bone and other materials. J Biomech 1989;22:503–515.
15. van Rietbergen B, Odgaard A, Kabel J, Huiskes R. Direct mechanics assessment of elastic symmetries and properties of trabecular bone architecture. J Biomech 1996;29:1653–1657.
16. Kabel J, van Rietbergen B, Dalstra M, Odgaard A, Huiskes R. The role of an effective isotropic tissue modulus in the elastic properties of cancellous bone. J Biomech 1999;32: 673–680.

17. Ladd AJ, Kinney JH, Haupt DL, Goldstein SA. Finite-element modelling of trabecular bone: comparison with mechanical testing and determination of tissue modulus. J Orthop Res 1998;16:622–628.
18. Odgaard A. Three-dimensional methods for quantification of cancellous bone architecture. Bone 1997;20:315–328.
19. Kabel J, Odgaard A, van Rietbergen B, Huiskes R. Connectivity and the elastic properties of cancellous bone. Bone 1999;24:115–120.
20. Mosekilde Li,Viidik A, Mosekilde Le. Correlation between the compressive strength of iliac and vertebral trabecular bone in normal individuals. Bone 1985;6:291–295.
21. Turner CH, Cowin SC, Rho JY, Ashman RB, Rice JC. The fabric dependence of the orthotropic elastic constants of cancellous bone. J Biomech 1990;23:549–561.
22. van Rietbergen B, Odgaard A, Kabel J, Huiskes R. Relationships between bone morphology and bone elastic properties can be accurately quantified using high-resolution computer reconstructions. J Orthop Res 1998;16:23–28.
23. Odgaard A, Linde F. The underestimation of Young's modulus in compressive testing of cancellous bone specimens. J Biomech 1991;24:691–698.
24. Keaveny TM, Pinilla TP, Crawford RP, Kopperdahl DL, Lou A. Systematic and random errors in compression testing of trabecular bone. J Orthop Res 1997;15:101–110.
25. Kabel J, van Rietbergen B, Odgaard A, Huiskes R. The constitutive relationships of fabric, density and elastic properties in cancellous bone architecture. Bone 1999;25: 481–486.
26. van Lenthe GH, Huiskes R. Can the mechanical trabecular bone quality be estimated reliably from mean intercept length or other morphological parameters? In: Pedersen P, Bendsøe MP, editors. Synthesis in Bio-Solid Mechanics. Dordrecht: Kluwer Academic, 1999:349–360.
27. Currey JD. The effect of porosity and mineral content on the Young's modulus of elasticity of compact bone. J Biomech 1988;21:131–139.
28. Choi K, Goldstein SA. A comparison of the fatigue behavior of human trabecular and cortical bone tissue. J Biomech 1992;25:1371–1381.
29. Mullender MG, Huiskes R, Versleyen H, Buma P. Osteocyte density and histomorphometric parameters in cancellous bone of the proximal femur in five mammalian species. J Orthop Res 1996;14:972–979.
30. Burr DB, Turner CH, Naick P, Forwood MR, Ambrosius W, Hasan MS, Pidaparti R. Does microdamage accumulation affect the mechanical properties of bone? J Biomech 1998;31:337–345.
31. Fazzalari NL, Forwood MR, Smith K, Manthey BA, Herreen P. Assessment of cancellous bone quality in severe osteoarthrosis: bone mineral density, mechanics, and microdamage. Bone 1998;22:381–388.
32. Marcus R. The nature of osteoporosis. In: Marcus M, Feldman D, Kelsey J, editors. Osteoporosis. San Diego: Academic Press, 1996:647–660.
33. Burnell JM, Baylink DJ, Chesnut CH, Mathews MW, Teubner EJ. Bone matrix and mineral abnormalities in postmenopausal osteoporosis. Metabolism 1982;31:1113–1120.
34. Mori S, Harruff R, Ambrosius W, Burr DB. Trabecular bone volume and microdamage accumulation in the femoral heads of women with and without femoral neck fractures. Bone 1997;21:521–526.
35. Riggs B, O'Fallon W, Chao E, Wahner H, Muhs J, Cedel S. Effect of fluoride treatment on the fracture rate in postmenopausal women with osteoporosis. N Engl J Med 1990;322:802–809.
36. Richards A, Mosekilde Li, Sogaard CH. Normal age-related changes in fluoride content of vertebral trabecular bone-relation to bone quality. Bone 1994;15:21–26.
37. Britton JM, Davie MWJ. Mechanical properties of bone from iliac crest and relationship to L5 vertebral bone. Bone 1990;11:21–28.
38. Rodan GA. Coupling of bone resorption and formation during bone remodelling. In: Marcus M, Feldman D, Kelsey J, editors. Osteoporosis., San Diego: Academic Press, 1996:647–660.

39. Frost HM. Vital Biomech. Proposed general concepts for skeletal adaptation to mechanical usage. Calcif Tissue Int 1987;45: 145–156.
40. Currey JD. The mechanical adaptation of bones. Princeton: Princeton University Press, 1984.
41. Cowin SC, Moss-Salentijn L, Moss ML. Candidates for the mechanosensory system in bone. J Biomech Engin 1991;113:191–197.
42. Mullender MG, Huiskes R. A proposal for the regulatory mechanism of Wolff's law. J Orthop Res 1995;13:503–512.
43. Dalsky GP, Stocke KS, Ehsani AA, Slatopolsky E, Lee WC, Birge SJ. Weight-bearing exercise training and lumbar bone mineral content in postmenopausal women. Ann Intern Med 1988;108:824–828.
44. Mullender MG, van Rietbergen B, Ruegsegger P, Huiskes R. Effect of mechanical setpoint of bone cells on mechanical control of trabecular bone architecture. Bone 1998;22:125–131.
45. Karlsson MK, Johnell O, Obrant KJ. Is bone mineral density advantage maintained long-term in previous weight lifters? Calcif Tissue Int 1995;57:325–328.
46. Heinonen A, Oja P, Kannus P, Sievanen H, Haapasalo H, Manttari A, Vuori I. Bone mineral density in female athletes representing sports with different loading characteristics of the skeleton. Bone 1995;17:197–203.
47. van Lenthe GH, van den Bergh J, Hermus A, Huiskes R. The prospects of estimating the trabecular-bone tissue properties from ultrasound, micro-CT and micro-FEA. Transact 45th ORS 1999;24:570.
48. Muller R, van Campenhout H, van Damme B, vander Perre G, Dequeker J, Hildebrand T, Ruegsegger P. Morphometric analysis of human bone biopsies: a quantitative structural comparison of histological sections and micro-computer tomography. Bone 1998;23:59–66.
49. Hodgskinson J, Currey JD. Young's modulus, density and material properties in cancellous bone over a large density range. J Mat Sci Mat Med 1992;3:377–381.
50. Yang G, Kabel J, van Rietbergen B, Odgaard A, Huiskes R, Cowin SC. The anisotropic Hooke's Law for cancellous bone and wood. J Elasticity 1999: 53:125–146.

6 Biochemical Markers and Bone

J.-E. B. Jensen, H. A. Sørensen and O. H. Sørensen

Introduction

It is well established that a low bone mass is associated with an increased risk of osteoporotic fractures. Peak bone mass and bone loss with aging are the major determinants of osteoporosis [1]. It has not been clearly established at what age the negative bone balance starts. An accelerated loss of bone is seen immediately after the menopause, continuing for 2–8 years [2,3]. Serum and urinary levels of biochemical markers of bone turnover are increased during that period and return to premenopausal levels during hormone replacement therapy (HRT). This has been shown in groups of patients treated with HRT [4,5]. Significant suppression of biochemical markers has also been demonstrated in groups of patients treated with other antiresorptive agents such as bisphosphonates [6,7] or raloxifene [8]. The clinical usefulness of monitoring the bone markers in an individual patient is, however, less evident.

Biochemical Markers of Bone Turnover

Bone is composed of hydroxyapatite crystals, which are laid down in a matrix consisting of about 90% type I collagen and 10% noncollagenous proteins including osteocalcin. The basic structure of collagen is a triple helix consisting of two alpha-1 and one alpha-2 chains with a high content of glycine, proline and hydroxyproline. Procollagen is formed in the osteoblasts and after secretion to the extracellular space the extension peptides are cleaved at the amino-terminals (N-) and carboxy-terminals (C-) before final fibril formation. These extension peptides can be measured in the blood as markers of bone formation, the so-called PINP and PICP. The collagen molecules aggregate to fibrils that are stabilized by covalent cross-links. By the action of lysyl-oxidase on lysine and hydroxylysine residues different types of cross-links are made. In the N- and C-terminal nonhelical telopeptide regions the pyridinium cross-links are formed from two telopeptides linked to a helical site on an adjacent molecule (Fig. 6.1). The pyridinium cross-links and the N- and C-terminal telopeptides (NTx and CTx, respectively) can be measured as markers of bone resorption.

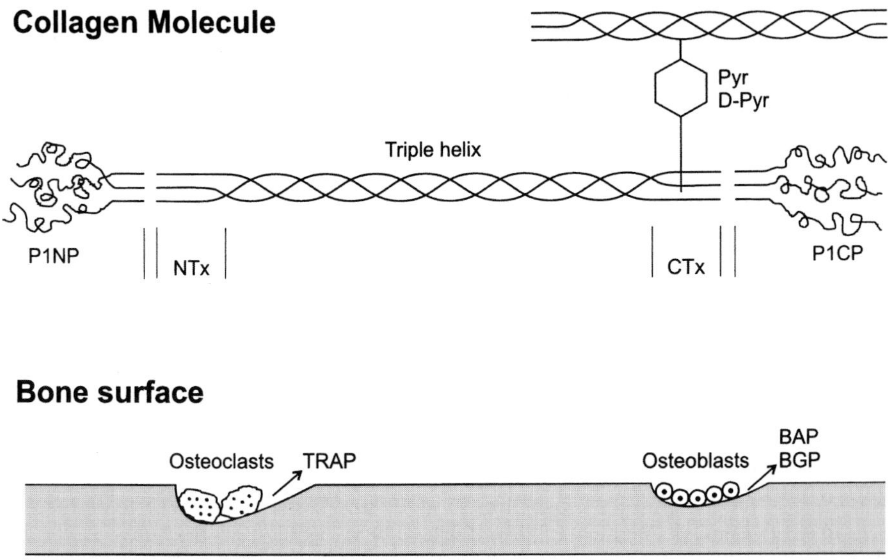

Figure 6.1. The biochemical markers of bone turnover in relation to the collagen molecule and the action of bone cells. Pyr, pyridinoline; D-Pyr, deoxypyridinoline; PINP, amino-terminal propeptide of type 1 collagen; PICP, carboxy-terminal propeptide of type I collagen; NTx, amino-terminal nonhelical telopeptide of the collagen molecule involved in cross-link formation; CTx, carboxy-terminal telopeptide of the collagen molecule; TRAP, tartrate-resistant acid phosphatase; BAP, bone-specific alkaline phosphatase; BGP, osteocalcin (bone GLA protein).

During formation of new bone the osteoblasts secrete small proteins which become incorporated in the matrix. One of these is osteocalcin (BGP) which, like the bone specific alkaline phosphatase (BSAP), can be measured in the blood as a marker of bone formation.

Traditionally the bone markers are divided into markers of bone formation and bone resorption. Several of the markers are produced during both resorption and formation and are thus simply markers of bone turnover. Most of them are not specific for bone but are also derived from other tissues. In Fig. 6.1 the most common markers are listed.

Biochemical Markers of Bone Resorption

Hydroxyproline

The estimation of hydroxyproline (OHP) in urine is a widely used method to estimate the degradation of bone collagen. Unfortunately OHP is present in all types of collagen and therefore is not specific for bone. Only about 10% of OHP products are excreted in the urine due to high resorption in the kidney followed by degradation in the liver. Hydroxyproline peptides arise from both formation and degradation of collagen and a major proportion of excreted OHP derives from collagen-rich food [9]. As it is not possible to distinguish between contribution from diet and endogenous collagen breakdown it is necessary to place the patient on a gelatine-poor diet before urine collection. Two different types of assays are used. One is based on colorimetric techniques involving a risk of interfering chromophores [10], the other is based on high-performance liquid chromatography (HPLC) and UV absorbance, which has a much lower analytical variation [11].

Pyridinium Cross-links and Telopeptides

The pyridinium cross-links comprise pyridinoline (Pyr) and deoxypyridinoline (D-Pyr) and are present in all mature collagen except the skin [12]. Pyr is the major cross-link in all collagen tissues, whereas D-Pyr is present in significant amounts only in bone. Hence, D-Pyr is more specific for bone than Pyr. The pyridinium cross-links are stable, not metabolically degraded or reutilized, and the urinary levels are not influenced by diet [13]. They are excreted in the urine: around 60% peptide bound and 40% in a free form. Since bone is the most abundant collagen source in the body and characterized by a high turnover, it is generally accepted that most of the pyridinium cross-links in blood and urine are derived from resorption of bone matrix. Furthermore the ratio of Pyr to D-Pyr in the urine is similar to that of bone, i.e., 3:1.

The pyridinium cross-links are measured as total pyridinolines, free pyridinolines, and as cross-linked telopeptides (NTx and CTx). Total pyridinolines in the urine are measured after hydrolysis, separation by HPLC, and measurement of the intrinsic fluorescence of the compounds [14]. Direct immunoassays have been developed to measure the free fractions of Pyr and D-Pyr in the urine. The obvious advantage of these assays is that no pretreatment of the urine is necessary [15]. It is important to recognize that there are clinical situations where the ratio between the pyridinoline fractions in the urine can change. It has thus been shown that bisphosphonate treatment of osteoporosis as well as vitamin D and calcium supplementation in vitamin D deficiency can induce different responses in urinary cross-links, with decreases in the peptide-bound fraction but without significant changes in the free forms [16,17].

The telopeptides are the peptide cross-linked fragments at the N- and C-terminals. Both can be measured with specific antibodies. In one of the first assays a large part of the C-terminal fragment was measured in the blood [18]. Other fragments were measured in the urine [19,20]. Recently assays to measure pyridinium cross-links as well as NTx and CTx in serum have been developed [21,22]. The peptide region of CTx is isomeric and exists in both an alpha and a beta form. The clinical relevance of these different forms has not yet been established.

Tartrate-Resistant Acid Phosphatase

During bone resorption osteoclasts secrete acids and enzymes. The tartrate-resistant acid phosphatase isoenzyme (TRAP) is produced by osteoclasts and the serum concentration of the enzyme has been used as a marker of bone resorption [23]. The enzyme is not specific for bone and is difficult to separate from isoenzymes deriving from other tissues such as platelets and erythrocytes. It is not stable in frozen serum, and measurements are further impeded by the occurrence of natural enzyme inhibitors in the blood. New immunoassays might improve the usefulness of measurements of TRAP [24], but the clinical value of TRAP measurements has yet to be established.

Biochemical Markers of Bone Formation

Alkaline Phosphatase

Alkaline phosphatase (AP) is highly represented in bone and seems to be involved in mineralization. Bone diseases with high turnover such as Paget´s disease and osteomalacia can easily be evaluated using the total AP as the majority of the enzyme activity in these situations is derived from bone. In low-turnover bone diseases such as osteoporosis measurement of the total AP is of less clinical value. Serum AP comprises several different isoforms that differ in their composition of the carbohydrate side chains, which makes separation possible. The most common sources of AP are the liver and bone, which deliver similar amounts of the enzyme to the blood. Several methods have been developed to separate the bone-specific alkaline phosphatase (BAP), including heat denaturation, gel electrophoresis, wheat germ lectin binding and different immunoassays. Most promising are the lectin binding assays and the newer immunoassays, although none of these is able to separate the bone isoenzyme completely [25,26].

Osteocalcin

Osteocalcin (BGP) is a small noncollagenous molecule consisting of 49 amino acids. It is produced by the osteoblasts and is thus a marker of bone formation. However, only a part of the newly synthesized BGP is released to the blood; part of it is incorporated into the bone matrix and thereby also released during bone resorption. BGP is rapidly degraded to several fragments in the blood. Garnero et al. [27] have shown that one-third of the immunoreactivity in serum is derived from the intact molecule, one-third from several small fragments and one-third from an N-terminal midfragment. The multiple fragments have created serious analytical problems, with discordant results between laboratories due to the use of different antibodies reacting with different parts of the molecule [28]. Masters et al. [29] evaluated results from eight commercial kits and concluded that results cannot be compared between assays even when normalized against healthy subjects. New assays use two monoclonal antibodies in order to measure only the intact molecule, but standardization is needed in order to compare results [30].

BGP is unstable at room temperature and does not tolerate repeated thawing and freezing [27]. It is dependent upon the presence of vitamin K, which is necessary for the carboxylation of three glutamate residues to gamma-carboxyglutamate. It has recently been shown that osteoporotic patients with hip fracture have increased serum levels of undercarboxylated BGP [31]. The results need confirmation. Gundberg et al. [32] recently evaluated the methods of measurement of undercarboxylated BGP and found that a number of precautions have to be taken to obtain reliable results.

Procollagen I Extension Peptides

As mentioned earlier,procollagen I extension peptides are released from the procollagen C- (PICP) and N- (PINP) terminals to the blood, where they are measured as markers of bone formation. Type I collagen, however, is present in many tissues, particularly the skin, and the relative contribution from these sites to circulating PICP and PINP has not been clarified. The metabolism of the peptides is unknown, which means that serum concentrations might depend upon unknown factors of degradation. Ebeling et al. [33] compared the utility of assays for PICP and PINP in different metabolic diseases including osteoporosis and came to the conclusion that these assays were generally inferior to those for serum BGP and BSAP.

Evaluation of Bone Markers in Individual Patients

There are several underlying factors that must be taken into consideration when interpreting the results of a bone marker measurement: diurnal rhythm, day-to-day variations, seasonal variations, menstrual variations, age and sex, diet, physical activity, alcohol and smoking, and diseases and medications.

Diurnal rhythm has been demonstrated in both formative and resorptive markers [34–37] with peak values in the night and declines in the early morning. Blood and urine samples are usually collected in the morning, when the values might change from hour to hour. The variations in the formative markers are generally around 20%, whereas more than a 50% variation has been observed in most of the resorptive markers.

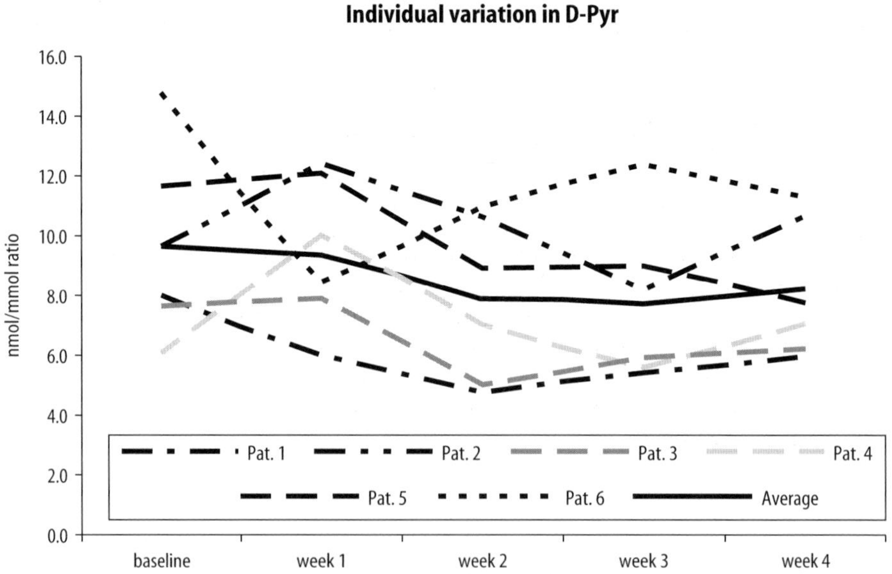

Figure 6.2. The week-to-week variability in double HPLC measurements of deoxypyridinoline (D-Pyr) excretion in relation to urinary creatinine excretion. Samples were obtained during 5 consecutive weeks in six randomly selected osteoporotic postmenopausal women.

Several of the resorptive markers can now be measured in the blood. The concentrations are lower than in the urine, but the diurnal variations are less pronounced. A variation of about 25 % has thus recently been demonstrated for serum NTx [21].

The day-to-day variability in biochemical markers is partly explained by imprecise timing of specimen collection. Variations in creatinine excretion also play an important role in the evaluation of the urinary resorptive markers. These are often based on values corrected for urinary creatinine, which is dependent upon muscle mass, age, diet, kidney function, and even circadian variations in creatinine excretion [38].

Seasonal variations have been described [34,39] as well as *variations with the menstrual cycle* [40]. The latter is of minor practical importance since most osteoporotic patients have passed the menopause.

Age- and gender-related changes have been demonstrated in a number of studies. Seibel et al. [41] found higher urinary Pyr and D-Pyr in the older than in the younger group of a population aged 50–81 years. Delmas et al. [42] described a linear increase with age in the urinary cross-links creatinine ratio, whereas Robins et al. [15] found no significant variations with age in adults but higher levels in men than in women. Several studies have shown that serum BGP varies with age and sex [43].

Alcohol and smoking were demonstrated in a large study by Woitge et al. [39] to suppress bone markers in women, whereas in males only alcohol has such an effect. It was shown in the same study that *physical activity* was associated with higher levels of formative markers and reduced levels of resorptive markers.

Diet with a high gelatine content has a pronounced effect on the urinary excretion of OHP, whereas urinary Pyr and D-Pyr are unaffected by gelatine intake [13]. Major changes in dietary calcium intake have an influence on both formative and resorptive bone markers [44].

Many *diseases* influence bone metabolism such as hyperthyroidism and hyperparathyroidism. Several *drugs* have marked influence on bone turnover for example glucocorticoids and thyroid hormones.

Suggested Use of Biochemical Markers of Bone Turnover

Biochemical markers are valuable in single patients with metabolic bone diseases with very high bone turnover such as Paget´s disease. The markers can, in these clinical situations, be used for both diagnosis and monitoring of treatment. It is less clear whether biochemical markers are useful to classify the single individual with osteoporosis. It is not possible to separate a large skeleton with a low turnover from a small skeleton with a high turnover. Nevertheless, use of biochemical markers has been suggested in single osteoporotic patients for: prediction of low bone mass, prediction of bone loss, estimation of future fracture risk, and monitoring of treatment.

Prediction of Low Bone Mass

Some studies have shown that measurement of a single marker of bone turnover or a combination of markers can identify groups of patients with low bone mass. No studies, however, have proved that such measurements have predictive power in the single patient.

Gertz et al. [45] thus found a relationship between urinary NTx and lumbar spine bone mineral density (BMD) in 65 early postmenopausal women ($r = -0.26$). The authors suggested that a larger population might yield better estimates of this correlation, but this would have no importance for the single case. Schneider and Barret-Connor [46] showed that the levels of urinary NTx could be used to discriminate between elderly persons with normal, osteopenic and osteoporotic BMD values of the hip and spine. The authors looked at mean values for large groups but not at the correlation between urinary NTx and BMD. Ravn et al. [47] measured a specific sequence of the C-telopeptide (CrossLaps) and serum BGP in large groups of pre- and postmenopausal women. They found correlations between BMD of the spine and the hip and the two bone markers with r values ranging from −0.13 to −0.32. As pointed out by Mazess [48], *r* values of that magnitude would explain only 5–10% of the variations in BMD, and he further demonstrated that body weight predicts bone density much better than markers of bone turnover.

Garnero et al. [49] investigated the association between a number of bone markers and bone mass in 653 normal pre-, peri- and postmenopausal women. In premenopausal women and in those up to 20 years after the menopause the markers could explain only 0–10 % of the BMD variance. In elderly women (mean 75 years) who were more than 20 years from menopause the markers could explain 19–30 % of the variance, and even more in the oldest population. There was, however, large overlap between the ranges of the markers in these groups. This supports the view that it is unlikely that bone mass can be predicted in the single patient by one or more biochemical markers of bone turnover.

Prediction of Bone Loss

Some studies indicate that future bone loss can be estimated by measurement of one or more biochemical markers of bone turnover.

Christiansen et al. [50] identified a group of so-called fast bone losers that could be identified by a single measurement of body mass, serum alkaline phosphatase, urinary calcium and hydroxyproline. A majority of the patients were investigated 12 years later [51]. The investigators found that previous fast losers remained fast losers, as evaluated by changes in bone mineral content of the distal forearm. It seems, however, that the initial bone mass accounted for the strong association.

Falch and Sandvik [52] followed the bone mineral content of the forearm in a group of premenopausal women who later entered the menopause. During 10 years of observation the investigators could not identify a subgroup of fast bone losers.

Hui et al. [1] in a similar way followed a large group of healthy women with measurement of the bone mass of the midshaft radius. In a group of these women they calculated the rates of change in bone mass during the first and second 5-year period after cessation of menses. The correlation between these two rates was only 0.22, which illustrates that only a small proportion of "fast losers" remains "fast losers" over a long period.

Cosman et al. [53] studied the usefulness of bone markers for prediction of longitudinal bone loss in the spine and hip, which are more relevant sites from a clinical point of view than the forearm. The formation markers (serum BGP, AP, BAP and PICP) were significantly correlated with changes in BMD of the lumbar spine, whereas the only resorption marker that correlated was urine OHP. Only one formation marker (PICP) but all resorption markers, except TRAP, correlated with changes in the hip. The correlations were, however, rather weak and the authors concluded that measuring individual serum and urine markers of bone turnover cannot accurately predict the bone loss rates in the spine and the hip.

Keen et al. [54] performed a 4-year prospective study in 141 postmenopausal women. The purpose was to investigate whether bone markers are predictive of bone loss from clinically important sites (lumbar spine and femoral neck). A series of biochemical markers (serum BGP, AP, urinary calcium, OHP, Pyr, and D-Pyr) as well as a battery of endogenous sex hormones were measured at baseline. Bone density was repeatedly measured at the two sites. There was no evidence of a fast loser subgroup as the bone loss was normally distributed without evidence of bimodality. Furthermore there were no significant correlations between the rate of change in bone density and any biochemical marker, either individually or in combination.

Reginster et al. [55] claimed that they were able to identify 100% of postmenopausal "fast bone losers" with a specificity of 76% by measuring serum phosphorus, estrone, androstendione and urinary calcium. These parameters were measured at baseline and again after 6 months. The changes were used to predict bone loss at the lumbar spine after 3 years. Those who exhibited the most pronounced decreases in serum estrone and androstendione, the most significant predictors, also had the largest loss of bone. The women had all had their last menses 6–36 months previously; so the so-called fast losers were those who had just entered the menopause and still had high levels of sex hormones. It is a well-known fact that the most rapid loss of bone is seen immediately after the menopause, so the findings have to be confirmed in women who are longer from the menopause if they are to be of practical use in other groups of postmenopausal women.

It thus still remains to be shown that a "fast loser" soon after the menopause will remain a "fast loser".

Prediction of Fractures

Long-term population studies are needed to evaluate the usefulness of biochemical markers of bone turnover to predict future osteoporotic fractures.

Åkesson et al. [56] studied retrospectively and prospectively 328 women aged 40–80 years. Serum levels of BGP, PICP and CTx were measured at baseline and all fractures were recorded for the following 5 years in the prospective part of the study. No significant correlations were seen between bone markers and fracture susceptibility, although there was a tendency to lower levels of serum BGP and PICP in the patients who sustained a fracture. The investigators could not find any evidence of an association between high bone turnover and fracture risk.

In a large prospective Dutch study (the Rotterdam Study) increased urinary pyridinoline, but not deoxypyridinoline, concentrations were associated with an increased risk of hip fracture [57]. The association between urinary pyridininium cross-links and fracture risk, however, appeared to be related to disability at baseline, indicating that decreased mobility will result in increased bone resorption and consequently increased bone fragility. The authors concluded that it remained to be proved whether simple measurements of risk factors for hip fracture are more cost-effective than measurement of relative expensive bone markers.

Garnero et al. [58] compared a panel of bone markers obtained at baseline from 109 elderly women with a hip fracture with those from 292 age-matched controls.

Both groups participated in a large French prospective study of women over the age of 75 years (the EPIDOS study). Urinary CTx and free D-Pyr levels, but not the other markers measured, i.e., serum BGP and BAP and urinary NTx, were significantly associated with increased fracture risk. Gait speed and femoral neck BMD were more closely related to hip fracture risk than the markers of bone turnover. The investigators demonstrated that urinary CTx and free D-Pyr in combination with measurement of hip BMD could predict hip fracture risk with odd ratios of 4.8 and 4.1, respectively.

However, the study also showed that the patients could be most significantly divided into risk groups according to the BMD of the femoral neck, with those in the lowest quartile of hip BMD having an odds ratio of 4.5 for a hip fracture.

It thus remains to be clarified whether measurement of bone markers will add to the predictive values obtained by BMD measurements alone.

Monitoring Treatment

It is well established that biochemical markers change significantly in groups of patients treated with inhibitors of bone resorption, such as estrogens [4,5], raloxifene [8], and bisphosphonates [6,7]. The critical difference ($p < 0.05$) is the difference between two measurements in a patient that is necessary to be statistically significant. It is calculated from the within-subject variation plus the analytical variation. The critical differences in 32 Danish postmenopausal women, 11 healthy subjects and 21 osteoporotic patients followed with weekly measurements for 4 weeks are shown in Table 6.1.

Several investigators have suggested that bone markers can be used to monitor response to therapy in the individual patient. It is important, however, to consider the circadian and day-to-day variability, which, expressed as the coefficient of variation, is typically 20–30% for formative and resorptive markers in an individual. This means that a change of 50–80% is necessary to conclude that a significant ($p < 0.05$) change has occurred in the individual patient. A change of that magnitude is larger than the mean changes usually observed in treated groups.

No studies have proved that biochemical markers can provide useful prognostic information about treatment response in the single patient. Hirsch et al. [59] estimated bone turnover rate by measurement of serum AP and urinary D-Pyr/creatinine in 994 women who were randomized to treatment with alendronate or placebo. They concluded that these bone markers could not be used to predict the

Table 6.1. Critical differences in biochemical markers of bone turnover in 32 Danish postmenopausal women followed with weekly measurements for 4 weeks

Biochemical marker	Critical difference[a] healthy subjects	Critical difference osteoporotic patients
Urinary OHP/creatinine	51.6%	82.8%
Urinary Pyr/creatinine	29.4%	41.3%
Urinary-Dpyr/creatinine	33.8%	45.7%
Serum AP	13.9%	17.5%
Serum BGP	18.0%	31.3%

[a]Critical difference is the smallest change in repeated measurements in a single patient at a 5% significance level.

changes in bone mass in the two groups. Greenspan et al. [60], on the other hand, followed 120 women randomized to treatment with alendronate or placebo. They measured urinary D-Pyr and NTx, both corrected for creatinine, as markers of bone resorption and serum levels of BGP and BAP as markers of formation. There were relatively few significant correlations between baseline levels of bone markers and subsequent changes in BMD. They did find, however, an association between the changes in some of the markers measured after 6 months and BMD changes after 2.5 years in women treated with alendronate. The most significant correlations showed r values of 0.3–0.4, which means that only 10–15 % of the changes in BMD could be explained by the changes in the biochemical markers. It is far from convincing that such values will be cost-effective in the single patient.

In the study by Cosman et al. [53], in which they followed estrogen-treated and untreated women for 3 years, they found that of 10 biochemical markers used, only serum BGP and serum PICP were predictive at all of the rate of BMD changes in estrogen-treated women. Together these variables could, however, predict only 4–5% of the variance in either the spine or the hip BMD.

A comprehensive study of long-term variability of bone markers was recently presented by Hannon et al. [61]. More than 200 untreated postmenopausal women were followed for up to 5 years. The critical difference for duplicate measurements was calculated for the three markers investigated and found to be 76%, 99% and 67% for serum BAP, urinary NTx and free D-Pyr, respectively. The investigators concluded that the intraindividual variability over 2–5 years precludes their use to monitor long-term response to treatment.

Biochemical markers of bone turnover might have a minor role in short-term monitoring of treatment, although there are no data showing that they can predict or identify treatment response in the individual patient.

Several investigators advocate the use of bone markers to identify noncompliance or nonresponse to treatment. In daily clinical routine, however, a treatment will rarely be changed or stopped if the biochemical markers do not exhibit a response that is larger than the critical difference after 1 or 3 months of treatment.

Until now the only sensitive method for evaluation of response to therapy is repeated bone mass measurements.

Conclusion

In recent years much effort has been expended to improve the specificity and sensitivity of biochemical markers of bone turnover. These markers have proved to be useful in epidemiological and intervention studies, where groups are studied. It has, however, not been proved that bone markers have any clinical utility in the single osteoporotic patient, to predict either bone mass, future bone loss or fracture risk. Some studies, but far from all, indicate that markers of bone turnover can be used to evaluate short-term response to antiresorptive therapy. It has to be better elucidated before their use can be recommended in daily clinical practice, where the individual variability is higher than in a research set-up.

Recent studies have demonstrated that biochemical bone markers can not be used to monitor the response to long-term treatment of osteoporosis. It is clear that they can not replace longitudinal measurements of bone mass.

References

1. Hui SL, Slemenda CW, Johnston CC, Jr. The contribution of bone loss to postmenopausal osteoporosis. Osteoporos Int 1990;1: 30–34.
2. WHO Study Group. Assessment of fracture risk and its application to screening for osteoporosis. WHO technical report series 843. Geneva: WHO, 1994.
3. Löfman O, Larsson L, Ross I, Toss G, Berglund K. Bone mineral density in normal Swedish women. Bone 1997;20:167–174.
4. Christiansen C, Riis BJ. Five years with continous oestrogen/progesteron therapy: effects on calcium metabolism, lipoproteins, and bleeding pattern. Br J Obstet Gynaecol 1990;97:1087–1092.
5. Fuleihan G E-H, Brown EM, Curtis K, et al. Effect of sequential and daily continuous hormone replacement therapy on indexes of mineral metabolism. Arch Intern Med 1992;152:1904–1909.
6. Harris ST, Gertz BJ, Genant HK, et al. The effect of short-term treatment with alendronate on vertebral density and biochemical markers of bone remodeling in early postmenopausal women. J Clin Endocrinol Metab 1993;76:1399–1406.
7. Adami S, Baroni MC, Broggini M, et al. Treatment of postmenopausal osteoporosis with continuous daily oral alendronate in comparison with either placebo or intranasal salmon calcitonin. Osteoporos Int 1993;3 (Suppl 3):S21–S27.
8. Delmas PD, Bjarnason NH, Mitlak BH, et al. Effects of raloxifene on bone mineral density, serum cholesterol concentrations, and uterine endometrium in postmenopausal women. N Engl J Med 1997;337:1641–1687.
9. Russell RG. The assessment of bone metabolism in vivo using biochemical approaches. Horm Metab Res 1997;29:138–144.
10. Kivirikko KI, Laitinen O, Prockop DJ. Modification of a specific assay for hydroxyproline in urine. Anal Biochem 1967;19:249–255.
11. Wilson PS, Kleerekoper M, Bone H, Parfitt AM. Urinary total hydroxyproline measured by HPLC:comparison of spot and timed urine collections. Clin Chem 1990;36:388–389.
12. Eyre DR. The specificity of collagen cross-links as markers of bone and connective tissue degradation. Acta Orthop Scand 1995;266(Suppl):166–170.
13. Colwell A, Russell RG, Eastell R. Factors affecting the assay of urinary 3-hydroxy pyridinium crosslinks of collagen as markers of bone resorption. Eur J Clin Invest 1993;23:341–349.
14. Kollerup G, Thamsborg G, Bhatia H, Sorensen H. Quantitation of urinary hydroxypyridinium cross-links from collagen by high-performance liquid chromatography. Scand J Clin Lab Invest 1992;52:657–662.
15. Robins SP, Woitge H, Hesley R, Ju J, Seyedin S, Siebel MJ. Direct, enzyme-linked immunoassay for urinary deoxypyridinoline as a specific marker for measuring bone resorption. J Bone Miner Res 1994;9:1643–1649.
16. Garnero P, Shih WJ, Gineyts E, Karpf DB, Delmas PD. Comparison of new biochemical markers of bone turnover in late postmenopausal osteoporotic women in response to alendronate treatment. J Clin Endocrinol Metab 1994;79:1693–1700.
17. Kamel S, Brazier M, Rogez JC, et al. Different responses of free and peptide-bound cross-links to vitamin D and calcium supplementation in elderly women with vitamin D insufficiency. J Clin Endocrinol Metab 1996;81:3717–3721.
18. Risteli J, Elomaa I, Niemi S, Novamo A, Risteli L. Radioimmunoassay for the pyridinoline cross-linked carboxy-terminal telopeptide of type I collagen: a new serum marker of bone collagen degradation. Clin Chem 1993;39:635–640.
19. Hanson DA, Weis MAE, Bollen AM, Maslan SL, Singer FR, Eyre DR. A specific immunoassay for monitoring human bone resorption: quantitation of type I collagen cross-linked N-telopeptides in urine. J Bone Miner Res 1992;7:1251–1258.
20. Bonde M, Qvist P, Fledelius C, Riis BJ, Christiansen C. Immunoassay for quantifying type I collagen degradation products in urine evaluated. Clin Chem 1994;40:2022–2025.

21. Gertz BJ, Clemens JD, Holland SD, Yuan W, Greenspan S. Application of a new serum assay for type I collagen cross-linked N-telopeptides: assessment of diurnal changes in bone turnover with and without alendronate treatment. Calcif Tissue Int 1998; 63:102–106.
22. Rosenquist C, Fledelius C, Christgau S, et al. Serum crosslaps one step ELISA. First application of monoclonal antibodies for measurement in serum of bone-related degradation products from C-terminal telopeptides of type I collagen. Clin Chem 1998;44: 2281–2289.
23. Minkin C. Bone acid phosphatase :tartrate-resistant acid phosphatase as a marker of osteoclast. Calcif Tissue Int 1982;34:285–290.
24. Kraenzlin M, Lau KHW, Liang L, et al. Development of an immunoassay for human osteoclastic tartrate-resistant acid phosphatase. J Clin Endocrinol Metab 1990;71: 442–451.
25. Woitge HW, Seibel MJ, Ziegler R. Comparison of total and bone-specific alkaline phosphatase in patients with nonskeletal disorder or metabolic bone diseases. Clin Chem 1996;42:1796–1804.
26. Kyd PA, Vooght KD, Kerkhoff F, Thomas E, Fairney A. Clinical usefulness of bone alkaline ohosphatase in osteoporosis. Ann Clin Biochem 1998;35:717–725.
27. Garnero P, Grimaux M, Seguin P, Delmas PD. Characterization of immunoreactive forms of human osteocalcin generated in vivo and in vitro. J Bone Miner Res 1994;9:255–264.
28. Blumsohn A, Hannon RA, Eastell R. Apparent instability of osteocalcin in serum as measured with different commercially available immunoassays. Clin Chem 1995;41: 318–319.
29. Masters PW, Jones RG, Purves DA, Cooper EH, Cooney JM. Commercial assays for serum osteocalcin give clinically discordant results. Clin Chem 1994;40:358–363.
30. Dessauer A. Analytical requirements for biochemical bone marker assays. Scand J Clin Lab Invest 1997;227:S84–S89.
31. Szulc P, Chapuy MC, Meunier PJ, Delmas PD. Serum undercarboxylated osteocalcin is a marker of the risk of hip fracture: a three-year follow-up study. Bone 1996; 18:487–488.
32. Gundberg CM, Nieman SD, Abrams S, Rosen H. Vitamin K status and bone health: an analysis of methods for determination of undercarboxylated osteocalcin. J Clin Endocrinol Metab 1998;83:3258–3266.
33. Ebeling PR, Peterson JM, Riggs BL. Utility of type I procollagen propeptide assays for assessing abnormalities in metabolic bone disease. J Bone Miner Res 1992;7:1243–1250.
34. Nielsen HK, Brixen K, Mosekilde L. Diurnal rhythm and 24-hour integrated concentrations of serum osteocalcin in normals: Influence of age, sex, season, and smoking habits. Calcif Tissue Int 1990;47:284–290.
35. Eastell R, Simmons PS, Colwell A, et al. Nyctohemeral changes in bone turnover assessed by serum bone Gla-protein concentration and urinary deoxypyridinoline excretion effects of growth and aging. Clin Science 1992;83:375–382.
36. Greenspan SL, Dresner-Pollak R, Parker RA, London D, Ferguson, L. Diurnal variation of bone mineral turnover in elderly men and women. Calcif Tissue 1997;60:419–423.
37. Aoshima H, Kushida K, Takahashi M, et al. Circadian variation of urinary type I collagen crosslinked C-telopeptide and free and peptide-bound forms of pyridinium crisslinks. Bone 1998;22:73–78.
38. Bollen A-M, Martin MD, Leroux BG, Eyre DR. Circadian variation in urinary excretion of bone collagen cross-links. J Bone Miner Res 1995;10:1885–1890.
39. Woitge HW, Scheidt-Nave C, Kissling C, et al. Seasonal variation of biochemical indexes of bone turnover: results of a population-based study. J Clin Endocrinol Metab 1998;83:68–75.
40. Nielsen HK, Brixen K, Bouillon R, Mosekilde L. Changes in biochemical markers of osteoblastic a tivity during the mentrual cycle. J Clin Endocrinol Metab 1990;70: 1431–1437.

41. Seibel, MJ, Woitge H, Scheidt-Nave C, et al. Urinary hydroxyoyridinium crosslinks of collagen in population-based screening for overt vertebral osteoporosis:results of a pilot study. J Bone Miner Res 1994;9:1433–1440.
42. Delmas PD, Gineyts E, Bertholin A, Garnero P, Marchand F. Immunoassay of pyridinoline crosslink excretion in normal adults and in Paget's disease. J Bone Miner Res 1993;8:643–648.
43. Tarallo P, Henny J, Fournier B, Siest G. Plasma osteocalcin: biological variations and reference limits. Scand J Clin Invest 1990;50:649–655.
44. Åkesson K, Lau K-H W, Johnston P, Imperio E, Baylink DJ. Effects of short-term calcium depletion and repletion on biochemical markers of bone turnover in young adult women. J Clin Endocrinol Metab 1998;83:1921–1927.
45. Gertz BJ, Shao P, Hanson DA, et al. Monitoring bone resorption in early postmenopausal women by an immunoassay for cross-linked collagen peptides in urine. J Bone Miner Res 1994;9:135–142.
46. Schneider DL, Barret-Connor EL. Urinary N-telopeptide levels discriminate normal, osteopenic, and osteoporotic bone mineral density. Arch Intern Med 1997;157:1241–1245.
47. Ravn P, Fledelius C, Rosenquist C, Overgaard K, Christiansen C. High bone turnover is associated with low bone mass in both pre- and postmenopausal women. Bone 1996;19:291–298.
48. Mazess RB. Body Weight predict bone density better than resorption markers. Arch Intern Med 1998;158:298–300.
49. Garnero P, Sornay-Rendu E, Chapuy M-C, Delmas PD. Increased bone turnover in late postmenopausal women is a major determinant of osteoporosis. J Bone Miner Res 1996;11:337–349.
50. Christiansen C, Riis BJ, Rødbro P. Prediction of rapid bone loss in postmenopausal women. Lancet 1987;I:1105–1108.
51. Hansen MA, Overgaard K, Riis BJ, Christiansen C. Role of peak bone mass and bone loss in postmenopausal osteoporosis: 12-year study. BMJ 1991;303:961–964.
52. Falch JA, Sandvik L. Perimenopausal appendicular bone loss: a 10-year prospective study. Bone 1990;11:425–428.
53. Cosman F, Nieves J, Wilkinson C, Schnering D, Shen V, Lindsay R. Bone density change and biochemical indices of skeletal turnover. Calcif Tissue Int 1996;58:236–243.
54. Keen RW, Nguyen T, Sobnack R, Perry LA, Thompson PW, Spector TD. Can biochemical markers predict bone loss at the hip and spine? A 4-year prospective study of 141 early postmenopausal women. Osteoporos Int 1996;6:399–406.
55. Reginster JY, Deroisy R, Collette J, Albert A, Zegels B. Prediction of bone loss rate in healthy postmenopausal women. Calcif Tissue Int 1997;60:261–264.
56. Åkesson K, Ljunghall S, Jonsson B, et al. Assessment of biochemical markers of bone metabolism in relation to the occurrence of fracture: a retrospective and prospective population-based study of women. J Bone Miner Res 1995;10:1823–1829.
57. Van Daele PLA, Seibel MJ, Burger H, et al. Case-control analysis of bone resorption markers, disability, and hip fracture risk:the Rotterdam study. BMJ 1996;312:482–483.
58. Garnero P, Hausherr E, Chapuy M-C, et al. Markers of bone resorption predict hip fracture in elderly women: the EPIDOS prospective study. J Bone Miner Res 1996;11: 1531–1538.
59. Hirsch L, Santora A, Kher U, Yates J, Bell N, Correa-Rotter R. Bone turnover rate does not predict BMD response to alendronate. Osteoporos Int. 1996;6 (Suppl 1):S262.
60. Greenspan SL, Parker RA, Ferguson L, Rosen HN, Maitland-Ramsey L, Karpf DB. Early changes in biochemical markers of bone turnover predict the long-term response to alendronate therapy in representative elderly women: a randomized clinical trial. J Bone Miner Res 1998;13:1431–1438.
61. Hannon RA, Blumsohn A, Ellison JV, Peel NF, Eastell R. Long-term variability of biochemical markers of bone turnover in postmenopausal women. Bone 1998;23:S159.

7 Identifying the Patient at Risk of Osteoporotic Fracture

H. Kröger and R. Honkanen

Introduction

Osteoporosis is a silent disease, without any preceding symptoms, until the first fracture occurs. Thus, the diagnosis of osteoporosis is often made in the orthopaedic wards after a low-energy fracture. Although orthopaedic surgeons know the frightful consequences of osteoporosis they may easily miss the diagnosis while concentrating on the technical aspects of fracture treatment. However, the identification of an osteoporotic patient with a fracture and her or his proper management is crucial, since several studies and recent trials have shown that a prevalent fracture increases the risk of subsequent fractures, and with pharmacological treatment of patients with established osteoporosis the risk of further fractures can be lowered. Identification of subjects at high risk of fracture constitutes the most rational approach to fracture prevention.

Prevalent fractures are strong predictors for subsequent fractures. In addition, several genetic, anthropometric and lifestyle factors as well as medical conditions are associated with an increased fracture risk. The occurrence of fracture depends on the exposure and propensity to trauma, level and attenuation of trauma energy and bone strength (Fig. 7.1). Thus, risk factors for fractures can be categorized into two main components: those related to trauma (e.g., falling tendency) and those related to bone strength (e.g., bone mineral density, BMD) [1]. However, several risk factors such as immobility or old age may operate through both skeletal and extraskeletal routes. In addition, several risk factors seem to be related to each other and part of this effect is associated with age-related bone loss. However, older subjects are at greater risk of fracture than younger subjects with the same level of bone density. Thus, factors associated with increased risk of falls with age must play a role.

Primary prevention of fractures requires the identification of individuals at high risk for osteoporosis prior to fracture. To promote this identification, a clinician should be aware of the risk factors in everyday practice. Bone mass is the major measurable determinant of fragility fractures. The determination of a patient's risk factor profile helps to select persons for bone densitometry, preventive measures and treatment.

Several risk factors for fractures have been identified in epidemiological studies [1–4]. Most of these studies have focused on risk factors for hip fracture and only

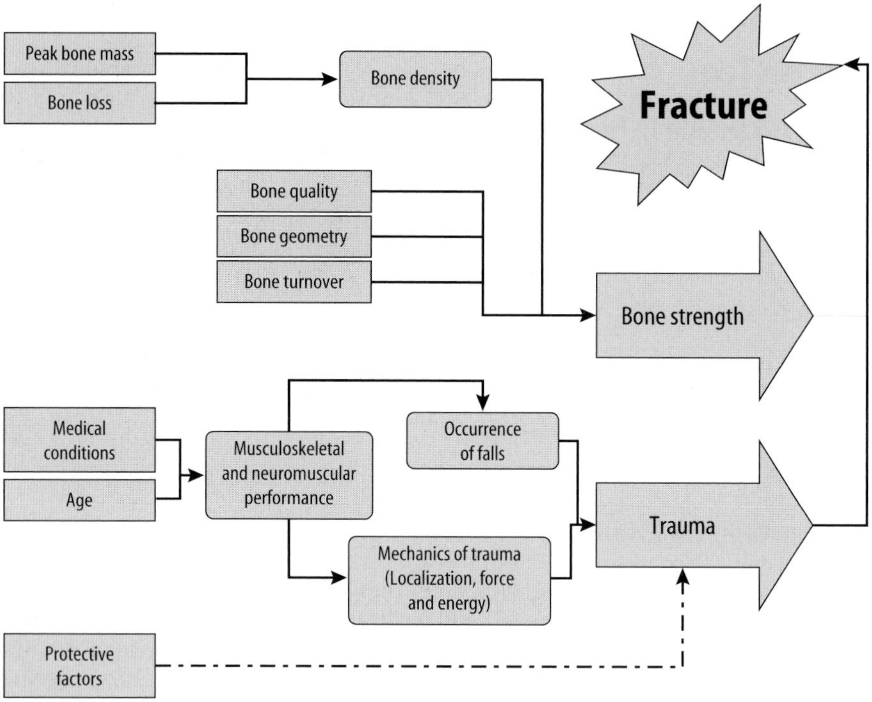

Figure 7.1. Components of fracture risk.

few deal with fractures in the perimenopausal and early postmenopausal period [3,5–7]. The studies concerning fracture risk in men are rare [3,8,9]. Risk factor profiles for fractures differ according to the skeletal site [2,7,10–12] and may differ also with age.

Bone Mineral Density

At present bone density is the best single surrogate measure for the breaking strength of bone. The diagnosis of osteoporosis is based on BMD measurement. Although other abnormalities in the skeleton and extraskeletal factors such as falls are important in the pathogenesis of osteoporotic fractures, only BMD can be measured with high precision and reasonable accuracy. The definition of osteoporosis includes disturbance in bone microarchitecture, i.e., bone quality, besides low bone mass and density. Trabecular perforations and accumulation of microdamage surely increase bone fragility. To date methods assessing bone quality in clinical practice are not available.

It should be borne in mind that fractures occur also in the absence of osteoporosis and that not all osteoporotic subjects will suffer from fracture. However, as bone mass decreases, fracture risk increases exponentially. There is no definite cutoff identifying cases with osteoporosis. In contrast, the risk of fracture increases with decreasing BMD and it is high in the presence of osteoporosis.

Methods for Assessing Bone

Several noninvasive methods of bone mass measurement have been applied since the 1960s. Single-photon absorptiometry (SPA) was developed for the measurement of bone mass and density in the peripheral skeleton (radius and calcaneus). Dual-photon absorptiometry (DPA) facilitated measurements of the axial skeleton. In the 1990s dual X-ray absorptiometry (DXA) became the most commonly used technique in the measurement of bone mass and density of the axial skeleton [13]. The new fan-beam DXA technology offers an option of using semiautomatic vertebral morphometry (MXA) for prescreening patients for vertebral deformities [14].

Quantitative ultrasound (QUS) measurements made on bones such as the calcaneus, tibia, digits and patella may provide new measures of bone fragility. It has been suggested that broadband ultrasound attenuation (BUA) is influenced not only by bone density but also by the microarchitectural characteristics of bone such as trabecular spacing and orientation. The speed of sound (SOS) may vary with the elasticity of bone [15].

BMD and Fracture Risk

Several cross-sectional and longitudinal studies have shown that bone density is inversely related to fracture risk. The initial study population in the Kuopio Osteoporosis Study consisted of all the 14 220 women aged 47–56 years residing in the Kuopio Province in 1989. A random stratified sample of 3222 women underwent DXA densitometry in 1990–1991. During the follow-up of 2 years, 183 validated low-energy nonspine fractures were recorded in 168 women. Women in the lowest quartile of spinal BMD had a relative fracture risk of 2.9 compared with women in the highest quartile. The respective risk by using the femoral neck BMD quartiles was 2.2. The relative fracture risk was 1.5 per 1 SD decrease in spinal BMD and

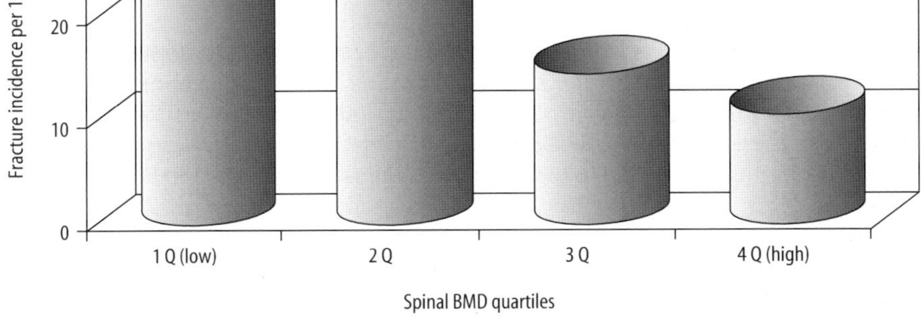

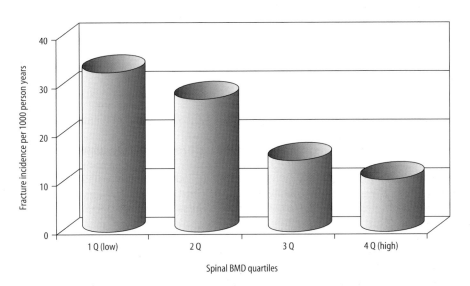

Figure7.2. Incidence of perimenopausal fractures by quartiles of spinal BMD.

1.4 per 1 SD decrease in femoral BMD. The conclusion was that the axial BMD measurement at the time of menopause could be of use in predicting subsequent fracture risk (Fig. 7.2) [16].

In another prospective study with a mean follow-up of 1.8 years among 8134 volunteer non-black American women over 65 years of age, the age-adjusted relative risk of hip fracture was 1.6 for each 1 SD decrease in bone density at the lumbar spine and 2.6 for each 1 SD decrease in BMD at the femoral neck [17]. Peripheral measurements of the radius and calcaneus have also shown a good predictive power for future incident fractures [18, 19].

Thus, the prospective studies show that for each standard deviation decline in BMD, the relative risk of fracture increases by about 1.5× in general but by at least 2.5× according to site-specific measurement. The ability of BMD to predict fracture is comparable to the use of blood pressure to predict stroke, and better than the ability of serum cholesterol to predict myocardial infarction.

Quantitative Ultrasound and Fracture Risk

Recent data suggest that BUA of the calcaneus predicts the risk of hip fracture in elderly women independently and as well as DXA. In the EPIDOS study 5662 elderly women (mean age 80.4 years) were measured at baseline with calcaneal US and femoral neck DXA. One hundred and fifteen hip fractures were recorded during 2 years of follow-up. The relative risk of hip fracture for a 1 SD reduction was 2.0 for BUA, 1.7 for SOS and 1.9 for femoral BMD. After controlling for BMD, QUS variables remained predictive of hip fracture [20]. Bauer, et al. [21] have also shown in a large prospective study on elderly women in the USA that each 1 SD reduction in BUA was associated with a doubling of the risk of hip fracture. Prospective validation using studies in peri- and early postmenopausal women and secondary forms of osteoporosis are needed before ultrasound of bone can be recommended for fracture risk assessment in these groups.

It should be noted, however, that although decreased BUA or SOS are independent risk factors for fractures in the elderly, QUS is not a surrogate for DXA in the diagnosis of osteoporosis. Although the discordance between QUS and axial BMD does not diminish the strength of the predictive value of QUS, the problem with false negatives (normal QUS but decreased axial BMD) still exists.

Indications for BMD Measurements

At present population screening for osteoporosis is not recommended because of unselected costs. Therefore, a so-called case finding policy has been widely applied [22]. Patients should be selected for bone densitometry on the basis of substantial risk factors. There are several well-established risk factors and causes of secondary osteoporosis in the presence of which further diagnosis by BMD, even among asymptomatic subjects, is indicated. Similarly, the diagnosis of osteoporosis may be confirmed with bone densitometry in patients with previous low-trauma fractures, radiological evidence of osteopenia or vertebral deformity. However, it should be borne in mind that bone densitometry is indicated only when its results could affect a treatment decision.

Table 7.1. Risk factors for osteoporosis, falls and fractures

Risk factor	Osteoporosis	Fall	Fracture
Low bone density			+
Age	+	+	+
Female gender	+	+	+
Postmenopausal status	+	+	+
Tallness		+	+
Low body weight	+		+
Long hip axis length			+
Previous fracture	+	+	+
Family history of fracture			+
Immobility/low physical activity	+	+	+
Current smoking	+	+	+
High caffeine intake			+
Alcohol abuse	+	+	+
High bone turnover	+		+
Osteomalacia/vitamin D deficiency	+	+	+
Chronic illnesses	+	+	+
Corticosteroids	+		+
Sedative medications		+	+
Visual impairment		+	+
Cognitive impairment		+	+
Neurological diseases		+	+
Lower limb disability	+	+	+
Hyperthyroidism	+		+
Hyperparathyroidism	+		+
Malabsorption	+		+
Celiac disease	+		+
Gastrectomy	+		+
Chronic arthritides	+	+	+
Chronic renal/liver diseases	+		+
Cushing syndrome	+		+
Malignancies	+		+
Organ transplantations	+		+
Living in a nursing home		+	+

Risk Factors for Low Bone Density

Several epidemiological cross-sectional studies and case–control studies have identified a large number of risk factors for low bone density (Table 7.1). As noted earlier, low bone density is a strong determinant of fracture, but few of these risk factors have been found to predict fractures independently of low BMD in prospective studies.

The amount of bone present later in life is determined by bone mass achieved during youth and the subsequent rate of bone loss. A vast majority of studies have investigated predictors of bone loss. On the other hand, studies on children may provide even more important information regarding bone accumulation. Exercise and adequate calcium intake during rapid growth period are important in optimizing of peak bone mass [23,24]. On the other hand, factors operating during the growth period may compromise the achievement peak bone mass. Some diseases (e.g., childhood malignancies and juvenile chronic arthritis) are associated with decreased bone density compared with that in age-matched healthy children [25,26].

The risk factors for low BMD have limited value in estimating a woman's actual bone density. At best only one-third of the variability of BMD can be predicted [27,28]. Thus, risk factor status cannot be used as a surrogate for bone densitometry, but rather as an aid when deciding the need for bone densitometry. There are certain groups in which the risk of osteoporosis is increased and bone densitometry is indicated as part of clinical evaluation and case finding. Analysis of risk factors is also helpful in defining the cause of osteoporosis.

Risk Factors for Falls

One-third of the elderly fall annually. Incidence of injurious falls increases with age [29] and is higher in the institutionalized than home-living elderly [30]. Falls are associated with a previous fall, disability, health disorders, and with the use of psychotropic drugs [31–33].

Besides the risk factors for low BMD and falls as noted above, several independent risk factors for fractures have been identified that can be used to assess individuals in everyday practice. Since hip fracture is the most devastating outcome of osteoporosis, most studies are concentrated on hip fractures (Table 7.1).

Personal History of a Fracture

A low-energy fracture in a woman after the age of 50 years is a usual cause for seeking medical care. A fall from standing height or lower is usually considered moderate trauma that is related to osteoporosis. Osteoporosis may play a role in up to 75% of fractures in people aged 45 years or older [34]. Consequently, perimenopausal women with fractures constitute a distinct risk group for osteoporosis.

Women who have had either vertebral fractures or nonspine fractures have an increased risk of recurrent vertebral fractures, independent of BMD [19,35]. Similarly, women who have had wrist fractures have an increased risk of hip fracture [36]. Among 9516 white women 65 years of age or older (mean age 72 years) (Study of Osteoporotic Fractures) low calcaneal BMD and a history of any type of fracture since the age of 50 years independently increased the risk of hip fracture by 50% [1]. Similarly, in perimenopausal women aged 47–56 years ($n = 3068$) a history of any type of fracture since the age 15 years independently predicted subsequent fractures during 3.6 years follow-up by 70% [37]. Because the risk is independent of BMD, fracture history may indicate an increased tendency to fall, the existence of another extraskeletal risk factor or a defect in bone strength other than low bone density. As regards the vertebral fractures, altered loading characteristics of vertebrae adjacent to the fracture site may play a role.

Only one-third of women with vertebral fractures come to medical attention. Spinal radiographs or vertebral morphometry with a MXA scan might be indicated in elderly women with low BMD. The detection of asymptomatic vertebral fracture puts the patient into a higher risk group than low BMD alone.

Age, Weight, Sex and Menopausal Status

Most risk factors associated with fractures become more prevalent with advancing age. Thus, it is not surprising that the risk of hip fracture increases by 1.5–2× for every 5 year increase in age [17,38]. During the perimenopausal years the risk of fracture is increased in postmenopausal women as compared with premenopausal women independently of femoral BMD [16]. Similarly, if bilateral oophorectomy is carried out under the age of of 45 years, the risk of fracture is increased [28]. Estrogen deficiency may predispose to an increased propensity to fall, but this hypothesis has not been established. On the other hand, women on long-term hormone replacement therapy have a decreased risk of fracture [37,39,40]. Female sex is a risk factor for fractures, as demonstrated by the higher prevalence of osteoporotic fractures in women than in men. Lower areal peak bone density, faster bone loss, smaller bone size and a higher prevalence of falls may explain the higher risk of fracture observed in women.

Low body weight is associated with low BMD [41] and increased risk of fracture [42,43], whereas gaining weight since 25 years of age is protective against hip fracture [1]. Low body weight may be a marker for poor heath and nutritional deficiency, which are common in elderly, institutionalized patients. Naturally, fat padding around the hip is also smaller in thin subjects.

Skeletal Geometry, Family History and Genetics

Mechanical properties of a bone are dependent not only on bone mass and its material properties, but also on its size, geometry and architecture (Fig. 7.1). Sex differences in the occurrence of fracture may partly be explained by the larger cross-sectional area of bones in men and differences in subperiosteal bone apposition [44].

There is increasing evidence that femoral neck geometry may play an important role in the risk of hip fracture. Faulkner and coworkers [45] reported that hip axis length (HAL), the measured distance along the femoral neck axis between the external border of the greater trochanter and inner pelvic rim, obtained from the image of DXA scan, is an independent predictor of hip fracture. An algorithm developed by Yoshikawa, et al. [46] using the principles of single plane engineering, makes an estimation of femoral neck mechanical strength from an anteroposterior DXA scan (so-called hip strength analysis, HSA), and preliminary results show that HSA may improve the prediction of hip fracture [47].

There is evidence that taller subjects are at increased risk of hip fracture [1,3]. This may be because they fall further [48].

Skeletal geometry is typically inherited. This may partly explain the finding that the risk of hip fracture in women with a maternal history of hip fracture is about twice that of women without such a history, independent of BMD [1]. However, shared environmental factors may play a role as well.

Twin studies and family studies indicate that genetic factors play an important role in the pathogenesis of osteoporosis. Recently, an association between vitamin D receptor gene (VDR) polymorphism and bone density was reported. Not all studies have shown this association, however. Polymorphism in and around other candidate genes (e.g., collagen type 1 alpha gene and estrogen receptor gene) have also been associated with bone density.

Lifestyle Risks

Although many lifestyle factors such as reduced dietary calcium intake, low physical activity, smoking, high alcohol consumption and caffeine intake have been associated with the risk of osteoporosis, the value of these lifestyle risk factors in predicting fracture is less well established [49,50]. Interactions between the lifestyle risks are likely to occur.

Studies in which the relationship between dietary calcium and hip fracture risk have been examined have given conflicting results [4,38,51–53]. Errors in the measurement of dietary calcium intake and slow changes in bone mineral may be the reason for negative findings. It is easier to show the association between calcium intake and fracture with a randomized clinical trial, which in fact has been done recently [54]. In conclusion, dietary calcium seems partially to protect from bone loss, though the effect in populations with a high calcium intake is small.

Impairment of mobility causes bone loss and constitutes a major risk factor for falls [55], whereas physical activity improves muscle strength and coordination and seems to preserve bone mass. Muscle strength may influence both BMD [41,56] and propensity to falls [57]. High body sway and low quadriceps strength have been shown to increase the risk of hip fracture in addition to low BMD in an Australian population-based study [58]. A recent study reported that women spending 4 h or less per day on their feet had an increased risk of hip fracture [1]. It is not known whether the adverse effects of physical inactivity and immobility are mediated by decreased BMD, coexisting illnesses, increased risk of falls or all of these. In most studies immobility may be a marker for impaired health in the elderly.

Several studies have suggested that current smokers have lower bone density. A recent meta-analysis suggested that smoking is a risk factor for osteoporotic fractures in postmenopausal women [59]. Current smoking might increase the risk of hip fracture by its adverse effects on health and neuromuscular fitness [1].

Some studies have reported that caffeine consumption is associated with increased fracture risk [1,60,61]. In perimenopausal women caffeine consumption did not increase the risk of fracture, however [6,37]. The adverse effect of caffeine on bone may be important in the elderly.

Subjects with alcohol abuse have increased risk of fracture, possibly owing to poor balance and associated illnesses [60], whereas moderate alcohol consumption may not be a risk factor for osteoporosis [41].

Medical Conditions

In general, health problems and chronic illnesses can predispose to fractures by impairing BMD and bone quality, by decreasing physical activity and increasing the likelihood of a fall.

Decreased visual acuity [43,62], poor depth perception [1], mental impairment or dementia [55] and impaired neuromuscular function (e.g., inability to rise from a chair without using the arms) [1,43,62] have been found to increase the risk of hip fracture. All these conditions are considered fall-related rather than BMD-related risk factors for fractures [31–33].

In the Study of Osteoporotic Fractures, elderly women who rated their health as fair or poor, had previous hyperthyroidism, had been treated with long-acting benzodiazepines or anticonvulsant drugs or spent 4 h a day or less on their feet showed increased risk of hip fracture that was independent of calcaneal BMD [1]. These conditions might be associated with existence of chronic illnesses, impaired health and increased likelihood of falls. In consistent with these findings, in the Kuopio Osteoporosis Study the presence of three or more chronic illnesses was found to be an independent predictor for fractures in perimenopausal women [37].

Long-term use of corticosteroids, hypercortisolism, hypogonadism, hyperparathyroidism, osteomalacia, renal and hepatic diseases, certain malignancies, rheumatoid arthritis, Paget´s disease, gastrectomy and organ transplantations are medical conditions usually associated with low bone density and increased risk of fractures [63]. Some of these are relatively rare in a population, but the individual fracture risk associated with them can be considerable.

As regards environmental factors which may predispose to fractures, residence in a home for the elderly or a nursing home seems to increase the risk of hip fracture by 6–8 times as compared with that of the independent elderly [64]. Institutionalized patients have many risk factors for both falls and osteoporosis, including poor physical and mental health, nutritional deficiencies (e.g., vitamin D deficiency predisposing to osteomalacia) and use of drugs interfering with alertness.

Bone Turnover

There is some evidence that a high rate of bone resorption assessed by biochemical markers may predict fracture risk. In the EPIDOS study baseline urinary excretion of type I collagen cross-linked C-telopeptide and free deoxypyridoline were higher in subjects who sustained a hip fracture during the 22 months of follow-up. Even after adjusting for femoral BMD the increased bone resorption measured using these markers predicted hip fracture [65]. Theoretically increased bone turnover and resorption rate may cause a deterioration in trabecular integrity and architecture, which in turn decreases bone strength more than could be anticipated on the grounds of BMD loss only. Thus some of the new biochemical markers of bone turnover might be used in combination with densitometry to improve the prediction of fracture in elderly women.

Conclusions

Early detection of a patient at risk for osteoporosis and fractures depends on the awareness among orthopaedic surgeons. Although the prevention of osteoporosis before irreversible bone loss has taken place is the primary aim, it is as important to prevent the subsequent fractures after the first one. The early diagnosis of osteoporosis is possible using bone densitometry. Risk factors should be used in selecting patients for bone densitometry. A combination of several risk factors seems reasonable since women with multiple risk factors and low BMD are at an especially high risk for hip fracture [1]. It should be borne in mind that most of the risk factors mentioned above apply with certainty only to white women. Studies on men and on women of other ethnic groups are scarce.

Several risk factors cannot be modified, including gender, height and family history. However, these risk factors can identify risk groups for bone densitometry and amenable to pharmacological intervention. Falls can also be prevented [66–68].

The prevention of falls requires a multifaceted strategy of risk assessment and intervention which includes environmental changes, improvement of functional ability, correction or treatment of health disorders including impaired vision and leg and foot problems, as well as avoidance of multiple medicines [69]. Prevention of hip fractures may include the use of hip pads [70].

It is also possible to modify some behavioral risk factors for low BMD such as smoking, inadequate calcium intake or physical inactivity, but the resulting benefits may be small. In contrast, the determination of BMD is important, since BMD represents the cumulative influence of multiple risk factors for bone loss and osteoporosis. Furthermore, effective treatments for bone loss are available.

Even if several risk factors for fractures have been identified in a patient, pharmacological treatment for osteoporosis should not be initiated based on their existence only. Namely, though fracture risk is increased in such persons, the risk may be mediated through factors not related to bone density. Thus, some of these individuals have a normal BMD and do not need drug therapy. Similarly, the initiation of bisphosphonate or other non-HRT antiresorptive therapy without BMD measurements for a 50-year-old woman with a wrist fracture or a mild vertebral deformity is not indicated, since not all these fractures are due to low-energy trauma and osteoporosis. In elderly individuals with multiple vertebral fractures, measurement of spinal BMD is not useful because of the frequent presence of artifacts. Similarly, bone densitometry is not required for the treatment decision in very elderly patients with hip fracture, since low bone mass is almost universal in such patients [71,72].

Orthopaedic surgeons are experts on bone injury and normally the first who meet patients with osteoporotic fractures. Unfortunately, after primary fracture care the diagnostic tests and treatment of the porous skeleton are seldom contemplated in orthopaedic wards. However, an orthopaedic surgeon could play an important role in the secondary prevention of fractures including drug treatment of osteoporosis. It is up to orthopaedic surgeons not only to repair fractured bones but also to identify the patients who need diagnostic test and other management for underlying bone pathology, i.e., osteoporosis.

References

1. Cummings SR, Nevitt MC, Browner WS, Stone K, Fox KM, Ensrud KE, et al. Risk factors for hip fracture in white women. Study of osteoporotic fractures research group. N Engl J Med 1995;332:767–773.
2. Kelsey JL, Browner WS, Seeley DG, Nevitt MC, Cummings SR. Risk factors for fractures of the distal forearm and proximal humerus. Am J Epidemiol 1992;135:477–489.
3. Meyer HE, Tverdal A, Falch JA. Risk factors for hip fracture in middle-aged Norwegian women and men. Am J Epidemiol 1993;137:1203–1211.
4. Johnell O, Gullberg B, Kanis JA, Allander E, Elffors L, Dequeker J, et al. Risk factors for hip fracture in European women: the MEDOS Study. Mediterranean Osteoporosis Study. J Bone Miner Res 1995;10:1802–1815.
5. Mallmin H, Ljunghall S, Persson I, Bergstrom R. Risk factors for fractures of the distal forearm: a population-based case-control study. Osteoporos Int 1994;4:298–304.
6. Torgerson DJ, Campbell MK, Thomas RE, Reid DM. Prediction of perimenopausal fractures by bone mineral density and other risk factors. J Bone Miner Res 1996;11: 293–297.

7. Honkanen R, Tuppurainen M, Kröger H, Alhava E, Saarikoski S. Relationships between risk factors and fractures differ by type of fracture. A population-based study of 12 192 perimenopausal women. Osteoporos Int 1998;8:25–31.
8. Hemenway D, Azrael DR, Rimm EB, Feskanich D, Willett WC. Risk factors for wrist fracture: effect of age, cigarettes, alcohol, body height, relative weight, and handedness on the risk for distal forearm fractures in men. Am J Epidemiol 1994;140:361–367.
9. Nguyen TV, Eisman JA, Kelly PJ, Sambrook PN. Risk factors for osteoporotic fractures in elderly men. Am J Epidemiol 1996;144:255–263.
10. Seeley DG, Browner WS, Nevitt MC, Genant HK, Scott JC, Cummings SR. Which fractures are associated with low appendicular bone mass in elderly women? The Study of Osteoporotic Fractures Research Group. Ann Intern Med 1991;115:837–842.
11. Seeley DG, Kelsey J, Jergas M, Nevitt MC:. Predictors of ankle and foot fractures in older women. J Bone Miner Res 1996;11:1347–1355.
12. Graafmans WC, Ooms ME, Bezemer PD, Bouter LM, Lips P. Different risk profiles for hip fractures and distal forearm fractures: a prospective study. Osteoporos Int 1996;6:427–431.
13. Blake GM, Fogelman I. Technical principles of dual energy x-ray absorptiometry. Semin Nucl Med 1997;27:210–228.
14. Lang T, Takada M, Gee R, Wu C, Li J, Hayashi-Clark C, et al. A preliminary evaluation of the Lunar Expert-XL for bone densitometry and vertebral morphometry. J Bone Miner Res 1997;12: 136–143.
15. Njeh CF, Boivin CM, Langton CM ()The role of ultrasound in the assessment of osteoporosis: a review. Osteoporos Int 1997;7:7–22.
16. Kröger H, Huopio J, Honkanen R, Tuppurainen M, Puntila E, Alhava E, Saarikoski S. Prediction of fracture risk using axial bone mineral density in a perimenopausal population: a prospective study. J Bone Miner Res 1995;10:302–306.
17. Cummings SR, Black DM, Nevitt MC, Browner W, Cauley J, Ensrud K, et al. Bone density at various sites for prediction of hip fractures. The Study of Osteoporotic Fractures Research Group [see comments]. Lancet 1993;341:72–75.
18. Hui SL, Slemenda CW, Johnston CC Jr. Baseline measurement of bone mass predicts fracture in white women. Ann Intern Med 1989;111:355–361.
19. Ross PD, Davis JW, Epstein RS, Wasnich RD. Pre-existing fractures and bone mass predict vertebral fracture incidence in women. Ann Intern Med 1991;114:919–923.
20. Hans D, Dargent-Molina P, Schott AM, Sebert JL, Cormier C, Kotzki PO, et al. Ultrasonographic heel measurements to predict hip fracture in elderly women: the EPIDOS study. Lancet 1996;348:511–514.
21. Bauer DC, Gluer CC, Cauley JA, Vogt TM, Ensrud KE, Genant HK, et al. Broadband ultrasound attenuation predicts fractures strongly and independently of densitometry in older women: a prospective study. Study of Osteoporotic Fractures Research Group [see comments]. Arch Intern Med 157: 1997;629–634.
22. Consensus development statement. Who are candidates for prevention and treatment for osteoporosis? Osteoporos Int 1997;7:1–6.
23. Kannus P, Haapasalo H, Sankelo M, Sievanen H, Pasanen M, Heinonen A, et al. Effect of starting age of physical activity on bone mass in the dominant arm of tennis and squash players. Ann Intern Med 1995;123:27–31.
24. Johnston CC Jr, Miller JZ, Slemenda CW, Reister TK, Hui S, Christian JC, et al. Calcium supplementation and increases in bone mineral density in children. N Engl J Med 1992;327:82–87.
25. Arikoski P, Komulainen J, Voutilainen R, Riikonen P, Parviainen M, Tapaninen P, et al. Reduced bone mineral density in long-term survivors of childhood malignancies. J Pediatr Hematol Oncol 1998;20:234–240.
26. Kotaniemi A, Savolainen A, Kautiainen H, Kröger H. Estimation of central osteopenia in children with chronic polyarthritis treated with glucocorticoids. Pediatrics 1993;91:1127–1130.

27. Cooper C, Shah S, Hand DJ, Adams J, Compston J, Davie M, et al. Screening for vertebral osteoporosis using individual risk factors. The Multicentre Vertebral Fracture Study Group. Osteoporos Int 1991;2:48–53.
28. Tuppurainen M, Kröger H, Saarikoski S, Honkanen R, Alhava E. The effect of gynecological risk factors on lumbar and femoral bone mineral density in peri- and postmenopausal women. Maturitas 1995;21:137–145.
29. Ryynänen O-P, Kivelä S-L, Honkanen R, Laippala P, Soini P. Incidence of falling injuries leading to medical treatment in the elderly. Soc Public Health 1991;105:373–386.
30. Luukinen H, Koski K, Honkanen R, Kivelä S-L. Incidence of injury-causing falls among older adults by place of residence: a population-based study. J Am Geriatr Soc 1995; 43:871–876.
31. Tinetti ME, Speechley M, Ginter SF. Risk factors for falls among elderly persons living in the community. N Engl J Med 1988;319:1701–7.
32. Myers AH, Baker SP, Van Natta ML, Abbey H, Robinson EG. Risk factors associated with falls and injuries among elderly institutionalized persons. Am J Epidemiol 1991;133:1179–1190.
33. Ryynänen O-P, Kivelä S-L, Honkanen R, laippala P, Saano V. Medications and chronic diseases as risk factors for falling injuries in the elderly. Scand J Soc Med 1993;21:264–271.
34. Cooper C, Melton LJ III. Magnitude and impact of osteoporosis and fractures In: Marcus R, Feldman D, Kelsey J, editors. Osteoporosis. San Diego: Academic Press, 1996:419–434.
35. Wasnich RD, Davis JW, Ross PD. Spine fracture risk is predicted by non-spine fractures. Osteoporos Int 1994;4:1–5.
36. Mallmin H, Ljunghall S, Persson I, Naessen T, Krusemo UB, Bergstrom R. Fracture of the distal forearm as a forecaster of subsequent hip fracture: a population-based cohort study with 24 years of follow-up. Calcif Tissue Int 1993;52:269–272.
37. Huopio J, Kröger H, Honkanen R, Alhava E, Saarikoski S. Risk factors for perimenopausal fractures. A prospective population-based study. Osteoporos Int 1998;8 (Suppl 3):6.
38. Paganini-Hill A, Chao A, Ross RK, Henderson B (). Exercise and other factors in the prevention of hip fracture: the Leisure World study. Epidemiology 1991;1:16–25.
39. Cauley JA, Seeley DG, Ensrud K, Ettinger B, Black D, Cummings SR. Estrogen replacement therapy and fractures in older women. Study of Osteoporotic Fractures Research Group. Ann Intern Med 1995;122:9–16.
40. Komulainen M, Kröger H, Tuppurainen MT, Heikkinen A-M, Alhava E, Honkanen R, et al. Effects of hormone replacement therapy and vitamin D on the prevention of non-vertebral fractures in early postmenopausal women: a 5-year randomized trial. Maturitas 1998;31:45–54.
41. Kröger H, Tuppurainen M, Honkanen R, Alhava E, Saarikoski S. Bone mineral density and risk factors for osteoporosis-a population-based study of 1600 perimenopausal women. Calcif Tissue Int 1994;55:1–7.
42. Gärdsell P, Johnell O, Nilsson BE. Predicting fractures in women using forearm bone densitometry. Calcif Tissue Int 1989;44:235–242.
43. Grisso JA, Kelsey JL, Strom BL, Chiu GY, Maislin G, O'Brien LA, et al. Risk factors for falls as a cause of hip fracture in women. N Engl J Med 1991;324:1326–1331.
44. Ruff CB, Hayes WC. Sex differences in age-related remodeling of the femur and tibia. J Orthop Res 1988;6:886–896.
45. Faulkner KG, Cummings SR, Black D, Palermo L, Gluer CC, Genant HK. Simple measurement of femoral geometry predicts hip fracture: the Study of Osteoporotic Fractures. J Bone Miner Res 1993;8:1211–1217.
46. Yoshikawa T, Turner CH, Peacock M, Slemenda CW, Weaver CM, Teegarden D, et al. Geometric structure of the femoral neck measured using dual-energy x- ray absorptiometry [published erratum appears in J Bone Miner Res 1995;10:510]. J Bone Miner Res 1994;9:1053–1064.

47. Crabtree NJ, Adams J, Pols H, Grazio S, Kroger H, Lorenc R, et al. Age, gender and geographical effects on hip geometry and bone mineral distribution: the EPOS study. Osteoporos Int 1997;7:291.
48. Hayes WC, Myers ER, Morris JN, Gerhart TN, Yett HS, Lipsitz LA. Impact near the hip dominates fracture risk in elderly nursing home residents who fall. Calcif Tissue Int 1993;52:192–198.
49. Cumming RG, Nevitt MC. Calcium for prevention of osteoporotic fractures in postmenopausal women. J Bone Miner Res 1997;12:1321–1329.
50. Joakimsen RM, Magnus JH, Fonnebo V. Physical activity and predisposition for hip fractures: a review. Osteoporos Int 1997;7:503–513.
51. Wickham CA, Walsh K, Cooper C, Barker DJ, Margetts BM, Morris J, et al. Dietary calcium, physical activity, and risk of hip fracture: a prospective study. BMJ 1989;299: 889–92.
52. Feskanich D, Willett WC, Stampfer MJ, Colditz GA. Milk, dietary calcium, and bone fractures in women: a 12-year prospective study. Am J Public Health 1997;87:992–997.
53. Honkanen R, Honkanen K, Valtola A, Kröger HP, Alhava E, Tuppurainen M, et al. Risk factors for perimenopausal distal forearm fracture: a prospective population-based cohort study. Abstract for the 2nd Joint Meeting of the American Society for Bone and Mineral Research and The International Bone and Mineral Society, San Francisco, 1–6 December 1998.
54. Dawson-Hughes B, Harris SS, Krall EA, Dallal GE. Effect of calcium and vitamin D supplementation on bone density in men and women 65 years of age or older. N Engl J Med 1997;337:670–676.
55. Graafmans WC, Ooms ME, Hofstee HM, Bezemer PD, Bouter LM, Lips P. Falls in the elderly: a prospective study of risk factors and risk profiles. Am J Epidemiol 1996; 143:1129–1136.
56. Nguyen TV, Kelly PJ, Sambrook PN, Gilbert C, Pocock NA, Eisman JA. Lifestyle factors and bone density in the elderly: implications for osteoporosis prevention. J Bone Miner Res 1994;9:1339–1346.
57. Koski K, Luukinen H, Laippala P, Kivela SL. Physiological factors and medications as predictors of injurious falls by elderly people: a prospective population-based study. Age Ageing 1996;25:29–38.
58. Nguyen T, Sambrook P, Kelly P, Jones G, Lord S, Freund J, Eisman J. Prediction of osteoporotic fractures by postural instability and bone density. BMJ 1993;307:11 11–1115.
59. Law MR, Hackshaw AK. A meta-analysis of cigarette smoking, bone mineral density and risk of hip fracture: recognition of a major effect. 1997;BMJ 315:841–846.
60. Hernandez-Avila M, Colditz GA, Stampfer MJ, Rosner B, Speizer FE, Willett WC. Caffeine, moderate alcohol intake, and risk of fractures of the hip and forearm in middle-aged women. Am J Clin Nutr 1991;54:157–163.
61. Kiel DP, Felson DT, Hannan MT, Anderson JJ, Wilson PW. Caffeine and the risk of hip fracture: the Framingham Study. Am J Epidemiol 1990;132:675–684.
62. Dargent-Molina P, Favier F, Grandjean H, Baudoin C, Schott AM, Hausherr E, et al. Fall-related factors and risk of hip fracture: the EPIDOS prospective study. Lancet 1996;348:145–149.
63. Kanis JA, Delmas P, Burckhardt P, Cooper C, Torgerson D. Guidelines for diagnosis and management of osteoporosis. The European Foundation for Osteoporosis and Bone Disease. Osteoporos Int 1997;7:390–406.
64. Ooms ME, Vlasman P, Lips P, Nauta J, Bouter LM, Valkenburg HA. The incidence of hip fractures in independent and institutionalized elderly people. Osteoporos Int 1994;4:6–10.
65. Garnero P, Hausherr E, Chapuy MC, Marcelli C, Grandjean H, Muller C, et al. Markers of bone resorption predict hip fracture in elderly women: the EPIDOS Prospective Study. J Bone Miner Res 1996;11:1531–1538.

66. Province MA, Hadley EC, Hornbrook MC, Lipsitz LA, Miller JP, Mulrow CD, et al. The effects of exercise on falls in elderly patients. A preplanned meta-analysis of the FICSIT Trials. Frailty and Injuries: Cooperative Studies of Intervention Techniques. JAMA 1995;273:1341–1347.
67. Tinetti ME, McAvay G, Claus E. Does multiple risk factor reduction explain the reduction in fall rate in the Yale FICSIT Trial? Frailty and Injuries Cooperative Studies of Intervention Techniques. Am J Epidemiol 1996;144:389–399.
68. Buchner DM, Cress ME, de Lateur BJ, Esselman PC, Margherita AJ, Price R, et al. The effect of strength and endurance training on gait, balance, fall risk, and health services use in community-living older adults. J Gerontol A Biol Sci Med Sci 1997;52:M218–224.
69. Tinetti ME, Baker DI, McAvay G, Claus EB, Garrett P, Gottschalk M, et al. A multifactorial intervention to reduce the risk of falling among elderly people living in the community. N Engl J Med 1994;331:821–827.
70. Lauritzen JB, Petersen MM, Lund B. Effect of external hip protectors on hip fractures. Lancet 1993;341:11–13.
71. Compston JE, Cooper C, Kanis JA. Bone densitometry in clinical practice. BMJ 1995; 310:1507–1510.
72. Kröger H, Reeve J. Diagnosis of osteoporosis in clinical practice. Ann Med 1998; 30:278–287.

Part II

Fracture Healing

8 Determinants for Consolidation or Deficient Fracture Healing in Osteoporotic Fractures

L. Nordsletten and J. E. Madsen

Introduction

Fracture healing has been assumed to be the same in osteoporotic and normal bone. However, fracture healing has hardly ever been compared in these two different patient groups since the fracture pattern also varies according to bone mass. Tibial shaft fractures may not heal equally easy in an old frail woman as in a young soccer player, but this has not been studied. While tibial fractures may represent a high proportion of fractures in the young age group they are totally overshadowed by the typical osteoporotic fractures in the old age group, and thus not the focus of interest.

Therefore, knowledge of the determinants of deficient fracture healing is mainly derived from studies of typical osteoporotic fractures. Fractures of the proximal femur have been extensively studied, as have distal radius fractures. In the distal radius malunion may be a problem, but the fractures nearly always unite.

Factors deciding the later fate of an osteoporotic fracture may be divided into intrinsic (biological and fracture type variations in the patient) and extrinsic (treatment of the fracture, either operative or non-operative) (Fig 8.1). This chapter will focus on the fractures of the upper end of the femur, as knowledge about these types of osteoporotic fractures is extensive. One should keep in mind, though, that the femoral neck fracture has special features different from other osteoporotic fractures. In displaced femoral neck fractures the head fragment may be more or less avascular, and healing may thus proceed only from the shaft fragment by creeping substitution until revascularization of the head takes place. Furthermore, the femoral neck is covered by synovium, not periosteum, and healing therefore usually proceeds without callus formation. With this slow type of fracture healing mechanical stability is mandatory, but in osteoporotic bone sufficiently stable constructs may be hard to obtain. Benterud et al. [1] showed that there was a high correlation between bone mass measured by computed tomography and the stability ($r^2 = 0.81$) and strength ($r^2 = 0.76$) of a femoral neck osteotomy fixed with screws , indicating that stable osteosynthesis may be impossible in severe osteoporosis. Experimental studies on fracture healing will also be discussed here where pertinent.

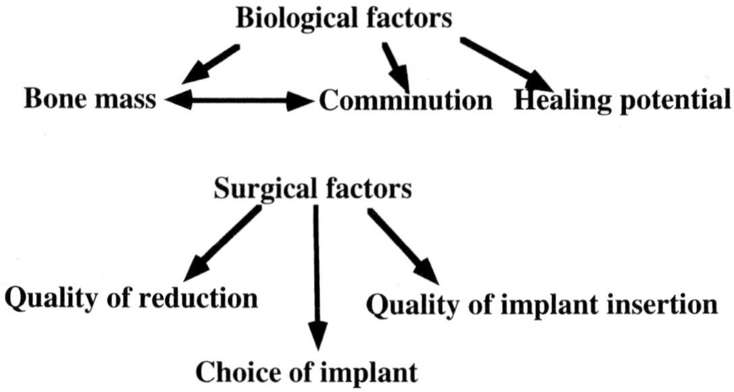

Figure 8.1. Schematic representation of determinants for consolidation or deficient fracture healing in osteoporotic fractures, divided into biological and surgical factors.

Biological Determinants for Deficient Fracture Healing

Hormonal and Cytokine Effects on Fracture Healing in Osteoporosis

Osteoporotic bone differs from normal bone mainly in its reduced mass. However, since osteoporosis is most frequent in postmenopausal women there are differences also in hormonal status that may significantly influence fracture healing. Estrogen receptors have been found in fracture callus tissue, and estrogen may therefore influence the healing process [2,3]. In experimental studies comparing fracture healing in estrogen-replete or estrogen-deplete animals fracture healing has been found to be delayed in ovariectomized animals [4]. In humans no such data exist at present.

Other hormones or cytokines may be altered in osteoporosis. Insulin-like growth factor 1 (IGF-1) has been found to be low in the plasma of men with osteoporosis [5], however, stimulation with IGF-1 in replete rats with tibial fracture has not shown any positive effect [6]. Immunohistochemical staining in a fibular fracture in diabetic and normal rats showed that endogenous basic fibroblast growth factor (bFGF) was widely distributed in the soft callus and periosteum in normal rats, whereas less bFGF was detected in diabetic rats [7]. Insulin treatment of diabetic rats restored the immunostaining for bFGF. The mere fact that many of the growth factors are bound in the bone substance [8], and thereby released during fracture, suggests that local stimulation due to release from the fractured bone may be diminished with low bone mass. Also, demineralized bone matrix from old and ovariectomized rats has been shown to have a low osteoinductive capacity, pointing to less growth factor activity in aged bone [9,10]. In 2-year-old compared with 3-month-old rats tibial fracture healing was delayed after 80 days; after 40 days the healing was similar [11]. In humans age has been found to be an independent risk factor for femoral neck fracture healing complications in some [12,13], but not all studies [14]. Age may in this instance be a marker for osteoporosis, but reduced healing capacity with age, as discussed above, may be another explanation.

Systemic Diseases

Several general diseases affect bone metabolism and probably also fracture healing in the osteoporotic skeleton. Rheumatoid arthritis, diabetes, renal failure and alcohol abuse may exemplify such conditions. Whether these diseases affect fracture healing has not been extensively studied. Zichner [15] claimed that fracture healing in renal failure may be disturbed, and found a high rate of nonunion after corrective osteotomies and fracture fixations in these patients.

Malnutrition has been known to delay fracture healing in humans. From experimental studies, protein deficiency seems to be the major cause for this, as protein deficiency caused lower ultimate distraction forces and lower callus stiffness despite adequate total calorie intake in rats [16].

Diabetics also seem to suffer delayed fracture healing, even though the clinical evidence for this may be sparse. Experimentally, however, evidence of decreased tensile strength and stiffness of healing bones in diabetic animals exists [17], and a decreased collagen content of the fracture callus during early healing was found. Treatment with insulin restored the bone strength, but no evidence exists on whether this corresponds to the human situation. In another rat study immunohistochemical staining showed that endogenous bFGF was widely distributed in normal rats 1 and 3 weeks after fracture, especially in the soft callus and periosteum, whereas much less bFGF was detected in diabetic rats. Insulin treatment of diabetic rats restored the immunostaining for bFGF [7].

Drug or alcohol abuse has been associated with osteopenia and increased risk of fracture. Also, it is generally accepted that abusers sustain a high rate of complications during fracture treatment, when treated both operatively and nonoperatively [18]. Whether fracture healing per se is impaired may, however, be difficult to establish. In tibial fractures it was shown that healing time was impaired in transverse but not in oblique fractures in a retrospective study on 49 alcoholics and 150 nonalcoholics in Malmö [19], but this study was not focusing on osteoporotic fractures. In a rat study of two groups with tibial fractures one of which was given alcohol, no differences in healing strength were found after 35 days, although the total bone mass was reduced in the alcohol group [20]. Further, the generally impaired nutritional state of drug abusers must be taken into account. Thus, substantial evidence for deficient fracture healing in drug or alcohol abusers is hard to find.

Radiological, Scintimetric and Bone Mass Determinants for Healing Complications

Several factors influencing the healing process or the stability of the fracture can be determined on radiographs or by scintimetry (Table 8.1).

Fracture configuration may determine eventual healing complications. Commonly used classifications for femoral neck fractures are Garden's and Pauwels'. Garden classified femoral neck fractures into undisplaced (I and II) or displaced (III and IV). The subgrouping of undisplaced and displaced fractures has not been shown to have prognostic value [21], while the grouping into displaced and undisplaced fractures reflects poor and good prognosis, respectively, with up to a 10-fold increased risk of healing complications in displaced fractures [13,14]. Pauwels' classification is based on the angle of the fracture line, the more vertical fracture lines indicating the more severe fractures. The prognostic value of Pauwels'

Table 8.1. Factors influencing fracture healing in femoral neck fractures as determined from radiographs, scintimetry or age of the patient. Risk ratio or odds ratio for healing complications are given where available

Determinants influencing fracture healing in femoral neck fractures	Risk/odds ratio
Fracture displacement [14,21]	10
Comminution [12,21,48]	3.8–8.7
Small head size [12]	3
Varus angulation [24]	6.5
Reduced scintimetric uptake [48]	4
Age [13,22)]	1.8

classification has not been reported despite its frequent use. Alho and co-workers [21] found that the fracture displacement in millimeters on the anteroposterior radiograph had a predictive value, while the Garden classification had not. In a later and larger study on mostly displaced fractures Alho et al. [22] found that other factors were more important, with varus angulation over 30° increasing the risk of later displacement 6-fold.

Bone mass has, unfortunately, usually been estimated by rather unreliable methods like the Singh-index [23], which has no predictive value for the healing of femoral neck fractures [13]. Only the study by Karlsson et al. [24] used dual-energy X-ray absorptiometry (DXA) measurement for evaluation of healing complications. Bone mineral density was measured within the first 10 days in 47 femoral neck fractures and 55 trochanteric fractures. Healing complications (pseudarthrosis or late segmental collapse in 16/47 femoral neck, 5/55 trochanteric fractures) could not be predicted by the DXA scan of the affected hip. The number of patients was, however, rather small in each group, and the authors warned against type 2 error. In a study of 249 patients with femoral neck fractures Arnold [25] analyzed iliac crest biopsies in 66 of these. Of the 9 with lowest trabecular bone volume (less than 10%), 7 had a displaced Garden type III or IV fracture, and of these 5 had a failure despite being properly reduced. Of the 28 patients with a well-reduced Garden III–IV fracture and higher bone volume healing disturbances occurred in only 4 hips.

Fracture comminution is correlated with poor bone mass. Elabdien et al. [26] found that the Barnett Nordin index could discriminate between stable (1- and 2-part) and unstable (3- and 4-part) trochanteric fractures. Comminution and hence instability of the fracture is therefore related to low bone mass (Fig. 8.1). The problem with comminuted fractures is therefore 2-fold in the osteoporotic patient: the fracture has a high degree of instability, and the bone in which to fix the osteosynthesis material is weak. Therefore, the osteosynthesis construct (the metal and bone) becomes weak. As patients are often incapable of unloading, the risk of secondary displacement is even higher. Comminution may, however, be difficult to detect during evaluation of the radiographs pre-operatively. Alho et al. [21] suggested that the length of the calcar should be measured divided into four parts, and that a missing part should be counted as comminution. Applying this method to the determination of comminution has been found to be predictive for healing complications [12,21].

Surgical Factors Affecting Fracture Healing

Quality of Surgery

A properly reduced fracture is mandatory for uncomplicated healing in osteoporotic fractures [27]. It has been shown experimentally that proper reduction is more important than type and placement of the osteosynthesis material [28]. The definition of good reduction may be summarized as the absence of the following signs on the anteroposterior view: (1) varus position, (2) valgus position $\geqslant 10°$, (3) lack of medial neb engagement and, on the side view, (4) tilting more than 5° [27]. In a prospective study on healing disturbances in 149 patients Alho et al. [12], using the same criteria as above, found a 3 times increased risk of failure with imperfect reduction, only exceeded by calcar comminution (odds ratio 3.8) and preoperative varus angulation more than 30° (odds ratio 6.5). In a prospective randomized study on 225 patients with displaced fractures we found that poor reduction increased the odds ratio for fixation failure 3 times with no difference between two Olmed screws or a sliding screw plate (SSP) with an additional cancellous screw [29]. In the same study there was an increased risk for healing failure in the SSP group when operated outside ordinary working time (odds ratio 6.6); this difference was not found in the Olmed group, probably pointing to larger difficulties with the more demanding SSP system when performed by inexperienced residents on call. In a prospective study on 98 femoral neck fractures fixed by a SSP more complications were found in patients operated on by a "less" compared with a "more" experienced surgeon [30]. The division between less and more experienced was made at 15 procedures undertaken, showing that training is of importance for the final result.

Choice of Implant

Several studies indicate that the choice of osteosynthesis material matters. Two hook pins were superior to a four-flanged nail in displaced femoral neck fractures [31], with reduced blood flow as determined by scintimetry as one possible causative factor [14]. We showed in a consecutive series that three Gouffon nails were inferior to three Mecron screws or two von Bahr screws [27], the probable explanation for the difference being a diameter less than 5 mm of the shaft of the Gouffon screws [32]. The diameter of the shaft should probably be larger than 6 mm, and screws with threads the same diameter as the shaft may reduce damage to the screw canal and thereby increase stability [1]. An alternative to two or more screws or pins are a SSP with one large-diameter screw. The SSP with an additional cancellous screw did, however, show marginally higher rates of fixation failure during the first 3 months compared with two Olmed screws in a randomized study of 225 displaced fractures ($p = 0.07$) [29]. After 3 years of follow-up there was no difference in reoperation rates between the two groups, both showing unacceptable high rates of 37% for the SSP and 29% for the Olmed screws. The differences between implants are probably dependent on the differences in initial stability [1], the additional damage caused to the already weak bone by inserting the device [33], and the damage to the blood supply of the femoral head [14]. The results from the inventors of an implant have usually been very good [34], compared with the results from other institutions [35]. In a meta-analysis of femoral neck fractures Parker

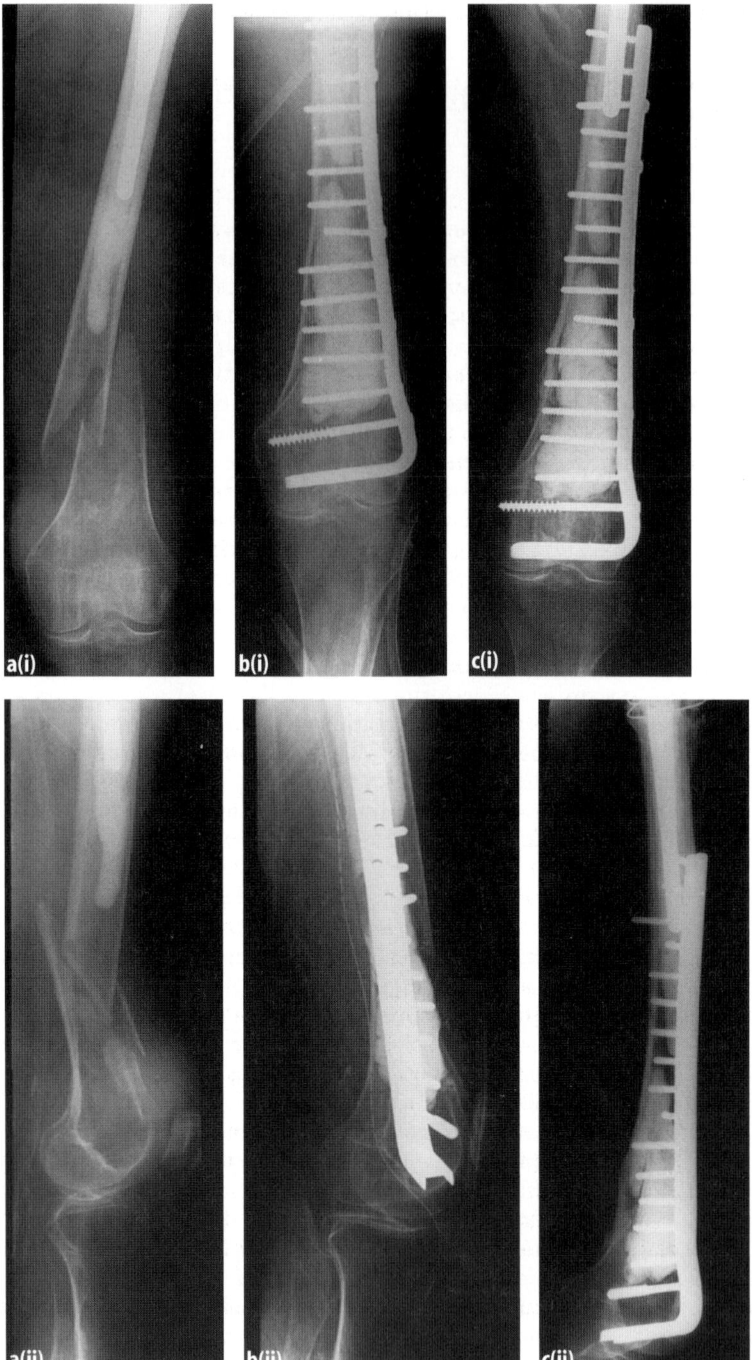

Figure 8.2. **a** Supracondylar femoral fracture in a 64-year-old female alcohol abuser with a long revision prosthesis in the hip after previous pertrochanteric fracture. Note the paper-thin cortical bone with comminution. (i) Anteroposterior; (ii) lateral. **b** Fracture fixed with an AO condylar plate augmented by bone cement. Note the large defect anteriorly on the lateral view. (i) Anteroposterior; (ii) lateral. **c** Uncomplicated fracture healing. After 4 years of follow-up note the cortical healing medially and no screw breakage. (i) Anteroposterior; (ii) lateral.

found screws to be superior to pins, whereas the optimum number of screws or pins could not be determined [36].

In trochanteric fractures a SSP was found to give fewer malunions than Ender nails in a randomized study of more than 200 patients with unstable fractures [37], although all fractures united. The introduction of the intramedullary gamma-nail in the treatment of trochanteric fractures has produced no reduction in healing complications compared with the SSP. Rather, the gamma-nail has consistently given new femoral fractures around the nail, an event rarely seen with the SSP [38]. In a review of all trochanteric fractures (n = 935) in Oslo during 2 years we found a 13-fold increased risk of a new peri-implant femoral fractures in patients treated by the gamma-nail compared with the SSP [39]. The lesson learned from the gamma-nail was already recognized by Schatzker et al. [40] in 1978, namely that: "Failures of fixation are due to failure of bone, usually not failure of the implant, and stronger implants may therefore not be the solution".

In supracondylar femoral fractures intramedullary fixation techniques have also emerged, and biomechanical studies have shown increased fixation strength in vitro compared with angled blade plates [41]. No reports of similar complications as seen with the gamma nail in the upper femur have been published so far.

Augmentation of Osteosynthesis

When bone quality is severely impaired, and a stable fracture fixation is impossible, augmentation of the osteosynthesis is an option (Fig. 8.2). Bone grafting is widely used, for instance in depression fractures of the tibial plateau. In severe osteoporosis, however, the available bone for autotransplantation may be limited, and allograft bone is of inferior value in fracture healing. For the fixation of screws bone cement has been used with success (Fig. 8.2). Uncontrolled studies have shown the beneficial effect of cementing in both supracondylar [42] and intertrochanteric fractures of the femur [40]. Unfortunately, no randomized study has been published to our knowledge. In a retrospective review of 56 intertrochanteric fractures in patients with osteoporosis according to the Singh index, 28 who had been operated on with cement augmentation and were compared with 28 operated on with the same method without augmentation [43]. In stable fractures no difference in outcome was found. In unstable comminuted fractures only 1 of 21 fixations failed when augmented, while 10 of 17 uncemented failed. Recently, augmentation of osteosynthesis by biological cements has been reported in both femoral neck and trochanteric hip fractures [44]. In 52 femoral neck fractures followed for an average of 6 months, 9 fractures had failed, while no failure of fixation was found in 39 trochanteric fractures. Extraosseous augmentation in trochanteric fractures is the addition of a stabilizing plate to the SSP system to reduce medialization of the distal fragment. This trochanteric stabilizing plate reduced the sliding of the screw in unstable trochanteric fractures, but without any impact on the number of reoperations [45].

Post-fracture osteopenia involves both fractured and other ipsilateral bones [46,47]. Karlsson et al. [24]found a bone loss of 29% after 3 months in the fractured femoral neck. This increased bone loss in the already compromised skeleton may jeopardize the fixation. In an experimental tibial fracture model in the rat we have shown that both pre- and post-treatment with the osteoclast inhibitor clodronate prevented the development of the accompanying osteopenia [48].

Whether prevention of post-fracture osteopenia is possible also in humans, and whether this will increase the strength of the fixation, remains to be shown.

References

1. Benterud JG, Alho A, Hoiseth A. Implant/bone constructs in femoral neck osteotomy: an autopsy study. Arch Orthop Trauma Surg 1994;113:97–100.
2. Boden SD, Joyce ME, Oliver B, Heydemann A, Bolander M. Estrogen receptor mRNA expression in callus during fracture healing in the rat. Calcif Tissue Int 1989;45:324–325.
3. Hoyland JA, Mee AP, Baird P, Braidman IP, Mawer EB, Freemont AJ. Demonstration of estrogen receptor mRNA in bone using in situ reverse- transcriptase polymerase chain reaction. Bone 1997;20:87–92.
4. Walsh WR, Sherman P, Howlett CR, Sonnabend DH, Ehrlich MG. Fracture healing in a rat osteopenia model. Clin Orthop 1997;342:218–227.
5. Ljunghall S, Johansson AG, Burman P, Kampe O, Lindh E, Karlsson FA. Low plasma levels of insulin-like growth factor-1 (IGF-1) in male patients with idiopathic osteoporosis. J Intern Med 1992;232:59–64.
6. Kirkeby OJ, Ekeland A. No effects of local somatomedin-C on bone repair: continuous infusion in rats. Acta Orthop Scand 1992;63:447–450.
7. Kawaguchi H, Kurokawa T, Hanada K, Hiyama Y, Tamura M, Ogata E, Matsumoto T. Stimulation of fracture repair by recombinant human basic fibroblast growth factor in normal and streptozotocin-diabetic rats. Endocrinology 1994;135:774–781.
8. Mohan S, Baylink DJ. Bone growth factors. Clin Orthop 1991;263:30–48.
9. Cesnjaj M, Stavljenic A, Vukicevic S. Decreased osteoinductive potential of bone matrix from ovariectomized rats. Acta Orthop Scand 1991;62:471–475.
10. Syftestad GT, Urist MR. Bone aging. Clin Orthop 1982;162:288–297.
11. Bak B, Andreassen TT. The effect of aging on fracture healing in the rat. Calcif Tissue Int 1989;45:292–297.
12. Alho A, Benterud JG, Rønningen H, Høiseth A. Prediction of disturbed healing in femoral neck fracture: radiographic analysis of 149 cases. Acta Orthop Scand 1992;63: 639–644.
13. Parker MJ. Prediction of fracture union after internal fixation of intracapsular femoral neck fractures. Injury 1994;25(Suppl 2):B3–6.
14. Nilsson LT, Johansson A, Strömqvist B. Factors predicting healing complications in femoral neck fractures: 138 patients followed for 2 years. Acta Orthop Scand 1993;64: 175–177.
15. Zichner L. [Therapy of bone and joint changes in renal osteodystrophy in adulthood]. Orthopade 1988;17:440–446.
16. Pollak D, Floman Y, Simkin A, Avinezer A, Freund HR. The effect of protein malnutrition and nutritional support on the mechanical properties of fracture healing in the injured rat. J Parenter Enteral Nutr 1986;10:564–567.
17. Macey LR, Kana SM, Jingushi S, Terek RM, Borretos J, Bolander ME. Defects of early fracture-healing in experimental diabetes. J Bone Joint Surg Am 1989;71:722–733.
18. Tonnesen H, Pedersen A, Jensen MR, Moller A, Madsen JC. Ankle fractures and alcoholism. The influence of alcoholism on morbidity after malleolar fractures. J Bone Joint Surg Am 1991;73:511–513.
19. Nyquist F, Berglund M, Nilsson BE, Obrant KJ. Nature and healing of tibial shaft fractures in alcohol abusers. Alcohol Alcohol 1997;32:91–95.
20. Nyquist F, Halvorsen V, Madsen JE, Nordsletten L, Obrant KJ. Ethanol and its effects on fracture healing and bone mass in male rats. Acta Orthop Scand 1999;70:212–216.
21. Alho A, Benterud JG, Ronningen H, Hoiseth A. Radiographic prediction of early failure in femoral neck fracture. Acta Orthop Scand 1991;62:422–426.

22. Alho A, Benterud JG, Ronningen H, Hoiseth A. Prediction of disturbed healing in femoral neck fracture: radiographic analysis of 149 cases. Acta Orthop Scand 1992;63:639–644.
23. Smith MD, Cody DD, Goldstein SA, Cooperman AM, Matthews LS, Flynn MJ. Proximal femoral bone density and its correlation to fracture load and hip-screw penetration load. Clin Orthop 1992;283:244–251.
24. Karlsson M, Nilsson JA, Sernbo I, Redlund-Johnell I, Johnell O, Obrant KJ. Changes of bone mineral mass and soft tissue composition after hip fracture. Bone 1996;18: 19–22.
25. Arnold WD. The effect of early weight-bearing on the stability of femoral neck fractures treated with Knowles pins. J Bone Joint Surg Am 1984;66:847–852.
26. Elabdien Zain BS, Olerud S, Karlström G. Ender nailing of pertrochanteric fractures: complications related to technical failures and bone quality. Acta Orthop Scand 1985; 56:138–144.
27. Husby T, Alho A, Nordsletten L, Bugge W. Early loss of fixation of femoral neck fractures: comparison of three devices in 244 cases. Acta Orthop Scand 1989;60: 69–72.
28. Hernefalk L, Messner K. In vitro femoral stiffness after femoral neck osteotomy and osteosynthesis with defined surgical errors. J Orthop Trauma 1996;10:416–420.
29. Benterud JG, Husby T, Nordsletten L, Alho A. Fixation of displaced femoral neck fractures with a sliding screw plate and a cancellous screw or two Olmed screws: a prospective, randomized study of 225 elderly patients with a 3-year follow-up. Ann Chir Gynaecol 1997;86:338–342.
30. Laursen JO, Husted H. Complications related to osteosynthesis with AO dynamic hip screws in femoral neck fractures. Orthopaedics 1997;5:319–323.
31. Strömqvist B, Hansson LI, Nilsson LT, Thorngren KG. Two-year follow-up of femoral neck fractures: comparison of osteosynthesis methods. Acta Orthop Scand 1984;55: 521–525.
32. Husby T. Biomechanical properties of the femoral neck relative to osteosynthesis methods and bone mineral content assessed by computed tomography. Thesis, University of Oslo, 1990.
33. Scott WA, Allum RL, Wright KW. Implant-induced trabecular damage in cadaveric femoral necks. Acta Orthop Scand 1985;56:145–146.
34. Strömqvist B, Hansson LI, Palmer J, Ceder L, Thorngren KG. Scintimetric evaluation of nailed femoral neck fractures with special reference to type of osteosynthesis. Acta Orthop Scand 1983;54:340–347.
35. Sernbo I, Johnell O, Baath L, Nilsson JA. Internal fixation of 410 cervical hip fractures: a randomized comparison of a single nail versus two hook-pins. Acta Orthop Scand 1990;61:411–414.
36. Parker MJ, Blundell C. Choice of implant for internal fixation of femoral neck fractures: meta-analysis of 25 randomized trials including 4925 patients. Acta Orthop Scand 1998;69:138–143.
37. Sernbo I, Johnell O, Gentz CF, Nilsson JA. Unstable intertrochanteric fractures of the hip: treatment with Ender pins compared with a compression hip-screw. J Bone Joint Surg Am 1988;70:1297–1303.
38. Aune AK, Ekeland A, Ødegaard B, Grøgaard B, Alho A. Gamma nail vs compression screw for trochanteric femoral fractures: 15 reoperations in a prospective, randomized study of 378 patients. Acta Orthop Scand 1994;65:127–130.
39. Osnes EK, Lofthus CM, Stensvold I, Falch JA, Meyer H, Kristisansen IS, Pike E, Nordsletten L. Bruk av gammanagle og plateskrue ved behandling av pertrochantære brudd i Oslo. In: Hofgaard H, editor. Proceedings of the Norwegian Surgical Society, 1998:150.
40. Schatzker J, Ha'eri GB, Chapman M. Methylmethacrylate as an adjunct in the internal fixation of intertrochanteric fractures of the femur. J Trauma 1978;18:732–735.
41. Strømsøe K, Alho A, Høiseth A. Retention of distal femoral osteotomy fixed with a

AO condylar plate and Grosse-Kempf locked nail in relation to bone mineral in cadavers. Arch Orthop Trauma Surg 1994;113:153–156.
42. Benum P. The use of bone cement as an adjunct to internal fixation of supracondylar fractures of osteoporotic femurs. Acta Orthop Scand 1977;48:52–56.
43. Bartucci EJ, Gonzalez MH, Cooperman DR, Freedberg HI, Barmada R, Laros GS. The effect of adjunctive methylmethacrylate on failures of fixation and function in patients with intertrochanteric fractures and osteoporosis. J Bone Joint Surg Am 1985;67:1094–1107.
44. Goodman SB, Bauer TW, Carter D, Casteleyn PP, Goldstein SA, Kyle RF, et al. SRS cement augmentation in hip fracture treatment: laboratory and initial clinical results. Clin Orthop 1998;348:42–50.
45. Madsen JE, Naess L, Aune AK, Alho A, Ekeland A, Stromsoe K. Dynamic hip screw with trochanteric stabilizing plate in the treatment of unstable proximal femoral fractures: a comparative study with the Gamma nail and compression hip screw. J Orthop Trauma 1998;12:241–248.
46. Obrant KJ. Trabecular bone changes in the greater trochanter after fracture of the femoral neck. Acta Orthop Scand 1984;55:78–82.
47. Madsen JE, Almaas R, Nordsletten L. Strength reduction of the femoral shaft and neck after ipsilateral tibial fracture in the rat. Eur J Exp Musculoskel Res 1995;4:65–68.
48. Madsen JE, Larsen TB, Falch J, Kirkeby OJ, Nordsletten L. No adverse effect of clodronate on fracture healing in rats. Acta Orthop Sacnd 1998;69:532–536.
49. Alho A, Benterud JG, Muller C, Husby T. Prediction of fixation failure in femoral neck fractures: comminution and avascularity studied in 40 patients. Acta Orthop Scand 1993;64:408–410.

9 Perspectives on Growth Factors, Bone Graft Substitutes and Fracture Healing

T. R. Johnson, E. Tomin, and J. M. Lane

Introduction

The decreased bone mass associated with osteoporosis reduces the load-bearing capacity of both cancellous and cortical bone resulting in an increased fracture risk among the affected population. This disease affects over 28 million men and women in the United States [1], which underscores the importance of understanding both the treatment of this common metabolic bone disease and the augmentation of normal fracture healing. Osteoporosis does not impair fracture healing, but diminished bone mass causes a decrease in surface contact between bone surfaces and may result in increased time restoring normal bone strength. The diminished bone mass also reduces the strength and stability between the bone and fixation devices, which can lead to delayed fracture healing and nonunion [2]. Thus, treatment of osteoporotic fractures may benefit from the enhancement and acceleration of the healing process. Other conditions implicated as risk factors for impaired fracture healing, delayed union, and nonunion include infection, distraction, instability, age, obesity, soft tissue trauma and fracture site.

Normal fracture healing is a specialized process in which structural integrity is restored through the regeneration of bone. Both endochondral ossification, the process by which bone is formed from a cartilaginous precursor, and intramembranous ossification, the process by which bone forms under a mesenchymal model, are subject to this unique process. This regeneration is a timely process that requires neoangiogenesis, recruitment of osteoprogenitor cells to the fracture site and induction of these cells to generate new bone [3]. This bone is then remodelled along the lines of stress according to the laws of Wolff. This process is affected by both systemic and local factors; however, local factors have been shown to be more important in autocrine and paracrine fashions for the augmentation of fracture healing [4].

Autogenous cancellous bone graft is considered the gold standard for the treatment of bone deficit. The components required to heal fractures are provided naturally by such a graft. These basic components are osteoinductive growth factors, an osteoconductive hydroxyapatite–collagen matrix and osteogenic stem cells present in bone marrow elements. Despite the effectiveness of autogenous bone graft, availability of the supply is limited to only a few donor sites in the skeletal system. Surgical morbidity, donor site pain, paresthesias, prolonged anesthesia time, infection and increased intraoperative blood loss are associated with autogenous bone graft harvesting (approximating 8–10 %) [5]. As an alternative substitute to autogenous graft, allografts are less desirable because of immunological rejection, potential of disease transmission, infections and biological inferiority.

To overcome these problems with autografts and allografts, investigators have attempted to develop synthetic composite grafts that are intended to simulate the natural course of components required by fracture healing. Developing a comparable bone graft substitute requires all the components provided by autogenous cancellous bone. The relationship between osteoinduction, osteoconduction and osteogenic stem cells are interdependent; each component requires the other two to maximize bone-forming ability. An idealized synthetic bone graft would contain: (1) osteoinductive growth factors, to recruit and stimulate osteoprogenitor stem cells as signalling molecules; (2) primitive osteoprogenitor stem cells with receptors that respond to these signals, by differentiating into osseous forming cells; (3) osteoconductive material to provide a favorable environment for cells and growth factors to function; and (4) structural integrity. Such matrix should be replaced by newly formed bone with full integration into the host bone.

As a limited alternative to cancellous bone graft, cortical bone is able to provide structural support. While both vascular and nonvascular cortical grafts supply graft sites with mechanical support and compressive strength, the contribution of osteoinductive osteoconductive, and osteogenic components is limited compared with cancellous grafts. Less than 5% of the cortical bone cells survive nonvascularized grafting [6].

In addition to the factors mentioned above, autogenous bone grafts are histocompatible, retain viable osteoblasts that participate in the formation of new bone, and do not transfer diseases such as hepatitis and HIV. Autogenous grafting has been used successfully for treating a variety of orthopaedic disorders, including reconstruction and replacement of skeletal defects, augmentation of fracture repair, arthrodesis fortification, and filling of defects created during the treatment of tumors, trauma and arthritis.

Despite proven efficacy, autogenous grafting is associated with several shortcomings and potential complications. The quantity of bone available for harvesting is limited and there is appreciable donor site morbidity. Biologically compatible bone graft substitutes have been developed in an attempt to limit these complications, while utilizing their resources to enhance fracture healing. Alternatives have been used in a wide range of pathological orthopaedic conditions, but no single graft substitute provides all the necessary components of bone regeneration.

Einhorn [7] provides an overview of osteoconduction, osteoinduction, osteogenesis, and methods used to capitalize on these constituents of fracture repair. Osteoconduction supports the ingrowth of capillaries, perivascular tissue and osteoprogenitor cells from the recipient host bed into the structure of either the graft or the graft substitute. Osteoconductive materials include calcium-based ceramic grafts, calcium–collagen composite grafts, bioactive glasses and biodegradable synthetic polymers.

Growth factors, such as transforming growth factor betas (TGF-βs), bone morphogenetic proteins (BMPs), fibroblast growth factors (FGFs), platelet-derived growth factor (PDGF) and insulin-like growth factors (IGFs), are extracted and isolated from bone matrix. These growth factors in combination orchestrate the recruitment, differentiation and mitogenesis of osteoprogenitor stem cells, leading to the formation of osteoblasts with the capacity to produce new bone. Demineralized bone matrix contains limited amount of these growth factors; therefore, it has limited ability to both provide osteoinduction and serve as an osteoconductive matrix.

Currently used osteogenic substances that support the formation of new bone include autogenous bone marrow and mesenchymal stem cells. The value of these methods is related to their ability to bring osteoprogenitor cells to a deficient grafting location.

Systemic approaches to bone regeneration including administering prostaglandins and circulating osteogenic cells have been attempted. Unfortunately, no exogenous systemic agents have been shown to chemically enhance fracture healing in a reproducible fashion.

Allografts

Allografts provide no osteoprogenitor cells and have limited osteoinductive potential, but are useful for structural support and osteoconduction. Nonstructural uses include reconstruction of defects related to removal of bone cysts and benign neoplasms, filling osteolytic cavities during revision of joint arthroplasty, and mixing with autogenous donor tissue to augment osteoinduction and osteogenesis. In terms of structural potential, allografts are used to replace defects during arthroplasty, stabilize arthrodesis and serve as segments during long bone reconstruction. Osteochondral allografts have been used to replace resected bone and provide a biological joint surface [8] (Fig. 9.1).

Bone allografts are available prepared as fresh, frozen and freeze-dried. Fresh grafts require no preservation, but clinical uses are limited to joint resurfacing due to the time required to transfer the graft, which decreases time available for screening of donor disease. Fresh allografts generate an intense immune response [6]. Therefore, frozen and freeze-dried allografts are currently the mainstay of treatment. Freezing the tissue and storing at −60 °C lowers enzymatic degradation and decreases immunogenicity without altering biomechanical properties. Freeze-drying reduces both antigenicity and biochemical changes even further, while allowing for up to 5 years of storage at room temperature. This is due to dehydration and vacuum packing. Unfortunately, the process of freeze-drying damages biomechanical properties, particularly hoop strength. On the other hand, all these techniques largely retain the osteoconductive properties of both cancellous and cortical bone.

Although the osteoconductive properties are retained, these treatment processes destroy osteoprogenitor cells and retain only minor amounts of the deeply bound osteoinductive growth factors. Current regulations have resulted in HIV infection risk at less than 1 per million [9], yet sterilization compromises both the structural and biochemical properties of the donor tissue. Nonunion (10%), fractures (5–15%) and infection (15%) have also been associated with use of allografts [10–13]. When used in unfavorable grafting beds, allografts should be augmented with either autograft or another substitute that provides osteoinductive growth factors and osteoprogenitor cells.

Ceramics

Ceramic products, composed of hydroxyapatite, tricalcium phosphate or a combi-

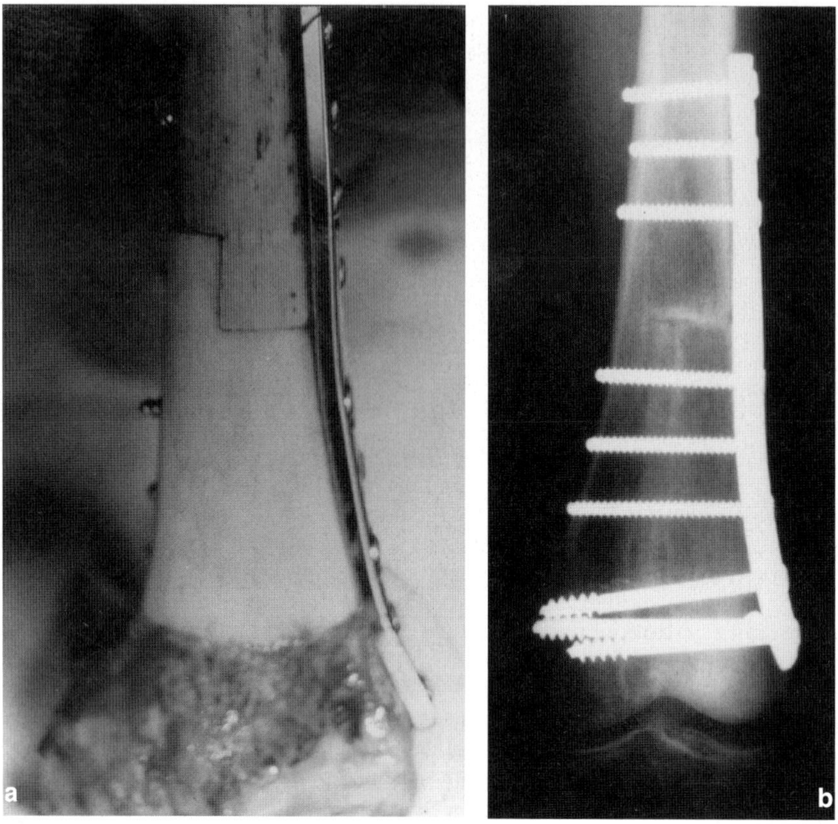

Figure 9.1. **a** Plated allograft. **b** Follow-up on a patient implanted with an allograft. From Gazdag et al. [8].

nation of both, are used solely for the purpose of providing an osteoconductive matrix. Biosynthetic ceramic products are manufactured using high-pressure compaction techniques and high-temperature sintering to produce a variety of porous, nonporous and granular porous particle implants. Unfortunately, these synthetic ceramic products fail to reproduce the interconnected network of pores found in cancellous bone and the ingrowing osteoblasts must resorb ceramic material before gaining access to the internal structure. Another type of ceramic material, replamineform, has interconnected porous networks that resemble those of human cancellous bone (Fig. 9.2). This product is produced from marine coral specimens using a process that replaces coralline calcium carbonate with calcium phosphate.

The mechanical properties of ceramic products are comparable to cancellous bone once they have been incorporated and remodelled. Hence, the shape, architecture and chemical composition of the product affect the utility. Tricalcium phosphate is partially converted to hydroxyapatite in the body and is resorbed at rates 10–20 times faster. It has been shown to remain in the body as segments for periods lasting up to 10 years [14–16]. In clinical applications, tricalcium phosphate remodels more quickly, but provides less compressive strength than hydroxyapatite.

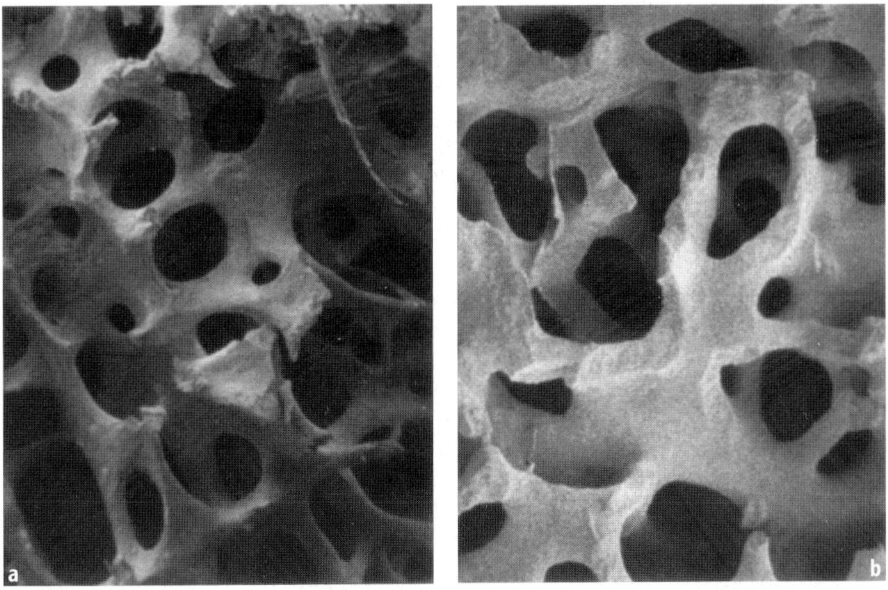

Figure 9.2. **a** Human bone. **b** Scanning electron micrographs of coral hydroxyapatite. Courtesy of Edwin Shore PhD, Interpore-Cross Inc., Irvine, CA.

Collectively, the ceramic products are brittle and lack tensile strength. This property limits their use in applications that require significant torsion, bending or shear stress. They must be shielded from loading forces using rigid stabilization and non-weightbearing until there is evidence of bony ingrowth. Clinically, they may be used as bone graft expanders and filler when combined with autograft or placed near rich bone marrow. Hydroxyapatite has osteoconductive properties that allow these products to bond well to bone. It has been suggested that hydroxyapatite has significant chemical affinity for local growth factors, but these products have no osteoinductive capabilities alone [8].

Despite consistently being found inferior to autogenous bone grafting in animal studies, certain studies with allografts have yielded favorable results. In tibial plateau fractures under compression, Bucholz et al. [17] reported no difference in functional outcome between coralline hydroxyapatite versus cancellous bone (Fig. 9.3). Recently, tricalcium phosphate has been used with corticocancellous bone in spinal fusion for scoliosis, yielding promising results [18]. It has also yielded similar results when used to fill defects due to benign tumors and trauma. In animal studies, bone marrow has been shown to grow well within ceramics and mesenchymal stem cells work best when used with ceramic hydroxyapatite [19,20]. Composites of human bone marrow and ceramics have not been reported to date.

Ceramics appear to have no early adverse effects, such as inflammation. The resorbing cell for hydroxyapatite is the foreign body giant cell and small granules of material have been shown to elicit a foreign body giant cell reaction, although this type of response is practically nonexistent when these products are in a structural block arrangement. The main limitations are due to their brittle nature. Ceramics must be protected by orthopaedic implant fixation or they may shatter.

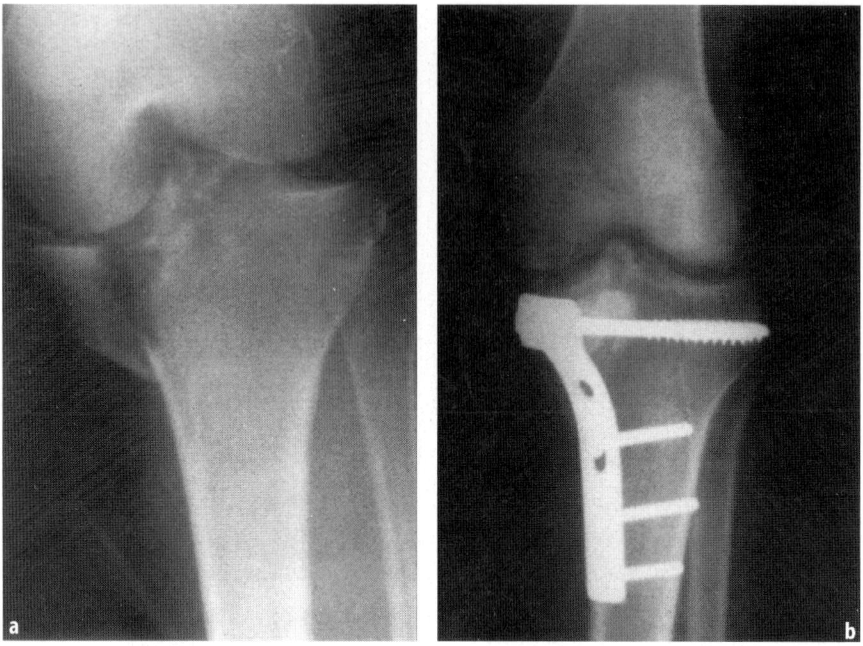

Figure 9.3. a Tibial plateau fracture. **b** The fracture after repair with coral hydroxyapatite. From Bucholz et al. [17].

There is currently an injectable ceramic in clinical trial that was developed for the in situ formation of the mineral phase of bone. When injected into the site of a fracture it creates a firm ceramic mass within hours and achieves most of its compressive strength by 24 h. Animal studies have shown that this material is more easily remodelled in vivo and can be replaced by host bone due to the inclusion of carbonate within the crystals [21]. More recently, initial clinical and laboratory results have shown potential for clinical augmentation of hip and distal radius fractures [22,23].

A calcium sulfate matrix has been reintroduced for grafting of defects. It is rapidly resorbed and may function as a non-osteoconductive filler that physiologically inhibits soft connective tissue proliferation into the defect. As it resorbs, bone forms rapidly in the developing void [24].

Demineralized Bone Matrix

Mild acid extraction of bone removes the mineral phase of bone, leaving collagen, growth factors and non-collagenous proteins. This demineralized bone matrix (DBM) has enhanced osteoinductivity due to retained BMP activity and has been used to promote bone regeneration in well-supported skeletal defects [8]. The available amount of BMP activity in the demineralized grafts is much lower than the amount used in recombinant BMP studies, however. This is due to preparation and sterilization techniques. Some types of DBM are processed using a technique that

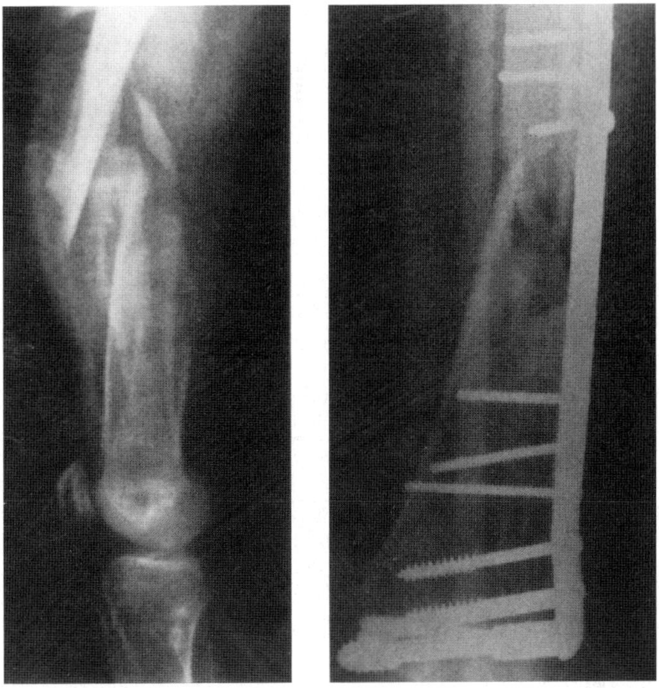

Figure 9.4. Repair of a femoral fracture using demineralized bone matrix (Grafton DBM). Courtesy of N. Scarborough.

does not expose the tissue to the ethylene oxide and gamma radiation, and this method may protect some of the native BMP activity.

Despite maintained osteoinductive potential, demineralized bone matrix has no structural strength. It is available freeze-dried as a powder, crushed granules and chips that have limited osteoconductive potential. DBM has been used to augment autogenous bone grafts while repairing cysts, fractures, nonunions and arthrodesis (Fig. 9.4) [25–27]. It is also available packaged into a syringe as a gel that may be used intraoperatively to augment internal fixation or as an adjunct to other graft substitutes. These products have been used to facilitate the development of bone with mechanical strength comparable to autografts [6,8]. Recent animal studies have indicated, however, that demineralized bone matrix may not be as effective in achieving stable spinal fusions, although successful results have been reported [28–30]. Presently, these freeze dried DBM products are satisfactory carriers of morphogenetic proteins [31].

Growth Factors

Growth factors appear to play many critical roles in the enhancement of fracture healing and future use is promising. Growth promoting substances identified at healing fracture sites include TGF-βs, BMPs, FGFs, IGFs and PDGFs [32]. These substances lead to new bone formation at extraskeletal locations. Although enhancement of tissue growth via exogenous growth factors is logical therapy, regeneration may be potentiated by other factors as well. Research on delivery systems and exogenous application of these molecules is presently under way. Development of a delivery system to release growth factors in a predictable and precise concentration is essential before these molecules can be implanted into patients [33].

TGF-βs are a superfamily of polypeptide growth factors that regulate the proliferation and expression of differentiated phenotypes for many cell populations, including chondrocyte, osteoblast, and osteoclast precursors. This superfamily consists of TGF-β_1, TGF-β_2, TGF-β_3, TGF-β_4, TGF-β_5, and other molecules, including BMPs and growth differentiation factors (GDFs). The extracellular matrix of bone is the largest source of TGF-β in the body [34]. Studies by Joyce et al. [35,36] have shown that TGF-β is synthesized by chondrocytes and osteoblasts during endochondral ossification and is initially released by platelets into the fracture hematoma. It seems to stimulate intramembranous bone formation by stimulating osteoblastic proliferation and activity. TGF-β also appears to regulate the proliferation of chondrocytes and synthesis of a cartilaginous matrix, depending on precursor cell maturity and differentiation stage [4]. Crichlow et al. [37] evaluated the effect of this molecule in rabbit fractures. Exogenous growth factor was injected into the developing callus of rat tibial fractures healing under both stable and unstable mechanical conditions. Large doses resulted in increased callus size of the stable fractures; however, in unstable fractures, callus bone and cartilage formation was retarded. These authors concluded that TGF-β does not stimulate callus formation during the initial phase of fracture healing. In addition, growth factors that stimulate cell proliferation in the callus may act to hinder bone remodelling.

PDGF has been shown to affect bone and cartilage cells in normally healing human fractures; however, its role in fracture healing is presently unclear [38]. Using immunohistochemistry, PDGF has been detected in various cell types during fracture repair and assumed to play an important role in fracture healing. In a rabbit tibial osteotomy model, a single injection of PDGF increased callus density, volume and possibly osteogenesis, yet mechanical testing showed no improvement in strength [39]. According to Einhorn and Trippel [32] the therapeutic potential of PDGF will be noticed in the presence of other growth factors.

FGF and IGF have also been demonstrated to participate in bone formation and fracture repair. IGF factor may also participate in endochondral fracture repair. Studies suggest IGF-I accelerates the repair of intramembranous bone defects [40]. IGF-II may also play a similar role in fracture repair. More studies are necessary before possible therapeutic potential may be realized [32]. IGF, PDGF and FGF are well-studied mitogenic factors that are produced in early phases of fracture repair and localized in the bone matrix [41]. Acidic and basic FGF (aFGF and bFGF) have been shown to both induce and inhibit bone repair, depending on the applied dose [42]. Basic FGF increases mitogenesis for fibroblasts [43], osteoblasts [44], and chondrocytes [45] and also stimulates angiogenesis and endothelial cell migration in a dose-dependent manner [46]. However, in vitro studies demonstrated that it reduces the synthesis of type I collagen and decreases alkaline phosphatase activity and mineralization [47]. Immunohistochemical analysis of the fractures demonstrated that bFGF was widely distributed in the soft callus and periosteum during the early stage of fracture repair. Daily injections of bFGF caused marked stimulation of endosteal bone formation in both cortical and secondary cancellous bone areas [44]. Another study indicated that bFGF increased the distribution of TGF-β in the endosteal cells [48]. Consequently, TGF-β may at least in part mediate the effects

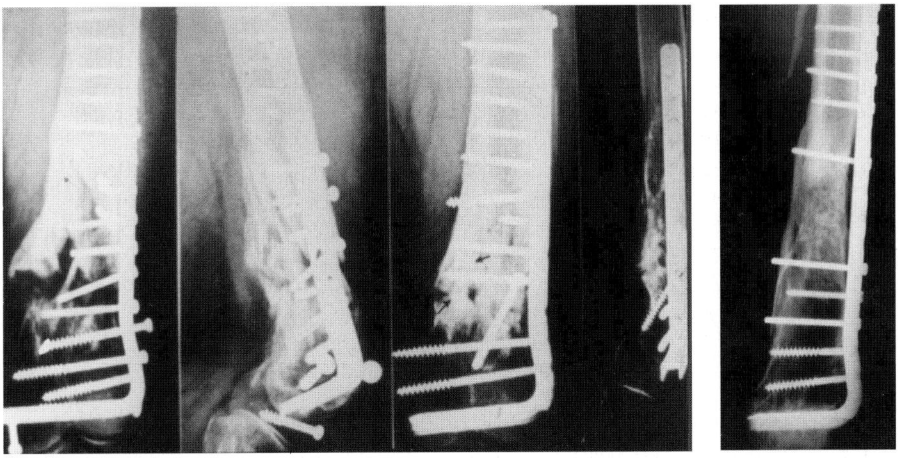

a b

Figure 9.5a,b. Repair of a nonunion using human bone morphogenetic protein (hBMP) extractions combined with cancellous bone graft. From Johnson et al. [55].

of bFGF. This is further supported by an in vitro study, which reported that the stimulation of osteoblastic cells by bFGF increased mRNA expression of TGF-β [49].

Perhaps most promising are the low-molecular-weightBMPs, with functions ranging from multitissue organogenesis to bone formation and regeneration [50]. More than 24 BMP peptides have been described [31] and some appear to have bone morphogenetic activity previously described by Urist [51]. The characterization, localization and chronology of BMP-2 and BMP-4 have been identified in both types of fracture healing by using immunolocalization techniques [52]. The presence of BMP-2 and -4 was dynamically altered during the fracture repair process, which suggests these molecules are important regulators in fracture repair. Additional supporting evidence for the critical role of BMPs as signalling molecules comes from in vitro studies. Wang et al. [53] demonstrated that BMP-2 causes commitment and differentiation of multipotential stem cell line into osteoblast-like cells.

A native preparation of human bone extract containing numerous growth factors (hBMP) has been used successfully for treating established nonunions and spine fusions, resulting in success rates of 93% and 100%, respectively [54–56] (Fig. 9.5) More recently, recombinant human BMPs (rhBMP-2 and rhBMP-7 [osteogenic protein 1, OP-1]) have become available in large amounts and shown to heal fractures and defects in various animal models. For example, in rats, implantation of rhBMP-2 has been shown to consummate de novo chondrogenesis and osteogenesis. (Fig. 9.6) BMP-4, -6, -7 and, to a lesser extent BMP-5, have also been shown to induce new bone formation [57]. Lane et al. [58] have shown that both rhBMP-2 alone and in composite with autogenous bone marrow is superior to either syngeneic bone graft or bone marrow in healing rat femoral defects. Similar results have been reported in other animal and primate models [59–65].

As osteoporotic patients are predisposed to vertebral body fractures, rhBMPs will eventually be used to improve spinal arthrodesis performance. It is estimated that more than 180 000 spine fusions were performed in the United States in 1983. There

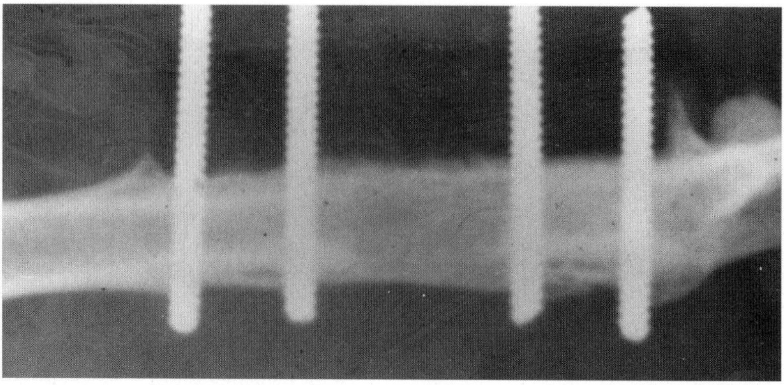

Figure 9.6. Repair of critical segmental bone defect in rat femur using recombinant human bone morphogenetic protein-2 (rhBMP 2). From Yasko et al. [60].

is now adequate evidence in animal models that both rhBMP-2 and -7 are superior to autogenous grafts in achieving spine fusions in animals [61,66–72]. In these models, rhBMP-2 and -7 used with various carrier systems have been superior to autogenous iliac crest bone for inducing transverse process arthrodesis.

Currently, none of the recombinant growth factors are approved by the United States Food and Drug Administration for clinical use; however, the clot associated with bone marrow and the noncollagenous mixture in demineralized bone matrix do contain small amounts of biologically active factors. Comprehensive clinical studies are currently under way to demonstrate efficacy of these factors in augmenting the healing process. Evaluation of these molecules must include side effects, toxicity, immunogenicity and efficacy of the delivery systems used.

Bone Marrow

Autogenous bone marrow contains osteoprogenitor cells and has been used alone and in combination with inorganic matrix to promote osteogenesis [73–75]. Presently, autogenous bone marrow offers the ability to augment both synthetic graft materials and allografts. In addition, it may be used to establish normal fracture hematomas following surgical irrigation. Although clinical applications are currently limited, animal models offer promising results. Marrow is advantageous because there is essentially no morbidity associated with harvesting.

Bone marrow has been grown in porous ceramic and used to bring osteoprogenitor cells to deficient grafting beds [19]. Using a rat model of femoral segmental defects, bone marrow produced rates of union comparable to those of autogenous cancellous bone [76]. This marrow-augmented bone demonstrated biomechanical properties similar to that produced by cancellous grafting. Autogenous bone marrow has been shown to be synergistic when used in combination with recombinant human BMP-2 [58]. Therefore, it is hypothesized that bone marrow osteoprogenitor stem cells have BMP receptors.

Clinically, when administered in sufficient quantities, bone marrow has been used to treat patients with nonunions [77–79] (Fig 9.7). It should be harvested in aliquots of approximately 2.5 ml per site and used immediately to maintain viability.

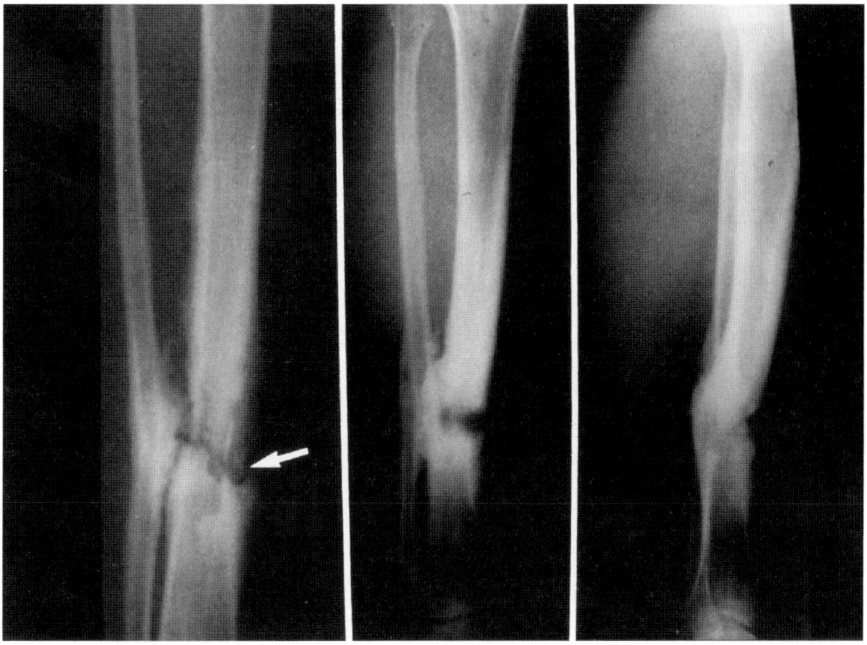

Figure 9.7. Autologous bone marrow injections as a substitute for tibial nonunions. From Connolly et al. [78].

Although marrow contains osteoprogenitor cells in concentrations ranging from 1/50 000 to 1/2 million nucleated cells, depending on the age of the patient, techniques exist to increase these numbers up to 5-fold [80]. Mesenchymal stem cells have been expanded by growing marrow in culture and used to heal osseous defects in combination with ceramics and collagen mixtures [20]. Use of these expanded stem cell populations for osteogenesis offers many future possibilities.

Composite Grafts

Composite grafts, i.e., any combination of materials that includes both an osteoconductive matrix with either osteogenic cells or osteoinductive growth factors, attempt to incorporate the favorable properties of the different materials, as no single substitute can provide all the components provided by autogenous bone graft. They are currently used in craniofacial reconstruction and appear to be useful as bone graft expanders or graft substitutes in stabilized fractures.

Collagraft is a composite of suspended, deantigenated, bovine fibrillar collagen and porous calcium phosphate ceramic (65% hydroxyapatite and 35% tricalcium phosphate) that is non-osteoinductive. This composite graft has been combined with autogenous bone marrow to provide osteoprogenitor cells and limited amounts of growth factors to produce results comparable to cancellous iliac bone grafts in acute long bone fractures [81] (Fig. 9.8). For traumatic defects, this composite reduces surgical complications and morbidity by decreasing the duration of surgery [82]. It is currently available in soft strips or paste form, which limits its use due

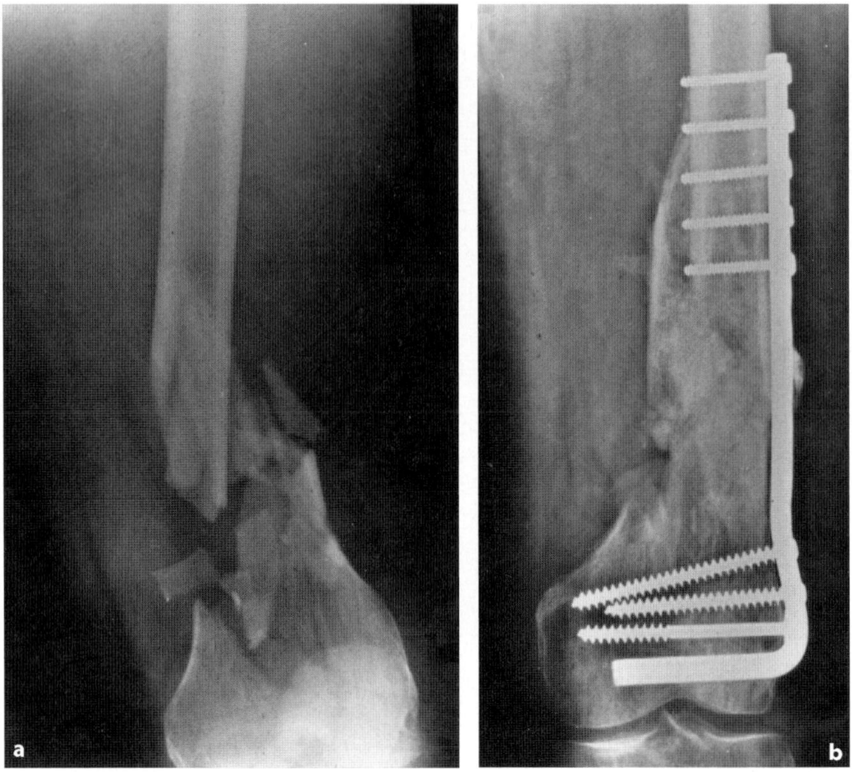

Figure 9.8a,b. Collagraft repair in a femoral fracture. From Cornell et al. [81].

to lack of structural integrity and a tendency for granules to migrate to ectopic sites in the absence of adequate hemostasis. For these reasons, the use of Collagraft is contraindicated for intra-articular fractures.

Animal studies have evaluated other composite graft substitutes. Recombinant human BMP-2 in combination with TGF-β in ceramic bovine bone has produced favorable results in mice[83]. Sciandini et al. [84] evaluated a composite of bovine-derived bone protein and natural calcium carbonate coral reconstituted with bovine collagen as a graft substitute in dogs. These authors concluded that the combination of bovine derived bone protein and a coralline carrier performed better than autogenous graft at delivering osteoinductive factors to defect sites [84]. Commercially available demineralized bone matrix has also demonstrated a capacity to serve as a carrier for recombinant human BMP [85]. This product potentially contains limited amounts of several BMPs as well as other mitogenic and angiogenic factors necessary for fracture healing. Such composites may have clinical implications in the future.

Summary

Bone regeneration is usually successful in fracture repair given a favorable host, appropriate fracture bed and osseous stability. When needed, augmentation is currently available for recalcitrant repair through autogenous bone grafting. New forms of biocompatible graft substitutes, including bone marrow cells, osteoconductive matrices and osteoinductive growth factors, can not only achieve results comparable to autogenous bone graft without morbidity, but also offer the promise of surpassing the well-established "gold standard".

References

1. Brunelli MP, Einhorn TA. Medical management of osteoporosis. Clin Orthop 1998; 348:15–21.
2. Buckwalter JA, Einhorn TA, Bolander ME, Cruess RL. Healing of the musculoskeletal tissues. In Rockwood, CA, Green DP, Bucholz RW, Heckman JD, editors. Rockwood and Green's fractures in adults, 4th ed. Philadelphia: Lippincott-Raven, 1996: 261–304.
3. Brighton CT. Principles of fracture healing. AAOS Instr Course Lect 1984;33:60.
4. Cornell CN, Lane JM. Newest factors in fracture healing. Clin Orthop 1992;277:297–310.
5. Younger EM, Chapman MW. Morbidity at bone graft donor sites. J Orthop Trauma 1989;3:192–195.
6. Lane JM, Bostrom MP. Bone grafting and new composite biosynthetic graft materials. AAOS Instr Course Lect 1998;47:525–534.
7. Einhorn TA. Current concepts review: enhancement of fracture healing. J Bone Joint Surg Am 1995;77:940–956.
8. Gazdag AR, Lane JM, Glaser D, Forster RA. Alternatives to autogenous bone graft: efficacy and indications. J Am Acad Orthop Surg 1995;3:1–8.
9. Buck BE, Malinin TI, Brown MD. Bone transplantation and human immunodeficiency virus: An estimate of risk of immunodeficiency syndrome (AIDS). Clin Orthop 1989; 240:129–136.
10. Berrey BH Jr, Lord CF, Gebhardt MC, et al. Fractures of allografts: frequency, treatment, and end results. J Bone Joint Surg Am 1990;72:825–833.
11. Tomford WW, Thongphasuk J, Mankin HJ, et al. Frozen musculoskeletal allografts: a study of the clinical incidence and causes of infection associated with their use. J Bone Joint Surg Am 1990;72:1137–1143.
12. Mankin HJ, Springfield DS, Gebhardt MC, et al. Current status of allografting for bone tumors. Orthopedics 1992;15:1147–1154.
13. Flynn JM, Springfield DS, Mankin HJ. Osteoarticular allografts to treat distal femoral osteonecrosis. Clin Orthop 1994;303:38–43.
14. Jarcho M. Calcium phosphate ceramics as hard tissue prosthetics. Clin Orthop 1981;157: 259–278.
15. Bucholz RW, Carlton A, Holmes RE. Hydroxyapatite and tricalcium phosphate bone graft substitutes. Orthop Clin North Am 1987;18:323–334.
16. Altermatt S, Schwobel M, Pochon JP. Operative treatment of solitary bone cysts with tricalcium phosphate ceramic: a 1 to 7 year follow up. Eur J Pediatr Surg 1992;2:180–182.
17. Bucholz RW, Carlton A, Holmes RE. Interporous hydroxyapatite as a bone graft substitute in tibial plateau fractures. Clin Orthop 1989;240:53–62.
18. Le Huec JC, Lesprit E, Delavigne C, et al. Tri-calcium phosphate ceramics and allografts as bone substitutes for spinal fusion in idiopathic scoliosis: comparative clinical results at four years. Acta Orthop Belg 1997;63:202–211.

19. Nakahara H, Goldberg VM, Caplan AI, et al. Culture expanded periosteal-derived cells exhibit osteochondrogenic potential in porous calcium phosphate ceramics in vivo. Clin Orthop 1992;276:291–298.
20. Bruder SP, Fink DJ, Caplan AI. Mesenchymal stem cells in bone development, bone repair, and skeletal regeneration therapy. J Cell Biochem 1994;56:283–294.
21. Constantz BR, Ison IC, Fulmer MT, et al. Skeletal repair by in situ formation of the mineral phase of bone. Science 1995;267:1797–1799.
22. Goodman SB, Bauer TW, Carter D, et al. Norian SRS cement augmentation in hip fracture treatment: laboratory and clinical results. Clin Orthop 1998;348:42–50.
23. Jupiter JB, Winters S, Sigman S, et al. Repair of five distal radius fractures with an investigational cancellous bone cement: a preliminary report. J Orthop Trauma 1997;11:110–116.
24. Pecora G, Andreana S, Magarone JE III, et al. Bone regeneration with a calcium sulfate barrier. Oral Surg Oral Med Oral Pathol Oral Radiol Endod 1997;84:424–429.
25. Killian JT, Wilkinson L, White S, Brassard M. Treatment of unicameral bone cyst with demineralized bone matrix. J Pediatr Orthop 1998;18:621–624,
26. Tiedeman JJ, Garvin KL, Kile TA, Connolly JF. The role of composite, demineralized bone marrow in the treatment of osseous defects. Orthopedics 1995;18:1153–1158.
27. Michelson JD, Curl LA. Use of demineralized bone matrix in hindfoot arthrodesis. Clin Orthop 1996;325:203–208.
28. Cook SD, Dalton JE, Prewet AB,: Whitecloud TS III. In vivo evaluation of demineralized bone matrix as a bone graft substitute for posterior spinal fusion. Spine 1995;20: 877–886,
29. Helm GA, Sheehan JM, Sheehan JP, et al. Utilization of type I collagen gel, demineralized bone matrix, and bone morphogenetic protein-2 to enhance autologous bone lumbar spinal fusion. J Neurosurg 1997;86:93–100.
30. Marone MA, Boden SD. Experimental posterolateral lumbar spinal fusion with a demineralized bone matrix gel. Spine 1998;23:159–167.
31. Reddi AH. Role of morphogenetic proteins in skeletal tissue engineering and regeneration. Nat Biotech 1998;16:247–252.
32. Einhorn TA, Trippel SB. Growth factor treatment of fractures. AAOS Instr Course Lect 1997;46:483–486.
33. Urist MR. Experimental delivery systems for bone morphogenetic protein. In: Wise DL, Altobelli DE, Schwartz ER, Gresser JD, Trantolo DJ, Yaszemski M, editors. Handbook of biomaterials and applications. Boston: Marcel Dekker, 1995:1093–1133.
34. Centrella M, McCarthy TL, Canalis E. Transforming growth factor-beta and remodeling of bone. J Bone Joint Surg Am 1991;73: 1418–1428.
35. Joyce ME, Roberts AB, Sporn MB, et al. Transforming growth factor-beta and the initiation of chondrogenesis and osteogenesis in the rat femur. Cell Biol 1990;110: 2195–2207.
36. Joyce ME, Jingushi S, Bolander ME. Transforming growth factor-beta in the regulation of fracture repair. Orthop Clin North Am 1990;21:199–209.
37. Crichlow MA, Bland YS, Ashhurst DE. The effect of exogenous transforming growth factor-beta 2 on healing fractures in the rabbit. Bone 1995;16:521–527.
38. Andrew JG, Hoyland JA, Freemont AJ, et al. Platelet derived growth factor expression in normally healing human fractures. Bone 1995;16:455–460.
39. Nash TJ, Howlett CR, Martin C, et al. Effect of platelet derived growth factor on tibial osteotomies in rabbits. Bone 1994;15:203–208.
40. Canalis E, McCarthy T, Centrella M. Growth factors and regulation of bone remodeling. J Clin Invest 1988;81:277–281.
41. Hauschka PV, Mavrakos AE, Iafrati MD, et al. Growth factors in bone matrix. J Biol Chem 1986;261:12665–12674.
42. Wang JS. Basic fibroblast growth factor for stimulation of bone formation in osteoconductive and osteoinductive implants. Acta Orthop Scand 1996;67(Suppl):269.

43. Gospodarowicz D, Moran JS. Mitogenic effect of fibroblast growth on early passage cultures of human and murine fibroblasts. J Biol Chem 1975;66:451–457.
44. Nagai H, Tsukuda R, Mayahara H. Effects of basic fibroblast growth factor (bFGF) on bone formation in growing rats. Bone 1995;16:367–373.
45. Wang JS, Aspenberg P. Basic fibroblast growth factor and bone induction in rats. Acta Orthop Scand 1993;64:557–561.
46. Ingber DE, Folkman J. Mechanochemical switching between growth and differentiation during fibroblast growth factor-stimulated angiogenesis in vitro: role of extracellular matrix. J Cell Biol 1989;109:317–330.
47. Hurley MM, Abreu C, Harrison JR, et al. Basic fibroblast growth factor inhibits Type I collagen gene expression in osteoblastic MC 3T3-E1 cells. J Biol Chem 1993;268: 5588–5593.
48. Nakamura T, Hanada K, Tamura M, et al. Stimulation of endosteal bone formation by systemic injections of recombinant basic fibroblast growth factor in rats. Endocrinology 1995;136:1276–1284.
49. Noda M, Vogel RM. Fibroblast growth factor enhances type β1 transforming growth factor gene expression in osteoblast-like cells. J Cell Biol 1989;109:2529–2535.
50. Wozney JM. The bone morphogenetic protein family and osteogenesis. Mol Reprod Dev 1992;32:160–167.
51. Urist MR. Bone: Formation by autoinduction. Science 1965;150:893.
52. Bostrom MP, Lane JM, Berberian WS, et al. Immunolocalization and expression of bone morphogenetic proteins 2 and 4 in fracture healing. J Orthop Res 1995;13:357–367.
53. Wang EA, Israel DI, Kelly S, Luxenberg DP. Bone morphogenetic protein-2 causes commitment and differentiation in C3H10T1/2 and 3T3 cells. Growth Factors 1993; 9:57–71.
54. Johnson EE, Urist MR, Finerman GA. Repair of segmental defects of the tibia with cancellous bone grafts augmented with human bone morphogenetic protein: a preliminary report. Clin Orthop 1988;236:249–257.
55. Johnson EE, Urist MR, Finerman GA. Bone morphogenetic protein augmentation grafting of resistant femoral nonunions: a preliminary report. Clin Orthop 1988;230: 257–265.
56. Johnson EE, Urist MR, Finerman GA. Resistant nonunions and partial or complete segmental defects of long bones: treatment with implants of a composite of human bone morphogenetic protein (BMP) and autolyzed, antigen-extracted, allogenic (AAA) bone. Clin Orthop 1992;277:229–237.
57. Wozney JM, Rosen V. Bone morphogenetic protein and bone morphogenic protein gene family in bone formation and repair. Clin Orthop 1998;346:26–37.
58. Lane JM, Yasko AW, Tomin E, et al. Bone marrow and recombinant human bone morphogenetic protein 2 in osseous repair. Clin Orthop, 1999;361:216–27.
59. Bostrom MP, Lane JM, Tomin E, et al. Use of bone morphogenetic protein in the rabbit ulnar nonunion model. Clin Orthop 1996;327:272–82.
60. Yasko AW, Lane JM, Fellinger EJ, et al. The healing of segmental bone defects, induced by recombinant human bone morphogenetic protein (rhBMP-2): A radiographic, histological, and biomechanical study in rats. J Bone Joint Surg Am 1992;74:659–670.
61. Cook SD, Baffes GC, Wolfe MW, et al. The effect of recombinant human bone morphogenetic protein-1 on healing large segmental bone defects. J Bone Joint Surg 1994;76A: 827–838.
62. Cook SD, Wolfe MW, Salked SL, et al. Effect of recombinant human osteogenic protein-1 on healing of segmental defects in non-human primates. J Bone Joint Surg Am 1995;77:734–750.
63. Cook SD, Baffes GC, Wolfe MW, et al. Recombinant human bone morphogenetic protein-7 induces healing in a canine long-bone segmental defect. Clin Orthop 1994;301: 302–312.

64. Sciandini MF, Dawson JM, Berman LM, Johnson KD. Dose-response characteristics of recombinant human bone morphogenetic protein-2 (rhBMP-2) in a canine segmental defect model. Trans Orthop Res Soc 1996;41:284.
65. Zdeblick TA, Ghanayem AJ, Rapoff AJ, et al. Cervical interbody fusion cages: an animal model with and without bone morphogenetic protein. Spine 1998;23:758–765.
66. Cook SD, Dalton JE, Tan EH, et al. In vivo evaluation of recombinant human osteogenic protein (rhOP-1) implants as bone graft substitute for spinal fusions. Spine 1994;19: 1655–1663.
67. Sandhu , Kanim LE, Kabo JM, et al. Evaluation of rhBMP-2 with an OPLA carrier in canine posterolateral (transverse process) spinal fusion model. Spine 1995;20: 2669–2682.
68. Sandhu HS, Kanim LE, Kabo JM, et al. Effective doses of recombinant human bone morphogenetic protein-2 in experimental spinal fusion. Spine 1996;21:2115–2122.
69. Boden SD, Schimandle JH, Hutton WC, et al. The use of an osteoinductive growth factor for lumbar spinal fusion. I. Biology of spinal fusion. Spine 1995;20:2626–2632.
70. Boden SD, Schimandle JH, Hutton WC, et al. The use of an osteoinductive growth factor for lumbar spinal fusion. II. Study of dose, carrier, and species. Spine 1995;20: 2633–2644.
71. Muschler GF, Hyodo A, Manning T, et al. Evaluation of human bone morphogenetic protein 2 in a canine spinal fusion model. Clin Orthop 1994;308:229–240.
72. Fischgrund JS, James SB, Chabot MC, et al. Augmentation of autograft using rhBMP-2 and different carrier media in the canine spinal fusion model. J Spinal Disord 1997;10:167–172.
73. Burwell RG. The function of bone marrow in the incorporation of a bone graft. Clin Orthop 1985;200:125–141.
74. Salama R, Weissman SL. The clinical use of combined xenografts of bone an autologous red marrow: a preliminary report. J Bone Joint Surg Br 1978;60:111–115.
75. Burwell RG, Friedlaender GE, Mankin HJ. Current perspectives and future directions: the 1983 invitational conference on osteochondral allografts. Clin Orthop 1985;197: 141–157.
76. Werntz J, Lane J, Piez K, et al. The repair of segmental defects with collagen and morrow. Orthop Trans 1986;10:262–263.
77. Connolly J, Guse R, Lippiello L, et al. Development of an osteogenic bone marrow preparation. J Bone Joint Surg Am 1989;71:684–691.
78. Connolly JF, Guse R, Tiedeman J, et al. Autologous marrow injection as a substitute for grafting of tibial nonunions. Clin Orthop 1991;266:259–270.
79. Healey JH, Zimmerman PA, McDonnell JM, Lane JM: Percutaneous bone marrow grafting of delayed union and nonunion in cancer patients. Clin Orthop 1990;256:280–285.
80. Morrison SJ, Wandycz AM, Akashi K, et al. The aging of hematopoietic stem cells. Nat Med 1996;2:1011–1016.
81. Cornell CN, Lane JM, Chapman M, et al. Multicenter trial of Collagraft as bone graft substitute. J Orthop Trauma 1991;5:1–8.
82. Chapman MW, Bucholz R, Cornell C. Treatment of acute fractures with a collagen-calcium phosphate graft material. J Bone Joint Surg Am 1997;79:495–502.
83. Si X, Jin Y, Yang L. Induction of new bone by ceramic bovine bone with recombinant human bone morphogenetic protein 2 and transforming growth factor beta.. Int J Oral Maxillofac Surg 1998;27:310–314.
84. Sciandini MF, Dawson JM, Johnson KD: Evaluation of bovine derived bone protein with a natural coral carrier as a bone-graft substitute in a canine segmental defect model. J Orthop Res 1997;15:844–857.
85. Niederwanger M, Urist MR. Demineralized bone matrix supplied by bone banks for a carrier of recombinant human bone morphogenetic protein (rhBMP-2): a substitute for autogeneic bone grafts. J Oral Implantol 1996;22:210–215.

Part III

Orthopaedic Management Options

10 Displaced Intracapsular Fractures

G. A. Pryor

Introduction

Low bone density generally [1], and proximal femoral bone density in particular [2], are strong risk factors for intracapsular fractures. In practice the majority of patients suffering this type of fracture are markedly osteoporotic and usually elderly. However, while low bone density is important in the etiology of this fracture, it is only one factor and usually acts in combination with a minor fall. Typically the patient will lose balance and fall the impact being close to the hip. The weakened osteoporotic bone is unable to absorb the residual energy of the impact and a fracture results.

The intracapsular fracture may also occur when a torsional strain is applied to a loaded femur. The axially loaded femur breaks at its weakest point, i.e., where it is most horizontal: the neck. Intracapsular fractures displace as the femoral head rolls off the back of the neck. This displacement force has two separate effects. First, there is disruption of the ascending cervical vessels carrying the main blood supply to the femoral neck. Second, comminution of the posterior aspect of the femoral neck occurs.

The variable degree of disruption to the blood supply of the femoral head may impair head viability. The comminution of the posterior aspect of the femoral neck combined with the osteoporotic nature of the bone will limit the chances of successful reduction and fixation of the fracture. Together these effects serve to reduce the long-term success of the treatment of this injury.

Management

With very few exceptions the displaced intracapsular fracture should be treated operatively. Even the demented, immobile patient should benefit from surgery, if only to relieve pain and make nursing easier. If the fracture is treated nonoperatively then nonunion will be inevitable. Although the pain may ease, the immobility will be permanent and thus conservative treatment is only appropriate if life expectancy is very short.

For operative treatment the choice is between preservation of the femoral head and its replacement by some form of arthroplasty. Both these options have benefits and drawbacks. The displaced intracapsular fracture is often still referred to as the unsolved fracture because neither of the two options has been clearly shown to be the better.

Reduction and fixation, while a less traumatic procedure, has a higher chance of re-operation. In a meta-analysis of 106 published reports [3] between 20% and 36% of patients required a second operation after reduction and fixation, compared with between 6% and 18% after hemiarthroplasty. Replacement arthroplasty means sacrificing viable femoral heads, but gives a more certain chance of a reasonable outcome.

In the younger patient, the femoral head should undoubtedly be preserved at all costs. However, it is the elderly osteoporotic patient who is most likely to sustain this fracture. For these patients femoral head preservation is certainly not a necessity and primary arthroplasty may allow the low-demand, elderly patient to mobilize sufficiently to resume their pre-injury level of mobility and independence.

Rather than labelling the fracture unsolved, perhaps a more logical approach is to consider reduction and fixation to be the most appropriate treatment, except in certain circumstances:

Indications for Primary Arthroplasty

Absolute indications:

- Abnormal joint – rheumatoid or osteoarthritis.
- Abnormal bone – Paget's disease of bone; metabolic bone disease – chronic renal failure, hyperthyroidism; pathological fracture.

Relative indications:

- Delayed presentation.
- The very elderly (although physiological age is more important than chronological, the risk of nonunion does increase with age [4]).

Reduction and Fixation of the Displaced Intracapsular Fracture

For reduction and fixation of the fracture, the following factors must considered:
Pre-operative care. Excessive movement of the limb should be avoided as this may further damage circulation to the femoral head. The use of preoperative traction has not been shown to be of value.
Timing of surgery. There is limited evidence to support the view that these fractures should be treated as emergencies and reduced and fixed within 6–8 h of injury. However, some studies suggest the incidence of nonunion and other healing complications increases the longer fixation is delayed [5,6], although this is not a universal finding. In the younger patient there is some evidence to support the view that the fracture should be reduced and fixed within 8 h [7].

In general, for the elderly osteoporotic patient the operative management of this fracture should be considered urgent but not an emergency and hence should be performed within 24 h, preferably on a planned daytime list – a Confidential Enquiry into Peri-operative Deaths [CEPOD] recommendation. After 2 days from injury there is a progressive increase in the risk of nonunion. By 1 week closed reduction becomes very difficult and nonunion is almost inevitable. Arthroplasty would then certainly be appropriate for the elderly osteoporotic patient.

Aspiration of the Hip Joint

Aspiration of the hip joint as soon as possible after injury has been advocated, in order to reduce intracapsular pressure and aid blood flow to the femoral head [8]. However, preoperative aspiration is probably of little value in the displaced fracture in the elderly. The displacement of the fracture is likely to have already torn the capsule, relieving the tamponade effect. Moreover, intracapsular pressure does spontaneously reduce with time and the avoidance of traction also limits intracapsular pressures [9]. Tearing or kinking of the ascending cervical vessels is probably a more potent cause of reduced blood flow.

Aspiration of the hip at the time of closed reduction and fixation is more likely to be helpful, if only to reduce postoperative pain. This can easily be performed by insertion of a needle under X-ray control once the fracture is reduced, prior to fixation.

Reduction of the Fracture

The intracapsular fracture should be internally fixed in an anatomical position if at all possible. However the presence of posterior neck comminution, variously reported in between 50% and 90% of fractures [10,11], may result in re-angulation posteriorly. Methods advocated to avoid this problem have included reduction into valgus, open reduction and bone grafting or resorting to arthroplasty. In the elderly osteoporotic patient, however, there would rarely be an indication to consider open reduction.

The quality of reduction is probably the most significant factor in determining a successful outcome. A satisfactory reduction can usually be obtained by the surgeon carefully positioning the patient on the fracture table and performing a gentle manipulation of the leg. Under X-ray control gentle traction is applied until the fracture ends are aligned on the anteroposterior view. The leg is then internally rotated to correct the angulation of the neck. A more forceful manipulation, as in the original techniques described by Leadbetter and Flynn, is rarely required and likely to damage the impaired circulation further.

The accuracy of the reduction can be judged by the Garden alignment index [12]. On the anteroposterior X ray this is a measure of the angle between the trabeculae of the femoral head and the axis of the femoral shaft. The normal angle is 160° and after fracture reduction it should be between 160° and 180°. An angle greater than 180° indicates an excessively valgus reduction, which may compromise the blood supply of the femoral head, while less than 160° leads to a higher risk of nonunion.

Occasionally, despite all efforts, an adequate reduction cannot be achieved. In this case the options are:

- Internal fixation in the best position attainable.
- Open reduction and internal fixation.
- Proceed to arthroplasty.

In the elderly patient, the best course of action will generally be to accept an inadequate reduction and insert the internal fixation in the best possible position. The fracture is then carefully monitored in the early postoperative period. If failure of fixation occurs, prompt reoperation and hemiarthroplasty can be performed before the patient's mobility and independence is seriously threatened.

Open reduction is inappropriate except in the younger patient (probably below the age of 60 years), where preservation of the femoral head is paramount. Proceeding directly to arthroplasty after attempts at reduction have failed will be likely to result in an excessively long anesthetic and theater time. The elderly patient is likely to be at greater risk of complications than if a second planned procedure has to be performed, should the fixation fail.

Choice of Implant

A considerable range of implants is available for fixation of intracapsular fractures, including various designs of nails, pins, screws and screw-plates. A meta-analysis of 25 randomized trials including a total of nearly 5000 patients [13], which considered fracture healing complication rate, found screws preferable to smooth pins. Moreover the use of a sliding screw plate design appeared unnecessary and was

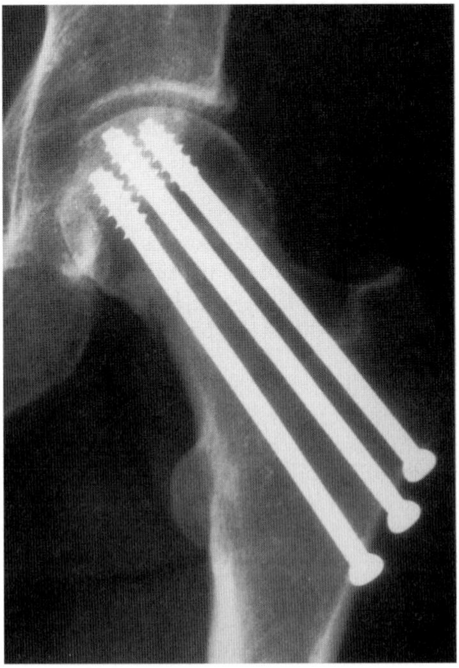

Figure 10.1. Correct reduction and position of internal fixation (three AO screws) on the anteroposterior view.

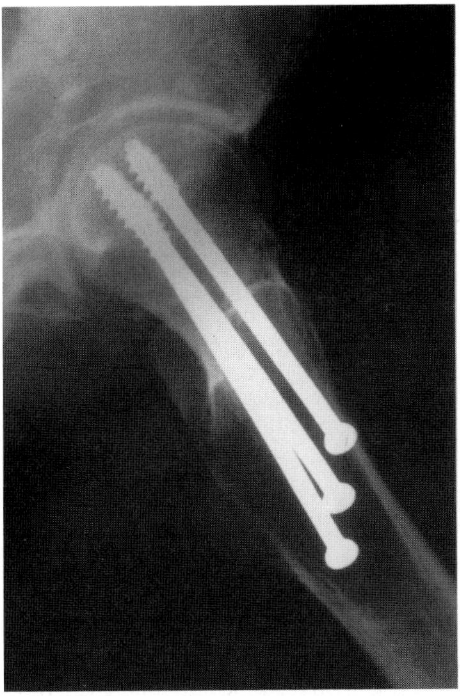

Figure 10.2. Correct reduction and position of internal fixation on the lateral view.

associated with increased operative blood loss, duration of surgery and possibly slightly higher infection rate. There was insufficient evidence to state conclusively whether two screws was more effective than three.

Position of the Fixation

Position of the fixation will to some extent depend on the design of implant used. However with the use of multiple screws, a reasonable summary of the optimum screw position is given below [14] and is illustrated in Figs. 10.1 and 10.2.

1. Lower screw inserted at the level of the lesser trochanter and in contact with the calcar femorale.
2. Angle between screws less than 10°.
3. At least 4 mm separation between screws.
4. The medial part of all screws to be within the central or inferior part of the femoral head on the anteroposterior view.
5. Where two screws are used, the distal portions, should on the lateral view, be placed centrally within the femoral head. Some scatter is advisable if more than two screws are used.
6. The tips of the screws to lie 2–10 mm from the joint surface.

Postoperative Management

For the postoperative care of proximal femoral fractures in the elderly there can only be one rule: mobilization without restrictions. There are important reasons why this policy should be followed after fixation of the displaced intracapsular fracture in the elderly. The limited functional reserve and upper limb strength makes true nonweight-bearing very difficult for most elderly patients. In addition to delaying efforts to rehabilitate the patient, there is no evidence to support the view that nonweight-bearing actually reduces the chances of re-displacement, nonunion or subsequent avascular necrosis.

Some authors have advocated non- or partial weight-bearing [15,16] on empirical grounds. Most authors, however, support early weightbearing as pain permits. A randomized trial of early versus late weightbearing revealed no significant difference in the failure rates [17]. Other large studies have found no difference or even poorer results when weight bearing is delayed after internal fixation [18,19].

Furthermore the forces applied across the hip joint during certain movements, such as rising from a chair or moving the leg in bed, are actually greater than those that occur with weightbearing [20,21].

Postoperative Complications

There is no doubt that the reoperation rate after reduction and internal fixation of a displaced intracapsular fracture is significantly higher than that after arthroplasty. However, the exact rate of fracture healing or complications is difficult to determine as many published series are highly selective and a significant proportion of patients will die before successful healing is apparent. The rate of nonunion and failure of fixation does increase with age, but in practice this does not become more apparent as the very elderly are at increased risk of early (within 3 months) death [22]. From a summation of 20 published studies [14], the average rate of nonunion after internal fixation of displaced intracapsular fractures was reported to be 21%.

Nonunion may become manifest early due to redisplacement of the femoral head (Fig. 10.3). In such cases in the elderly osteoporotic patient, a further operation will be indicated provided the patient's overall condition permits. This will generally be arthroplasty as in the elderly osteoporotic patient further attempts to preserve the femoral head are inappropriate. Methods of refixation, open reduction and bone grafting and osteotomy with the risk of further failure are outside the scope of this chapter.

Although most elderly patients in this position will stand a second planned procedure, the paramount consideration must be restoration of mobility and independence. Repeated surgical procedures necessitating prolonged hospital stays may eventually produce a healed fracture and viable femoral head, but if the patient has lost his or her independence and resides in a nursing home, the price has probably not been worth paying.

Nonunion may not always result in displacement of the fracture with marked consequent pain and disability. On occasions the fixation remains secure, but an obvious radiological nonunion occurs. In such cases the surgeon may be faced with the dilemma of whether to recommend further surgery. The judgment must consider the state of health and independence of the patient, but generally reoperation is best left until hip becomes symptomatic.

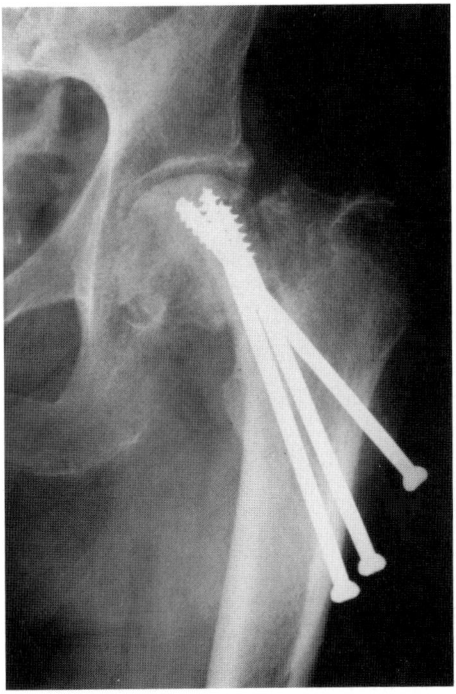

Figure 10.3. Nonunion and redisplacement of intracapsular fracture.

Once the fracture has united there remains the risk of avascular necrosis developing from disruption of the femoral head blood supply at the time of fracture. The risk of this occurring is broadly related to the initial degree of displacement [18], but the reported incidence varies widely with length of follow-up and method of diagnosis. The most accurate method is histological and figures as high as 84% of all cases have been reported [23].

What is of more practical relevance in the elderly is symptomatic late segmental collapse secondary to the avascular necrosis. Once established it is usually easy to diagnose on plain radiographs, but may be difficult to identify in the early stages. Moreover the presence of the internal fixation can make CT imaging difficult and prevent magnetic resonance imaging. In such cases removal of the fixation may be appropriate provided it is certain that union has occurred. This may also produce pain relief in addition to allowing better diagnostic imaging.

In the elderly osteoporotic patient, functional assessment is essential and once increasing pain and disability become apparent, arthroplasty should be performed. Even in the younger patient other measures such as core decompression are of little value in post-traumatic avascular necrosis. Furthermore muscle pedicle grafting is unlikely to be of value once collapse of the femoral head has begun. In the older patient, the need to preserve mobility and hence independence, rather than to preserve the femoral head is paramount.

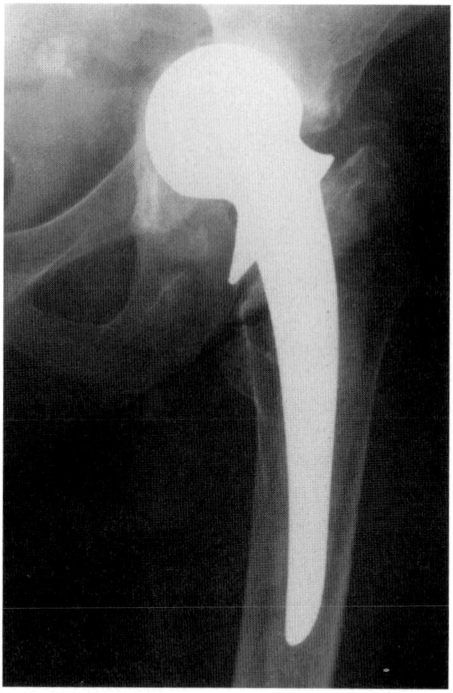

Figure 10.4. The Thompson hemiarthroplasty, also illustrating acetabular erosion.

Arthroplasty for the Displaced Intracapsular Fracture

Ever since the advent of the first effective designs of hemiarthroplasty for intracapsular fractures in the 1950s, there has been debate over when to use the prosthesis as primary treatment.

Moore, in the original report on the use of his femoral head replacement [24], advocated hemiarthroplasty as a primary treatment for older and infirm patients. Thompson, who developed the other most commonly used prosthesis, was adamant that it should only be used once internal fixation had failed and nonunion become apparent. This is reflected in an important design difference of these two implants which are still widely used today.

The angle of the collar of the Thompson stem is steeper as it is designed to sit at the level of the intertrochanteric line, the neck having become absorbed as the nonunion developed (Fig. 10.4). Whereas the Moore stem, on the other hand, is designed to sit on the calcar, which is still present in the fresh fracture (Fig. 10.5).

The indications for arthroplasty are given in the introduction to this chapter. Once the decision has been made, the next issues to address are: the approach to the hip joint, the design of prosthesis and the use of bone cement. As with the original decision there are no certainties with any of these aspects.

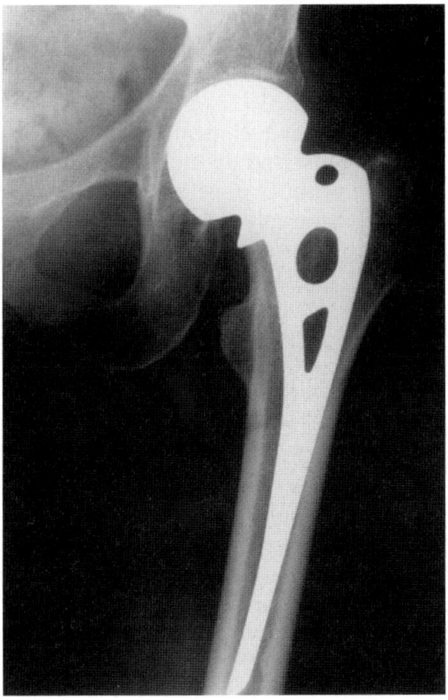

Figure 10.5. The Austin Moore hemiarthroplasty.

Surgical Approach

For any surgical approach there is inevitably a compromise between tissue dissection and the adequacy of the exposure. For the osteoarthritic patient undergoing total hip replacement, both sides of the joint must be clearly visualized to ensure adequate preparation and accurate fixation of the components, necessary to maximize the longevity of the prosthesis.

For the average patient undergoing replacement of the femoral head after intracapsular fracture, although technically accurate surgery is obviously essential, the demands are very different. Most will be frail patients in their late seventies or eighties who usually have other medical problems and little functional reserve of muscle strength. In these individuals surgery should be rapid, and cause as little disruption to the muscles of the hip as is consistent with correct insertion of a stable implant.

The commonly used surgical approaches are either posterior or one of the modifications of the anterolateral approach, which involves dissection to a greater or lesser extent of gluteus medius and vastus lateralis. The less impairment of muscle function the better and the posterior approach by preserving the abductor mechanism is the least disruptive.

The risk of certain surgical complications is considered to be influenced by the surgical approach, although much of the evidence for this is somewhat conflicting.

The dislocation rate is often stated to be higher with the posterior approach as the confused elderly patient will often draw the leg up into flexion and adduction. This will put added strain on the disrupted posterior capsule. However, although some authors have supported this view [25, 26] this is not a universal finding [27,28]. Probably of more significance is the technical accuracy of the surgery. It has been rightly stated that "a correctly inserted prosthesis seldom dislocates" [29].

The risk of postoperative wound infection has also been reported to vary depending on the approach. The argument that a posterior approach has a greater risk of wound infection because the wound is more easily contaminated by an incontinent patient [30] is not supported by any scientific evidence. Several studies have reported higher infection rates with the posterior approach [25,30]. However, this seems to be related to postoperative dislocation and other authors have reported a higher infection rate after an anterior approach [32].

The surgical approach has also been implicated in postoperative mortality [32] although again this appears to be related to dislocation, which has an associated increased risk of mortality as well as wound infection.

One complication that does appear conclusively to be related to approach is intra-operative fracture and/or penetration of the femoral shaft by the prosthesis. The increased fragility of osteoporotic bone in these fracture patients means there is a greater risk of periprosthetic fracture at the time of insertion. This was recognized by early authors [24,33] as being more likely when an anterior approach is used due to poorer visualization and the difficulty of inserting a straight stem prosthesis. Later reports have confirmed this additional risk with the anterior approach [25,29,34].

In summary, the best approach is the one the surgeon is most familiar with, although each has its own associated problems which the surgeon should recognize. For the frail elderly patient the least disruption to muscle function the better.

Choice of Prosthesis

The options for femoral head replacement or hemiarthroplasty are:

1. Solid hemiarthroplasty –in practice either the Moore or the Thompson.
2. Bipolar hemiarthroplasty – femoral head containing an inner mobile bearing.
3. Total hip arthroplasty.

The solid or unipolar hemiarthroplasties of Moore and Thompson were developed nearly half a century ago and are still in common use. They involve articulation of the metal head against the articular cartilage of the acetabulum. Articular cartilage has been shown to undergo degeneration when in contact with a hemiarthroplasty, with virtually complete loss after 5 years [35]. An earlier radiological study in humans found a progressive loss of joint space and acetabular erosion, with one reason suggested for these changes being underlying osteoporosis [36].

The exact cause of acetabular erosion, protrusion of the prosthetic head through the floor of the acetabulum, as illustrated in Fig. 10.4, is not known for certain and is not the inevitable consequence of using a solid head prosthesis. Various etiological factors have been suggested including damage to the acetabulum at the time of the fracture, excessive pressure secondary to a tight reduction, inaccurate matching of head size and osteomalacia.

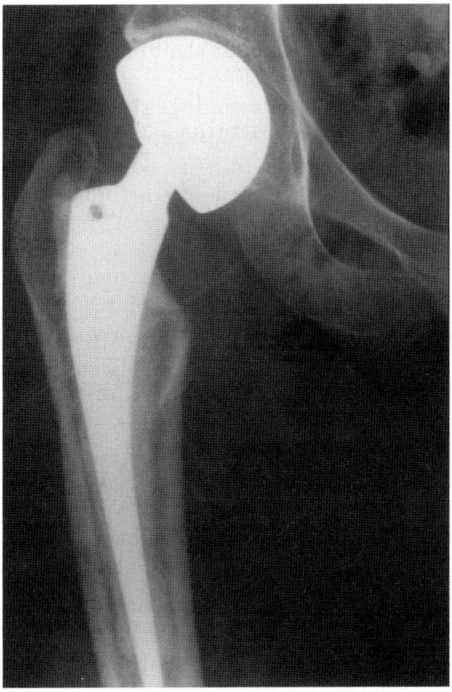

Figure 10.6. A cemented bipolar hemiarthroplasty.

The bipolar prosthesis was developed in an attempt to prevent acetabular erosion. By means of an inner bearing the acetabular surface is protected as movement takes place at the inner bearing, in preference to that between the prosthetic head and the acetabulum (Fig. 10.6).

A number of different designs are available and have been claimed to reduce or eliminate the risk of acetabular erosion. These include the Charnley–Hastings [37], Bateman [38], Monk [39] and Exeter [40]. However, reports must be considered carefully as there are a number of important variables that may influence the function of the inner bearing. These include the time from insertion, whether the limb is load-bearing when movement is assessed and the diameter of the inner bearing. As regards the last, the 22 mm diameter inner bearing appears to function most effectively [41].

Of more significance in the typical elderly hip fracture patient is whether there is any real benefit in using what is a more expensive implant on a routine basis. A number of studies have considered this issue. A comparison of cemented Thompson unipolar and Monk bipolar prostheses in patients over 80 years found no significant difference in the rate of complications between the two groups at 2 years [42]. Similarly the short-term results of a randomized trial of cemented unipolar and bipolar prostheses found no difference in hip rating outcomes for the two groups [43].

Other studies have failed to show any difference in the functional ability after unipolar and bipolar hemiarthroplasty as well as emphasizing the lower cost of unipolar prostheses [44]. Moreover in addition to the lack of benefits, long operating times and increased complications have been reported with bipolar prostheses [45]. Dislocation of a bipolar prosthesis can be difficult to manage and will usually require open reduction.

In summary there is very little justification for routine use of a bipolar prosthesis in the primary treatment of the displaced intracapsular fracture in the elderly. There may be a use in certain circumstances, such as younger patients with late presentation or failed reduction, or as an alternative to other forms of arthroplasty in pathological fractures, or in the arthritic hip.

The third form of arthroplasty that may be considered is total hip replacement. First, however, it must be appreciated that the results of this so-called gold standard for the treatment of the arthritic hip cannot in any way be compared with its use in the elderly fracture patient. Unlike the relatively younger and fitter arthritic patients, those who sustain a displaced intracapsular fracture are generally older, sicker and, having been admitted as an emergency, are unprepared for major surgery.

Retrospective reviews of selected patients undergoing total hip arthroplasty for an acute fracture have reported satisfactory clinical results although with higher perioperative complications [46,47]. Most notable of the complications is dislocation which occurs in about 10% of cases – substantially higher than most reports of primary arthroplasty for arthritis. It has been suggested that this higher rate may be due to a greater range of movement of the hip joints in fracture patients, as there is no pre-existing soft tissue contraction, such as develops in an arthritic hip joint [48].

In addition to the short-term complications a higher revision rate of up to 32% at 6 years has been reported [49]. However, this is not a consistent finding, with one retrospective study comparing cemented and uncemented hemiarthroplasty with total hip replacement reporting lower mortality, dislocation and revision rates for total hip replacement [50].

What is certain is that to perform total hip arthroplasty on all elderly patients with a displaced intracapsular fracture would be to overtreat a very considerable proportion of them. Moreover to consider it more appropriate in the younger more active patient is to ignore the fact that these are the very patients in whom the femoral head should if possible be preserved and who are most likely to cope with a second planned procedure, should the fixation fail.

The role of total hip replacement should be considered as largely a salvage procedure, after other forms of surgical treatment have failed. It should only be used in the primary treatment where there is pre-existing damage to the joint or if there is a high risk of nonunion, such as after delayed presentation (Figs. 10.7, 10.8).

The Use of Cement

Since Charnley's pioneering work in the 1960s there has been no doubt that stabilization of the prosthetic stem within the femoral shaft is more reliable and secure with the use of polymethylmethacrylate bone cement. Furthermore in the elderly osteoporotic patient, the wide femoral canal and thin brittle cortex means that the stable press-fit interlock between bone and prosthetic stem necessary for primary stability and subsequent osseous integration is unlikely to occur.

This is confirmed by the several retrospective reviews but more conclusively by two randomized control trials. These found improved gait, less pain and less

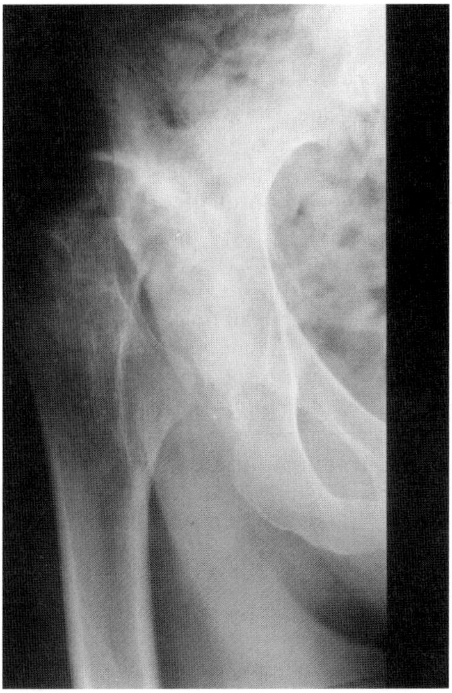

Figure 10.7. Delayed presentation of displaced intracapsular fracture. There is damage to the superior rim of the acetabulum.

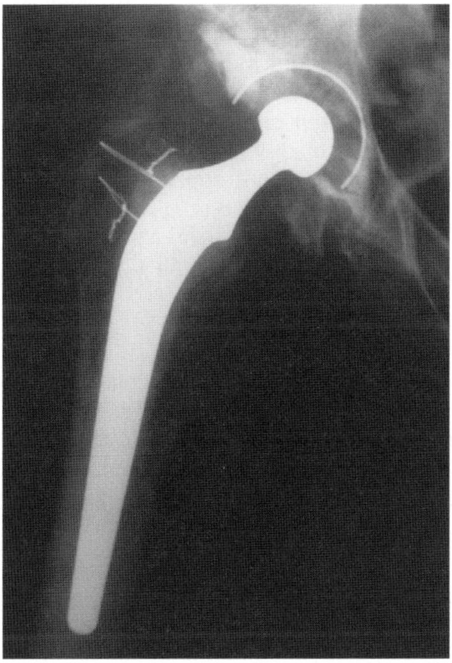

Figure 10.8. Primary treatment with Charnley total hip replacement.

dependence on walking aids in patients with a cemented stem in comparison with those who had received an uncemented stem [51,52].

Despite these findings, the use of cement is far from universal and there are some important disadvantages to its use in the frail elderly fracture patients, that do not appear to be so apparent in the osteoarthritic patient undergoing cemented total hip replacement.

Early reports indicated serious problems in patients undergoing cemented hemiarthroplasty that did not occur in hip fracture patients who underwent an uncemented procedure. Four intraoperative cardiac arrests in 22 patients undergoing cemented Thompson hemiarthroplasty were reported by Dandy in 1971 [53]. Post-mortem studies revealed evidence of fat embolism in patients who had died soon after cemented hemiarthroplasty, but not in similar patients who had undergone nail plate fixation [54].

More recent studies have continued to highlight the problem despite improvements in anesthetic technique. Transesophageal echocardiography has revealed thromboembolic showers passing through the atrium when cement is used in hemiarthroplasty. These were larger and far more extensive than when an uncemented hemiarthroplasty was used [55].

The episodes of hypotensive collapse and even cardiac arrest that may be precipitated by this embolic phenomenon are likely to be less well tolerated in these fracture patients than in arthritic patients as the former very commonly have coexisting medical pathology [56]. A recent CEPOD report in the UK highlighted the risks associated with use of cement in hip fracture patients, with up to six deaths thought to be related to its use [57].

The use of cement does not eliminate loosening of the prosthesis although revision rates are certainly lower for cemented stems. However, low-demand, very elderly, frail patients may tolerate a certain degree of weight-related pain from their uncemented stem. On the other hand the universal use of cement in this group is likely in practice to increase the mortality by about 1–2%. In conclusion, therefore, cement may achieve better fixation of the femoral stem, but at a price of greater morbidity and mortality. It is probably best reserved for the fitter, higher-demand patient for whom internal fixation is not appropriate or has failed.

Displaced Intracapsular Fracture: Management Summary

The primary treatment of the fracture should be considered reduction and internal fixation. Three screws of the AO type or similar are sufficient; a sliding hip screw is unnecessary. The majority of femoral heads are viable and will go on to unite. Where this does not occur, in the older patient hemiarthroplasty as a secondary procedure is a safe effective salvage procedure. In the younger patient in whom femoral head retention is still desirable, refixation with vascularized bone grafting is a reasonable alternative.

The indications for primary hemiarthroplasty are:

- *Absolute*:
  Abnormal joint, i.e., osteoarthritis or rheumatoid arthritis.
  Abnormal bone, i.e., metabolic bone disease, Pagets disease, pathological fractures.

- *Relative*:
  Delayed presentation, after 1 week successful internal fixation is unlikely.
  The very elderly, osteoporotic patient: although nonunion rate increases with age, the requirement for reoperation does not increase, due to the higher mortality rate.

Where primary hemiarthroplasty is performed:
- A unipolar prosthesis is adequate and this is probably best cemented in the higher-demand patient.

Alternative implants have a very limited role:
- Bipolar hemiarthroplasty: intermediate prosthesis possible use for secondary procedures.
- Total hip replacement: very few primary indications; arthritic joint, pathological fracture if life expectancy justifies, late presentation in the younger patient.

References

1. Cummings SR, Black DM, Nevitt MC, Browner WS, Cawley JA, Genant HK, et al. Appendicular bone density and age predict hip fracture in women. JAMA 1990;263: 665–68.
2. Cummings SR, Black DM, Nevitt MC, Browner WS, Cauley JA, Ensrud K, et al. Bone density at various sites for the prediction of hip fractures. Lancet 1993;341:72–75.
3. Lu-Yao GL, Keller RB, Littenberg B, Wennberg JE. Outcomes after displaced fractures of the femoral neck: a meta-analysis of 106 published reports. J Bone Joint Surg Am 1994;76:15–25.
4. Parker MJ. Prediction of fracture union after internal fixation of intracapsular femoral neck fractures. Injury 1994;25(Suppl 2):SB3–SB6.
5. Brown JT, Abrami G. Transcervical femoral fractures; a review of 195 patients treated by sliding nail plate. J Bone Joint Surg Br 1964;46:648–663.
6. Manninger J, Kazar G, Fekete G, Fekete K, Frenyo S, Gyarfas F, et al. Significance of urgent (within 6 hours) internal fixation in the management of fractures and the neck of the femur. Injury 1989;20:101–105.
7. Swinontkowski MF, Winquist RA, Hansen ST Jr. Fractures of the femoral neck in patients between the ages of twelve and forty nine years. J Bone Joint Surg Am 1984;66:837–846.
8. Crawfurd EJP, Emery RJH, Hansell DM, Phelan M, Andrews BG. Capsular distension and intracapsular pressure in subcapital fractures of the femur. J Bone Joint Surg Br 1988;70:195–198.
9. Melberg P-E, Korner l, Lansinger O. Hip joint pressure after femoral neck fracture. Acta Orthop Scand 986;57:501–504.
10. Klenerman L, Marcuson RW. Intracapsular fractures of the neck of the femur. J Bone Joint Surg Br 1970;52:514–517.
11. Meyers MH, Harvey JP, Moore TM. Treatment of displaced subcapital and transcervical fractures of the femoral neck by muscle-pedicle-bone graft and internal fixation: a preliminary report on one hundred and fifty cases. J Bone Joint Surg Am 1973;55:257–274.
12. Garden RS. Low angle fixation in fractures of the femoral neck. J Bone Joint Surg Br 1961;43:630–647.
13. Parker MJ, Blundell C. Choice of implant for internal fixation of femoral neck fractures. Acta Orthop Scand 1998;69:138–143.
14. Parker MJ, Pryor GA. Hip fracture management. Oxford: Blackwell Scientific, 1993:124.

15. Fielding JW, Wilson SA, Ratzan RE. A continuing end-result study of displaced intracapsular fractures of the neck of the femur treated with the Pugh nail. J Bone Joint Surg Am 1974;56:1464–1472.
16. Deyerle WM. Multiple-pin peripheral fixation in fractures of the neck of the femur: immediate weight bearing. Clin Orthop 1965;39:135–156.
17. Graham J. Early or delayed weight bearing after internal fixation of transcervical fracture of the femur: a clinical trial. J Bone Joint Surg Br 1968;50:562–569.
18. Barnes R, Brown JT, Garden RS, Nicoll EA. Subcapital fractures of the femur: a prospective review. J Bone Joint Surg Br 1976;58:2–24.
19. Nieminen S. Early weight bearing after classical internal fixation of medial fractures of the femoral neck. Acta Orthop Scand 1975;46:782–794.
20. Rydell N. Biomechanics of the hip joint. Clin Orthop 1973;92:6–15.
21. Norden M, Frankel VH. Biomechanics of the hip. In: Frankel VH, Norden M, editors. Basic biomechanics of the skeletal system,. Philadelphia: Lea & Febiger, 1980.
22. Parker MJ. Prediction of fracture union after internal fixation of intracapsular femoral neck fractures. Injury 1994;25(Suppl 2):SB3–SB6.
23. Sevitt S. Avascular necrosis and revascularisation of the femoral head after intracapsular fractures: a combined arteriographic and histological necropsy study. J Bone Joint Surg Br 1964;46:270–296.
24. Moore AT. The self-locking metal hip prosthesis. J Bone Joint Surg Am 1957;39:811–827.
25. Chan RN-W, Hoskinson J. Thompson prosthesis for fractured neck of femur: a comparison of surgical approaches. J Bone Joint Surg Br 1975;57:437–443.
26. Keen GS, Parker MJ. Hemiarthroplasty of the hip: the anterior or posterior approach? A comparison of surgical approaches. Injury 1993;24:611–613.
27. Stewart HD, Papagiannopoulos G. Hemiarthroplasty: a progression in treatment? J R Coll Surg Edinb 1986;31:345–350.
28. Salvati EA, Wilson PD. Long term results of femoral head replacement. J Bone Joint Surg Am 1973;55:516–524.
29. D'arcy J, Devas M. Treatment of fractures of the femoral head by replacement with the Thompson prosthesis. J Bone Joint Surg Br 1976;58:279–286.
30. Devas M. Geriatric orthopaedics. In: Surgery for the aged. Ann R Coll Surg Engl 1976;58: 15–24.
31. Lunt HRW. The role of prosthetic replacement of the head of the femur as primary treatment for subcapital fractures. Injury 1971;3:107–113.
32. Sikorski JM, Barrington R. Internal fixation versus hemiarthroplasty for displaced subcapital fracture of femur: a prospective randomised study. J Bone Joint Surg Br 1981;63:357–361.
33. Anderson LD, Hamsa WR, Waring TL. Femoral head prostheses: A review of 356 operations and their results. J Bone Joint Surg Am 1964;46:1049–1065.
34. Wood MR. Femoral head replacement following fracture: an analysis of surgical approach. Injury 1979;11:317–320.
35. Dalldorf PG, Banas MP, Hicks DG, Pellegrini VD. Rate of degeneration of human acetabular cartilage after hemiarthroplasty. J Bone Joint Surg Am 1995;77:877–882.
36. Drinker H, Murray WR. The universal proximal femoral endoprosthesis. J Bone Joint Surg Am 1979;61:1167–1174.
37. Devas M, Hinves B. Prevention of acetabular erosion after hemiarthroplasty for fractured neck of femur. J Bone Joint Surg Br 1983;65:548–551.
38. LaBelle LW, Colwill JC, Swanson AB. Bateman bipolar hip arthroplasty for femoral neck fractures. A five to ten year follow up study. Clin Orthop 1990;251:20–25.
39. Leyshon RL, Matthews JP. Acetabular erosion and the Monk "hard top" hip prosthesis. J Bone Joint Surg Br 1984;66:172–174.
40. Pearse MF, Bande S, O'Dwyer KJ, Ling RSM. The Exeter bipolar prosthesis in the active elderly patient: the results at 7 years. Int Orthop [SICOT] 1992;16:344–348.
41. Brueton RN, Craig JSJ, Hinves BL, Heatley FW. Effect of femoral component head size on movement of the two component hemiarthroplasty. Injury 1993;24:231–235.

42. Calder SJ, Anderson GH, Jagger C, Harper WM, Gregg PJ. Unipolar or bipolar prosthesis for displaced intracapsular hip fracture in octogenarians. A randomised prospective study. J Bone Joint Surg Br 1996;78:391–394.
43. Cornell CN, Levine D, O'Doherty J, Lyden J. Unipolar versus bipolar hemiarthroplasty for the treatment of femoral neck fractures in the elderly. Clin Orthop 1998;348:67–71.
44. Wathne RA, Koval KL, Ahranoff GB, Zuckerman JD, Jones DA. Modular unipolar versus bipolar prosthesis: a prospective evaluation of functional outcome after femoral neck fracture. J Orthop Trauma 1995;9:298–302.
45. Rosen LL, Miller BJ, Dupuis PR, Hadjipavlou A. A prospective randomised study comparing bipolar hip arthroplasty and hemiarthroplasty in elderly patients with subcapital fractures. J Bone Joint Surg Br 1992;74(Suppl III):282.
46. Lee BPH, Berry DJ, Harmsen WS, Sim FH. Total hip arthroplasty for the treatment of an acute fracture of the femoral neck. J Bone Joint Surg Am 1998;80:70–75.
47. Gregory RJH, Wood DJ, Stevens J. Treatment of displaced subcapital femoral fractures with total hip replacement. Injury 1992;23:168–170.
48. Gregory RJH, Gibson MJ, Moran CG. Dislocation after primary arthroplasty for subcapital fracture of the hip: wide range of movement is a risk factor. J Bone Joint Surg Br 1991;73:11–12.
49. Greenough CG, Jones JR. Primary total hip replacement for displaced subcapital fracture of the femur. J Bone Joint Surg Br 1988;70:639–643.
50. Gebhard JS, Amstutz HC, Zinar DM, Dorey FJ. A comparison of total hip arthroplasty and hemiarthroplasty for treatment of acute fracture of the femoral neck. Clin Orthop 1992;282:123–131.
51. Emery RJH, Broughton NS, Desai K, Bulstrode CJK, Thomas TL. Bipolar hemiarthroplasty for subcapital fracture of the femoral head. A prospective randomised trial of cemented Thompson and uncemented Moore stems. J Bone Joint Surg Br 1991;73:322–324.
52. Sonne-Holm S, Walter S, Jensen JS. Moore hemiarthroplasty with and without bone cement in femoral neck fractures:a clinical controlled trial. Acta Orthop Scand 1982;53:953–956.
53. Dandy DJ. Fat embolism following prosthetic replacement of the femoral head. Injury 1971;2:85–88.
54. Gresham GA, Kucznski A, Rosborough D. Fatal fat embolism following replacement arthroplasty for transcervical fractures of the femur. BMJ 1971;II:617–619.
55. Christie J, Burnett R, Potts HR, Pell ACH. Echocardiography of transatrial embolism during cemented and uncemented hemiarthroplasty of the hip. J Bone Joint Surg Br 1994;76:409–411.
56. Ceder L, Elmqvist D, Svensson S-E. Cardiovascular and neurological function in elderly patients sustaining a fracture of the neck of the femur. J Bone Joint Surg Br 1981;63:560–566.
57. The Report of the National Confidential Enquiry into Perioperative Deaths 1993/1994. London: NCEPOD (35–43 Lincoln's Inn Fields, London WC2A 3PN), 1996.

11 Trochanteric Fractures

M. R. Baumgaertner and C. M. Wahl

Introduction

Trochanteric hip fractures are, in many ways, the paradigm for treatment of musculoskeletal illness in the elderly. These fracture types occur rarely in those younger than 65 years old, and then, usually under circumstances of severe trauma or neoplasm. The challenges presented to the orthopaedic surgeon in the treatment of pertrochanteric hip fractures are many, both in and out of the operating room. Not only does the surgeon contend with osteoporosis and significant fracture comminution in attempting to achieve a stable osteosynthesis in a weightbearing limb, but he or she must be cognizant of the impact of the fracture on the patient with regard to medical well-being, mental vigor, rehabilitation and the potential for ultimate independence.

Special considerations apply to the hip fracture in elderly populations, notably osseous atrophy and anatomy. Osteoporosis greatly affects the trabecular network of bone that acts as a scaffold to transmit forces from the femoral head through the femoral neck to the shaft of the femur. Ward eloquently described these trabeculae in his paper of 1838 [1]. These are distributed into a primary compressive group (fanning from the dome of the femoral head to the medial femoral neck or calcar), the primary tensile group (arching from the fovea of the head to the lateral femoral cortex just distal to the greater trochanter), secondary compressive and tensile groups, and a greater trochanteric group (orienting along stress lines in the lateral femur). There is relatively little trabecular bone peripherally in the head and centrally in the neck. Singh used the presence and absence of these groups to develop a radiographic classification of osteopenia [2]. This grading system runs from I to VI, with VI representing normal bone (all trabeculae present) and grade I representing severe osteopenia with evident bone loss in all groups. Inter- and intra-observer error complicate the use of the Singh classification [3], but some studies have correlated the lower grades with a higher incidence of loss of fixation

Another difference in the normal anatomy of the elderly population involves a gradual decrease in the angle portended by the femoral neck and shaft. In the normal adult population, this angle varies between 120° and 135°. Noble and associates [4] recognized a gradual decrease in this angle with age, and an average neck-shaft angle of 125° in those over 70 years of age. This gradual reduction of the neck-shaft angle effectively lengthens the bending moment acting against the trochanteric region and acts in concert with a relative paucity of trabecular bone to predispose the elderly patient to fracture.

Diagnosis and Classification

The presentation of a patient with a trochanteric hip fracture is predictable and rarely subtle. Almost all fractures are due to direct or indirect twisting forces imparted to the proximal femur during a fall. The elderly population is at high risk for such falls, given the gait disturbances, muscle weakness, decreased visual and hearing acuity and other medical illness that can accompany aging. Although most patients present with isolated injuries, 10% will have coincident fractures. Most commonly these occur in other bones affected greatly by osteopenia: the wrist, shoulder, elbow, ribs, pelvis and spine. The history and examination must exclude these additional diagnoses.

The patient usually gives a history of a slip and fall, or other low-energy trauma. It is important to secure a reasonable explanation for the fall, to rule out syncope, cerebral or cardiac ischemia, hypoglycemia, or other common but potentially life-threatening medical problems that could complicate surgery. A directed interview of the patient's internist, relatives or caregivers should address particular medical problems, allergies, previous laboratory studies or hospitalizations, and especially the patient's pre-injury ambulatory and functional level – as these issues will become important during the recovery and rehabilitation phases of care. On physical examination, the injured leg appears shortened and externally rotated. Care should be taken to note local skin conditions, as well as evidence of decubiti at the heels, buttocks or sacrum which could complicate surgery or the postoperative course.

Most trochanteric fractures can be accurately diagnosed on a good-quality anteroposterior view of the pelvis and a cross-table lateral view. When possible, the affected limb should be held in gentle traction and internal rotation to allow comparison of the injured and uninjured sides. In addition, fragment overlap is kept to a minimum, and the deforming muscular forces are somewhat neutralized – creating a clearer image of the fracture pattern. The anteroposterior view will often reveal the fracture obliquity, number of fragments, and indicate whether or not the posteromedial cortex will be stable to compression once reduced. The lateral view will clarify any posterior displacement of the shaft and flexion of the proximal head neck fragment.

Rarely, a computed axial tomographic (CT) scan may be useful in understanding complex fracture patterns. In patients who present with hip pain and a mechanism consistent with the diagnosis of a fracture but radiographs that are equivocal, a technetium bone scan or magnetic resonance imaging (MRI) may serve to make or exclude the diagnosis. Bone scans are relatively inexpensive, but they subject the patient to significant radiation and require a 72 h delay from injury to be adequately sensitive. MRI has been shown to be superior to the bone scan for the elucidation of occult hip fractures [5], and should be considered the study of choice.

Several classification systems have been advocated since Evans' original attempt in 1949 [6–8]. None has been universally accepted. Most surgeons, and many authors, simply separate fractures into stable or unstable patterns. A stable fracture is usually only two parts, and once reduced can tolerate compressive loads across the neck without loss of neck shaft alignment. The implant functions primarily as a tension band. Unstable fracture patterns have intermediate or multiple

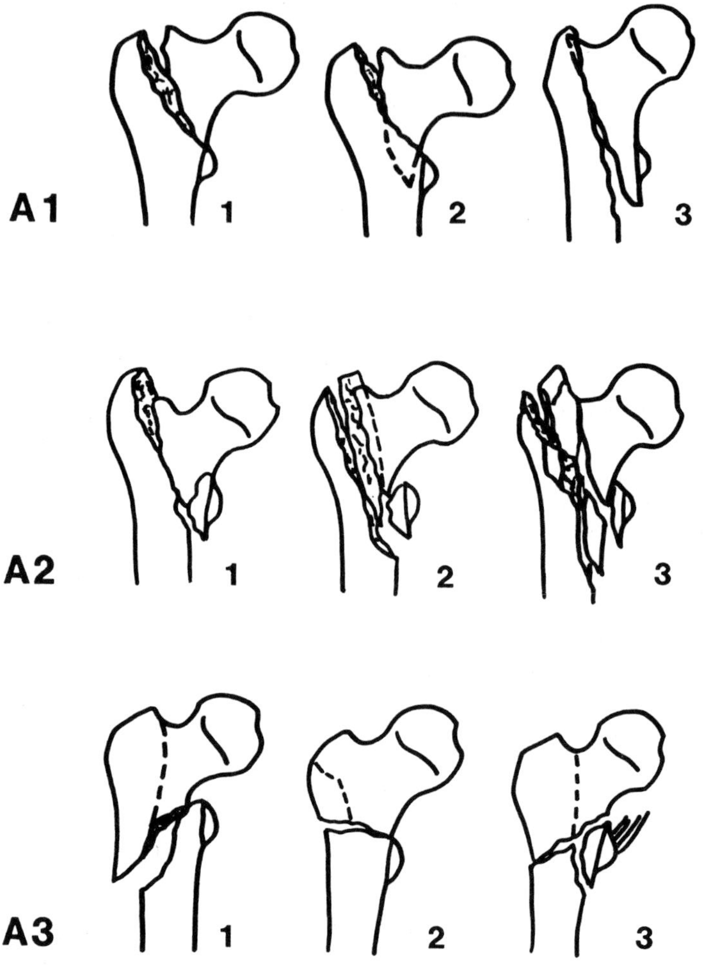

Figure 11.1. The AO classification for trochanteric fractures. *A1* simple pertrochanteric; *A2* multifragmentary pertrochanteric; *A3* intertrochanteric.

fragments, usually posteromedially, but they can instead have so-called reverse oblique fracture lines that run from proximal medial to distal lateral. In these fractures, reduction is more difficult and resistance to medial compression is not re-established. Given the poor bone quality of the patient who sustains these fractures, mechanical failure with complete varus collapse of the proximal fragment is much more likely.

The Müller/AO classification of fractures for the hip has been adopted by the Orthopaedic Trauma Association as part of a coordinated description of all skeletal fractures [9]. As seen in Fig. 11.1 there are three types of trochanteric fracture patterns (two-part peritrochanteric, multipart peritrochanteric, and intertrochanteric fractures), and each group has three subtypes. This system has the distinct advantage of being alphanumerically formatted, but it also maintains the concept of stability. All type 1 fractures are stable two-part fractures, type 3 fractures are unstable by fracture line geometry, and most type 2 fractures are unstable because of significant and multiple fragmentation.

Treatment Options

Surgical stabilization allows the potential to re-establish near-normal anatomy and immediately mobilize and begin rehabilitating the patient. Nonoperative treatment of pertrochanteric fractures is only appropriate for patients who will not benefit from surgical stabilization and therefore should not be subject to its antecedent risks. Hornby and coworkers [10] prospectively compared skeletal traction with sliding hip screw fixation. Although they appreciated no significant differences in mortality, pain or complications from decubiti, the nonoperative group were hospitalized significantly longer, had more malunions and were less likely to return to an independent level of functioning. Patients who are in the final stages of a terminal illness and unlikely to survive the rehabilitation period and individuals who were bed-bound prior to injury should be treated humanely without concern for functional outcome. In such persons, analgesics are administered and the patient is allowed to sit up as tolerated. A low-pressure bed should be used in the immediate period after injury to avoid complications from decubiti. Within 10–14 days the fracture may become organized enough to allow the patient to transfer with support. One can expect a decreasing need for analgesic support at this time. At least one study suggests that in the nonambulatory, senile patient, nonoperative treatment in a nursing home setting was more humane, less costly and put the patient at less risk [11]. For patients temporarily too medically ill to undergo an operation, skeletal traction adequate to maintain a normal neck-shaft angle should be employed. This avoids problems associated with skin traction, and should allow for closed or minimally invasive reduction even when surgery is delayed.

The primary goal of treatment for the previously ambulatory patient with a trochanteric fracture is the establishment of a functional, painless extremity as quickly as possible. The elderly patient will not tolerate long periods of immobilization and bedrest. As a general rule their capacity for rehabilitation with regard to strength, stamina and coordination is perhaps optimal shortly after injury, before depression, muscle atrophy, pneumonia and the other known complications of bedrest and pain can occur and dominate treatment. To facilitate successful surgery and allow early rehabilitation, the surgeon should consider the following:

1. Any surgical intervention chosen must take into account the difference in density and distribution of bone present in the osteoporotic individual compared with the young patient.
2. A dynamic device that maintains the neck-shaft angle and facilitates postoperative fracture impaction at the expense of a slightly shortened extremity is preferred in this population.
3. The fixation construct envisioned must allow for the complete mobilization of the patient, preferably stable enough to allow immediate weightbearing to tolerance.
4. Surgery should be only as invasive (in terms of anesthesia, blood loss and muscle dissection) as necessary to achieve the goals described above.

Zuckerman et al. [12] found that delay more than 48 h from admission to surgery was an important predictor of mortality at 1 year. It is generally accepted that the fixation of trochanteric fractures is a surgical urgency, not emergency, and delays for medical reasons are prudent in the elderly population, although delays greater than 72 h are associated with a higher cost of treatment, and significantly higher complication rate [13]. There is no consensus concerning the safest anesthetic technique for these patients.

Kaufer [14] defined five factors upon which the stability of any instrumented fracture depend. These include the quality of bone, the fracture pattern, the reduction achieved, the implant's design features, and the positioning of the implant within the bone. The first two factors have been discussed already, and although they must be fully appreciated, they are not within the surgeon's control. However, the reduction, implant selection and operative technique are determined by the surgeon, and consequently so is the ultimate quality of the bone-implant construct and the success of treatment.

Fracture Reduction

No single variable plays as great a role in the expeditious and successful management of a trochanteric fracture as the fracture reduction. With the development and widespread use of dynamic hip screws that allow fractures with gaps to collapse and impact postoperatively, absolute anatomical reduction of fragments is not necessary and actually discouraged in light of the additional surgical trauma required. However, axial and translational reduction of the major proximal and distal fragment in both the anteroposterior and lateral planes is mandatory if the implant is to guide the fragments into stable opposition. No device can improve upon a poor reduction.

The fracture table is a tool that greatly facilitates the safe and effective management of patients with trochanteric fractures. Perhaps most importantly, it allows the surgeon to position the torso and both lower extremities so that adequate, orthogonal anteroposterior and lateral fluoroscopic images of the fracture zone and femoral head can be consistently and repeatedly obtained. Additionally, if skeletal traction is used, or the foot is secured to the traction apparatus, length and rotation of the distal fragment can be continuously maintained from closed reduction to final implant placement.

Stable fracture patterns rarely present a problem for reduction and can be successfully managed with different surgical techniques [8,15]. Fracture impaction with detectable extremity shortening can be expected in up to 25% of patients with apparently stable fractures treated with dynamic screws [16], but it is rarely of functional significance. Most fractures can be reduced with gentle longitudinal traction (to regain length), abduction (to correct varus) and internal rotation of the shaft. Stable two-part fractures that involve the base of the neck or bisect the lesser trochanter are occasionally not able to be reduced in a closed fashion [17]. Open reduction demonstrated the psoas tendon flexing and impaling the neck in the soft tissue; releasing the tendon allowed reduction.

Unstable fracture patterns may present a more difficult task to the surgeon. The initial reduction maneuvers are similar to those for stable fractures, but slight valgus overcorrection is to be encouraged. Not only does an increased neck-shaft angle reduce offset and bending forces, the slight resultant increase in limb length minimizes the limb shortening effect of fracture site collapse that is expected as the fracture settles into a position of stability. After adequate longitudinal traction has re-established leg length, the extremity is slowly abducted under fluoroscopic guidance until there is no apparent varus angulation at the principal fracture site. Finally, the distal fragment is rotated until it aligns with the proximal fragment. Not uncommonly, fracture instability is so severe that indirect techniques are futile and formal open reduction is indicated. The lateral fluoroscopic view is critical to confirm that posterior translation of the shaft has been corrected (an external support can be used if necessary) and the neck version has been re-established. Rotational reduction must be assessed carefully, both clinically and fluoroscopically by comparing the transcondylar axis and neck version. Frequently the trochanter fragments will not fully reduce, but as long as the anatomical axis is restored, appropriate placement of a sliding hip screw will allow for stability to be achieved postoperatively. Unless the posteromedial fragment is singular and quite large it is usually best to treat it indirectly.

Previously, fixed length nails and screws had exceedingly high failure rates when fracture stability could not be achieved at surgery. To manage these unstable fractures, surgeons performed displacement osteotomies to convert the unstable fracture pattern into a nonanatomical but stable one [18–20]. The development of dynamic devices that allowed for fracture collapse but maintained axial alignment obviated the need to achieve absolute stability intraoperatively. Recently, two randomized prospective clinical trials demonstrated that osteotomy and fixation with a sliding hip screw was associated with significantly longer surgery and more blood loss, but no advantages when compared with anatomical reduction of unstable fractures [21,22]. Another report shows no biomechanical advantage [23]. Currently, osteotomies are rarely, if ever indicated for acute fractures, but the principles behind these techniques are often useful for fixation failures and nonunions in the trochanteric region.

Implant Options and Insertional Techniques

Compression Hip Screws

The evolution of devices and techniques used for fixation of pertrochanteric hip fractures has concerned itself primarily with complications associated with loss of fixation in osteoporotic bone. The "first generation" devices that were employed included the Jewett and Holt nails. These were angled nail plate devices of fixed length that could not accommodate the collapse and settling required of an unstable fracture to stabilize and unite. If the nail was placed too deeply, it would perforate the joint; if positioned too shallowly into the osteoporotic areas of the head and neck, varus collapse and cut-out would occur. Additionally, if union was not prompt, fatigue failure of the implant or pull-out of the screws were common problems. The current design of the compression hip screw (CHS) can be placed very deeply into the head because the proximal screw retracts into the barrel as the fracture impacts. These devices have large outside diameters, blunt edges and broad contact surface area to discourage migration or penetration, and refinements in biomaterials have made them extremely strong. Implant breakage secondary to fatigue is rare.

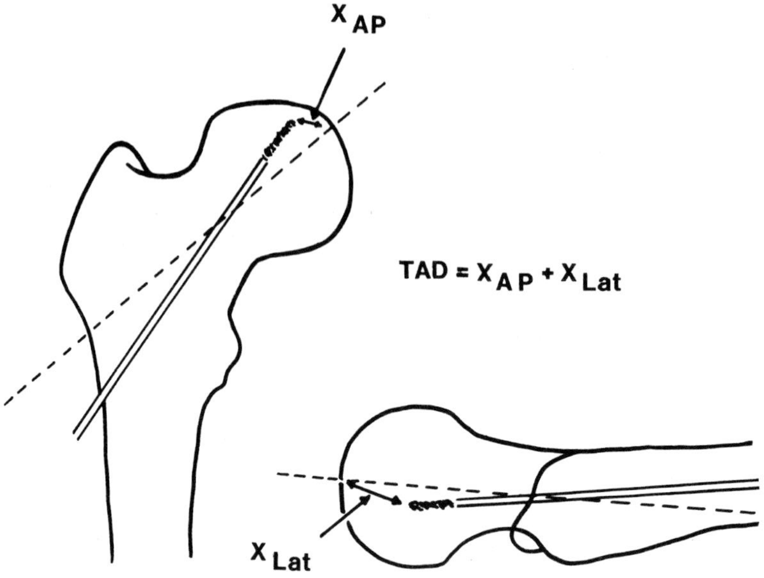

Figure 11.2. The tip-apex distance (TAD) summarizes implant depth and location on the anteroposterior and lateral images into a single number that is predictive of cut-out (see text). After Baumgaertner and Solberg [39].

The first step in successful insertion of the CHS is an anatomically aligned fracture. Although it is preferable to achieve this by a closed reduction, there should be no hesitation to formal open manipulation if necessary. In rare instances with extremely unstable fractures, the proximal fragment may be manipulated into physiological position with a guide pin and then temporarily stabilized by advancing the pin through the head into the acetabulum. The distal fragment is then reduced routinely. It is always advisable to place an additional guide pin across the fracture well superior to the planned course of the hip screw to guard against rotational torque during reaming and screw placement, and to help hold the reduction in the case of accidental guide pin removal.

Following reduction, the next (and perhaps most critical) step is to seat the guide pin centrally and to the level of subchondral bone in both planes. Recent work at our institution has confirmed the reports of multiple authors that this position is ideal for construct stability and offers a simple technique to record and grade implant position. The distance from the tip of the screw to the true apex of the femoral head on both the anteroposterior and lateral views are summed to generate a tip-apex distance (TAD). This measurement takes into account but does not specifically define peripheral or shallow malposition (Fig. 11.2). A TAD less than 25 mm is required to minimize the risk of failure. As the value increases we have shown failure by cut-out to increase exponentially [24].

The screw length is determined, taking into account the amount of acute collapse expected with the release of intraoperative traction, so that the distal end of the screw shaft is within 5–8 mm of the lateral extent of the barrel. A 135° angled four-hole plate is selected for the great majority of fractures. It is aligned and held to the shaft with a pointed clamp that avoids damage to the medial periosteal tissues. With unstable fractures it is very helpful to release some traction temporarily and encourage impaction in the axis of the shaft at this time. Assess the reduction, the potential for fracture stability and the length and position of implants in both planes. It may be necessary to redistract the screw barrel assembly and reposition the plate slightly distally on the shaft to facilitate the establishment of a posteromedial buttress.

Recently, modifications to the CHS plate have been presented to facilitate management of severely unstable fractures. An additional trochanteric stabilizing plate abuts the greater trochanter proximally and is attached distally to the shaft by sandwiching it between a conventional sideplate and its screws. The plate prevents excessive collapse of the fracture and medialization of the shaft but a hole in the plate allows free lag screw sliding. In one study, operations and hospital stays were longer, but lag screw sliding more than 20 mm was decreased from 20% to 4% of unstable fractures [25].

Another design modification, the Medoff plate, allows collapse in the axis of the shaft in addition to, or instead of, the sliding screw. This is achieved by a second sliding mechanism within the sideplate. This may be advantageous for fixation of severely unstable trochanteric fractures or those with subtrochanteric extension. Although an increased operative intervention and blood loss appears necessary, and the potential for excessive extremity shortening exists, reports have demonstrated a reduced rate of mechanical failure compared with a conventional CHS [26,27]. This may be of particular value in severely osteoporotic patients.

Intramedullary Fixation

Intramedullary nails are often preferred over plates for fixation of osteoporotic fractures because wide intramedullary canals allow placement of an adequate-sized nail without additional trauma, and the problem of screw pull-out from thin cortices is largely avoided. For trochanteric fractures, additional mechanical advantages include a decreased moment of inertia of the more medial, intramedullary location of the nail compared with the sideplate as well as its tendency to act as a buttress against excessive shaft medialization. Lastly, and perhaps most attractive, the ability to place these devices percutaneously offers potential improvements in perioperative complications and the rate of complications (Fig. 11.3).

Multiple flexible intramedullary nails, such as those designed by Ender, to be inserted percutaneously just proximal to the femoral condyles and driven retrograde across the fracture zone to fan out in the head, have repeatedly offered clinical results inferior to the CHS [15,28]. Indications for their use are relative and rare. Occasionally, a debilitated patient too ill to undergo more extensive surgery, or patients in which soft tissue considerations prevent a hip incision, may benefit from this approach.

The gamma nail (Howmedica; Rutherford, NJ) was the first widely marketed rigid intramedullary nail indicated for fixation of pertrochanteric fractures. A short nail with a valgus bend facilitated insertion through the tip of the trochanter and a large, partially threaded proximal interlock screw was designed to allow for fracture impaction. Numerous comparative studies failed to show any definite advantage of this nail over the CHS, but the complication and reoperation rates were higher [29]. Femoral shaft fracture, due at least in part to surgical technique errors and the stress riser effect of the nail ending at the midshaft and impinging on the anterior cortex, were reported in all series.

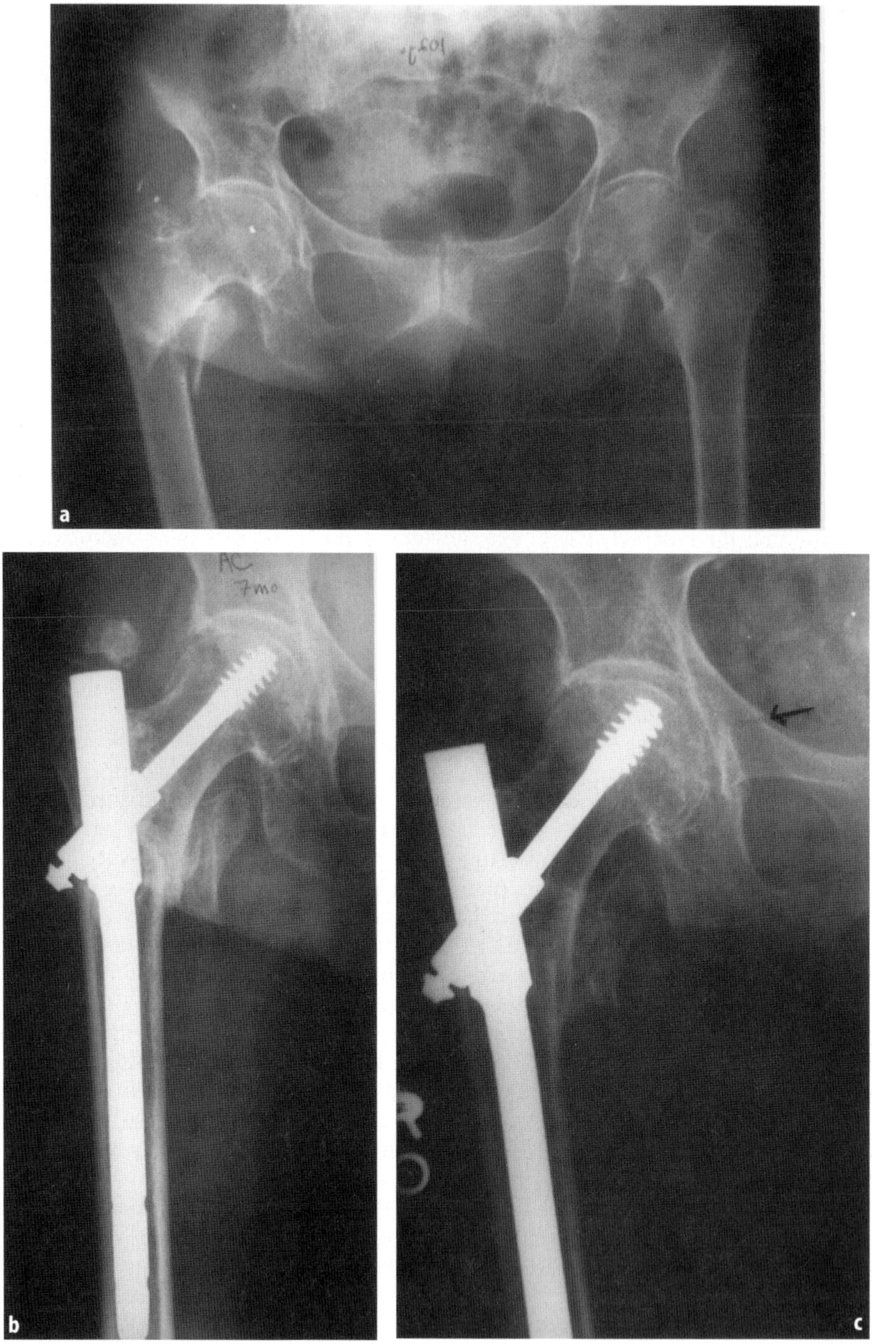

Figure 11.3. **a** Radiograph of 102-year-old woman with unstable trochanteric fracture. **b** Seven months following fixation with intramedullary hip screw. **c** At age 105 years following another fall resulting in pelvic rami fractures (*arrow*) but no periprosthetic complication.

A different device, the Intramedullary Hip Screw (Smith+Nephew & Richards, Memphis, TN) allows a standard compression hip screw to slide within a barrel-shaped sleeve that is attached to a nail. Other design modifications include smaller distal interlocking screws and a decreased valgus bend to facilitate a less traumatic insertion. Early reports suggest more efficient surgery and faster rehabilitation, especially for unstable fractures, reverse obliquity fractures and fractures with subtrochanteric extension, but complications continue to be higher with this device compared with a screw and sideplates [30–32].

There is little question that intramedullary fixation of trochanteric fractures is more technique dependent than open management with a sideplate, and most all studies to date have acknowledged a surgical "learning curve". Nonetheless the surgeon who appreciates the nuances of this technique can offer a more efficient operative intervention to his or her always osteoporotic and often ill patient.

A successful nailing can not occur unless a closed reduction can be achieved. If formal open reduction is required, many of the advantages of nailing are lost and plate fixation may be preferred. Since the adduction required to insert the nail tends to worsen a varus deformity at the hip, it is critical to secure well the foot in the holder to allow for the aggressive traction occasionally necessary. Following percutaneous placement of a guide pin that enters just medial to the tip of the trochanter and crosses the fracture to lie in the canal, the fracture zone must be over-reamed with the dedicated entrance reamer. Medial-directed pressure on the trochanter ensures that a channel is actually reamed in the osteoporotic bone rather than simply displacing the fragments as the reamer passes. Reaming of the canal itself is rarely necessary. The nail is positioned in the canal without force and without the mallet. If resistance is met, confirm that the tip of the straight nail is not binding on the anterior cortex of the bowed femoral shaft. Occasionally, the entrance site needs to be enlarged, a smaller nail chosen, or the canal itself is reamed. Once the nail is seated, if traction has not corrected varus malalignment, the limb can be abducted to increase the neck-shaft angle slightly. Central and deep screw placement is equally critical with this device, but since the location and direction of the guide pin is determined by a jig attached and aligned with the femoral shaft, the technique of pin placement is different. Advancing the nail, increasing traction and abducting the limb will all bring the guide pin inferiorly in the head. To correct lateral plane alignment, jig rotation as well as actual anterior/posterior translation of the device and femoral shaft is performed. Do not accept a suboptimal pin position. The appropriate length cannulated screw is placed after reaming. After locking the screw to the nail with the set screw, the fracture should be assessed for rotational and axial stability with traction released. Only rarely will distal interlocking be necessary, and if indicated one screw is usually adequate. Hardy et al. [31] noted thigh pain and cortical hypertrophy when two screws were used. Another, newer device uses two proximal screws to minimize the chance of rotational instability at the fracture and a smaller, potentially less stiff distal tip to minimize risk of shaft fracture (Fig. 11.4). The insertional technique is very similar to previously mentioned devices.

Cement Augmentation

Injectable biomaterials such as polymethylmethacrylate (PMMA) and calcium phosphate cements (CPC) can be used to improve screw purchase in osteoporotic bone

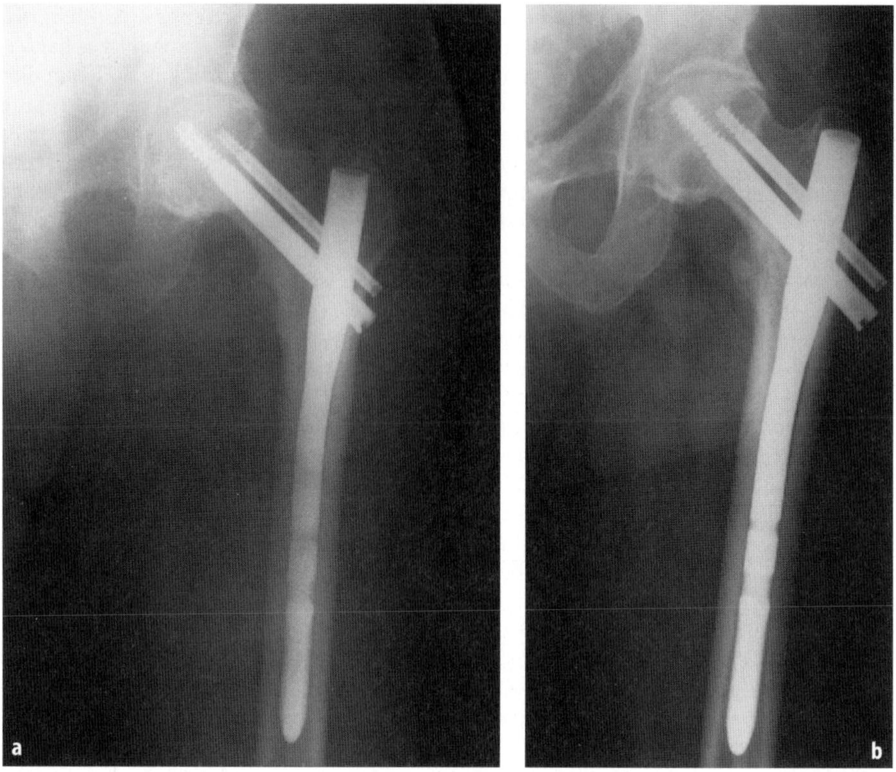

Figure 11.4. Proximal femoral nail used to treat trochanteric fracture. **a** Immediate postoperative radiograph; **b** 3-month follow-up showing impaction and healing.

[33,34]. For this technique, the surgeon injects liquid-phase cement into the screw hole and reinserts the screw. Depending on material and protocol, the screw may be tightened further after the material solidifies [35]. PMMA, although easy to work with, has several disadvantages. As a foreign body, it can not be remodelled or replaced by native bone, and if it is inadvertently placed in the fracture site it can prevent union. Lastly, the heat generated by curing (especially of large masses of cement) may cause thermonecrosis of surrounding bone and tissues.

The calcium phosphate cements address many of the difficulties encountered with PMMA, but their chalk-like texture and longer set-up time makes them less user-friendly. Calcium phosphates are osteoconductive materials which can be remodelled, incorporated, and eventually replaced by bone. Like PMMA, these cements have been shown to augment pull-out strength in stripped screw holes [36]. Goodman et al. [34] have reported favorably on the initial laboratory and clinical results using osteoconductive cements for the temporary augmentation of hip fracture fixation during bone healing. The design of another type of dynamic hip implant, the Alta hip bolt (Howmedica) facilitates the easy injection of liquid-phase biomaterials through the cannulated and vented plunger-shaped proximal fixation [33]. Prospective studies proving the benefits of such constructs are still necessary. The surgeon is best advised to place his or her implant deep and central in the head, where generally very good purchase can be obtained, even in patients with severe osteopenia.

Prosthetic Replacement

Rarely, prosthetic replacement may be indicated for peritrochanteric fractures [37,38]. If pre-existing symptomatic osteoarthrosis is significant, total joint replacement is warranted. If the fracture involves the head or severely involves the subtrochanteric zone, cemented hemiarthroplasty with possible calcar reconstruction is indicated. The length of the prosthesis should extend beyond the most inferior fracture by at least a length of three canal diameters to limit stress concentration and refracture at the tip of the prosthesis. The complication rates of prosthetic replacement are higher than that of elective replacement (particularly with regard to rate of dislocation and leg length discrepancy) but patient outcome is generally better than when repair of these truly severe fractures is attempted and unsuccessful. Additionally, immediate weightbearing is usually well tolerated.

Difficult Fracture Types in the Elderly

The reverse obliquity intertrochanteric fracture (AO type A3, 1–3) represents a peculiar challenge to the orthopaedist. Because these fractures are generally distal and nearly parallel to the screw placed within the femoral neck, the fragments will not impact into a load-sharing configuration with typical 135° constructs. In fact, the shaft tends to medialize excessively, shortening the extremity without closing the fracture gap. All loads at the fracture zone must be carried by the implant and the tenuous bone-implant interface. Failure rates secondary to cut-out, plate separation from the femoral shaft, and implant fatigue are unacceptable (Fig. 11.5).

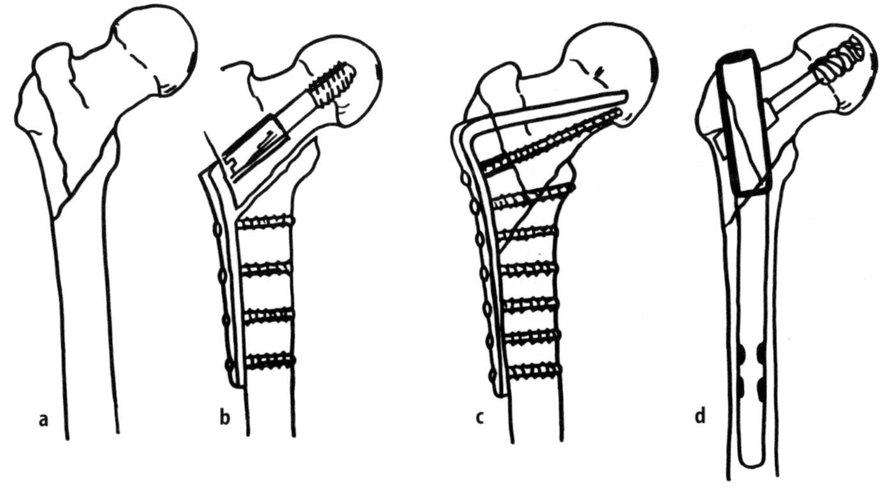

Figure 11.5. **a** Reverse oblique intertrochanteric fracture. Fixation with: **b** compression hip screw, **c** 95° blade plate and **d** an intramedullary hip screw. After Browner et al. Skeletal trauma, vol 2, 2nd edn. Philadephia: Saunders, 1998.

Pertrochanteric fractures with significant subtrochanteric extension are also problematic when a CHS is used. Although traction can usually re-establish anatomical alignment, since the medial cortex is completely incompetent to tolerate compression loads acute, complete collapse of the sliding screw can occur once traction is released. A long plate is required to gain adequate cortical purchase distal to the fracture zone. Cerclage wiring or independent lag screw placement can be attempted, but this has the tendency to further devitalize compromised subtrochanteric vascularity.

Intramedullary devices appear to offer clear advantages for both reverse obliquity and peritrochanteric fractures with subtrochanteric extension. The implant, by virtue of its intramedullary location, buttresses the proximal fragment and limits medial displacement of the shaft as well as offering superior fatigue properties compared with the CHS. In a simple reverse oblique fracture, generally no distal interlocking is required, and this allows for some dynamic impaction in the axis of the shaft. For fractures with subtrochanteric extension, the zone of injury is not violated, and the nail is simply interlocked distally to maintain length and rotational reduction. Full-length versions of intramedullary hip screws are preferred for fractures approaching the isthmus or for any pathological fractures. These semipercutaneous techniques, although challenging, spare the patient the significant dissection required to implant a long enough sideplate to fix the unstable fracture, and generally allow for immediate weightbearing as tolerated.

If an open plating technique is preferred, fixation should be performed with a 95° angled blade plate or dynamic compression screw (DCS). Unlike the CHS, these devices allow for additional screws to be placed into the medial cortex of the proximal fragment as well as a lag screw across the reverse obliquity fracture. They do not allow for any postoperative impaction, however, and therefore if there is moderate medial bone deficiency or devitalization, bone grafting is indicated and weightbearing should be limited to minimize the risk of implant fatigue or failure of the implant-bone interface. Although more technically demanding to insert, there are advantages to fixation with the 95° blade plate over the DCS. The implant is inserted without removing additional bone, and the blade's broad surface resists rotation. This difference may be far more critical in the osteopenic cancellous bone of the elderly person, where fixation failure and proximal fragment migration is often the result of poor screw purchase.

Whether a fracture table is used or the extremity is positioned freely, a preoperatively planned surgical tactic is of critical importance when selecting a 95° device. The surgeon must achieve intraoperative stability without devitalizing the fracture zone, and this demands awareness and consideration of fragments that might better be managed without direct manipulation. Using the normal side as a template, draw the fracture planes of the reduced fragments and the position and appropriate direction of the implant. The sequence of insertion and direction of critical screws should be noted. Is there a greater trochanteric component that requires reduction before seating the blade? A well-conceived and well-drawn plan minimizes the difficulties encountered when the fracture distorts normal surgical landmarks.

Surgical Complications

The vast majority of failures after the fixation of trochanteric fractures with sliding screws are due to screw cut-out and varus collapse. Failure is almost always evident within 3 months, and rates of 10–15% are usually reported [24–26]. Although bone quality, fracture geometry and the accuracy of the reduction achieved have been shown to influence cut-out, appropriate positioning of the screw very deeply and in the center of the head and neck appears to minimize or prevent this mode of failure. In at least one prospective study, cut-out was eliminated by emphasizing the critical step of appropriate screw placement [39]. The frequency of other modes of mechanical failure, such as implant fatigue, disassociation of the screw from the plate, and pull-out of the screws from the femoral shaft when combined, rarely exceed 2–3%. Similarly, low rates of nonunion and infection are to be expected, due to the rich vascularity of the region and the near universal use of effective antibiotic prophylaxis. Femoral shaft fracture at or near the distal tip of the implant is exceedingly rare in hips fixed with sideplates, but is a frequently reported complication when using the Gamma nail [29,40,41]. Treatment invariably requires reoperation, usually with exchange to a full-length nail. It is thought that abnormally high stresses concentrated at the tip of the nail, combined with technical errors inserting the device, are responsible (poor entrance site, excessive force driving the nail, cortical perforations due to missed distal interlocking) [29,32]. Design modifications in the other types of intramedullary hip screws appear to have substantially reduced, but not eliminated this mode of failure [30–32].

Postoperative Management and Outcome

No one has ever shown convincingly that postoperative weightbearing recommendations influence results. Recent work by Koval et al. [42]. suggests that mentally competent patients will self regulate the forces across the fracture zone, increasing load as the fracture unites. They recommended allowing weightbearing as tolerated. In noncompetent patients it may be best simply to limit activity (e.g., bed to chair transfers only) rather than attempt to enforce weightbearing restrictions. Patients should be examined at about 2 weeks after surgery to exclude wound problems, and should have clinical and radiographic checks at 6, 12 and 24 weeks.

The outcomes of patients with trochanteric hip fractures have been extensively studied. Mortality rates range between 14% and 36% within the first year after fracture [43], which exceed the rates for patients with femoral neck fractures. The ambulatory status patients achieve after treatment of their trochanteric hip fracture is a primary determinant of their quality of life. In many cases, the injury presents an insurmountable obstacle to independence that leads to institutionalization. In one study by Koval et al. [44], 92% of 336 patients who were community ambulators before hip fracture regained ambulatory status after treatment. However, despite adequate follow-up, less than half (41%) were able to return to their preoperative level of functioning, with the remainder losing some degree of independence. Outcomes even less favorable are to be expected if only considering severely osteoporotic patients with unstable trochanteric fractures.

There are numerous obstacles to the successful management of the osteoporotic patient with an unstable trochanteric fracture. The surgeon must consider the effect that the particular fracture pattern and bone quality will have on the strength of the proposed bone/implant construct. Mental or physical comorbidities may influence the patient's ability to undergo repair and actively engage in rehabilitation. Nonetheless, current implants and techniques, carefully selected and implanted with attention to surgical detail, can be expected to achieve and maintain anatomically aligned mechanical stability long enough for surviving patients to heal their fractures.

References

1. Ward FO. Human anatomy. London: Renshaw, 1838.
2. Singh M, Nagrath AR, Maini PS. Changes in trabecular pattern of the upper end of the femur as an index of osteoporosis. J Bone Joint Surg Am 1970;52:457–467.
3. Khairi MRA, Cronin JH, Robb JA, Smith DM, Yu PL, Johnston CC. Femoral trabecular pattern index and bone mineral content measurment by photon absorption in senile osteoporosis. J Bone Joint Surg Am 1976;58:221.
4. Noble PC, Alexander JW, Lindahl LJ. The anatomic basis of femoral component design. Clin Orthop 1988; 235:148.
5. Rizzo PF, Gould ES, Lyden JP, Asnis SE. Diagnosis of occult fractures about the hip. Magnetic resonance imaging compared with bone-scanning [see comments]. J Bone and Joint Surg Am 1993;75:395–401.
6. Jensen JS, Michaelsen M. Trochanteric femoral fractures treated with McLaughlin osteosynthesis. Acta Orthop Scand 1975;46:795–803.
7. Evans EM. Trochanteric fractures. J Bone and Joint Surg Br 1951;33:192–204.
8. Kyle RF, Gustilo RB, Premer RF. Analysis of 622 intertrochanteric hip fractures. J Bone and Joint Surg Am 1979;61:216–221.
9. Müller ME, Nazarian S, Koch P, Schatzker J. The comprehensive classification of fractures of long bones. Berlin Heidelberg New York: Springer, 1990.
10. Hornby R, Evans JG, Vardon V. Operative or conservative treatment for trochanteric fractures of the femur. A randomised epidemiological trial in elderly patients. J Bone Joint Surg Br 1989;71:619–623.
11. Lyon LJ, Nevins MA. Nontreatment of hip fractures in senile patients. JAMA 1977; 238:1175–1176.
12. Zuckerman JD, Skovron ML, Koval KJ, Aharonoff G, Frankel VH. Postoperative complications and mortality associated with operative delay in older patients who have a fracture of the hip. J Bone Joint Surg Am 1995;77:1551–1556.
13. Rogers FB, Shackford SR, Keller MS. Early fixation reduces morbidity and mortality in elderly patients with hip fractures from low-impact falls. J Trauma 1995;39:261–265.
14. Kaufer H. Mechanics of the treatment of hip injuries. Clin Orthop 1980;146:53–61.
15. Levy RN, Siegel M, Sedlin ED, Siffert RS. Complications of Ender-pin fixation in basicervical, intertrochanteric, and subtrochanteric fractures of the hip. J Bone Joint Surg 1983;65:66–69.
16. MacEachern AG, Heyse-Moore GH. Stable intertrochanteric femoral fractures: a misnomer? J Bone Joint Surg Br 1983;65:582–583.
17. Moehring HD, Nowinski GP, Chapman MW, Voigtlander JP. Irreducible intertrochanteric fractures of the femur. Clin Orthop 1997;339:197–199.
18. Dimon JHD. The unstable intertrochanteric fracture. Clin Orthop 1973;92:100–107.
19. Sarmiento A, Williams EM. The unstable intertrochanteric fracture: treatment with a valgus osteotomy and I-beam nail-plate. A preliminary report of one hundred cases. J Bone Joint Surg Am 1970;52:1309–1318.
20. Roberts A, Rooney T, Loone J. A comparison of the functional results of anatomic and medial displacement valgus nailing of intertrochanteric fractures of the femur. J Trauma 1972;12:341.
21. Desjardins AL, Roy A, Paiement G, Newman N, Pedlow F, Desloges D, et al. Unstable intertrochanteric fracture of the femur. A prospective randomised study comparing anatomical reduction and medial displacement osteotomy. J Bone Joint Surg Br 1993;75: 445–457.
22. Gargan MF, Gundle R, Simpson AH. How effective are osteotomies for unstable intertrochanteric fractures? J Bone Joint Surg Br 1994;76:789–792.
23. Chang WS, Zuckerman JD, Kummer FJ, Frankel VH. Biomechanical evaluation of anatomic reduction versus medial displacement osteotomy in unstable intertrochanteric fractures. Clin Orthop 1987;225:141–146.

24. Baumgaertner MR, Curtin SL, Lindskog DM, Keggi JM. The value of the tip-apex distance in predicting failure of fixation of peritrochanteric fractures of the hip. J Bone Joint Surg Am 1995;77:1058–1064.
25. Madsen JE, Naess L, Aune AK, Alho A, Ekeland A, Stromsoe K. Dynamic hip screw with trochanteric stabilizing plate in the treatment of unstable proximal femoral fractures: a comparative study with the gamma nail and compression hip screw. J Orthop Trauma 1998;12:241–248.
26. Watson JT, Moed BR, Cramer KE, Karges DE. Comparison of the compression hip screw with the Medoff sliding plate for intertrochanteric fractures. Clin Orthop 1998; 348:79–86.
27. Lunsjo K, Ceder L, Stigsson L, Hauggaard A. One-way compression along the femoral shaft with the Medoff sliding plate. The first European experience of 104 intertrochanteric fractures with a 1-year follow-up. Acta Orthop Scand 1995;66:343–346.
28. Jensen JS, Sonne-Holm S. Critical analysis of Ender nailing in the treatment of trochanteric fractures. Acta Orthop Scand 1980;51:817–825.
29. Parker MJ, Pryor GA. Gamma versus DHS nailing for extracapsular femoral fractures. Meta-analysis of ten randomised trials. Int Orthop 1996;20:163–168.
30. Rantanen J, Hannu TA. Intramedullary fixation of high subtrochanteric femoral fractures: a study comparing two designs, the gamma nail and the intramedullary hip screw. J Orthop Trauma 1998;12:249–252.
31. Hardy DC, Descamps PY, Krallis P, Fabeck L, Smets P, Bertens CL, et al. Use of an intramedullary hip-screw compared with a compression hip-screw with a plate for intertrochanteric femoral fractures. A prospective, randomized study of 100 patients. J Bone Joint Surg Am 1998;80:618–630.
32. Baumgaertner MR, Curtin SL, Lindskog DM. Intramedullary versus extramedullary fixation for the treatment of intertrochanteric hip fractures. Clin Orthop 1998;348: 87–94.
33. Choueka J, Koval KJ, Kummer FJ, Crawford G, Zuckerman JD. Biomechanical comparison of the sliding hip screw and the dome plunger. J Bone Joint Surg Br 1995;77: 277–283.
34. Goodman SB, Carter D, Goldstein SA, Larsson S, Swiontkowski MF, Yetkinler DN. Norian SRS cement augmentation in hip fracture treatment. Clin Orthop 1998;348: 42–50.
35. Schatzker J, Ha'eri GB, Chapman M. Methylmethacrylate as an adjunct in the internal fixation of intertrochanteric fractures of the femur. J Trauma 1978;18:732–735.
36. Mermelstein LE, Chow LC, Friedman C, Crisco JJ III. The reinforcement of cancellous bone screws with calcium phosphate cement. J. Orthop Trauma 1996;10:15–20.
37. Haentjens P, Casteleyn PP, De Boeck H, Handelberg F, Opdecam P. Treatment of unstable intertrochanteric and subtrochanteric fractures in elderly patients. Primary bipolar arthroplasty compared with internal fixation. J Bone Joint Surg Am 1989;71: 1214–1225.
38. Vahl AC, Dunki Jacobs PB, Patka P, Haarman HJ. Hemiarthroplasty in elderly, debilitated patients with an unstable femoral fracture in the trochanteric region. Acta Orthop Belg 1994;60:274–279.
39. Baumgaertner MR, Solberg BD. Awareness of tip-apex distance reduces failure of fixation of trochanteric fractures of the hip. J Bone Joint Surg Br 1997;79:969–971.
40. Radford PJ, Needoff M, Webb JK. A prospective randomised comparison of the dynamic hip screw and the gamma locking nail. J Bone Joint Surg Br 1993;75:789–793.
41. Bridle SH, Patel AD, Bircher M, Calvert PT. Fixation of intertrochanteric fractures of the femur. A randomised prospective comparison of the gamma nail and the dynamic hip screw. J Bone Joint Surg 1991;73:330–334.
42. Koval KJ, Sala DA, Kummer FJ, Zuckerman JD. Postoperative weight-bearing after a fracture of the femoral neck or an intertrochanteric fracture. J Bone Joint Surg Am 1998;80:352–356.

43. White BL, Fisher WD, Laurin CA. Rate of mortality for elderly patients after fracture of the hip in the 1980s. J Bone Joint Surg Am 1987;69:133540.
44. Koval KJ, Skovron ML, Aharonoff GB, Meadows SE, Zuckerman JD. Ambulatory ability after hip fracture. A prospective study in geriatric patients. Clin Orthop 1995;310: 150–159.

12 Subtrochanteric Fractures of the Femur

R. Hoffmann and S. Kolbeck

Introduction

Fractures of the proximal femur occur predominantly in elderly patients and have a tremendous impact on the health care system. Approximately 250 000 fractures of the proximal femur occur in the United States each year [1], and this number is projected to double by the year 2050 as the population ages [2]. Osteoporosis, higher age, vestibular disease, vertigo, dementia, malignant tumor and cardiopulmonary disease are all associated with an increased risk of fractures of the proximal femur. With a rising prevalence of these fractures in a population of a growing average age, the incidence of these fractures in young people is also increasing. In the elderly these fractures are generally the result of low-energy trauma caused by a single fall. In young patients, in contrast, fractures around the hip and proximal femur fractures mainly occur with high-energy trauma and are generally associated with multiple injuries. Despite marked improvements in implant designs and surgical techniques, these fractures consume a substantial proportion of the health care resources. These facts demonstrate the importance of proximal femoral fractures both for the single patient and for society in general.

General Considerations

The subtrochanteric region of the femur extends from the lesser trochanter to the proximal third of the femoral shaft. It is an area of high mechanical stress concentration on a small area of bone [3]. Eccentric loads act on the proximal femur with high compressive forces on the medial and high tensile forces on the lateral cortex. In addition the abductor muscles [gluteal muscles] increase these stress values and create together with the hip flexor muscles [iliopsoas] and the external rotators the typical displacement of the proximal fragment resulting in abduction, external rotation and flexion. The distal fragment is typically displaced to the medial side by the strong pull of the adductors [4].

Subtrochanteric fractures occur both in young and in elderly patients. The mechanism of injury is usually direct trauma to the proximal femur. Older patients often suffer from a minor fall in which the subtrochanteric fracture may occur through osteoporotic bone. In addition, these fractures often occur without any adequate trauma in metastatic bone disease of geriatric patients. To sustain a subtrochanteric fracture of the femur younger patients with normal bone densitiy are typically involved in high-energy trauma, such as a fall from a great height or a motor vehicle accident. These patients then have a high incidence of multiple-system injuries.

Conservative treatment of subtrochanteric fractures is lengthy, prone to systemic complications, and overall unsatisfactory because of the high mechanical stresses which predispose to a high rate of failure. Allis [5], already in 1891, recognized the complications of shortening, angular deformity and rotational malalignment that often result after conservative treatment of these fractures.

Different systems of classification of subtrochanteric fractures have been described. The most common are the Seinsheimer classification [6], based on the number of fragments and the location and number of fractures lines, and the AO/ASIF classification [7], based on the degree of comminution. Seinsheimer included four types, with type I being the most proximal and type IV the most distal. Each type is divided into subtypes A, B and C, with A being the most stable and C the most unstable subtype. In the AO/ASIF classification the subtrochanteric fractures are part of the classifaction for the femur diaphysis. These fractures are divided into simple A fractures (spiral, oblique and transverse), wedged B fractures (spiral wedge, bending wedge, fragmented wedge) and comminuted C fractures (complex and segmental fractures).

The timing of any procedure depends on the patient's overall condition and in young patients, especially in polytrauma, surgery has to be performed on an emergency basis. In some cases a temporary external fixator may be indicated prior to a secondary definitive treatment. In a single injury definitive surgery should be carried out without further delay. In geriatric patients with low-energy trauma special care has to be taken with regard to hydration and cardiac disregulation. These patients are best put into traction initially and prepared for surgery on an intensive care unit. Surgery should usually then be possible within 24 h.

Surgical Treatment

Anteroposterior and lateral radiographs of the whole femur are necessary to assess and classify the fracture completely. Additional radiographs of the pelvis are mandatory to rule out associated dislocations of the hip or pelvic fractures. For exact operative planning radiographs of the contralateral femur may be very helpful, especially for C-type fractures to assess the real length of the femur [8].

A great variety of intra- and extramedullary implants is available for internal fixation of subtrochanteric fractures. Condylar blade plate systems or Dynamic Condylar Screw (DCS) systems are still in use in many places [9–11]. Modern implantation techniques of these devices preserve the vascularity of the medial wall fragments using a "no touch" approach, avoiding any attempt at anatomical reduction of these intermediate fragments [9]. This leads to a "biological" bridging of the fracture zone with favorably longer plates and spares the need for bone grafting of the medial cortex. However, the application of angled blade plate systems is technically very demanding and asks for advanced surgical skills and experience [12].

This is a main cause for a steady increase in the use of intramedullary fixation devices, since a majority of surgeons feel more comfortable with this type of implant for these difficult fractures [8]. Also, intramedullary nail systems usually preserve the fracture vascularity better and offer marked biomechanical advantages over

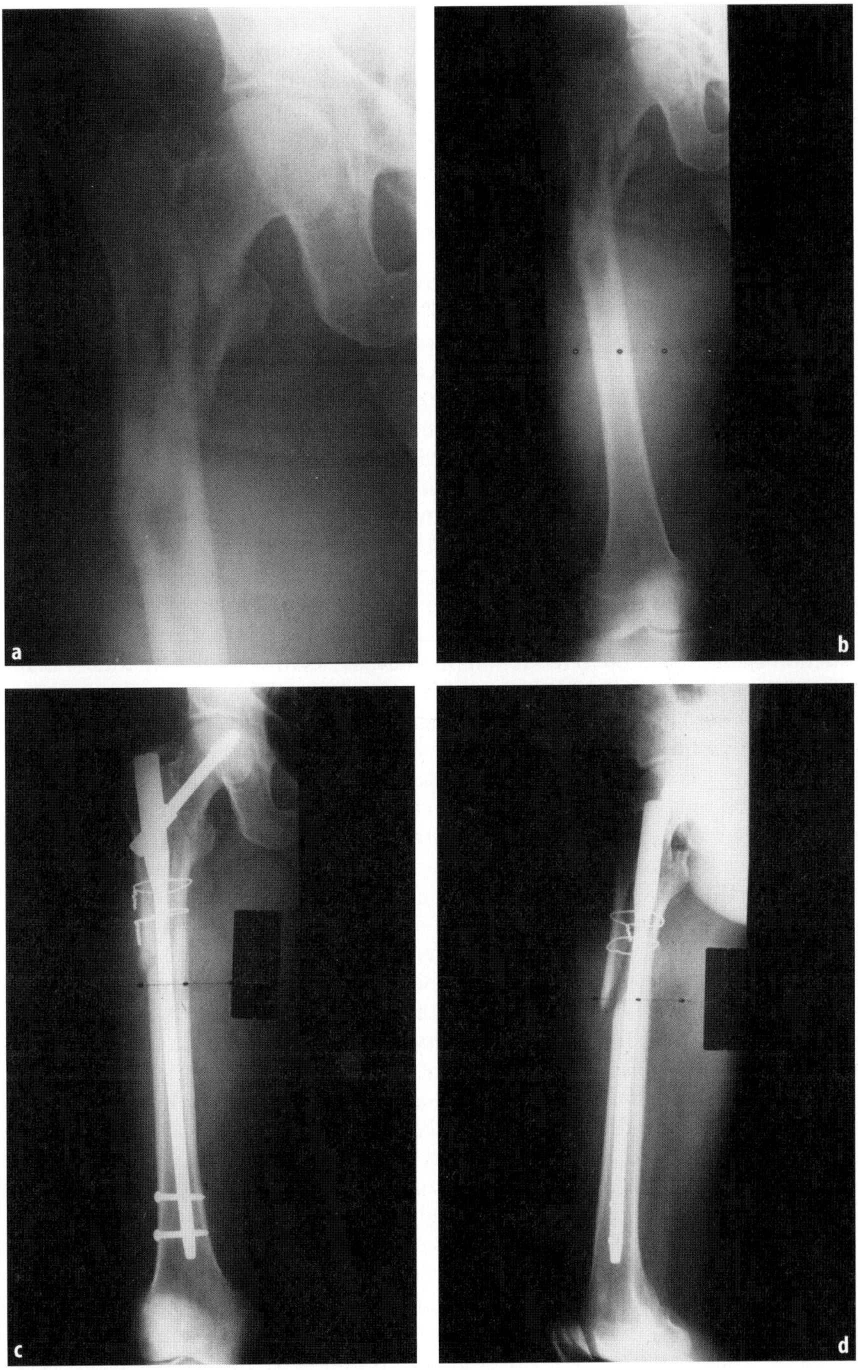

Figure 12.1a–d. Comminuted proximal femur fracture (inter-/subrochanteric] in a 72-year-old man: internal fixation with IMHS (Classic Nail) and cerclage wires through a limited open approach.

plates [13,14]. According to the anatomy of the fracture regular interlocking rods, reconstruction nails or regular or long-shaft intramedullary hip screw (IMHS) devices may be used (Fig.12.1). Usually strong solid nail systems such as the second generation reconstruction nails or the IMHS that offer a proximal locking option into the femoral neck-head area are preferable [15–23]. However, proper implantation of these devices in subtrochanteric fractures is far from easy, and the demands on the operative technique are often underestimated. Mistakes in surgical technique or indication combined with suboptimal implant design or biomechanics may lead to intraoperative or postoperative failure of fixation [24–30].

The AO/ASIF offers five implants for fixation of subtrochanteric fractures. Standard extramedullary devices are the 95° condylar blade plate or the DCS. The Dynamic Hip Screw (DHS) may be considered in few selected cases but carries potential dangers and techincal problems, especially in presence of comminution in the area of the greater trochanter or the entry point of the hip screw [8]. Operation is best carried out on a regular radiolucent operating table with the complete extremity draped sterile and flexible. Preoperative planning is indispensable and includes a sketch of the osteosynthesis with the help of the radiographs and special templates. Also the steps in reduction and the surgical tactic have to planned in advance. The lateral approach to the femur must be as limited as possible and care must be taken to preserve the vascularity of medial wall and intermediate fragments. Fracture reduction is performed indirectly by manipulation of the leg. Temporary Schanz screws in the main fragments, a distractor and carefully used reduction clamps may aid in reduction. In marked osteoporosis of the elderly manipulation has to be especially subtle to avoid cutting out or breaking in of the reduction aids. Careful soft tissue handling is paramount, avoiding surgical bone stripping and minimizing the insertion of soft tissue retractors whenever possible. The intraoperative use of an image intensifier usually proves very helpful. Simple fracture types must be reduced anatomically. In comminuted fractures the principles of a bridging osteosynthesis apply with restoration of length, axis and rotation of the femur. This can be checked for intraoperatively without major effort if the methods described by Krettek et al [31] are applied. No attempt is made to reduce intermediate fragments anatomically. Thus, there is no need for primary bone grafting. The proximal main fragment should safely be engaged by the blade/screw of the system. An additional large fragment screw into the proximal fragment through the plate is indispensable. The distal shaft fragment has to be fixed to the plate with four bicortical screws. In poor bone quality the use of cancellous screws may sometimes be more appropriate than the use of cortical screws. The use of bone cement in the screw holes may add to the purchase of the screws in severe osteoporosis. Disadvantages of the extramedullary devices in comparison with the intramedullary devices are the usually more extensive surgical approach and a longer operation time, both resulting in a higher blood loss. Furthermore, in contrast to the nail systems postoperative unrestricted weightbearing is not achievable with plate systems in most cases. This is clearly an advantage for the intramedullary devices, especially in uncompliant or geriatric patients.

AO/ASIF intramedullary devices for subtrochanteric fractures are the AO-Titanium Nail (UFN) (Fig. 12.2), a reconstruction nail with modular proximal locking options, and the Proximal Femoral Nail (PFN) (Fig. 12.3), which is a second-generation IMHS system. Both systems come in different lengths, diameters and angles for proximal locking into the femoral neck-head area. The UFN has a proximal spiral blade locking option into the femoral neck. The spiral blade is fixed into the

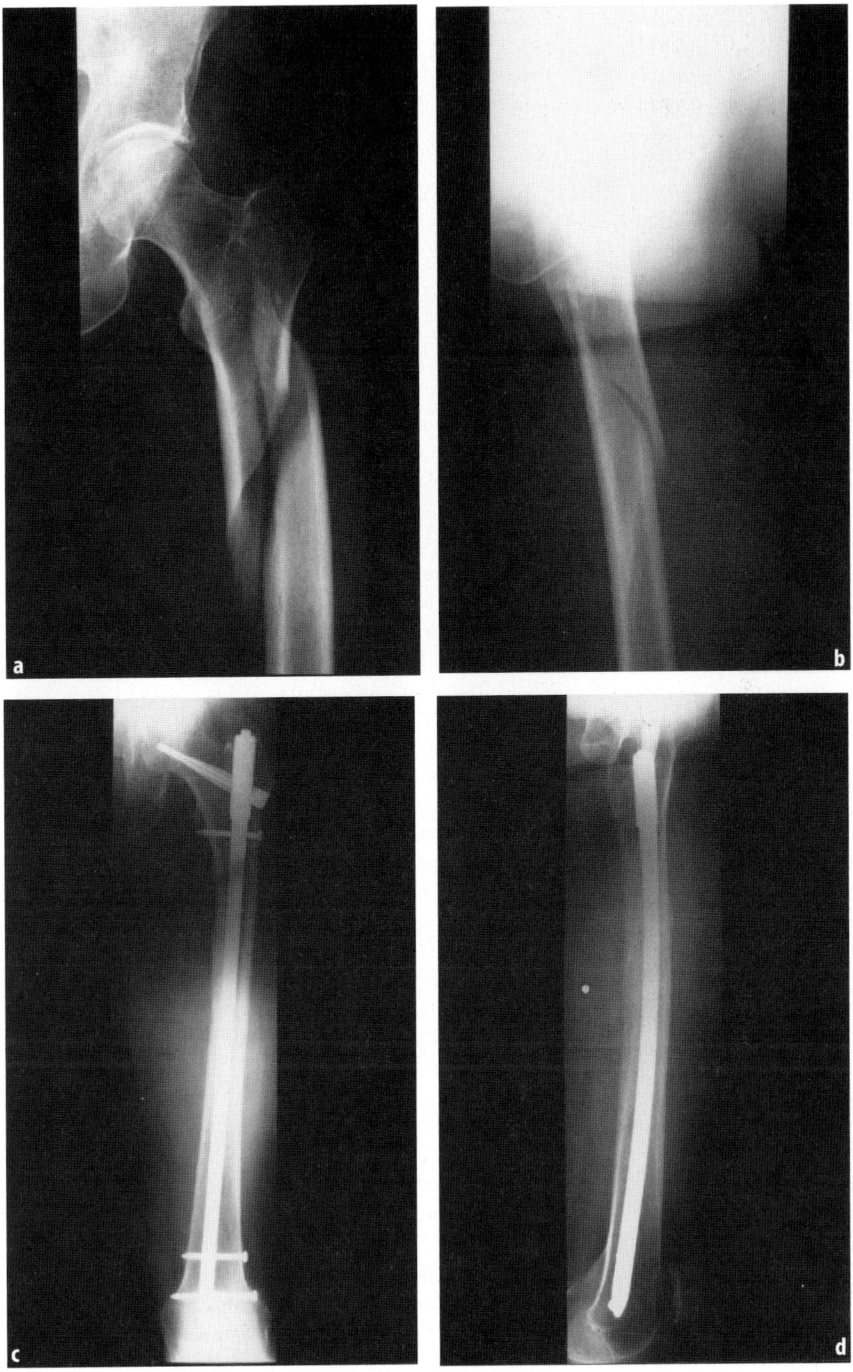

Figure 12.2a–d. Subtrochanteric spiral fracture of the femur in an 82-year-old man: internal fixation with an Unreamed Femoral Nail (UFN) plus proximal spiral blade locking.

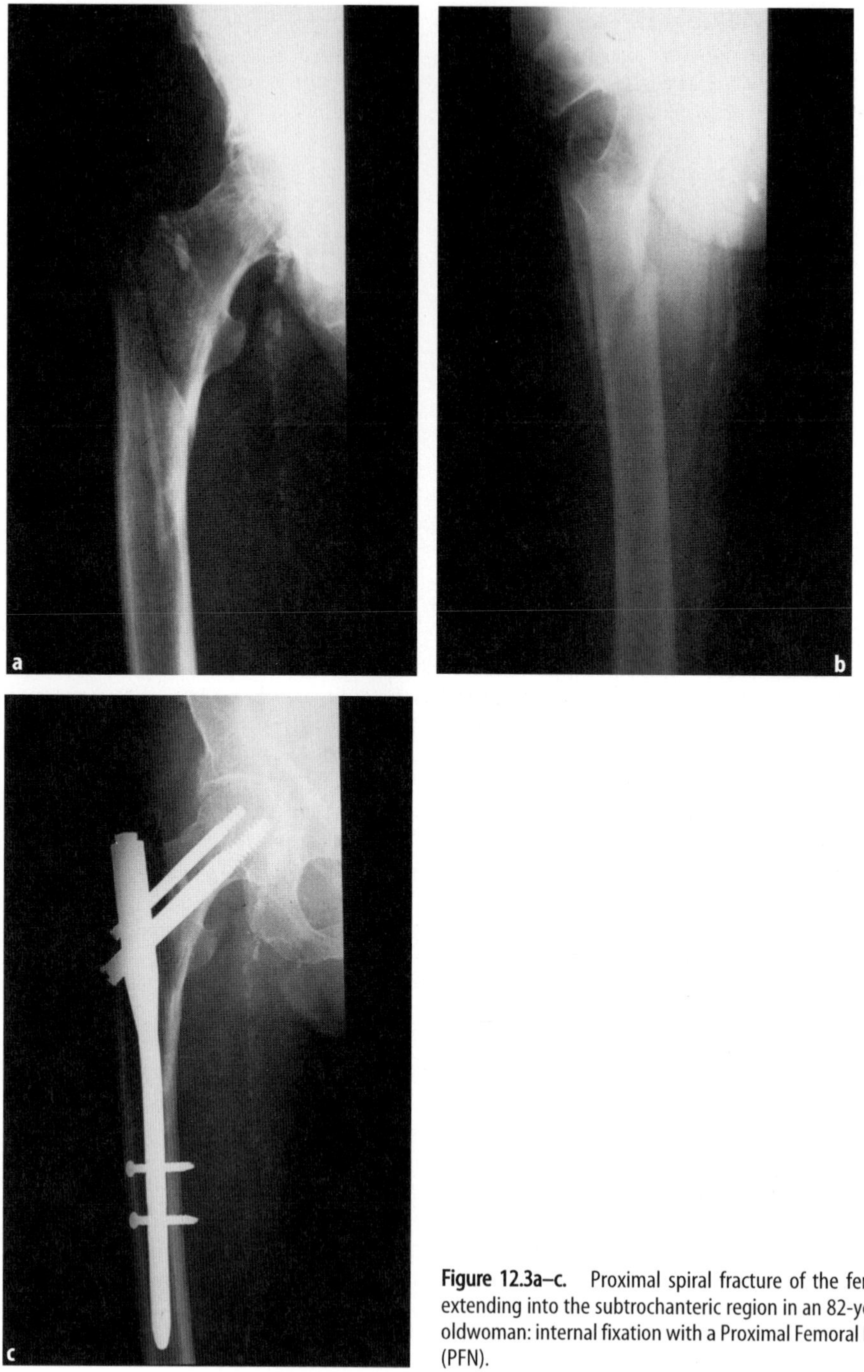

Figure 12.3a–c. Proximal spiral fracture of the femur extending into the subtrochanteric region in an 82-year-oldwoman: internal fixation with a Proximal Femoral Nail (PFN).

nail by special sleeves that are pushed over the end of the nail prior to nail insertion. These sleeves determine the angle of blade insertion and provide angular stability to the spiral blade in the nail. The handling of the implant is facilitated by radiolucent insertion and targeting handles. The PFN features a proximal double screw locking mode into the femoral neck. Both canulated screws are inserted parallel through radiolucent targeting handles. Thus rotational stability and a potential for dynamic gliding of the neck fragment is insured. For both implants preoperative planning with, in particular, determination of the proximal locking angles, nail length and diameter is strongly advisable. In elderly patients with marked osteoporosis and a wide medullary cavitiy of the shaft, a large-diameter nail is preferable.

Although preliminary results with the UFN and spiral blade locking in subtrochanteric fractures have been favorable [8,16], some concerns regarding indications and biomechanical characteristics of the device exist [24,32]. In addition the PFN seems to be easier to apply for most surgeons. In particular, the proximal entry point of the nail is much easier to hit with the PFN than with the UFN. Also postoperative weightbearing seems to be safer with the biomechanically stronger PFN, which is especially important in geriatric patients. For these reasons the PFN is increasingly becoming the AO/ASIF implant of choice for most surgeons who treat subtrochanteric fractures of the femur.

Operation for both implants can be carried out on a fracture table with some traction to the leg or on a radiolucent regular operating table. The latter is preferred in the authors' own practice. Preoperatively undisturbed intraoperative X-ray control with the image intensifier has to be checked before draping the patient sterile. Since the proximal main fragment is usually malaligned in external rotation, flexion and abduction, correct opening of the medullary canal is not easy. Great care must be taken not only to hit the entry point correctly but also to open the medullary canal in its exact axis. This must be checked for under image intensification in both planes and is one of the crucial parts of the whole procedure since it will mainly determine further correct or malalignment. Nail insertion can be accomplished over small or limited lateral approaches to the proximal femur. A limited approach down to the tip of the proximal fragment may aid in reduction und thus in correct opening of the medullary canal. In addition temporary Schanz screws inserted as "joysticks" into the main fragments can help in fragment manipulation and fracture reduction. The fracture can also be reduced with the help of the nail. The proximal fragment can be manipulated with the partially inserted nail and be aligned to the distal shaft fragment. In osteoporosis or marked comminution this may be dangerous, since especially the posterior wall fragments might break out of the proximal fragment. Reduction will then be far more difficult. It seems more appropriate to manipulate the proximal fragment only lightly with the nail and rather realign the distal shaft fragment to the tip of the nail. Blown-out proximal medial wall fragments may be realigned with the help of cerclage wires (Fig. 12.1, 12.4). This can easily be accomplished if the leg has been draped flexible. As with the extramedullary implants, simple fracture types should be reduced anatomically, while comminuted fractures should be realigned with restoration of length, axis and rotation [31]. This can easily be controlled intraoperatively if the contralateral leg is also draped sterile and flexible. The distal locking of the implants is routinely performed with two locking bolts.

In conclusion, intramedullary devices offer marked advantages in the fixation of subtrochanteric fractures. They are preferable not only in osteoporosis but also in metastatic bone disease of the femur shaft and the subtrochanteric region [33,34].

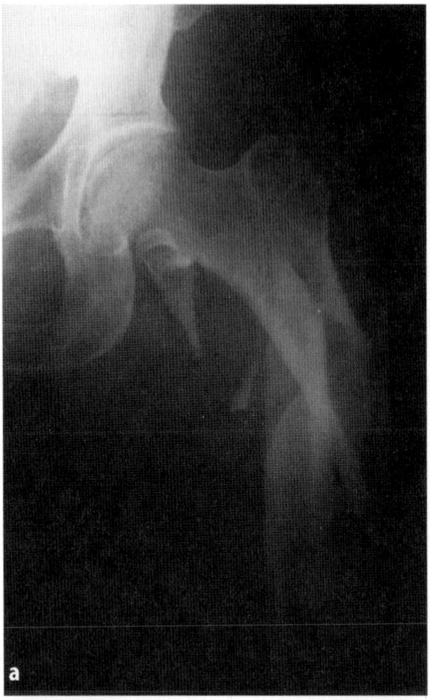

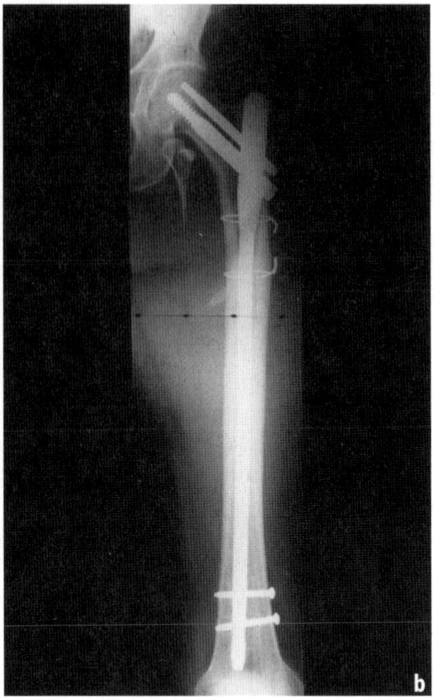

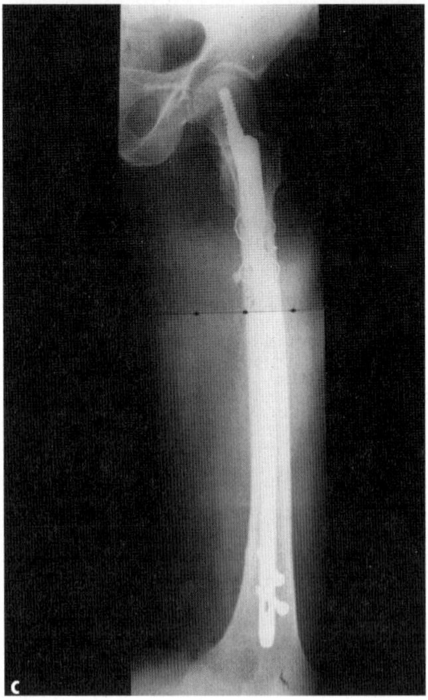

Figure 12.4a–c. Subtrochanteric fracture of the femur in a 64-year-oldwoman: internal fixation with a long Proximal Femoral Nail (PFN) and cerclage wires through a limited open approach.

Postoperative Treatment

Depending on the general condition of the patient remobilization starts on the first or second postoperative day with bedside sitting, followed by walking in a walker or on crutches. In elderly patients the stability of fixation achieved should allow for unrestricted weightbearing since such patients have the most limited compliance. This is better achieved with intramedullary devices rather than with extramedullary plate systems. Isometric muscle exercises should be started as soon as possible and special attention paid to the abductor muscle function. CPM machines can aid in preventing muscular adhesions in the femur shaft area. Analgesic drugs should be provided to facilitate mobilization. Bone healing should be completed after 3–5 months. If the implants are used correctly, all work properly even in marked osteoporosis. If failure of fixation or loss of reduction occurs, however, the choice of how to proceed is related to the mode of failure, the bone quality and the age and demands of the patient. In younger patients a repeated internal fixation is considered when the head still has good bone stock and intact cartilage, and is still vital. In geriatric patients a re-osteosynthesis may be considered on a case-by-case basis; however, an arthroplasty with long stem shaft components is often the more appropriate salvage procedure.

References

1. Praemer A, Furner S, Rice DP, editors. Musculoskeletal conditions in the United States. Park Ridge, IL: The American Academy of Orthopaedic Surgeons, 1992.
2. Frandsen PA, Kruse T. Hip fractures in the county of Funen, Denmark. Implications of demographic aging and changes in incidence rates. Acta Orthop Scand 1983;54:681–686.
3. Koch JC. The laws of bone architecture. Am J Anat 1917;21:177–298.
4. Froimsen AI. Treatment of comminuted subtrochanteric fractures of the femur. Surg Gynecol Obstet 1970;131:465–472.
5. Allis OH. Fractures in the upper third of the femur exclusive of the neck. Med News 1891;59:585–590.
6. Seinsheimer F III. Subtrochanteric fractures of the femur. J Bone Joint Surg.Am 1978;60:300–306.
7. Müller ME, Allgöwer M, Schneider R, Willenegger H.. Manual of internal fixation, 3rd ed. Berlin Heidelberg New York: Springer, 1991.
8. Hoffmann R, Südkamp NP, Schütz M, Raschke M, Haas NP. [Update on internal fixation of subtrochanteric fractures]. Unfallchirurg 1996;99:240–248.
9. Kinast C, Bollhofner BR, Mast JW, Ganz R. Subtrochanteric fractures of the femur. results of treatment with the 95° condylar blade plate. Clin Orthop 1989;238:122–130.
10. Nungu KS, Olerud, C., Rehnberg L. Treatment of subtrochanteric fractures with the AO dynamic condylar screw. Injury 1993;24:90–92.
11. Warwick DJ, Crichlow TPKR, Langkamer VG, Jackson M. The dynamic condylar screw in the management of subtrochanteric fractures of the femur. Injury 1995;26:241–244.
12. Schatzker J, Wadell JP. Subtrochanteric fractures of the femur. Orthop Clin North Am 1980;11:539–554.
13. Tencer AF, Johnson KD, Johnston DWC, Gill K. A biomechanical comparison of various methods of stabilization of subtrochanteric fractures of the femur. J Orthop Res 1984;2:297–305.
14. Pugh KJ, Morgan RA, Gorczyca JT, Pienkowski D. A mechanical comparison of subtrochanteric femur fracture fixation. J Orthop Trauma 1998;5:324–329.

15. Aronoff PM, Davis PM, Wickstrom JK: Intramedullary nail fixation as treatment of subtrochanteric fractures of the femur. J. Trauma 1971;11:637–650.
16. Hoffmann R, Südkamp NP, Müller CA, Schütz M, Haas NP. [Internal fixation of proximal femur fractures with the modular interlocking device of the ASIF unreamed femoral nail: first clinical results]. Unfallchirurg 1994;97:568–574.
17. Chi-Chuan W, Chun-Hsiung S, Zhon-Liau L. Subtrochanteric fractures treated with interlocking nailing. J Trauma 1991;31:326–333.
18. Wiss DA, Brien WW. Subtrochanteric fractures of the femur. results of treatment by interlocking nailing. Clin Orthop 1992;283:231–236.
19. Kang S, McAndrew MP, Johnson KD. The reconstruction locked nail for complex fractures of the proximal femur. J Orthop Trauma 1995;9:453–463.
20. Ratanen J, Aro HT. Intramedullary fixation of high subtrochanteric femoral fractures: a study comparing two implant designs, the gamma nail and the intramedullary hip screw. J Orthop Trauma 1998;12:249–252.
21. Chevally F, Gamba D. Gamma nailing of pertrochanteric and subtrochanteric fractures: clinical results of a series of 63 consecutive cases. J Orthop Trauma 1997;11: 412–415..
22. Alvarez JR, Gonzolez RC, Aranda RL, Blanco MF, Dehesa MC. Indications for use of the long gamma nail. Clin Orthop 1998;350:62–66.
23. Parker MJ, Dutta BK, Sivaji C, Pryor GA. Subtrochanteric fractures of the femur. Injury 1997;28:91–95.
24. Broos PLO, Reynders P, Vanderspeeten K. Mechanical complications associated with the use of the unreamed AO femoral intramedullary nail with spiral blade: first experience with 35 consecutive cases. J Orthop Trauma 1998;12:186–189.
25. Lindsey RW, Teal P, Probe RA, Rhoads D, Davenport S, Schauder K. Early experience with the gamma interlocking nail for peritrochanteric fractures of the proximal femur. J Trauma 1991;31:1649–1658.
26. Stapert JWJL, Geesing CLM, Dunki Jacobs PB, de Wit RJ. First experience and complications with the long gamma nail. J Trauma 1993;34:394–400.
27. Zickel RE. An intramedullary fixation device for the proximal part of the femur. Nine years′ experience. J Bone Joint Surg Am 1976;58:866–872.
28. Bergman GD, Winquist RA, Mayo KA, Hansen Jr ST. Subtrochanteric fracture of the femur. fixation using the zickel nail. J Bone Joint Surg Am 1987;69:1032–1040.
29. Ovadia DN, Chess JL. Intraoperative and postoperative subtrochanteric fracture of the femur associated with removal of the Zickel nail. J Bone Joint Surg Am 1988;70:239–243.
30. Yelton C, Low W. Iatrogenic subtrochanteric fracture: a complication of Zickel nail. J Bone Joint Surg Am 1986;68:1237–1240.
31. Krettek Ch, Miclau T, Grün O, Schandelmaier P, Tscherne H. Intraoperative control of axes, rotation and length in femoral and tibial fractures. Technical note. Injury 1998;Suppl 3:29–39.
32. Wheeler DL, Croy TJ, Woll TS, Scott MD, Senft DC, Duwelius PJ. Comparison of reconstruction nails for high subtrochanteric femur fracture fixation. Clin Orthop 1997;338: 231–239.
33. Karachalios T, Atkins RM, Sarangi PP, Crichlow TPKR, Solomon L. Reconstruction nailing for pathological subtrochanteric fractures with coexisting femoral shaft metastases. J Bone Joint Surg Br 1993;75:119–122.
34. Hoffmann R, Melcher I, Wichelhaus A, Haas NP. Surgical treatment of bone metastases in breast cancer. Anticancer Res 1998;18:2234–2250.

WRIST FRACTURE

13 Colles' and Dorsal Barton's Fractures

S. L. Olmsted and R. M. Szabo

Introduction

The Colles' fracture, first described in 1814 by Abraham Colles [1], is one of the most common injuries seen in the elderly osteoporotic patient. Much has been published on this injury, yet predicted outcome and treatment remain controversial. Historically authors have considered all fractures of the distal radius as a single entity. More recently, careful examination of the injury has led us to appreciate several different groups of patients that require different treatment, as well as several fracture patterns, which may behave differently. The specific group of patients addressed in this chapter is that of the elderly severely osteoporotic patient.

Epidemiology

Distal radius fractures are the most common fracture involving the upper extremity and comprise 15% of all fractures [2]. Postmenopausal osteoporosis has been implicated as a significant risk factor for sustaining distal radius fractures; however, some studies have challenged this idea, claiming the mineral content of age-matched controls is similar [3,4]. Recent studies have demonstrated a significant difference in bone density using the second metacarpal index comparing age-matched controls [5,6]. Bone mineral density values of the spine, hip and distal forearm of 111 patients with distal radius fractures were compared with those of age-matched controls and found to be significantly lower at all sites [7]. There is also a significant increase in the incidence of distal radius fractures in women over 50 years of age, and almost 85% of all distal radius fractures occur in women [8]. Epidemiological studies in Scandinavia have demonstrated an age-related increase in distal radius fractures in women; however, there is only a slightly increased incidence in men [9,10]. Several factors other than osteoporosis have been offered as explanations for the age-related increase in fractures, including gait disturbances, poor vision, diminished muscle strength, decreased range of motion and reaction time. All of these may contribute to the frequency of falls [11–13]. Fractures seen in the osteoporotic patient frequently result from ordinarily minor fall. Bone strength depends not only on the bone mass, but also on a variety of qualitative aspects of bone structure and architecture [14]. The two ultimate determinants of fracture occurrence are *bone strength* and the *propensity for trauma.* Because elderly patients with severe osteoporosis may have other comorbidities which place them at risk for falls, fractures of the distal radius have been endemic to this patient population [13].

Clinical Presentation

The most common mechanism of injury in this patient population is a fall onto an outstretched upper extremity from a standing or sitting height. Typically, a patient lands with the wrist extended, striking their palm as they attempt to break their fall. Clinical evaluation should include a thorough history of the fall to rule out underlying metabolic, cardiovascular or neurological causes for the fall. A history of head trauma or loss of consciousness should be inquired about. The examination should include the entire patient and particularly the entire upper extremity, as the energy of the fall is transmitted proximally and patients with osteoporosis can often have concomitant fractures. The distal forearm will typically have dorsal swelling and may have gross deformity represented by dorsal angulation, radial deviation and shortening. Careful neurovascular examination should be included since patients with distal radius fractures may sustain nerve contusions or develop compression neuropathies. Patients with median nerve dysfunction may require carpal tunnel pressure measurements to differentiate nerve contusion from acute carpal tunnel syndrome. Nerve contusions may be observed, while acute carpal tunnel syndrome requires immediate operative decompression. Untreated nerve compression or injury is a major factor in the later development of reflex sympathetic dystrophy [15,16].

Radiographic Examination

The radiographic examination should include a true lateral and posteroanterior (PA) view of the distal forearm and wrist. Oblique views may also provide valuable information. Additional radiographs of the elbow and shoulder may be necessary if injury is suspected or cannot be ruled out. In order to assess true ulnar variance and thus the amount of radial shortening, the PA radiographs are taken with the shoulder abducted to 90° and the elbow flexed 90° in neutral pronosupination. The PA film is assessed for radial inclination and radial length. The lateral film is assessed for palmar tilt. The oblique view may expose additional comminution or articular displacement; however, all views are used to assess the articular surface.

Many classification systems have been developed for distal radius fractures. To date, there is no universally accepted classification system, nor has any one been found to be consistently of prognostic value. Eponyms are continually being used, although often erroneously. Radiography had not been developed when Colles first described his own injury of the wrist so we really do not know the exact nature of his fracture. Nevertheless, the *Colles' fracture* is known as a complete extra-articular fracture with dorsal displacement or apex volar angulation, created by a bending moment and axial compression. Smith's fracture is the palmarly displaced counterpart to the Colles' fracture. Barton's fractures are intra-articular shear fractures and can be dorsal or palmar in direction. Regardless of the eponyms or classifications used, the important factors to be examined radiographically are the degree of comminution, the articular involvement, and the amount of displacement or shortening relative to the normal position. These factors determine the *stability* of the fracture, which is key in determining the method of treatment.

Treatment

The preferred method of treatment for distal radius fractures remains controversial. Abraham Colles wrote in 1814 that although "the deformity will remain undiminished throughout life, the limb will at some remote period again enjoy perfect freedom in all its motions and be completely exempt from pain" [1]. In spite of this optimistic view, many studies over the years have demonstrated significant limitations and disability of the upper extremity as long-term sequelae of distal radius fractures [17–19]. Most authors agree that achieving and maintaining an anatomical reduction until union is the best way to obtain a satisfactory result. In the young healthy patient this is the primary objective of treatment methods. In the elderly patient, final deformity may be accepted and well tolerated due to lower demands on the limb. The primary treatment goal for the elderly osteoporotic patient is early functional restoration of the limb, allowing the patient to return to their pre-injury level of functioning [20].

The method of treatment to achieve this objective is directed not only by careful study of the fracture but also by considering the needs of the patient. The varying levels of activity and independence in the geriatric population may necessitate individualizing the method of treatment. Patients maintaining a high level of independence and activity will benefit from more aggressive attempts at achieving an anatomical reduction, while patients with a very low level of functioning may not tolerate certain treatment methods because of medical or cognitive problems. For example, a patient who has multiple medical problems and residual neurological deficits from a stroke will easily be returned to their pre-injury level of functioning even with moderate residual deformity at the distal forearm. One must remain cognizant of the multitude of complications that can occur using the various methods of treatment, at any phase of treatment.

Historically there has been a trend toward more aggressive treatment of distal radius fractures. To date, however, there is little evidence that more aggressive treatment of this injury in the elderly patient with severe osteoporosis provides better overall functional results.

Predicting the behavior of distal radius fractures can be challenging. Abbaszadegan et al. [21] found that fractures treated by closed reduction and casting tended eventually to heal in a position near that of the original injury radiograph. Dias et al. [5] studied 127 fractures in patients over 50 years of age and found that 74.8% were classified as osteoporotic based on the second metacarpal cortical width, and those with osteoporosis ultimately healed with greater deformity. When severe osteoporosis results in minimal remaining bone stock, the behavior of the fracture is predictably unstable and options for treatment become more limited.

The mode of failure of internal fixation is from bone failure rather than implant failure. Osteoporotic bone typically has more extensive comminution and lacks adequate strength or purchase to hold plates and screws securely. In general, internal fixation devices that serve to impact the fracture site fare best in treating fractures in osteoporotic bone (e.g., dynamic hip compression screw) [22]. Unfortunately, shortening of the distal radius is a consistent risk factor predictive of a poor result [2,18,21,23–25]. Devices or treatment allowing impaction at the distal radius would leave significant shortening, and thus a predictably poor result. Frequently used methods of obtaining radial length attempt to distract the fracture leaving a void or cavity in the already osteoporotic metaphyseal bone. Additional considerations include the fact that the inadequate skeletal calcium reserves present in most individuals leads to a deficit in mineralization, and regardless of treatment method one can expect an additional 15% decrease in mineral content of the forearm bones in patients with distal radius fractures [26]. One method proposed to prevent further mineral loss is the administration of calcitonin and calcium. A prospective randomized placebo-controlled clinical trial demonstrated that administration of calcitonin and calcium not only impeded bone loss but also increased the metacarpal index, indicating increased cortical bone mass [27]. This protocol has not, however, become widely adopted.

Nonoperative Treatment: Nondisplaced Fractures

A majority of Colles' fractures in the elderly and osteoporotic patient can be treated nonoperatively with cast or brace immobilization. Patients with nondisplaced fractures should initially be placed into a well-padded splint. After 7–10 days, radiographs should be obtained to verify no further displacement. A short arm cast can then be applied with the wrist in neutral or slight extension to promote finger motion. The cast should end proximal to the metacarpal heads (proximal palmar crease) to allow full and early range of motion of the fingers. The thumb should also be left free for motion.

Elderly patients tend to have friable skin and adequate padding is necessary to prevent pressure ulceration or abrasions, particularly over the distal ulna and around the edges of the cast. Many prefabricated and custom braces have been designed for treatment of distal radius fractures and typically will be satisfactory for treating nondisplaced or stable fracture patterns. Functional braces, which allow immediate radiocarpal motion, have also been developed [28,29]. Ledingham et al. [28] reported on 60 patients in a randomized prospective study that demonstrated better early wrist function compared with casting. Immobilization of the fracture should continue for 4–6 weeks followed by the use of a removable splint and protected motion at the wrist.

Displaced Fractures

The definition of an "acceptable" reduction varies among authors. A satisfactory reduction of the Colles' and dorsal Barton's fractures can most often be achieved by closed means. The difficulty in treating patients with severe osteoporosis lies in the ability to *maintain* a satisfactory reduction until the fracture unites. Studies have shown that fractures tend to collapse back to the position seen on the initial injury radiographs in spite of reduction and immobilization [21,30–32]. Re-manipulation in patients over 60 years of age has been shown to result in *no* reduction of the final deformity [33]. Factors which tend to predict the ability to maintain the reduction are the degree of comminution and the amount of radial shortening seen on the initial injury radiographs [8,21,34]. Long-term outcome studies are lacking for the functional results in the elderly and osteoporotic patients. In general, an acceptable reduction should have less than 10° change in palmar tilt, less than

3 mm shortening, less than 5° change in radial inclination and less than 1 mm intra-articular incongruity. These general guidelines have evolved from studies looking at all age groups [35]. Elderly patients with low demands can usually tolerate more deformity. Deformity of up to 30° in the sagittal plane and 5 mm of shortening may be well accepted by elderly individuals [36].

The technique used for reduction of the fracture typically uses either a hematoma block with 1% lidocaine or regional anesthesia with or without sedation. Longitudinal traction is applied manually or using finger traps with counter-traction on the proximal arm. The deformity is reproduced allowing disimpaction of the fracture and the palmar cortex is reduced back into position with palmarly directed pressure on the dorsum of the distal fragment. Excessive traction or exaggeration of the deformity during reduction should be avoided as this may lead to additional soft tissue injury. Once the reduction is performed, a well-padded long arm cast or sugar tong splint can be applied. Many different wrist and forearm positions have been described for closed treatment of distal radius fractures. The Cotton-Loder position of excessive wrist flexion and ulnar deviation should be condemned as it increases pressure on the median nerve and inhibits finger motion [37]. Slight flexion of 10–20° is an acceptable position of immobilization. Gupta et al. [38] reported an interesting study demonstrating better results with casting the wrist in extension. An "S"-shaped mold to the cast provides three-point pressure on the fracture, while allowing wrist extension to neutralize deforming forces and promote finger motion. Above-elbow versus below-elbow casting remains controversial. Initial application of an above-elbow cast or sugar tong splint may improve patient comfort by reducing motion through the distal radioulnar joint and may promote elevation of the limb in the first 2 weeks. Immobilization above the elbow beyond this time increases the risk of elbow and shoulder stiffness, and the added weight of the cast and restricted elbow motion may significantly limit a patient's independence. The position of pronation or supination has not been shown to have any significant effect on the final result [39]. Neutral or slight pronation may be a more functional position and better accepted by the patient.

The use of functional braces for Colles' fractures in the elderly has been advocated dating back to Abraham Colles and traditional Chinese medicine [12,29]. Prefabricated braces have been designed employing three-point pressure yet allowing radiocarpal motion [40]. Moir et al. [41] reported results of a randomized prospective study of 85 patients with displaced distal radius fractures treated with functional bracing that allowed radiocarpal motion. Patients treated in the brace group showed better functional results at 6 months. Sarmiento et al. [29] advocated functional bracing in supination, and allowed palmar flexion of the wrist and flexion and extension of the elbow. It should be borne in mind, however, that in severe osteoporosis it is not uncommon for seemingly benign, mildly displaced fractures to have more extensive comminution resulting in late collapse and deformity (Fig. 13.1).

Closed Reduction and Percutaneous Pinning

Several techniques have been described using various numbers and directions of pins [41–45]. Kapandji described a technique of intrafocal pinning, in which the Kirschner wires are inserted into the fracture and used to reduce the fracture. The pins are then advanced through the far cortex for fixation and function as a buttress.

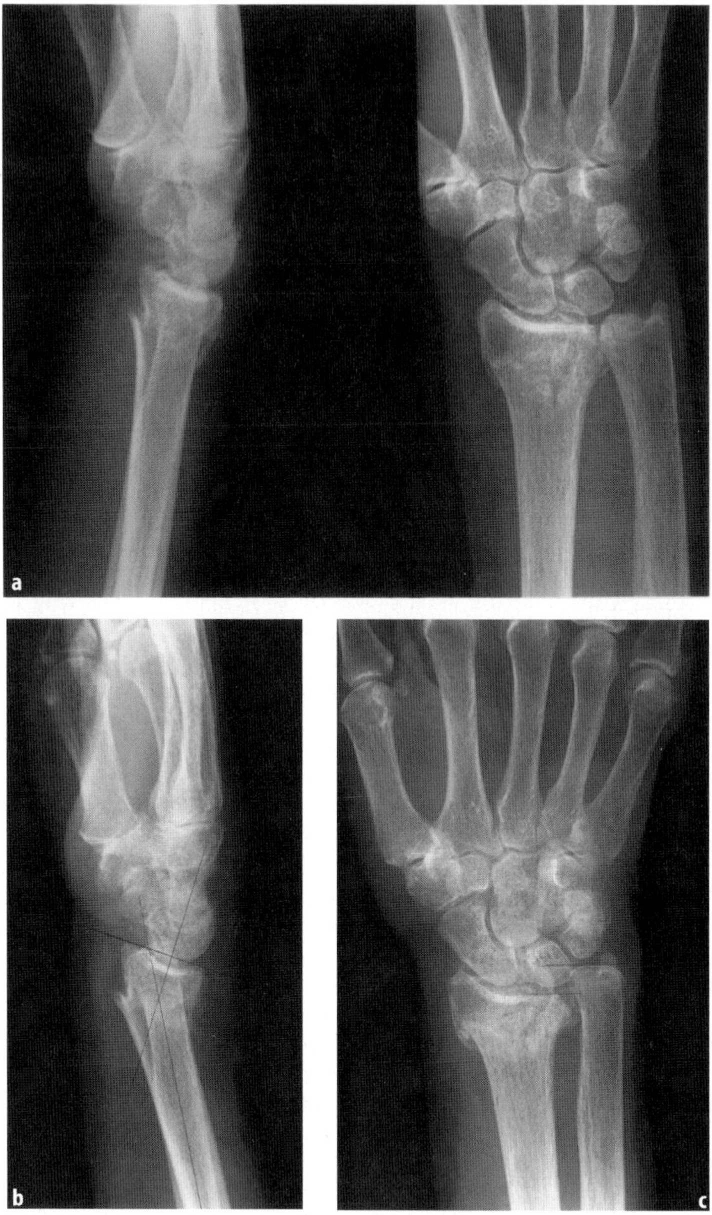

Figure 13.1a-c. A 78-year-old woman with multiple medical problems fell and sustained an extra-articular distal radius fracture of her left non-dominant hand. **a** Lateral and anteroposterior radiographs on the day of injury. The fracture appears stable. She was treated with closed reduction and casting. **b** Lateral and **c** anteroposterior radiographs at 12 weeks after casting. Osteoporosis and unappreciated dorsal comminution led to late collapse and deformity with a residual 30° loss of palmar tilt and 8 mm of positive ulnar variance. Despite these radiographic findings the patient returned to pre-injury activity levels with only mild ulnar-sided wrist pain. She did not desire further treatment.

Other techniques employ Kirschner wires across the fracture in a parallel or crossing pattern [42]. In severely osteoporotic bone, fixation is typically poor and percutaneous pinning may help to prevent re-displacement of the dorsal angulation in the sagittal plane by functioning as a buttress; however, it will not prevent radial shortening or displacement in the presence of comminution[35,43]. Following a closed reduction, Kirschner wires can be advanced under radiographic guidance. Small incisions followed by blunt dissection down to bone and the use of soft tissue guides can help prevent injury to sensory nerves or incarceration of tendons. Percutaneous pinning techniques are often used in combination with external fixation, plate fixation or cement fixation techniques.

External Fixation

Often a trial of closed treatment will be followed by application of an external fixator after the fracture has demonstrated re-displacement. Many studies have shown external fixation to be an effective treatment for distal radius fractures [46–55]. These studies, however, include the entire adult age spectrum in their patient groups. Two prospective randomized trials comparing external fixation with cast treatment in the elderly have failed to demonstrate superior clinical results [48,56]. Horne et al. [48] reported a series of 37 patients over 60 years old treated with external fixation who did not have better clinical results but did have increased complications. Roumen et al. [56] reported similar results in 101 distal radius fractures in patients over 55 years old. In both studies there was no correlation between the final radiographic result and the clinical outcome. External fixation should probably be reserved for patients maintaining a high level of activity and independence, and who have good cognitive function to participate in the care and management of the fixator (Fig. 13.2).

Following closed reduction, the reduction, fracture pattern and stability are reassessed. If severe comminution is present and significant shortening is predicted, the application of an external fixator may be considered. We prefer the open technique for pin placement through 3–4 cm incisions to reduce the complications of soft tissue injury and radial sensory nerve injury. Percutaneous technique has resulted in up to 25% incidence of radial sensory nerve complications [55]. External fixators use ligamentotaxis to restore anatomical alignment of the fracture. This is an effective technique for extra-articular fractures and many intra-articular fractures. The external fixator, however, is capable of maintaining only a reduction already achievable by manual techniques. There are a variety of available external fixators. All use the same principle of ligamentotaxis for reduction. The Agee WristJack allows multiplanar "adjustments" in the fixator, including palmar tilt in the sagittal plane, once the fixator is applied. It is important to remember, however, that the principal reduction must be performed *before* the application of any fixator, including the WristJack. Distraction and flexion across the wrist can cause excessive tension on the extrinsic extensor tendons producing "clawing" of the fingers while preventing full motion across the metacarpophalangeal and interphalangeal joints. The fixator allows the wrist to be positioned in the neutral position or extension, promoting finger motion while maintaining fracture reduction [57]. A prospective study of 20 consecutive distal radius fractures treated with a WristJack demonstrated maintenance of an anatomical reduction with 95% finger motion. Patients began motion of their fingers the day of surgery [47].

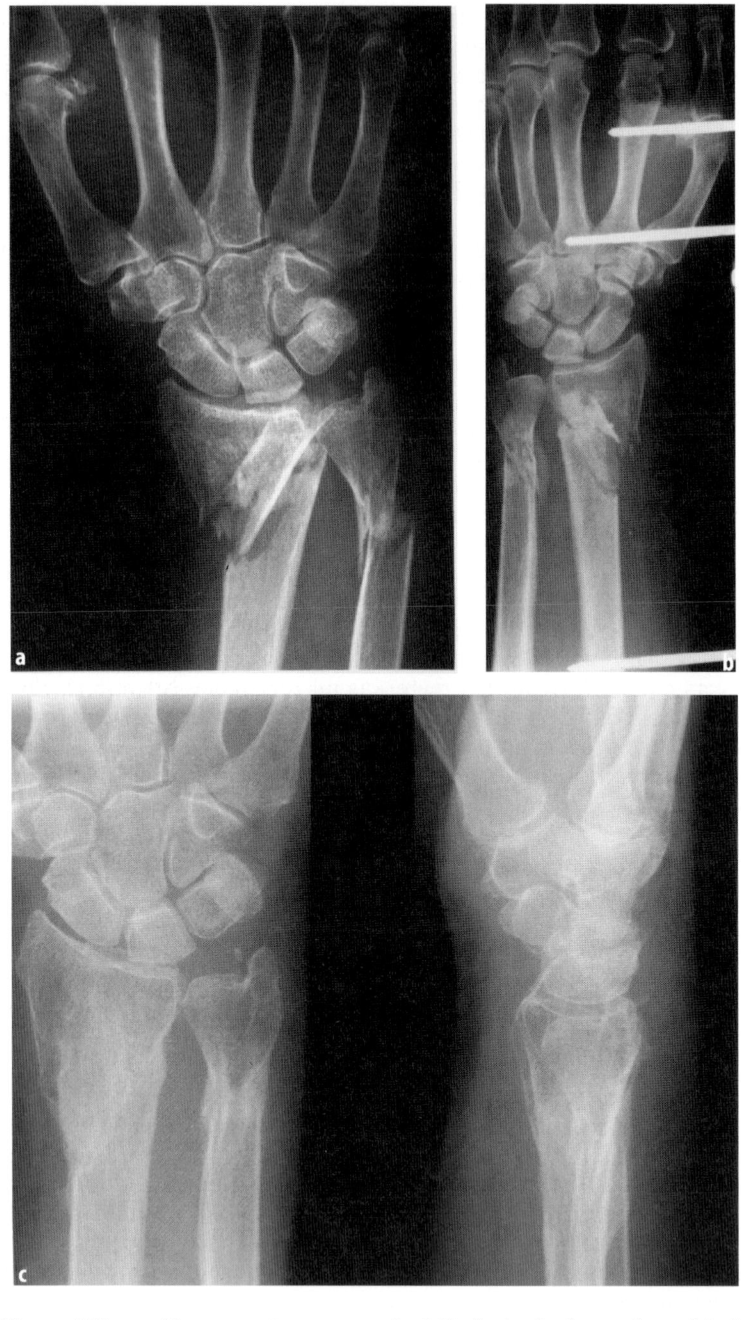

Figure 13.2a-c. A 76-year-old osteoporotic woman sustained this distal radius fracture from a fall while playing in a tennis tournament. **a** Initial injury. **b** This anteroposterior radiograph shows the patient treated with open reduction, autogenous iliac crest bone grafting and application of a WristJack external fixator. **c** Final anteroposterior and lateral radiographs demonstrate near anatomical restoration. The patient had nearly a full range of wrist motion and returned to playing tennis.

The external fixator is a stress-shielding device and also distracts across the fracture site often leaving a void in the metaphyseal bone. The addition of autogenous bone graft is recommended to fill the void in the metaphysis for its osteoinductive and osteoconductive properties as well as its ability to add inherent stability to the fracture. Synthetic bone graft material or allograft bone may reduce donor site morbidity, while still providing scaffolding for healing and some inherent stability [58]. Removal of the fixator will often be followed by collapse of the fracture if the metaphyseal void is ignored.

Instructions for pin care for the external fixator must be given in detail to the patient, family members and/or caregivers. Motion or tenting of the skin around the pins promotes pin tract infections. Releasing incisions and pin site dressings that reduce skin motion around the pins should be used to reduce the incidence of infection.

The external fixator is kept in place for approximately 6 weeks. Based on radiographic evidence for healing and the nature of the fracture and patient, the fixator may be required for 8–10 weeks. Following removal of the fixator, a removable splint is applied and protected motion is initiated for the wrist and forearm.

Cement Fixation

Recommendations for treating injuries in the elderly have included immediate rigid fixation to allow early mobilization and functional restoration. Severely osteoporotic bone leaves a comminuted shell of bone around a metaphyseal void that has little inherent stability. Methylmethacrylate cement has been used effectively for providing rigid fixation and stability in the Colles' fracture [59–61]. When Schmalholz [61] compared external fixation and cement fixation there was no difference in the clinical result, but a 24% complication rate in the external fixation group and no complications in the cement group [61]. Kiyoshige, reporting the results in 24 patients over 75 years of age, found that cement allowed immediate use of the affected hand and produced no complications [60].

The reduction of the fracture is performed as described above. A dorsal incision allows exposure to the dorsal comminution and access to the metaphyseal defect by hinging open the fragments. Reduction of the fracture can also be performed using elevators through the fracture void. Provisional fixation using Kirschner wires helps to maintain the reduction. Radial joint angles and ulnar variance are assessed radiographically. Cancellous bone around the defect is impacted out into the periphery. This serves to enlarge the cavity for greater surface area of fixation and add bone and stability to the porotic bone in the periphery. The cavity is irrigated thoroughly, then filled with high-viscosity bone cement (dough-like) with impaction into the metaphyseal bone for fixation (Fig. 13.3). Low-viscosity injected cement can leak into surrounding soft tissues. The dorsal cortical shell is replaced and periosteum is repaired. The Kirschner wire is removed prior to final curing of the cement. Patients are splinted for comfort until the incision is stable. Finger motion is encouraged immediately. Wrist motion is initiated at the time of suture removal.

Criticism of the bone cement technique includes thermal necrosis and the potential for infection. Clinical use of bone cement for distal radius fractures, however, has not resulted in significant increased infection rates or nonunions [59–61]. Complications from thermal necrosis are related to the volume of cement and the exothermic reaction. For the distal radius fracture this problem remains theoretical.

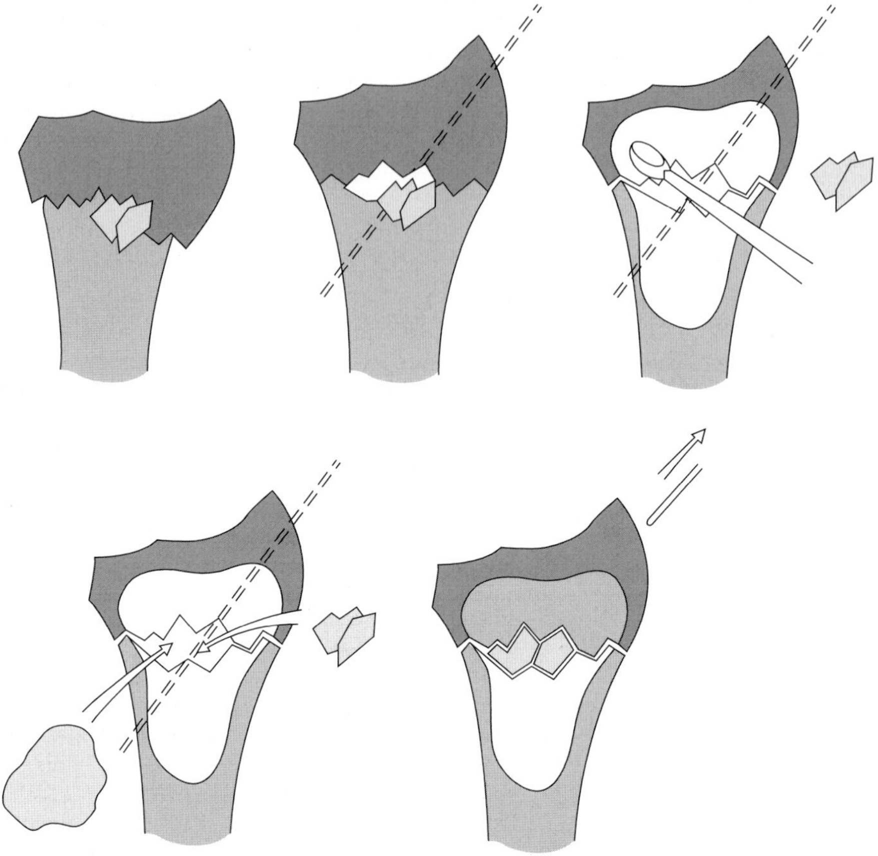

Figure 13.3. Under axillary block, the fracture is reduced and temporarily fixed with a Kirschner wire. The fracture area is exposed between the extensor carpi radialis and extensor pollicis longus tendons. The dorsal cortex of the fracture area is opened with a bone window and the medullary cavity is enlarged with a curette so that a sufficient amount of bone cement can be introduced. The medullary deficiency is then filled with the cement. Before the bone cement hardens the dorsal cortical bone is placed back on top of the cement and the Kirschner wire is removed. Reprinted with permission from Kiyoshige [60].

Norion SRS

The development of biocompatible bone cement materials is a new and exciting area. Norion SRS is a fast-setting high-strength calcium phosphate bone cement that has been used effectively to treat both intra and extra-articular distal radius fractures. Monocalcium phosphate, monohydrate, tricalcium phosphate and calcium carbonate are dry mixed. A sodium phosphate solution is added to form a paste [62]. The Norion SRS is an injectible paste which crystallizes to carbonate hydroxyapatite in situ via a non-exothermic crystallization reaction. The metaphyseal defect is filled and stability achieved in a similar fashion to that of the methylmethacrylate method. The surgical technique involves a closed or limited open reduction.

Through a small dorsal incision the dorsal comminution is hinged open exposing the metaphyseal defect cavity. Kirschner wires can be used for provisional fixation or to augment fixation. The mixing time of the reactants is 2 min with a working time of 5 min. Under physiological conditions the cement setting time is 10 min. During this time there should be no manipulation of the limb so that crystallization can occur. Patients have been protected by external splinting or casting for 2–6 weeks [63,64]. Early motion, however, is the goal, relying on the adhesive properties and the compressive strength of the cement restoring stability across the fracture site [63]. The new biomaterial appears to be remodelled in a manner similar to that of normal bone remodelling by osteoblasts and osteoclasts [62].

Plate Fixation

In patients with severe osteoporosis, plate fixation may be of limited value. The poor bone quality and small, comminuted fragments often prohibit stable fixation. Distal radius fractures with large fragments and little comminution, or those in conjunction with radius or ulnar shaft fractures, may benefit from plate fixation.

Barton's fractures are shear fractures of the dorsal or palmar rim of the distal radius. The carpus tends to follow the distal fragment and subluxates [65]. Buttress plates, with fixation only in the proximal fragment, are effective for treatment of dorsal Barton's fractures. The use of a buttress plate can reduce the subluxation and displacement of the fracture fragment [66,67]. Dorsal Barton's fractures are approached through a dorsal longitudinal incision entering the interval between the third and fourth extensor compartment. Reduction of the fracture is achieved with longitudinal traction and manipulation of the fragments. Provisional fixation with Kirschner wires may be useful. The buttress plate is contoured to maintain the reduction of the distal fragment. Bicortical fixation screws are placed in the proximal end of the plate. By pre-bending the plate, a buttress effect maintains the reduction of the distal fragment. Patients with severe osteoporosis will frequently have associated comminution or metaphyseal impaction. The addition of an external fixator to prevent dorsal displacement or radial shortening may be needed for the initial 4–6 weeks. Fractures with severe metaphyseal impaction associated with a shear fracture may require the articular surface to be elevated with insertion of bone graft, synthetic bone graft or cement to fill the resulting defect. If bone graft is used, an external fixator may be applied to prevent collapse.

Cement fixation in combination with a buttress plate may be used to augment screw fixation, maintain the elevated joint and add inherent stability. This construct makes the use of an external fixator and bone graft unnecessary and reduces the morbidity of these other procedures. The technique is similar to that described above; however, once the plate is applied, it is then removed. The reduction is maintained while cement is inserted into the metaphyseal defect, and the plate is reapplied as the cement cures. Cement can also be inserted into the screw holes to enhance their fixation. Caution must be used to avoid cement entering the joint or soft tissues. Distal screws may also be placed to augment fixation.

Postoperative Therapy

Mobilization of the fingers should begin immediately. Casts, splints, external fixators and postoperative dressings should allow maximum finger motion. Significant joint contractures can occur at the metacarpophalangeal and proximal interphalangeal joints if finger motion is restricted. Instructions should be given to the patient and family members for specific exercises to move the fingers and for edema control. Early involvement of a hand therapist can reduce complications associated with these injuries, particularly when patients need guidance or supervision. Once mobilization of the wrist is initiated, gentle active and active assisted motion should be started for all ranges of motion including flexion, extension, pronation, supination, radial and ulnar deviation. Progressive resistance exercises should be delayed until union is certain. Patients having difficulty with stiffness may also benefit from dynamic splinting.

Complications

Many complications can occur from this injury as well as from the different treatment methods. Most common complications that lead to poor results include malunions, neuropathies, joint contractures, algodystrophy, pin tract infections and post-traumatic arthrosis. Other less frequent complications include tendon ruptures and nonunions.

Loss of reduction is a common event and requires the physician, patient and family members to make a cooperative decision regarding further management based on the predictable outcome and the patient's level of functioning. Re-reduction is felt by many authors to be of little value, particularly if significant initial displacement, dorsal comminution and shortening are encountered [8,33]. Furthermore, the final radiographic result does not always correlate with the final functional result in the older patients. Typically dorsal angulation up to 30° and radial angle below 10° is tolerated, although grip strength may be reduced by 30%. Radial shortening of more than 5 mm can lead to distal radioulnar joint incongruency and ulnar impingement which can best be treated later with a distal radioulnar joint procedure (see below).

Although cadaver studies show a significant change in loads across the radiocarpal joint with malunited fractures, few malunions in the elderly ultimately go on to require an osteotomy. In elderly patients the demands placed on the wrist are relatively low, and often other medical problems or other painful arthritic joints may be the limiting factor in the patient's life. A common source of pain from a symptomatic malunion with positive ulnar variance is from the distal radioulnar joint. If ulnar-sided wrist pain or pain with forearm rotation becomes limiting, procedures to address the distal radioulnar joint are effective. Ulnar shortening may be insufficient if joint incongruency and arthrosis are present. There are several described arthroplasties for the distal radioulnar joint: Darrach, Darrach-Dingman, Darrach-Zancolli, Watson ulnar resection, Bowers' hemiresection interposition arthroplasty, and the Sauvé-Kapandji arthrodesis (Fig. 13.4) [35].

When a malunited distal radius fracture becomes symptomatic in a patient with severe osteoporosis, an osteotomy may be indicated. Fernandez [68] advocated the use of an opening wedge osteotomy with tricortical autogenous bone graft in combination with a distal radioulnar joint arthroplasty. Following an opening wedge osteotomy in the face of severe osteoporosis, however, the bone is slow to incorporate and there is a tendency for collapse or graft resorption. Posner and Ambrose [69] described a biplanar closing wedge osteotomy with resection of the ulnar head. The closing wedge osteotomy results in a more stable construct in osteoporotic

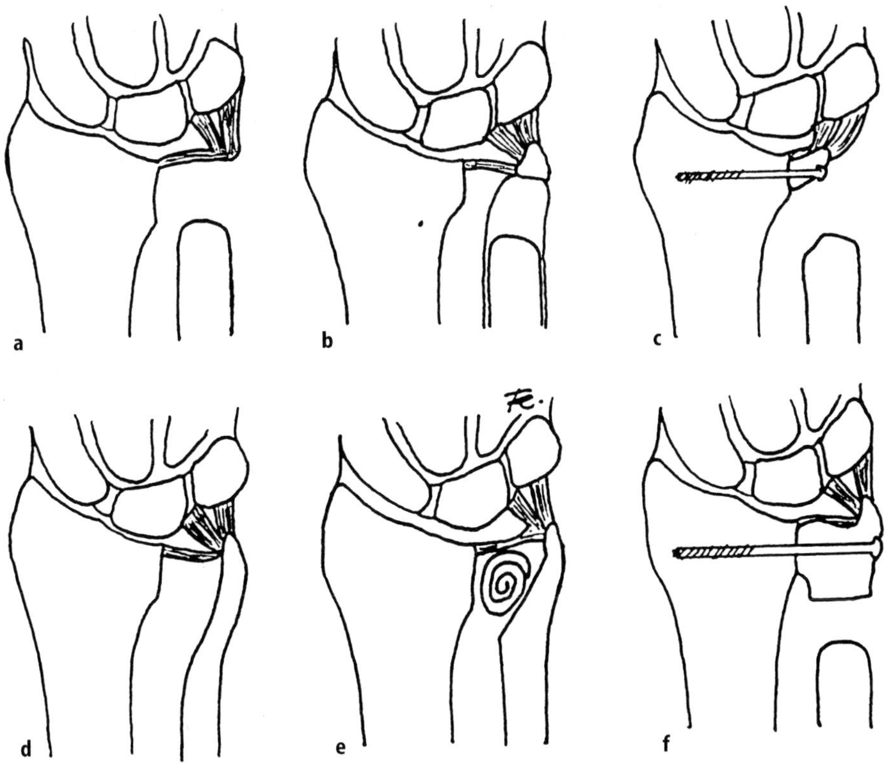

Figure 13.4a-f. Schematic of the various procedures for the distorted distal radioulnar joint. **a** Darrach, **b** Darrach-Dingman, **c** Darrach-Zancolli, **d** Watson ulnar resection, **e** Bowers' hemiresection, interposition arthroplasty, **f** Sauvé-Kapandji arthrodesis. Reprinted with permission from Fernandez and Jupiter [35].

bone. Union may be more certain without relying on the tricortical graft and donor site morbidity is eliminated. A closing wedge osteotomy will result in additional ulnar positive variance and therefore should be performed in combination with a procedure addressing the distal radioulnar joint. Posner described resection of the distal ulna; however, we have preferred a Sauvé-Kapandji procedure [70].

Neuropathies related to distal radius fracture can occur early or late. The incidence of median neuropathy has been reported to be as high as 22% [71]. The neuropathy may be transient from a contusion, acute carpal tunnel syndrome or a late carpal tunnel syndrome related to malunited fractures. The incidence of late median neuropathy has been reported to be 8% while ulnar neuropathy is seen in only 4% [72]. Radial sensory nerve injuries, reported to occur in up to 25% of cases, are most often iatrogenic from tight casts or braces, and percutaneous pin placement of Kirschner wires or external fixation pins [55]. This complication can be significantly reduced using the open pin placement method and careful dissection.

Algodystrophy has a reported incidence of 0.1% [17] to 26% [73]. Signs of algodystrophy can be detected as early as 1 week, and early recognition and aggressive treatment are key factors in reducing long-term sequelae from this complication [15]. Factors associated with the development of algodystrophy include constricting dressings or casts, excessive or prolonged distraction using external fixators and untreated neuropathies. This complication results in significant functional limitation of the upper extremity, impairing the elderly patient's ability to return to their pre-injury level of function.

In summary, the distal radius fracture is a common injury often seen in patients with severe osteoporosis. The injury can typically be treated nonsurgically with immobilization. The fractures are characteristically comminuted and predictably unstable leading to late collapse and deformity. The final radiographic position, however, does not necessarily correlate with the final functional result in this particular patient population. Treatment should be individualized, corresponding to the patient's level of activity and function. Preservation of upper extremity function and hand sensibility, and prevention of complications remain the primary goals of treatment.

References

1. Colles A. On the fracture of the carpal extremity of the radius. Edinb Med Surg J 1814;10:182–186.
2. Altissimi M, Antenucci R, Fiacca C, Mancini GB. Long-term results of conservative treatment of fractures of the distal radius. Clin Orthop Rel Res 1986;4:202–210.
3. Krølner B, Tøndevold E, Toft B, Berthelsen B, Nielsen SP. Bone mass of the axial and the appendicular skeleton in women with Colles' fracture: its relation to physical activity. Clin Physiol 1982;2:147–157.
4. Horsman A, Nordin BE, Simpson M, Speed R. Cortical and trabecular bone status in elderly women with femoral neck fracture. Clin Orthop Rel Res 1982;35:143–151.
5. Dias JJ, Wray CC, Jones JM. Osteoporosis and Colles' fractures in the elderly. J Hand Surg. [Br] 1987;12:57–59.
6. Dai LY, Chen DY, Wu DS, Wen Y. Osteoporosis in Colles fracture. Arch Orthop Trauma Surg 1998;117:65–67.
7. Mallmin H, Ljunghall S. Distal radius fracture is an early sign of general osteoporosis: bone mass measurements in a population-based study. Osteoporos Int 1994;4:357–361.
8. Schmalholz A. Closed rereduction of axial compression in Colles' fracture is hardly possible. Acta Orthop Scand 1989;60:57–59.
9. Bengnér U, Johnell O. Increasing incidence of forearm fractures. A comparison of epidemiologic patterns 25 years apart. Acta Orthop Scand 1985;56:158–160.
10. Schmalholz A. Epidemiology of distal radius fracture in Stockholm 1981–82. Acta Orthop Scand 1988;59:701–703.
11. Crilly RG, Delaquerrière Richardson L, Roth JH, Vandervoort AA, Hayes KC, Mackenzie RA. Postural stability and Colles' fracture. Age Ageing 1987;16:133–138.
12. Sharma JC, MacLennan WJ. Causes of ataxia in patients attending a falls laboratory. Age Ageing 1988;17:94–102.
13. Winner SJ, Morgan CA, Evans JG. Perimenopausal risk of falling and incidence of distal forearm fracture. BMJ 1989;298:1486–1488.
14. Cooper C. The epidemiology of fragility fractures: is there a role for bone quality? Calcif Tissue Int 1993;53(Suppl 1):S23–26.
15. Field J, Atkins RM. Algodystrophy is an early complication of Colles' fracture. What are the implications? J Hand Surg [Br] 1997;22:178–182.
16. Stern PJ, Derr RG. Non-osseous complications following distal radius fractures. Iowa Orthop J 1993;13:63–69.
17. Bacorn RW, Kurtzke, J.F. Colles' Fracture. A study of two thousand cases from the New York State Workmen's Compensation Board. J Bone Joint Surg Am 1953;35: 643–658.

18. Field J, Warwick D, Bannister GC, Gibson AG. Long-term prognosis of displaced Colles' fracture: a 10-year prospective review. Injury 1992;23:529–532.
19. Warwick D, Field J, Prothero D, Gibson A, Bannister GC. Function ten years after Colles' fracture. Clin Orthop 1993;45:270–274.
20. Steinberg DR, Szabo RM. Decision making in upper extremity problems in the elderly. Clin Orthop 1995;21:63–69.
21. Abbaszadegan H, Jonsson U, von Sivers K. Prediction of instability of Colles' fractures. Acta Orthop Scand 1989;60:646–650.
22. Cornell CN. Management of fractures in patients with osteoporosis. Orthop Clin North Am 1990;21:125–141.
23. Hagert CG. [Distal radius fractures are treated improperly. Our most common fracture is a complicated injury and deserves higher status]. Lakartidningen 1998;95: 3311–3313.
24. Hutchinson F III. Decision making in distal radius fractures. J South Orthop Assoc 1995;4:290–306.
25. Trumble TE, Schmitt SR, Vedder NB. Factors affecting functional outcome of displaced intra-articular distal radius fractures. J Hand Surg [Am] 1994;19:325–340.
26. Abbaszadegan H, Adolphson P, Dalén N, Jonsson U, Sjöberg HE, Kalén S. Bone mineral loss after Colles' fracture. Plaster case and external fixation equivalent. Acta Orthop Scand 1991;62:156–158.
27. Crespo R, Revilla M, Crespo E, Villa LF, Rico H. Complementary medical treatment for Colles' fracture: a comparative, randomized, longitudinal study. Calcif Tissue Int 1997;60:567–570.
28. Ledingham WM, Wytch R, Goring CC, Mathieson AB, Wardlaw D. On immediate functional bracing of Colles' fracture. Injury 1991;22:197–201.
29. Sarmiento A, Zagorski JB, Sinclair WF. Functional bracing of Colles' fractures: a prospective study of immobilization in supination vs pronation. Clin Orthop 1980;92: 175–183.
30. Dias JJ, Wray CC, Jones JM. The radiological deformity of Colles' fractures. Injury 1987;18:304–308.
31. Hove LM, Fjeldsgaard K, Skjeie R, Solheim E. Anatomical and functional results five years after remanipulated Colles' fractures. Scand J Plastic Reconstr Surg Hand Surg 1995;29:349–355.
32. Hove LM, Solheim E, Skjeie R, Sörensen FK. Prediction of secondary displacement in Colles' fracture. J Hand Surg [Br] 1994;19:731–736.
33. Collert S, Isacson J. Management of redislocated Colles' fractures. Clin Orthop 1978;50: 183–186.
34. Aro HT, Koivunen T. Minor axial shortening of the radius affects outcome of Colles' fracture treatment. J Hand Surg [Am] 1991;16:392–398.
35. Fernandez DL, Jupiter JB, Fractures of the distal radius: a practical approach to management. Berlin Heidelberg New York: Springer, 1996.
36. Kelly AJ, Warwick D, Crichlow TP, Bannister GC. Is manipulation of moderately displaced Colles' fracture worthwhile? A prospective randomized trial. Injury 1997;28: 283–287.
37. Gelberman RH, Szabo RM, Mortensen WW. Carpal tunnel pressures and wrist position in patients with colles' fractures. J Trauma 1984;24:747–749.
38. Gupta A. The treatment of Colles' fracture. Immobilisation with the wrist dorsiflexed. J Bone Joint Surg B 1991;73:312–315.
39. Stewart HD, Innes AR, Burke FD. Functional cast-bracing for Colles' fractures. A comparison between cast-bracing and conventional plaster casts. J Bone Joint Surg Br 1984;66:749–753.
40. Ferris BD, Thomas NP, Dewar ME, Simpson DA. Brace treatment of Colles' fracture. Acta Orthop Scand 1989;60:63–65.
41. Moir JS, Murali SR, Ashcroft GP, Wardlaw D, Matheson AB. A new functional brace for the treatment of Colles' fractures. Injury 1995;26:587–593.

42. Clancey GJ. Percutaneous Kirschner-wire fixation of Colles fractures. A prospective study of thirty cases. J Bone Joint Surg Am 1984;66:1008–1014.
43. Greatting MD, Bishop AT. Intrafocal (Kapandji) pinning of unstable fractures of the distal radius. Orthop Clin North Am 1993;24:301–307.
44. Mah ET, Atkinson RN. Percutaneous Kirschner wire stabilisation following closed reduction of Colles' fractures. J Hand Surg [Br] 1992;17:55–62.
45. Oskam J, Kingma J, Bart J, Klasen HJ. K-wire fixation for redislocated Colles' fractures. Malunion in 8/21 cases. Acta Orthop Scand 1997;68:259–261.
46. Abbaszadegan H, Jonsson U. External fixation or plaster cast for severely displaced Colles' fractures? Prospective 1-year study of 46 patients. Acta Orthop Scand 1990;61: 528–530.
47. Agee JM, Szabo RM, Chidgey LK, King FC, Kerfoot C. Treatment of comminuted distal radius fractures: an approach based on pathomechanics. Orthopedics 1994;17: 1115–1122.
48. Horne JG, Devane P, Purdie G. A prospective randomized trial of external fixation and plaster cast immobilization in the treatment of distal radial fractures [see comments]. J Orthop Trauma 1990;4:30–34.
49. Kaukonen JP, Karaharju E, Lüthje P, Porras M. External fixation of Colles' fracture. Acta Orthop Scand 1989;60:54–56.
50. Kongsholm J, Olerud C. Comminuted Colles' fractures treated with external fixation. Arch Orthop Trauma Surg 1987;106:220–225.
51. Kongsholm J, Olerud C. Plaster cast versus external fixation for unstable intraarticular Colles' fractures. Clin Orthop 1989;60:57–65.
52. Leung KS, Shen WY, Tsang HK, Chiu KH, Leung PC, Hung LK. An effective treatment of comminuted fractures of the distal radius. J Hand Surg [Am] 1990;15:11–17.
53. Ludvigsen TC, Johansen S, Svenningsen S, Saetermo R. External fixation versus percutaneous pinning for unstable Colles' fracture. Equal outcome in a randomized study of 60 patients. Acta Orthop Scand 1997;68:255–258.
54. Riis J, Fruensgaard S. Treatment of unstable Colles' fractures by external fixation. J Hand Surg [Br] 1989;14:145–148.
55. Solgaard S. External fixation or a cast for Colles' fracture. Acta Orthop Scand 1989; 60:387–391.
56. Roumen RM, Hesp WL, Bruggink ED. Unstable Colles' fractures in elderly patients. A randomised trial of external fixation for redisplacement. J Bone Joint Surg Br 1991; 73:307–311.
57. Agee JM. Distal radius fractures. Multiplanar ligamentotaxis. Hand Clin 1993;9:577–585.
58. Cornell CN, Lane JM, Chapman M, Merkow R, Seligson D, Henry S, et al. Multicenter trial of Collagraft as bone graft substitute. J Orthop Trauma 1991;5:1–8.
59. Kofoed H. Comminuted displaced Colles' fractures. Treatment with intramedullary methylmethacrylate stabilisation. Acta Orthop Scand 1983;54:307–311.
60. Kiyoshige Y. Intramedullary bone-cement fixation for Colles fractures in elderly patients. Tech Hand Upper Extrem Surg 1997;1:89–94.
61. Schmalholz A. Bone cement for redislocated Colles' fracture. A prospective comparison with closed treatment. Acta Orthop Scand 1989;60:212–217.
62. Constantz BR, Ison IC, Fulmer MT, Poser RD, Smith ST, VanWagoner M, et al. Skeletal repair by in situ formation of the mineral phase of bone [see comments]. Science 1995;267:1796–1799.
63. Jupiter JB, Winters S, Sigman S, Lowe C, Pappas C, Ladd AL, et al. Repair of five distal radius fractures with an investigational cancellous bone cement: a preliminary report. J Orthop Trauma 1997;11:110–116.
64. Kopylov P, Jonsson K, Thorngren KG, Aspenberg P. Injectable calcium phosphate in the treatment of distal radial fractures. J Hand Surg [Br] 1996;21:768–771.
65. Barton JR. Views and treatment of an important injury of the wrist. Med Exam Rec Med Sci 1838;1:365–368.
66. Oliveira JCD. Barton's fractures. J Bone Joint Surg Am 1973;55:586–594.

67. Almquist EE. Compression plate fixation for Barton's or Smith's type II fractures. Handchirurgie 1973;5:29–31.
68. Fernandez DL. Radial osteotomy and Bowers arthroplasty for malunited fractures of the distal end of the radius. J Bone Joint Surg Am 1988;70:1538–1551.
69. Posner MA, Ambrose L. Malunited Colles' fractures: correction with a biplanar closing wedge osteotomy. J Hand Surg Am 1991;16:1017–1026.
70. Slater RR, Szabo, R.M. The Sauve-Kapandji procedure. Tech Hand Upper Extrem Surg 1998;2:1–10.
71. Knirk JL, Jupiter JB. Intra-articular fractures of the distal end of the radius in young adults. J Bone Joint Surg Am 1986;68:647–659.
72. Aro H, Koivunen T, Katevuo K, Nieminen S, Aho AJ. Late compression neuropathies after Colles' fractures. Clin Orthop 1988;96:217–225.
73. Field J, Warwick D, Bannister GC. Features of algodystrophy ten years after Colles' fracture. J Hand Surg [Br] 1992;17:318–320.

14 Smith's and Volar Barton's Fractures

M. D. Putnam

Introduction

Fractures of the distal radius are common. Epidemiological studies have identified the largest at-risk population to be older women [1]. A smaller but also large at-risk population is older men. The two populations begin to appear more similar as age increases. It has been speculated that this age-related change is related to bone density [2–5]. Multiple articles have examined the issue of bone density in the distal radius as regards fracture risk and it is clear that at least three issues are present: (1) diminishing absolute bone mineral density, (2) changing likelihood of "falling" due to changes in coordination and strength, (3) changes in geometric measurements of the cortical outline. It has been demonstrated that the first two of these three variables may be subject to manipulation [6]. Nevertheless, it seems likely that the number of fractures occurring in the distal radius will continue to increase as the number of older adults increases. Because of the associated age related osteoporosis, the relative complexity of this problem may increase.

Diagnosis and Classification

Drs Barton and Smith separately observed fracture patterns before the advent of radiography. It is not possible to be certain that all the fractures described by Dr Barton in his original series or by Dr Smith in his were in fact exactly as they have been subsequently proposed radiographically [7,8]. Nonetheless, Smith and Barton are credited with the original observation of fractures involving the distal radius in a pattern different from that described by Mr Colles [9]. The most important distinguishing difference between the two fractures for our modern purpose is the direct disturbance of intra-articular joint congruity in the presence of a volar Barton's fracture as compared with the extra-articular position of Smith's fracture. As our understanding has evolved, it is clear that both fractures can result in a secondary disturbance of joint function either by malalignment of the bony elements or by disturbance of ligamentous origin/function or both of the foregoing. Thus, the volar Barton's fracture and Smith's fracture share a common ability to disturb intercarpal alignment as well as distal radial to ulnar joint function. Separately, the volar Barton's fracture can result in articular surface malunion with the lunate resting

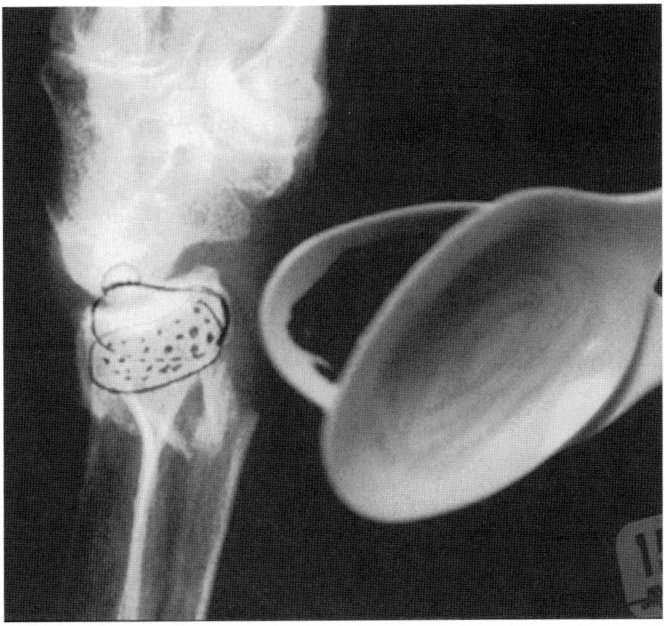

Figure 14.1. A "spoon model" is used to demonstrate the effect of changing the rotational positioning of two concave surfaces. As one concave surface alters its position relative to the other, they become incongruent. This model is felt to simulate the changes which occur in the distal radioulnar joint as the signoid notch of the distal radius falls either into palmar flexion or into dorsal flexion, thereby changing the relationship of the joint surfaces.

between a dorsal and palmar half of the distal radius fragments causing gross intra-articular incongruity. Fig. 14.1 illustrates the author's conception of the difficulty posed by extra-articular angle change. In this figure, the joint becomes progressively asymmetric as the tilt of the distal radius fragment changes.

Accurately diagnosing a Smith's or volar Barton's fracture can be accomplished, as was done by Dr. Smith and Barton, with reasonable accuracy without radiographs. However, radiographs assist in assessing the degree of comminution, fracture fragment alignment, and joint congruity. A new radiographic view of particular value as regards assessing the lunate fossa is termed by ourselves a fossa lateral (Fig. 14.2) [10]. The fossa lateral allows an accurate determination to be made as regards dorsal or volar tilt of the distal fragment end, and allows a clear view of the articular surface. The view can be completed before reduction, after reduction, and at follow-up to assess stability of the fracture and maintenance of reduction.

The potential role of computed tomography (CT) scans or magnetic resonance imaging (MRI) in management of these fractures acutely is limited [11]. Fractures which have healed in a malunited position could be assessed more completely using MRI and/or CT technology. This is particularly true as regards the stability of the distal radioulnar joint (DRUJ) itself as well as the alignment of articular surface malunion and/or early degenerative change. MRI is of particular value in situations where ligament assessment is required [11,12].

A more meaningful question which cannot be answered at this time is the validity of measures to assess bone density in the presence of acute fracture. The relationship

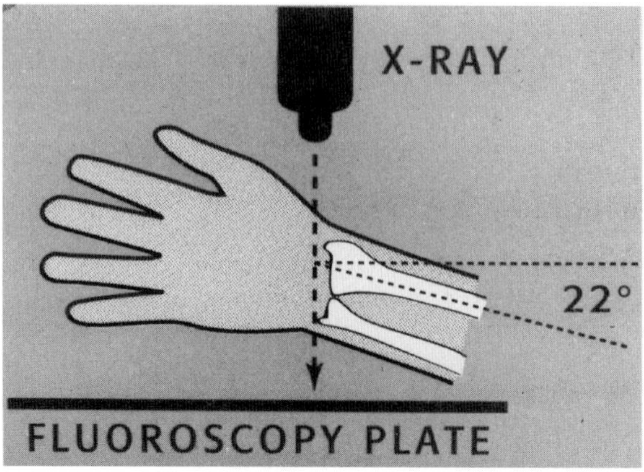

Figure 14.2. The fossa lateral is a radiographic view obtained from the lateral projection by lifting the hand away from the X-ray plate. Dependent upon the degree of radial inclination (normal equals 22°), the lunate fossa will be clearly visualized. In this manner it is possible to determine an accurate degree of dorsal or volar tilt as well as clearly visualizing the articular surface of the lunate fossa. A similar view can be obtained of the scaphoid fossa by placing the hand in an oblique position while at the same time maintaining the appropriate degree of radial inclination.

of uninjured limb bone density to injured bone density is unknown. For purposes of discussion, it can be assumed that the two would be similar. What is problematic is the exact relationship of injured bone density to cortical fixation and treatment methodologies most likely to be successful. It is generally accepted that osteoporotic bone will offer less fixation strength than normal bone. But, fixation preferences related to bone density are not quantified. Hence, although it is known that several tools are available to assess the relative density of bone, that these measurements relate to fracture risk, and that some methods can be used to alter the rate of bone density change in a favorable manner, it is not known what benefit, if any, this information lends to the acute management of unstable fractures.

Multiple classification mechanisms have been used to describe fractures of the distal radius. By design, this chapter deals with fractures previously described by specific surgeons. Thus, the chapter is utilizing an eponymous means of fracture classification. For the purposes of discussing treatment of each of these fracture types it is useful to comment on classification schemes and rationale. However, classification schemes as regards distal radius fractures have been found to be suboptimal as related to inter- and intraobserver reliability [11,13,14]. Kreder et al. [15] found that the only scheme with a reasonable predictive value and interexaminer agreement was the front end of the AO scheme wherein the fractures are divided into extra-articular, marginal – articular and intra-articular [14]. In this chapter, fractures will be described by eponymous type and OTA (Orthopaedic Trauma Association) type [16].

Goals of Treatment

It is obvious that the goal of fracture treatment is a healed fracture. The relative importance of "follow-on" goals is not known. But, in this author's experience, pain-free function ranks as the second goal with "no adjacent sequelae" (shoulder stiffness, CTS, RSD) a close third. Motion ranks fourth, but should be separated into forearm rotation and wrist motion [17–19]. Of these two, forearm rotation is decidedly more important to patient function. Finally, cosmesis is of some importance. But, with no exception has the author met a patient who truly valued form over pain-free function. Thus, all treatment should aim to gain pain-free forearm rotation in conjunction with a healed fracture without comorbid sequelae. In the elderly osteoporotic patient group full wrist motion can be considered desirable but should not be ranked as a high priority.

Available Fixation Tools

The list of available fixation tools seems endless by product number, but, makes more sense when divided into product type. In this manner, treatment tools which can be considered are: cast treatment, pin fixation with cast support, external fixation, internal fixation, combined internal and external fixation, and augmentation tools such as bone graft, bone graft substitutes (inert and variably active) and electrical stimulation. Each of these treatments has some value for the fractures discussed in this chapter and this book. However, because the fracture types being discussed are less stable, "weaker" fixation tools, such as casting, have less applicability as the primary treatment. Several of the above methods will be further discussed in case examples.

Concerns Regarding Fixation Methods

All fixation methods have three common fixation stress points or modes of failure. Fig. 14.3a details these three points as: (1) screw to bone interface, (2) screw device (fixation screw, external fixation screw/pin) to fixation device (external fixation bar, plate) interface, and (3) fixation device spanning the fracture region. As bone density declines, it is obvious that the first of these fixation points is less able to deliver support from the whole construct to the bone. Although this method of describing device function is simple it is useful when considering fixation plans and even has some applicability to understanding cast function. When considering cast application as a means of fracture management, it should be obvious that the cast will not provide direct skeletal support. But if the distance between solid cortices at point 3 in Fig. 14.3a, is small, and the general alignment of the bone can be maintained, then direct cortical apposition at point 3 may be sufficient to maintain an acceptable reduction. Notwithstanding the numerous "ifs and maybes" contained in the foregoing sentence, cast support of some distal radius fractures is sufficient. A more essential point to take away from Fig. 14.3a is the need to understand the fixation strength/quality achieved by the method which the surgeon has chosen to employ. Fig. 14.3b shows the relative strength of several methods of plate fixation [20]. Three points deserve emphasis.First, different plate designs will withstand different forces before failing in compression in like-density bones.Second, it is possible to use a bone grouting substance to enhance "screw to bone" fixation thereby "restoring" plate function in simulated osteoporotic bone.Third, using an "interference fit tine" may be equal to or better than screw fixation, particularly when the tine is secured to the plate. Fig. 14.3a shows a tined plate supporting the distal radial fragment. In this plate the distal screws play a lesser role in load transmission. The purpose in understanding the strength of fixation is at least twofold. First, it can be assumed that the surgeon will ask the patient to undertake finger motion during the immediate postoperative period. Does the fixation method employed impede finger function and is it "strong" enough to resist the forces which will be seen? Second, is the fixation sufficiently "strong" to allow early AROM (active range of motion) and/or AAROM (active-assisted range of motion) of the forearm and wrist? Fig. 14.3c shows a linear relationship between grip activity and load transmitted to the distal radius (M.D. Putnam et al., unpublished work). Although the exact load will vary dependent on ulnar length and wrist position, the essential fact is the grip activities constitute a balance between wrist extensors and flexors, as well as finger and thumb motors, such that a load 2–5 times as great as observed grip force may be transmitted to the distal radius. The degree to which any fixation construct can withstand and distribute such loads should be known to best plan rehabilitation (M.D. Putnam et al., unpublished work) [21,22].

Case Examples

Cast

In general, cast treatment of Smith's or volar Barton's fractures is not appropriate. The fractures are usually too comminuted and too oblique to be stabilized by cast support. However, an occasional exception may occur. An 81-years-old woman presented with the fracture seen in Fig. 14.4a. This extra articular fracture was initially shifted in a palmar direction. Gentle pressure restored neutral, perhaps even dorsal, position. Because the fracture was felt to be comminuted both dorsally

---

Figure 14.3. **a** Any fixation utilized to stabilize a fracture has at least three points of potential failure. *Point 1* is the interface between the screw threads and bone. This interface will be affected by fracture comminution, bone quality and thread size. The next point of possible device failure, *point 2*, is seen at the interface between any screw support mechanism and its interaction with the plate or supporting device. Utilizing an external fixator this would be the interaction between the pin and pin coupler. Regardless, direct incorporation of an interface at this location would reduce the likelihood of failure between these two supporting structures. This type of device, commonly referred to as blade-type device, is sometimes more difficult to employ. The third potential area of device weakness or failure, *point 3*, is where the device crosses the most comminuted section of the fracture. In a plate model this would represent the point where the plate crosses the comminuted section of the fracture, whereas in an external fixation model this would represent where the rod crossed the fracture. **b** Relative strengths of various fixation models utilized to support a distal radius osteotomy model. Horizontal brace indicate homogeneous groups identified by Tukey's Honest Significant Difference test at $p = 0.05$ level. As can be seen, some models would support more than 2 times the load of the weakest model. That is, the newtons resisted prior to device failure can be altered by the shape of the device considered separately from the quality of the bone. **c** The risk of failure after device fixation is related not only to the strength of the device itself but also to the load transmitted to the device during the early healing phase. If one assumes that a fracture itself cannot bear load, then the device used to stabilize the fracture is assumed to bear load during the healing period. Put differently, rehabilitation forces should be considered when planning a rehabilitation program and these should be designed not to exceed the strength of the device utilized to support the fracture. In our model, it is estimated that rehabilitation forces as low as 10 pounds of grip strength can produce loads as high as 300 newtons in the distal radial metaphysics. This may exceed the strength of some devices utilized to support distal radius fractures. ▶

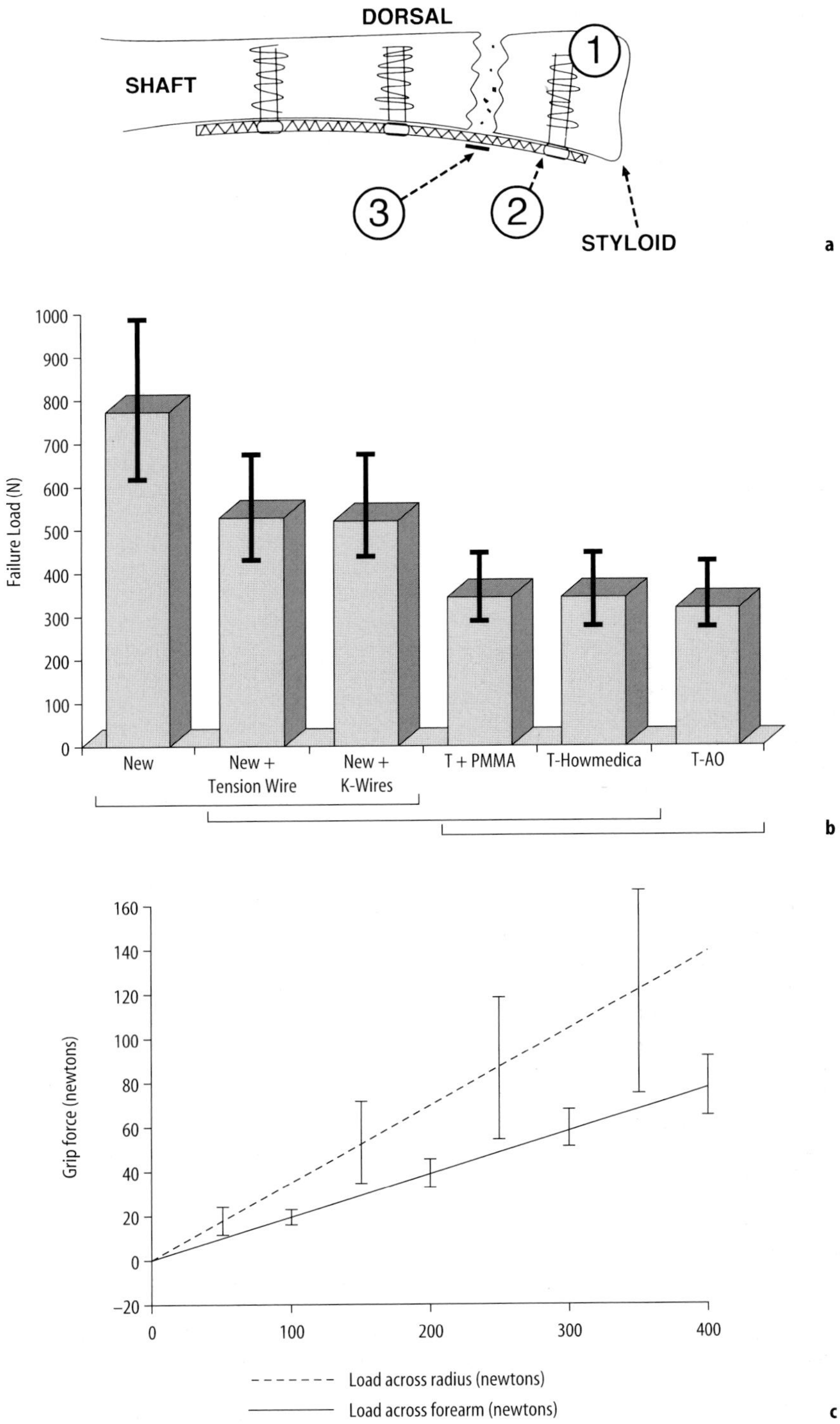
DORSAL
SHAFT
STYLOID
1
2
3
a
1000
900
800
700
600
500
400
300
200
100
0
Failure Load (N)
New
New + Tension Wire
New + K-Wires
T + PMMA
T-Howmedica
T-AO
b
160
140
120
100
80
60
40
20
0
−20
Grip force (newtons)
0
100
200
300
400
Load across radius (newtons)
Load across forearm (newtons)
c

Figure 14.3

and volarward it was felt that it would collapse in a direct proximal direction. Two additional key facts were identified. First, the patient had no specific need for full wrist or forearm motion. Second, at the time of initial presentation she was able to supinate and pronate the forearm with minimal pain. Thus, she was casted for 3 weeks using a short arm cast in neutral rotation. Fingers were free and the shoulder was mobilized immediately. At 3 weeks minimal fracture pain was present and the patient was changed to a support splint and allowed to remove the same for

---

Figure 14.4. **a** This patient demonstrates a fracture which at the time of original evaluation was displaced slightly palmarward. General pressure restored the fracture into a neutral position and the patient was noted to have functional rotation of her forearm after this reduction. We have decided to support the patient in neutral position utilizing a cast support for 3 weeks after which she was rehabilitated in a splint. The patient's final forearm rotation is shown in the clinical photographs and there was no complaint of pain or loss of function described by the patient. She had retained excellent finger motion and had no complaints related to treatment intervention. This patient is presented to demonstrate the utility of assessing the patient's needs and realizing the same by simply allowing fracture consolidation in the originally injured or minimally manipulated position. Although this situation is uncommon in our practice, it is important that the surgeon remembers same so as to not provide overtreatment which can lead to complication. **b** This combined intra-plus extra-articular fracture was identified as unstable and the ulnar shaft fracture was also noted. Unfortunately, the treatment selected seen in Fig. 4b2 was not sufficiently "strong" to resist the forces that were present in the postoperative period. In fact, although this fixator is designed to be used dynamically, it collapsed around the pin sites, which did not maintain a strong interface distally. The case is shown to illustrate the fact that external fixators alone may not be sufficient to support the most comminuted distal radius fractures. This is particularly true in the case of bone of lesser quality. In this situation, it may have been more reasonable to complete an original fixation of the distal radius fracture in slightly shortened position while at the same time excising the ulnar head and utilizing the same as bone graft. In any event, attempting to regain length of bone of poor quality is difficult and the strength of any external fixator must be considered as well as the interface strength between the external fixator pins and the bone. **c** A fracture similar to that seen in **b**. The bone is of fair quality and the metaphysical comminution is substantial although the intra-articular component of the fracture is not displaced. The patient was felt to represent a poor candidate for external fixation alone and the decision was made to proceed with reduction and internal fixation. A dorsal approach was chosen utilizing a "bladed plate". The ulnar styloid/head fragment was stabilized with a single pin which, based upon C-arm fluoroscopic inspection of the wrist at the time of surgical fixation, provided sufficient stability. The patient was noted to have stable rotation of the distal radioulnar joint at the completion of operative intervention and the healed radiographs (4c3, 4c4) demonstrate maintenance of operative reduction, healing of the fracture, and maintained joint space betwen the radius and carpal elements. At this time the patient had regained full forearm rotation and had painless radial-carpal motion. The plate has been left in place and the patient has had no complications related to plate placement or the longitudinal intramedullary pin. **d** Combined fixation utilizing internal and external fixation techniques is sometimes the most appropriate method for distal radius fractures. This patient presented with a combined intra- plus extra-articular fracture displaced in a palmarward fashion. Substantial comminution was present at the fracture site and Fig. 4d4 demonstrates the operative exposure as well as the degree of comminution originally visualized. The bone was noted to be of poor quality and although screw fixation was possible both proximal and distal to the fracture site, the fixation worked primarily as a buttress support. The interoperative radiograph demonstrates the combined presence of external fixation utilized at OR to insure original distraction of the fracture fragments. This was relaxed at the time of surgery after the internal fixation had been placed and utilized postoperatively as a neutralization device for 4 weeks. The fixator was removed when early evidence of fracture consolidation was verified and minimal tenderness was present by clinical palpation/compression about the original injury. Follow-up radiographs obtained at 3 months demonstrated maintained reduction of the fracture without joint incongruity. The internal fixation plate was left in place without evidence of loosening or metal fatigue. The patient regained full supination and functional dorsal flexion and complained of no undue discomfort. Utilization of this combined method is particularly valuable in fractures wherein one fixation method alone cannot achieve either fracture fragment reduction or complete stabilization (*see following pages for parts c–d).*

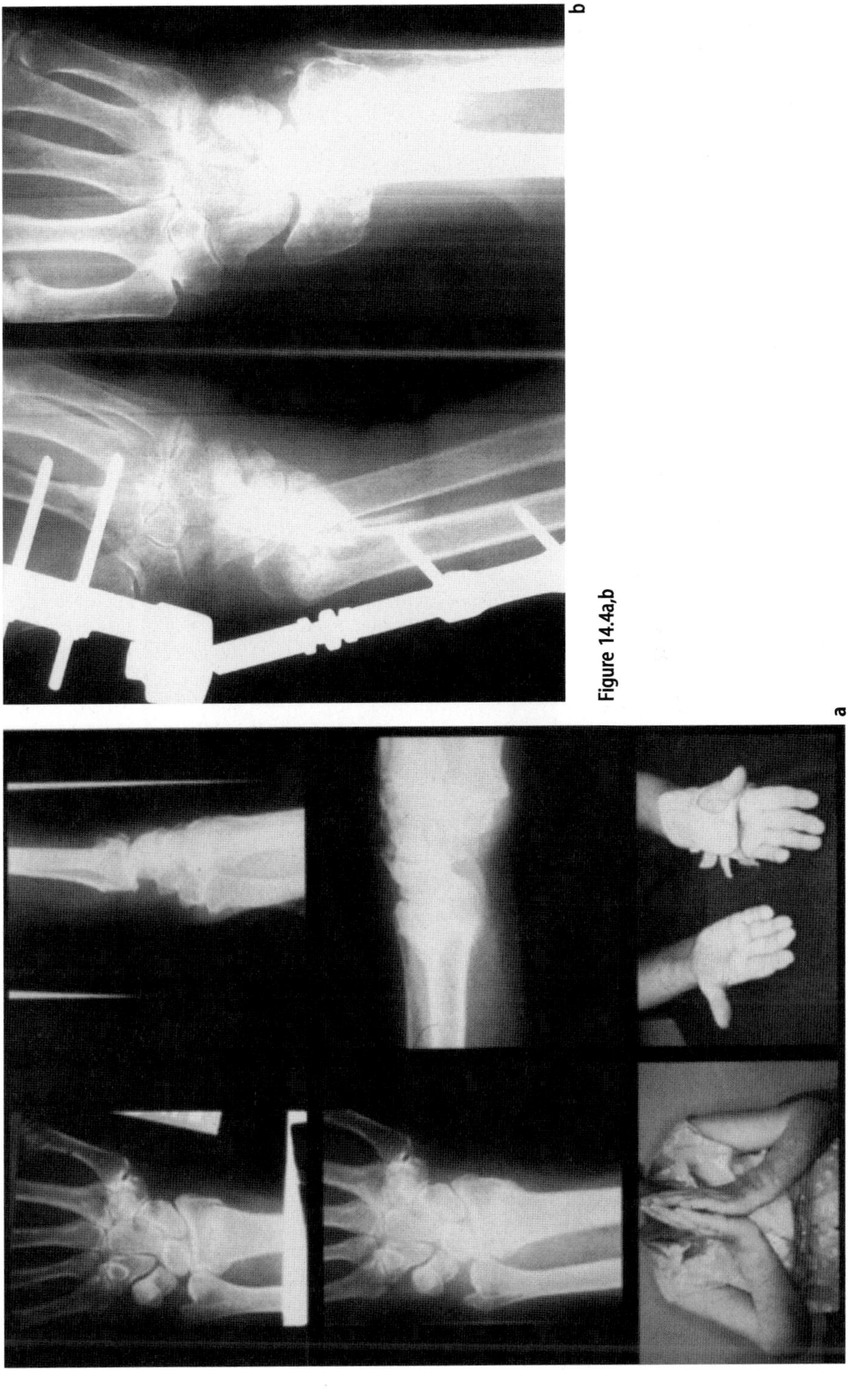

Figure 14.4a,b

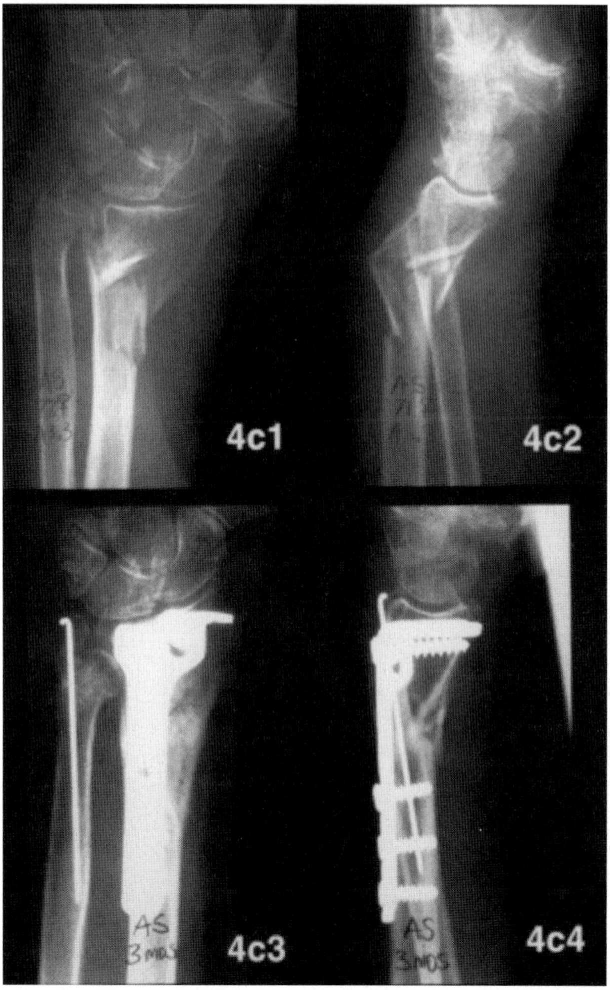

c

Figure 14.4. (*continued*)

showering. By 8 weeks she had regained useful function without pain. This case demonstrates a relatively uncommon situation as regards distal radius fractures, but it serves to emphasize the need to tailor the treatment to the patient's needs and not the needs of the surgeon or radiologist.

External Fixation

Although external fixation does offer direct control of bone elements, it may not be sufficient to resist the rotational collapse forces which will be seen after application [19,20,23,24]. A patient presented for care of a comminuted fracture with palmar displacement, associated joint involvement and an ulnar head fracture. The initial oblique radiograph and the 2 week follow-up radiograph after placement of

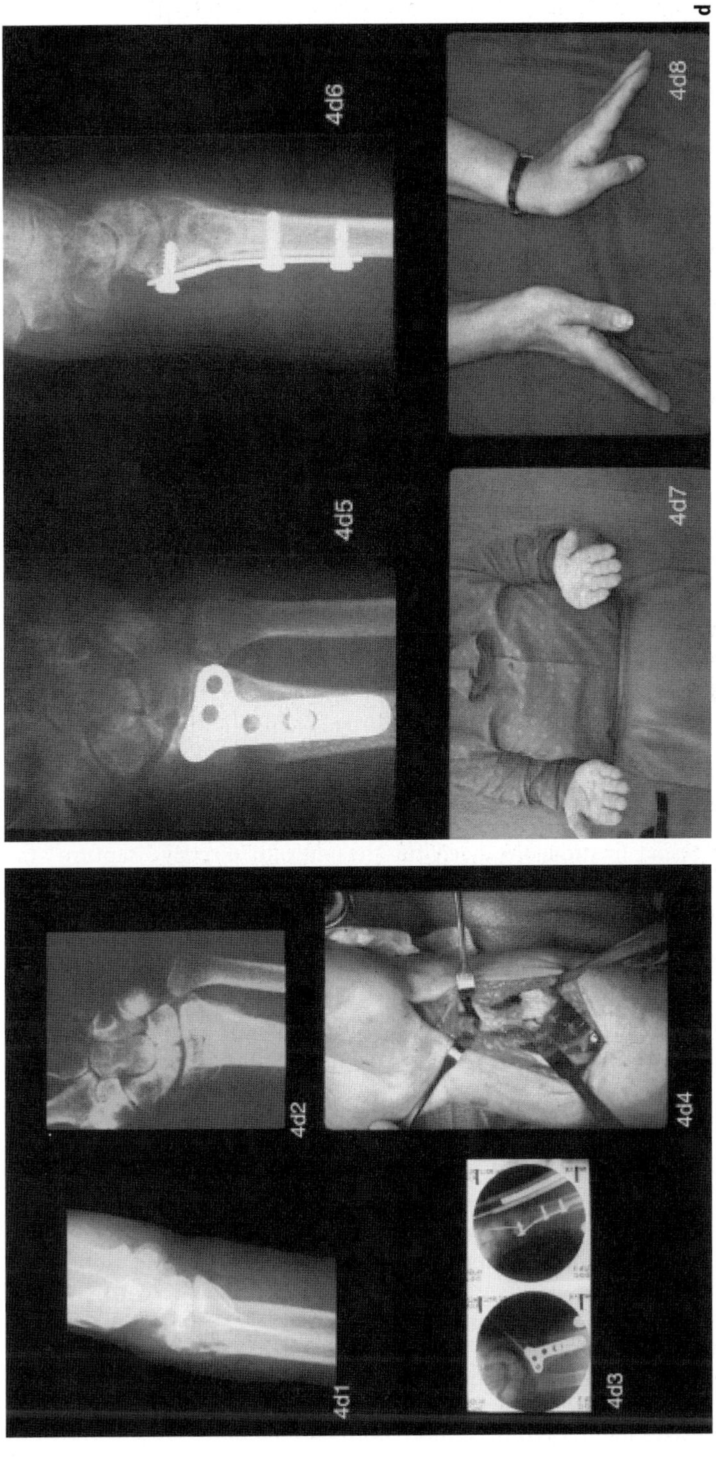

Figure 14.4. *(continued)*

an external fixateur are seen in Fig. 14.4b. The fixateur is noted to be a type which would allow dynamization. However, it was not used in this manner. Rather, it appeared, at the time of referral to our practice, that the loads exceeded the strength of the distal bone-to-pin interface, which had then rotated in the metacarpals. Data is available similar to that in Fig. 14.3b regarding the compression resistance of external fixation devices. Several are as able as the "strongest" commercially available plates. However, the number of proximal and distal attachment points to bone for most external fixateurs is no greater than, and usually less than, that for most plates. Perhaps more important, the attachment points are further from the fracture. So as rotational load is applied to the fracture the load which must be resisted by the pin or screw is magnified. Recalling the equation of Load = Force × Distance, it should be obvious that the external fixateur is at a mechanical disadvantage the further removed it is from the fracture site. This mechanical disadvantage is made worse in patients whose bone is weakened secondary to osteoporosis, which theoretically reduces the strength of the bone-to-pin interface.

Hence, although external fixation is important in the management of distal radius fractures, and the author and others have both written articles detailing principles to be followed when using external fixateurs, including in the elderly, and completed laboratory tests detailing the utility of external fixation combined with internal support, the case in Fig. 14.4b and this brief summary should emphasize the risks of external fixation in the elderly [23–26]. In the author's opinion, Fig. 14.4d is a better example of the role of external fixation in these unstable fractures in an osteoporotic patient.

Internal Fixation

Ellis originally described internal fixation of distal radius fractures in 1965 [27]. This article focused on Barton's fractures [27]. In this application, the plate was used as a buttress. However, as surgeons have attempted to repair other distal radius fractures using internal fixation, the need for the plate to directly "capture" the distal fragments has become obvious. As described earlier, plates offer some advantages over external fixation. However, the ability of screws to "hold" osteoporotic bone may be minimal.Thus, the surgeon can use grouts or other methods to increase the effective support offered by the plate [28,29]. If the plate is designed to "capture" the bone directly it may reduce the need for screw support distally and allow plates to be safely used in osteoporotic bone. A 72-year-oldwoman, is a case example. She presented after falling at home with a closed, comminuted, Smith's type fracture seen in Fig. 14.4c. The associated fracture of the ulnar head was found to be unstable at surgery. It was felt that this case could be treated by an attempt at internal fixation utilizing a plate system which did not rely solely on screw support for stabilization of the distal fragment. The fracture was approached dorsally because a plate of sufficient length was only available in a dorsal configuration. Because the fracture did not extend into the joint, it probably could have been approached from the volar side if the fracture were shorter or a longer plate was available. At surgery, the bone quality was judged as good proximally. Each of the proximal screws achieved tightness to chuck pinch. However, the distal screws were only fair-tip pinch tightness. But the stability of the radius construct was judged as good with the tines in place. That is, no fracture site motion was seen during observation while loading the radius either with direct vision or by C-arm fluoroscopy. The ulnar head was pinned longitudinally. Stability of the entire construct was felt sufficient to began AROM of all joints in the arm the day after surgery. Strengthening was begun at 6 weeks. The patient's radiographs at 3 months demonstrated healing of the fracture without change from the operatively reduced position. Importantly, she had painless motion of the forearm and wrist with no evidence of irritation from the fixation plate (excepting the ulnar pin, which was removed at 3 months), which has remained in place beyond 1 year.

The issues to emphasize with this case example are: (1) internal fixation can play a role in managing Smith's and Barton's fractures, (2) internal fixation plates are available which utilize tines or pegs and that these change the relative importance of the screw-to-bone interface in Osteoporotic bone, and (3) that regardless of the plate type employed, the surgeon must assess the quality of the fixation interfaces and rigidity of the overall construct as regards its ability to withstand early rehabilitation and design the therapy program for the patient after determining the construct strength.

Combined Fixation

Putnam and Fischer [30]have described a combined method of stabilizing distal radius fractures with plate and external fixation. This paper was an outgrowth of earlier work by the senior author and has also been reported on by others [31]. The critical facts to be gleaned from these works are: (1) that prolonged external fixation results in greater wrist stiffness, (2) combined external fixation and internal fixation can safely shorten the duration of external fixation, and (3) the ultimate outcome following this combined methodology is nearly equal to best outcomes after internal fixation.

A 68-year-old woman is an example of a patient managed using this methodology. She presented after slipping on ice. The closed fracture was felt to be best described as a Barton's fracture with extension to the dorsal metaphysis. The presentation radiographs are seen in Fig. 14.4d. This patient represents the possible best example of the difficulties faced by the surgeon in treating these unstable fractures in functional adults who have substantially diminished bone quality. Intraoperative exposure revealed substantial volar comminution of the metaphysis with reduced bone quality apparent based on the tightness of screw fixation which was achieved proximally (fair) and distally (poor). Intraoperative fluoroscopic views demonstrated restoration of length and fracture alignment as well as support of the reduction using an external fixateur. The patient began mobilization of all joints except the wrist but including the forearm/DRUJ the day after the injury. The fixateur was removed at 6 weeks. The patient's result at 6 months was remarkable for nearly symmetric forearm rotation and full finger motion with functional motion of her wrist in all planes without any residual pain.

This case represents the author's and others' preferred method of fracture management in bone too osteoporotic to be stabilized by fixation with modern plate/tine fixation devices [30,32].The author prefers the above method, which relies upon the patient healing their own bone, to those which would employ bone grouting substances in an attempt to provide fracture stabilization. Bone grouting agents may play a role in enhancing screw fixation but the use of these agents (active or inert) has not been shown to be superior for management of any fracture to date and should be considered with marked caution in the presence of osteoporosis. Schmaltz [33] reported on the use of PMMA for support of Colle's fractures in 1988.

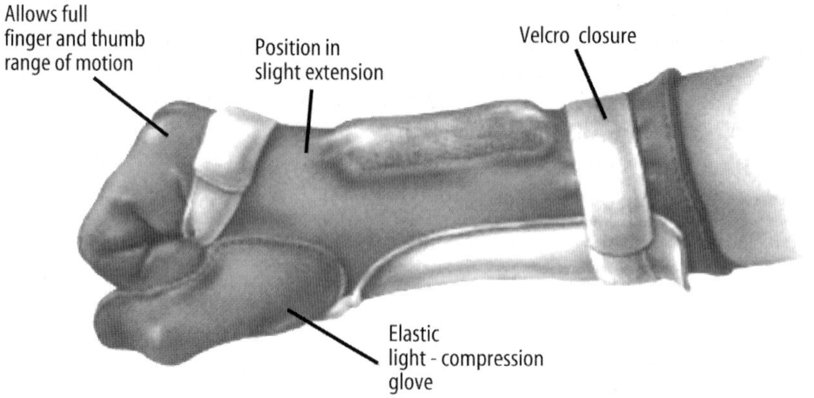

Figure 14.5. One of the most important component of post-fracture care is reduction of swelling. This can be achieved through a variety of means. Typically we utilize a compressive glove applied directly over the surgical incision site within the first 1–3 days after surgery. We make a custom glove in the presence of an external fixator and utilize Velcro straps to provide satisfactory compression around the external fixation pin sites. As a general rule, we allow patients to begin open care of the external fixation pin sites within the first several days after surgery, to include shower, careful pin tract cleaning and a light, sterile dressing. This is completed in conjunction with our active range of motion program to promote forearm rotation, finger motion and, when possible, gentle active range of motion of the radial-carpal articulation.

In this low-energy injury, sufficient support may be offered by the grout to allow healing around the agent. Norian and other agents may have a similar future utility [21,28]. But, again, grouting agents are not appropriate primary treatment agents in higher-energy distal radius fractures and/or in osteoporotic bone.

Post-fracture Management

This chapter has attempted to emphasize the relationship between fracture construct strength and the type of rehabilitation to be pursued postoperatively.

The need to relate the rehabilitation to fixation strength is most important if the patient will be undertaking motions which involve activation of any hand or wrist motors. Beyond building sufficient construct strength for the patient to begin mobilization, it is the role of the surgeon to prescribe the exercises and methods for the patient and/or therapist to use in promoting recovery from the injury [21,22,34,35]. In our experience, three factors are most important for the surgeon to emphasize in the immediate postoperative period: (1) avoidance and reduction of edema, (2) mobilization of the shoulder and (3) control of pain. These three factors are interrelated [38]. That is, a patient who feels unable to move the shoulder because of arm pain will in fact develop more dependent edema and more pain and then more edema. This can be the beginning of RSD, a frozen shoulder and/or a stiff hand. Other authors have also emphasized these points [37,38]. As seen in Fig. 14.5 we use an edema control glove in the immediate postoperative period. These are individually made in cases where a external fixateur has been used. The therapists also instruct the patient in finger, shoulder and elbow mobilization to begin the day after surgery. These exercises are in addition to whatever motions are allowable in the wrist and forearm based on fixation construct strength. An extra effort is needed to begin these programs early in this age of outpatient surgery and immediate hospital discharge, but it is our and others' experience that the end result is highly dependent upon patient acceptance and completion of the prescribed therapy, more so than the number of therapy visits [39].

The patient's activities should be advanced relative to bone healing and tissue swelling. Generally, we have been able to start strengthening by 6–8 weeks and discharge to unrestricted activity by 12–16 weeks.

Summary

Fractures of the distal radius are common and often difficult. Age-related weakening of the bone structure does make management of higher-energy and/or unstable fracture patterns more difficult. Newer plate support systems may offer these patients some enhanced outcomes with fewer treatment-related difficulties. However, one must remember the importance of intraoperative assessment of fracture construct repair strength and use the tool of external fixation for neutralization when the fracture construct strength is only fair or poor. Additionally, the need to balance fracture repair against planned rehabilitation and patients goals cannot be overstated. Finally, the surgeon is reminded of her or his important role in managing the rehabilitation as it applies to the injury as well as the whole arm. By following these guides, the desired outcome of a pain-free useful extremity should be obtained.

References

1. Falch JA. Epidemiology of fractures of the distal forearm in Oslo, Norway. Acta Orthop Scand 1983;54:291–301.
2. Düppe HG, Nilsson B, Johnell O. A single bone density measurement can predict fractures over 25 years. Calcif Tissue Int 1997;60:171–174.
3. Huang C, Ross DD, Wasnich RD. Short-term and long-term fracture prediction by bone mass measurements: a prospective study. J Bone Miner Res 1988;13:107–113.
4. Majumdar S, Genant HK, Gramp S, et al. Correlation of trabecular bone structure with age, bone mineral density, and osteoporotic status: in vivo studies in the distal radius using high resolution magnetic resonance imaging. J Bone Miner Res 1997;12:111–118.
5. Wapniarz M, Lehmann R, Reincke M, Schonau E, Klein K, Allolio B. Determinants of radial bone density as measured by PQCT in pre and postmenopausal women: the role of bone size. J Bone Miner Res 1997;12:248–254.
6. Kronhed AC, Mollerim M. Effects of physical exercise on bone mass, balance skill and aerobic capacity in women and men with low bone mineral density, after one year of training – a prospective study. Scand J Med Sci Sports 1998;8:290–298.
7. Barton JR. Views and treatment of an important injury of the wrist. Med Exam 1838; 1:365.
8. Smith RW. A treatise on fractures in the vicinity of joints and on certain forms of accidental and congenital dislocations. Dublin: Hodges & Smith, 1847.
9. Colles A. On the fracture of the carpal extremity of the radius. Edinb Med Surg J 1814;10:182–186.
10. Gesensway D, Putnam MD, Nelson EW, Mente PL, Lewis JL. Biomechanics of dorsal plating of the distal radius. Helsinki: Monduzzi Editore, 1995.

11. Flikklia T, Nikkola-Sihto A, Kaarela O, Paakko E, Raatikainen T. Poor interobserver reliability of AO classification of fractures of the distal radius additional tomography is of minor value. J Bone Joint Surg [Br] 1998;80:670–672.
12. Peicha G, Seibert F, Fellinger M, Grechenig W, Schippinger G. Lesions of the scapholunate ligaments in acute wrist trauma-arthroscopic diagnosis and minimally invasive treatment. Knee Surg Sports Traumatol Arthrosc 1997;5:176–183.
13. Illarramendi A, Gonzalez Della Valle A, Segal E, De Carli P, Maignon G, Gallucci G. Evaluation of simplified Frykman and AO classifications of fractures of the distal radius assessment of interobserver and intraobserver agreement. Int Orthop 1998;22:111–115.
14. Jupiter JB, Fernandes DL. Comparative classification for fractures of the distal end of the radius. J Hand Surg [Am] 1997;22:563–571.
15. Kreder HJ, Hanel DP, McKee M, Jupiter J, McGillivary G, Swiontkowski MF. X-ray film measurements for healed distal radius fractures [published erratum appears in J Hand Surg [Am] 1996;21:532]. J Hand Surg [Am] 1996;21:31–39.
16. Orthopaedic Trauma Association. Fracture and dislocation compendium orthopaedic trauma association. J Orthop Trauma 1996;10(Suppl 1):26–30.
17. Lidstrom A. Fractures of the distal end of the radius: a clinical and statistical study of end results. Acta Orthop Scand 1959;Suppl 41:1–118.
18. Hurov JR. Fractures of the distal radius: what are the expectations of therapy: a two-year retrospective study. J Hand Ther 1997;10:269–276.
19. Frykman G. Fracture of the distal radius including sequelae-shoulder-hand-finger syndrome, disturbance in the distal radio-ulnar joint and impairment of nerve function: a clinical and experimental study. Acta Orthop Scand 1967;Suppl 108:3–153.
20. Gesensway D, Putnam MD, Mente PL, Lewis JL. Design and biomechanics of a plate for the distal radius. J Hand Surg [Am] 1995;20:1021–1027.
21. Wehbe MA. Early motion after hand and wrist reconstruction. Hand Clin 1996;12:25–29.
22. Margles SW. Early motion in the treatment of fractures and dislocations in the hand and wrist. Hand Clin 1996;12:65–72.
23. Anderson R, O'Neil G. Comminuted fractures of the distal end of the radius. Surg Gynecol Obstet 1944;78:434.
24. Putnam MD, Seitz WH Jr. Advances in fracture management in the hand and distal radius. Hand Clin 1989;5:455–470.
25. Seitz WH Jr, Putnam MD, Dick HM. Limited open surgical approach for external fixation of distal radius fractures. J Hand Surg [Am] 1990;15:288–293.
26. Putnam MD, Walsh TM. External fixation for open fractures of the upper extremity. Hand Clin 1993;9:613–623.
27. Ellis J. Smith's and Barton's fractures: a method of treatment. J Bone Joint Surg Br 1965;47:724–7.
28. Jupiter JB, Winters S, Sigman S, et al., Repair of five distal radius fractures with an investigational cancellous bone cement: a preliminary report. J Orthop Trauma 1997; 11:110–116.
29. Yetkinler DN, Ladd AL, Poser RD, Constantz BR, Carter D. Biomechanical evaluation of fixation of intra-articular fractures of the distal part of the radius in cadavera: Kirschner wires compared with calcium-phosphate bone cement. J Bone Joint Surg Am 1999;81:391–399.
30. Putnam MD, Fischer MD. Treatment of unstable distal radius fractures: methods and comparison of external distraction and ORIF versus external distraction-ORIF neutralization. J Hand Surg [Am] 1997;22:238–251.
31. Kaempffe FA, Wheeler DR, Peimer CA, Hvisdak RS, Cervavolo J, Senall J. Severe fractures of the distal radius: effect of amount and duration of external fixator distraction on outcome. J Hand Surg [Am] 1993;18:33–41.
32. Wolfe SW, Swigart CR, Grauer J, Slade JF, Panjabi MM. Augmented external fixation of distal radius fractures: a biomechanical analysis. J Hand Surg [Am] 1998;23:127–134.
33. Schmaltz A. External skeletal fixation versus cement fixation in the treatment of redislocated Colles' fracture. Clin Orthop 1990;254:236–241.

34. Tubiana R. Early mobilization of fractures of the metacarpals and phalanges. Ann Chirurg Main 1983;2:293–297.
35. Bryan BK, Kohnke EN. Therapy after skeletal fixation in the hand and wrist. Hand Clin 1997;13:761–776.
36. Miller DS. Medical management of pain for early motion in hand and wrist surgery. Hand Clin 1996;12:139–147.
37. Zyluk A. [Algodystrophy after distal radius fractures.] Chir Narzadow Ruchu Ortop Pol 1996;61:349–355.
38. Zyluk A. [Latrogenic causes of post-traumatic reflex sympathetic dystrophy.] Wiad Lek 1998;51:173–178.
39. Oskarsson GV, Hjull A, Aaser P. Physiotherapy: an overestimated factor in after-treatment of fractures in the distal radius. Arch Orthop Trauma Surg 1997;116:373–375.

15 Cervical Spine Fractures and Osteoporosis

U. Berlemann and P. F. Heini

General Considerations

Osteoporosis as a generalized bone disease appears to affect the cervical spine differently from other spinal regions. Failure of the anterior column, i.e., vertebral body osteoporosis fractures, is typically seen in the thoracolumbar junction and the midthoracic region and is virtually unknown above the T4 level [1]. This may be related to biomechanical and histomorphological differences between the various spinal regions. Edmonston et al. [2] have shown for the thoracolumbar region up to the level T1 that vertebral body failure load strongly correlates with bone mineral density (BMD) and much less with vertebral dimensions. Biomechanical compressive tests, however, have shown that cervical spine segments may withstand considerable forces without apparent failure, even in old-aged specimens (P.A. Cripton, unpublished data). It may therefore be possible that force flows in the cervical spine differ from those in other spinal regions, such that the anterior column and thereby the vertebral bodies are less loaded. The different anatomical dimensions and relations between the anterior column and the posterior elements in the cervical spine may be a reflection of these force flows. The principal loading of the cervical spine results from dynamic rather than static processes as in the lumbar spine.

Another explanation could be a relatively smaller BMD decrease in the cervical spine. A recent investigation at our institution showed that BMD values of vertebral bodies actually increase caudally [3]. However, these data involved thoracic and lumbar vertebrae only. Furthermore, the "factor of risk" for an osteoporotic vertebral fracture depends on both the ratio of the load on the spine and the failure load of the bone [4]. Indeed, histomorphometric studies have shown, that (a) the vertebral cortical shell in the cervical spine is relatively thick compared with the thoracic spine, and (b) the decrease in cortical thickness with age was only significant below vertebral body T8 [5].

However, if in our context "cervical spine and osteoporosis" is seen as "cervical spine in the elderly", several important issues have to be considered and differentiated from the cervical spine at younger ages.

Cervical Spine Injuries in the Elderly

Fractures of the cervical spine usually result from major trauma, such as car or traffic accidents, falls from great heights or dives into shallow water. In elderly patients severe cervical spine injuries may already result from simple falls. Experimental studies have shown that with higher patient ages lower force values to the cervical spine are sufficient to cause the same failure probability as in younger people [6]. Aging and degeneration lead to a marked decrease in the range of motion of the cervical spine [7] and this additional stiffness also results in an altered response to trauma and force absorption. Patients typically present with minor head injuries and few complaints of neck pain only. A considerable number of fractures are therefore initially missed. In consequence, any elderly patient with even a minor trauma to the head or neck should be suspected of having cervical spine damage.

There is very little information available on treatment and outcome of cervical spine injuries in the elderly, especially regarding the subaxial spine. Any management may be complicated by pre-existing comorbidities such as cardiopulmonary compromise. These additional risk factors and limited physiological reserve may affect conservative treatment options as well as tolerance to surgical interventions. Also, the aims of treatment may be defined differently in the elderly and younger population. Whereas in the young the maximum functional result may be the principal aim, the elderly have to keep or regain their general mobility as soon as possible. Therefore, general implications of treatment options have to be considered to a much higher degree, which is frequently reflected in a reluctance towards surgery in the elderly [8]. It has been stated that bony union is not always necessary in the elderly, and a stable fibrous union may be an acceptable result [9]. Although classification of injuries and technical surgical principles are similar in the various age groups [10], the indications for surgical intervention in the elderly are somewhat restricted.

In the general population, about 50% of fractures involve the C5–6 and C6–7 level, with dens fractures being the second most frequent localization. The incidence of lower cervical spine injuries continuously declines with age. However, in cases of spinal canal narrowing due to osteophytic degeneration severe neurological symptoms may be observed even without any major dislocation of the cervical spine and sometimes even without any fractures (Fig. 15.1). These "central cord syndromes" usually occur with hyperextension injuries of the spine causing rupture of the anterior longitudinal ligament and discs. Focal hemorrhages are seen in the central portion of the spinal cord. Conservative treatment with immobilization of the cervical spine is recommended; a decompressive laminectomy is usually not indicated [11]. Depending on the degree of neurological damage, the prognosis of such injuries in the elderly is rather critical due to a high rate of complications, i.e., infections and respiratory problems.

In contrast, the incidence of upper cervical spine injuries rises in the elderly. Fractures of the dens are the most common location in patients above the age of 70 years [12]. Therefore, this injury deserves specific attention, especially as treatment options are discussed controversially [13].

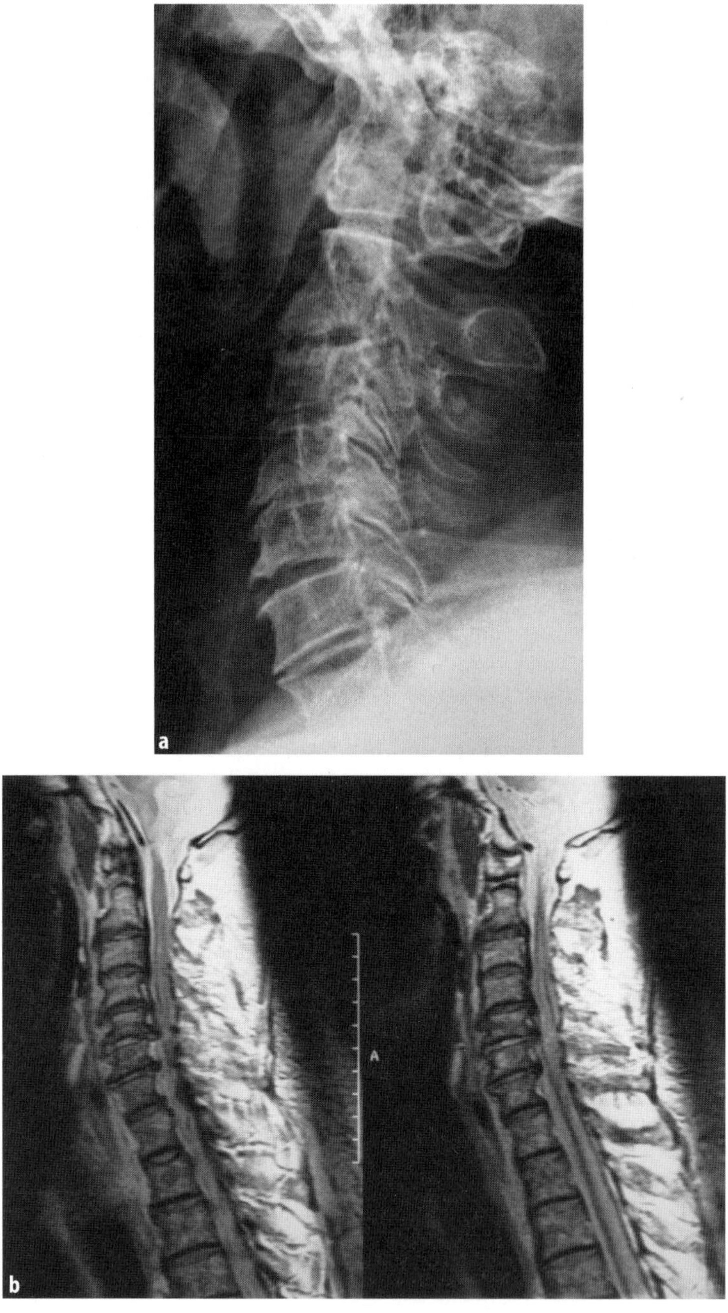

Figure 15.1a,b. A 68-year-old patient, presenting with incomplete tetraplegia after falling from a tree. **a** The lateral radiograph shows no apparent fracture, but there is advanced multilevel degeneration. **b** MRI confirms severe spinal canal stenosis, mainly at levels C4–5 to C6–7. The patient died a few days later due to pulmonary complications.

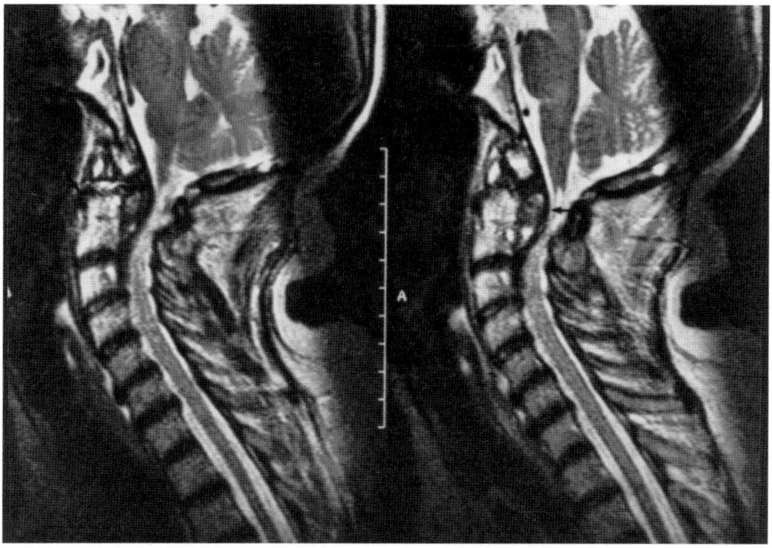

Figure 15.2. A 62-year-old patient presenting with cervical myelopathy 2 years after an initially missed dens fracture. MRI shows the pseudarthrosis (*arrow*, picture left) and a bulging tissue mass posterior to the dens (*arrow*, picture right). The patient is planned for an initial C1–2 transfacet stabilization followed by, if required, a transoral dens resection.

Fractures of the Dens Axis

Dens fractures are commonly classified according to Anderson and D'Alonzo [14]. A type 1 lesion is rare, represents an apical fracture of the upper part of the dens itself, and requires no surgical treatment. Type 3 is a fracture through the body of the atlas. In type 2 injuries the fracture line lies at the junction of the dens with the central body of the atlas. This injury accounts for two-thirds of all dens fractures, is difficult to treat and bears a substantial risk for nonunion, specifically in the elderly. External immobilization for several weeks is associated with high morbidity and mortality [15]. Patient tolerance towards rigid external immobilization with a halo-vest may also be limited. Furthermore, motion of the cervical spine even in a properly placed halo device remains considerable [16], a fact which may contribute to the observed nonunion in most patients over 60 years of age. Even though a stable fibrous union may give an acceptable result in the elderly [9,15], residual C1-2 instability may cause pain and late myelopathy (Fig. 15.2). Therefore, surgical stabilization for dens fractures has been proposed. The classical option is the posterior C1-2 arthrodesis [17] with high rates of bony union and good clinical results in some studies [18]. However, particularly in the elderly and high-risk patients unsatisfactory results with a considerable morbidity and mortality have also been reported [19]. Bone-graft donor site complications may also occur.

Direct posterior C1-2 interfacet screw fixation as described by Magerl [20] has also been advocated for cases of atlantoaxial instability. Although this stabilization results in a biomechanically very rigid construct, especially for lateral bending and rotation [21], severe osteoporosis does count as a contraindication of this technique, as there is a risk of screw breakage when solid bony fusion does not occur [22]. Furthermore, cervical rotation will be severely impaired after any kind of C1-2 arthrodesis as 50% of the rotational capacity of the cervical spine takes place at the atlantoaxial joint.

Anterior fracture stabilization using cannulated screws has been advocated as an alternative, initially with high success rates in younger patients [23]. In our clinic these experiences initiated a generous indication for this kind of fixation in the elderly also [24].

Own Material of Anterior Screw Fixation of Dens Fractures

Nineteen patients (9 women, 10 men) with an average age at the time of surgery of 75 (65–87) years were treated between 1985 and 1995. Seventeen patients could be contacted with an average clinical follow-up of 4.5 (1–11) years and radiological follow-up of 2.5 years (3 months to 11 years). Two patients had died 4 months and 5 years respectively after surgery from unrelated causes.

In 18 patients the injury was sustained by a fall, 11 of which were of low energy, e.g., a fall from a chair. One patient was involved in a motor vehicle accident. All patients sustained type 2 injuries, of which 4 were combined with a fracture of the C1 arch.

Fourteen patients had no initial neurological deficit, and none had any lasting symptoms. The number of associated injuries and the degree of neurological symptoms usually is low [15]. In 2 patients the diagnosis was initially overlooked but established and made after 1 week. One patient did not seek medical treatment until 2 weeks after sustaining the injury. Six patients had initially mild symptoms only.

Clark and White [25] defined a displacement of the dens of more than 5 mm or an angular deformity of more than 10° as significant. According to this definition our cases were classified as severely displaced in 13 cases, with a maximum of 15 mm displacement and 45° angulation. All fractures but two were displaced posteriorly and all but one in extension. Other studies have also shown that in the elderly displacement typically occurs posteriorly in contrast to the younger population [26].

The duration of surgery was between 45 min and 2 h. Five postoperative complications were noted. One hematoma required revision and 1 patient suffered from postoperative phases of apnea also due to the sustained contusio cerebri. All complications resolved without serious sequelae. Radiologically, the intraoperatively achieved position of the dens was maintained in 13 patients. In 6 cases the reduction was lost (maximum 4 mm and 10°). In one of these cases the dens fragment returned to its preoperative position. Sixteen fractures united within 3–6 months. In 2 cases a pseudarthrosis was diagnosed, but as the patients were free of symptoms no further surgical intervention was regarded as necessary in spite of residual instability in one case. It was frequently noted that the anterior cortex of the dens healed slower than the posterior part.

At follow-up 2 patients complained of occasional pain relating to the cervical spine that required analgesics, but 17 were pain-free. All patients returned to normal activities appropriate to their age and condition. There was no neurological impairment.

No relation could be found between long-term outcome and initial degree of fracture dislocation, time of surgery, or additional C1 injury.

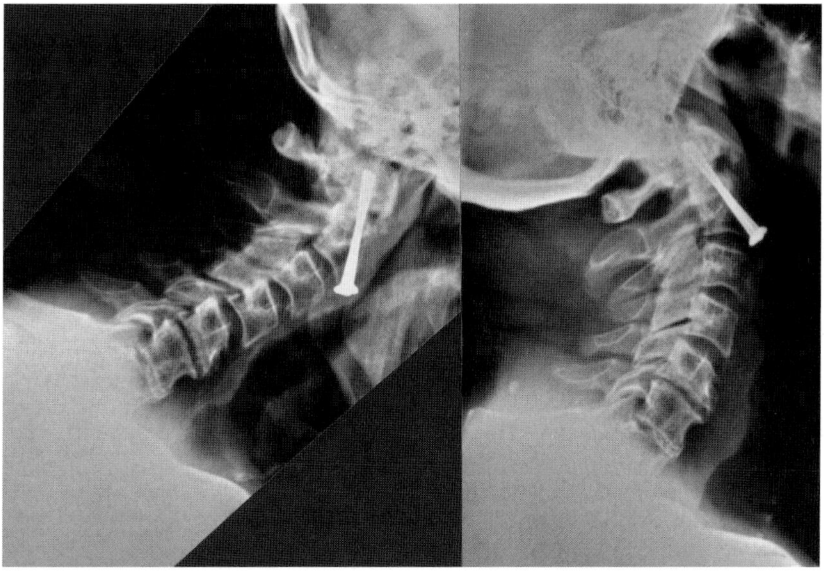

Figure 15.3. A 66-year-old patient with anterior dens stabilization of a type 2 fracture with a small anterior cortical defect. The anterior cortex has failed to heal, but a stable result is achieved. The patient is symptom-free.

Dens Fractures, Osteoporosis and Technical Pitfalls

Histomorphometric analysis of the dens has revealed very interesting data [27]. The base of the dens is a region of least resistance for fractures due to a reduced trabecular bone volume, poorer trabecular interconnections and reduced cortical thickness. These characteristics are markedly increased in osteoporotic bone, such that the resulting deficiency of bone mass in the base of the dens is considered responsible for the excessive fragility of the dens base in elderly patients. A high susceptibility to insufficiency fractures of the dens is also known in rheumatoid patients, where erosion and osteoporosis due to synovitis and steroid therapy can even cause spontaneous fractures [28].

Chiba et al. [29] analyzed a group of 62 type 2 fractures in patients of all ages and compared different treatment protocols. They concluded that anterior screw fixation was the therapy of choice, but emphasized the necessity of reasonable bone quality for adequate screw-hold. This is somewhat contradictory as osteoporotic changes at the dens base contribute to the fracture etiology. It is therefore important to gain a good screw-hold in the upper posterior dens cortex.

There are some critical surgical and technical issues which have to be considered. Before surgery the fracture has to be reduced using traction by Mayfield tongs, allowing good repositioning in the sagittal plane controlled by fluoroscopy with two orthogonal C-arm views. A very rigid cervical spine, as sometimes seen in elderly patients, may make reduction with clearance of the sternum impossible. In consequence, there may not be enough access for anterior fixation. This occurred in one of our patients who subsequently underwent posterior C1-2 fusion. Care has to be taken concerning the entry point of the screw at the body of C2; an entry too proximal into the anterior surface of C2 may result in an unstable fixation of the screw in the C2 body.

We observed delayed or even failed healing of the anterior cortex in about half the cases. This may be related to the high degree of injury to the local bone trabeculae with corresponding defects in the anterior cortex (Fig. 15.3) and/or to the compromised anterior blood supply [30].

Especially in the elderly a screw entry point relatively distal in the anterior portion of the C2–3 disc seems necessary to provide good fixation. Later, osteophytes may be observed in this segment, but this does not seem to cause any problems. Care also has to be taken not to distract the fracture site when the screw is inserted. This could contribute to pseudarthrosis and loss of reduction.

Conclusion

Cervical spine fractures in the elderly are characterized by a high proportion of upper cervical spine injuries, i.e., fractures of the dens axis, and associated rigidity of the spine due to aging and degeneration. In lower cervical spine injuries, little radiographic damage may be associated with severe neurological impairment. However, typical osteoporosis insufficiency fractures of the vertebral bodies are a rarity in the cervical spine.

General treatment principles do not differ from those in other age groups, but associated comorbidities play a major role. Immobilization is frequently not well tolerated, whereas surgical options may also be hampered by impaired general medical conditions.

However, for fractures of the dens axis anterior screw fixation is usually well tolerated and with few complications in the elderly. Considering some technical issues anterior screw fixation is therefore our therapy of choice for the dens fracture in the elderly patient. In cases of technical problems or nonunions the C1-2 transfacet screw fixation according to Magerl [20] represents a valuable alternative.

References

1. Wasnich RD. Vertebral fracture epidemiology. Bone 1996;18:S179–183.
2. Edmondston SJ, Singer KP, Day RE, Price RI, Breidahl PD. Ex vivo estimation of thoracolumbar vertebral body compressive strength: the relative contributions of bone densitometry and vertebral morphometry. Osteoporosis Int 1997;7:142–148.
3. Kaufmann M. Transpedikuläre Vertebroplastik zur Prophylaxe von Wirbelfrakturen bei schwerer Osteoporose. MD thesis, University of Bern, (submitted) 1998.
4. Myers ER, Wilson SE. Biomechanics of osteoporosis and vertebral fracture. Spine 1997;22:25S-31S.
5. Ritzel H, Amling M, Pösl M, Hahn M, Delling GG. The thickness of human vertebral cortical bone and its changes in aging and osteoporosis: a histomorphometric analysis of the complete spinal column from thirty-seven autopsy specimens. J Bone Miner Res 1997;12:89–95.
6. Pintar FA, Yoganandan N, Voo L. Effect of age and loading rate on human cervical spine injury threshold. Spine 1998;23:1957–1962.
7. Dvorak J, Antinnes JA, Panjabi MM, Loustalot D, Bonomo M. Age and gender related normal motion of the cervical spine. Spine 1992;17:S393–398.

8. Bohlman HH, Anderson PA. Anterior decompression and arthrodesis of the cervical spine: long term improvement. II. Improvement in incomplete traumatic quadriparesis. J Bone Joint Surg Am 1992;74:671–682.
9. Lieberman IH, Webb JK. Cervical spine injuries in the elderly. J Bone Joint Surg Br 1994;76:877–881.
10. Aebi M, Nazarian S. Klassifikation der Halswirbelsäulenverletzungen. Orthopäde 1987;16:27–36.
11. Kinoshita H, Hirakawa H. Pathological studies and pathological principles on the management of extension injuries of the cervical spine. Paraplegia 1989;27:172–181.
12. Ryan MD, Henderson JJ. The epidemiology of fractures and fracture-dislocations of the cervical spine. Injury 1992;23:38–40.
13. Seybold EA, Bayley JC. Functional outcome of surgically and conservatively managed dens fractures. Spine 1998;23:1837–1846.
14. Anderson LD, D'Alonzo RT. Fractures of the odontoid process of the axis. J Bone Joint Surg Am 1974;56:1663–1674.
15. Hanigan WC, Powell FC, Elwood PW, Henderson JP. Odontoid fractures in elderly patients. J Neurosurg 1993;78:32–35.
16. Koch RA, Nickel VL. The halo vest: an evaluation of motion and forces across the neck. Spine 1978;3:103–107.
17. Brooks AL, Jenkins EB. Atlanto-axial arthrodeses by the wedge compression method. J Bone Joint Surg Am 1978;60:279–283.
18. Weller SJ, Malek AM, Rossitch E. Cervical spine fractures in the elderly. Surg Neurol 1997;47:274–281.
19. Fried LC. Atlanto-axial fracture dislocations: failure of posterior C1 to C2 fusion. J Bone Joint Surg Br 1973;55:490–496.
20. Magerl F, Seemann P. Stable posterior fusion of the atlas and axis by transarticular screw fixation. In: Kehr P, Weidner A, editors. Cervical spine I, Strassbourg 1985. Wien: Springer, 1987:322–327.
21. Grob D, Crisco JJ, Panjabi MM, Wang P, Dvorak J. Biomechanical evaluation of four different posterior atlantoaxial fixation techniques. Spine 1992;17:480–490.
22. Weidner A. Application of the posterior interfacet screw for atlantoaxial pathology. In: Fessler RG, Haid RW, editors. Current techniques in spinal stabilization, New York: McGraw-Hill, 1996:93–99.
23. Aebi M, Etter C, Coscia M. Fractures of the odontoid process: treatment with anterior screw fixation. Spine 1989;14:1065–1070.
24. Berlemann U, Schwarzenbach O. Dens fractures in the elderly: results of anterior screw fixation in 19 elderly patients. Acta Orthop Scand 1997;68:319–324.
25. Clark CR, White AA. Fractures of the dens: a multicenter study. J Bone Joint Surg Am 1985;67:1340–1348.
26. Pepin JW, Bourne RB, Hawkins RJ. Odontoid fracture, with special reference to the elderly patient. Clin Orthop 1985;193:178–183.
27. Amling M, Wening VJ, Pösl M, Grote HJ, Hahn M, Delling G. Die Struktur des Axis-Schlüssel zur Ätiologie der Densfraktur. Chirurgie 1994;65: 964–969.
28. Toyama Y, Hirabayashi K, Fujimura Y, Satomi K. Spontaneous fracture of the odontoid process in rheumatoid arthritis. Spine 1992;17:436–441.
29. Chiba K, Fujimura Y, Toyama Y, Fujii E, Nakanishi T, Hirabayashi K. Treatment protocol for fractures of the odontoid process. J Spinal Disord 1996;9:267–276.
30. Schatzker J, Rorabeck CH, Waddell JP. Fractures of the dens: an analysis of thirty-seven cases. J Bone Joint Surg Br 1971;53:392–405.

16 Thoracic and Lumbar Spine Fractures

With Emphasis on Osteoporotic-Posttraumatic Vertebral Collapse

K. Kaneda and M. Ito

Introduction

Primary management aims in thoracolumbar osteoporotic-fragile fractures should be alleviation of pain, early ambulation, preservation of the physiological spinal balance with stability, and prevention of late neurological complications. There has been a general concensus that low-energy osteoporotic compression fractures in the thoracic and lumbar spine generally cause only localized pain and kyphosis without significant neurological complications. Therefore, urgent surgery is rarely indicated. Conservative treatment has been chosen for its ability to relieve back pain. Usually these fractures can be treated with a corset or hyperextension brace if tolerated. Early ambulation and avoidance of prolonged bed rest are important. Late onset of vertebral collapse can occur in these patients treated conservatively. Therefore, clinical and radiographic follow-up is mandatory. In this chapter, the management of osteoporotic/post-traumatic vertebral collapse with increasing kyphosis with or without neurological complications is described.

Late Neurological Compromise after Osteoporotic Fractures

In some patients with an osteoporotic-fragile fracture of the thoracolumbar spine treated conservatively, gradually increasing kyphosis and late complications of the spinal cord or the cauda equina can occur. This devastating neurological compromise is brought about by anterior impingement of the neural tissues in the anterior spinal canal by the retropulsed bony mass of the collapsed vertebra(e) [1–6].

Osteoporotic/Post-traumatic Vertebral Collapse

The cause of delayed post-traumatic vertebral collapse and the mechanism of the late neurological sequalae are not completely clear, but it seems to be the secondary bone ischemia associated with non-healing fractures of the vertebral trabeculae. Massive fibrous union of the fractured fragile trabeculae would bring about disturbance of the blood supply in the vertebral body, resulting in bone ischemia and finally vertebral collapse [7,8].

There has been no prospective study of osteoporotic vertebral fractures of the thoracolumbar spine. A retrospective review of patients who have required decompressive and reconstructive surgery for late neurological deficits following osteoporotic insufficiency fracture suggests that the risk factors include involvement of the thoracolumbar region (T11–L2) with either compromise of the anterior and middle column (burst fracture) or severe wedge compression, vacuum shadow within the fractured body, implying ischemic necrosis of bone, and/or the presence of segmental instability or hypermobility, combined with MRI evidence of retropulsed vertebral segments.

Reconstructive Surgery of Osteoporotic-Post-traumatic Vertebral Collapse

Materials and Methods

Between January 1987 and December 1995, a total of 92 patients (23 male, 69 female) with osteoporotic/post-traumatic vertebral collapse of the thoracic and lumbar spines were treated surgically in our department. The average age at surgery was 67.7 years (range 43–89 years).

Indications for surgery were devastating neurological compromise or increasingly unstable kyphosis at the fracture site. Seventy-six (83%) of the 92 patients suffered late devastating neurological deficits, and the other 16 (17%) had severe back pain with increasing thoracolumbar kyphosis. The intervals between neurological compromise and fracture were within 3 months in 43%, 3–6 months in 22%, 6–12 months in 9% and over 1 year in 13%; the interval was unknown in 13%. The neurological symptoms in 76 patients were a lesion of the spinal cord (lesion above the epiconus) in 5 patients, a lesion of the epiconus/conus medullaris with the cauda equina in 40, pure conus medullaris syndrome in 9, lesion of the cauda equina in 21 and lesion of the nerve roots in 1. The causes of injury were a fall while walking in 41 patients, a fall from a chair onto the floor in 23, lifting a heavy weight in 8 and no history of trauma in 20. The energy of trauma was thought to be low. Such low-energy trauma would not have resulted in compression fracture of the thoracolumbar spine in bone of normal quality and strength. The levels of the collapsed vertebra(e) were 28% at T12, 33% at L1, 14% at L2, 5% at L3, 5% at T12 and L1, 2% at L1 and L2, 2% at T11 and T12, and 11% at other levels. Seventy-three of the 92 patients had osteoporotic post-traumatic vertebral collapse at the thoracolumbar junction of T12 and L1. Their initial treatment was bracing with or without bed rest and prescription of nonsteroidal anti-inflammatory drugs in 75%. The other 25% did not receive any treatment.

Surgical Procedures (Fig. 16.1) [9]

Principles in the treatment of osteoporotic/post-traumatic vertebral collapse of the thoracolumbar spine are anterior spinal canal decompression by resection of the collapsed vertebra(e), correction of kyphosis and reconstruction of anterior column support using a vertebral spacer and the anterior instrumentation (Kaneda-SR).

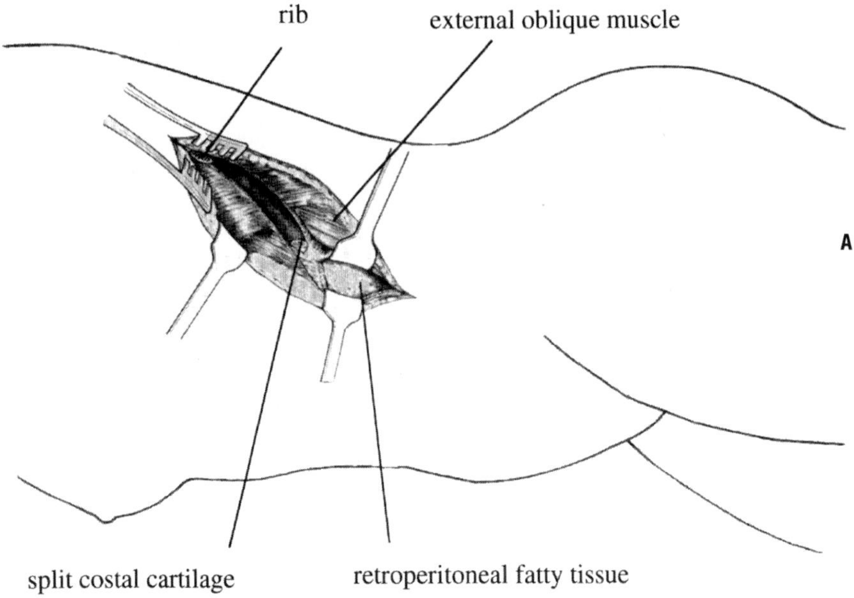

A

(a) (b)

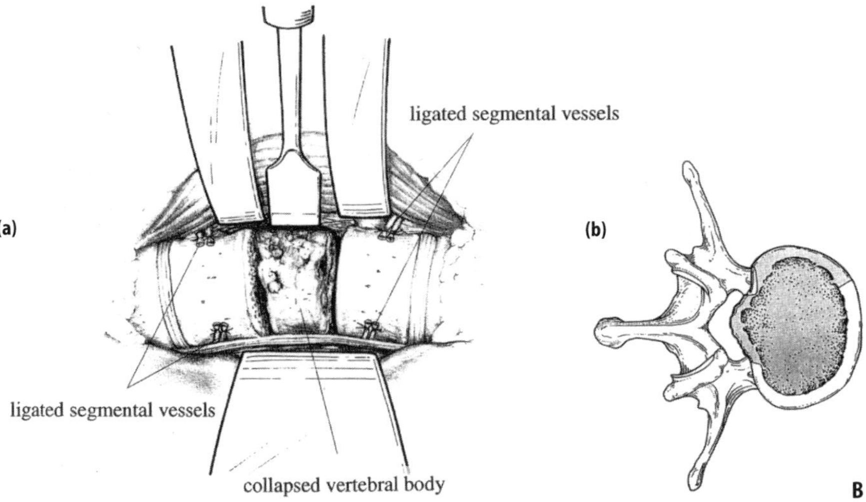

B

Fig. 16.1. **A** Extrapleural retroperitoneal approach. The tenth or eleventh rib is usually resected for an extrapleural retroperitoneal approach. After splitting the costal cartilage, retroperitoneal fatty tissue can be seen. The abdominal muscles are divided after separating the retroperitoneal fat and peritoneal contents from the anterior abdominal muscles. **B** Resection of collapsed vertebral body. **a** After removing adjacent intervertebral discs, the collapsed vertebral body is resected using flat or curved osteotomes. For the decompression of spinal canal, curved osteotome, curettes and 360° Kerrison rongeurs are utilized. **b** resection area in the axial plane is shown. (*continued next page*)

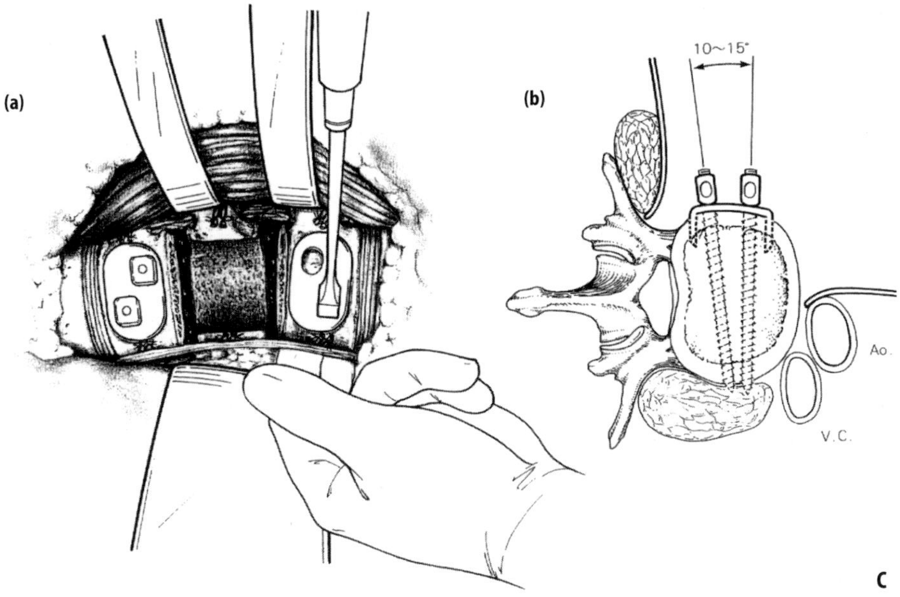

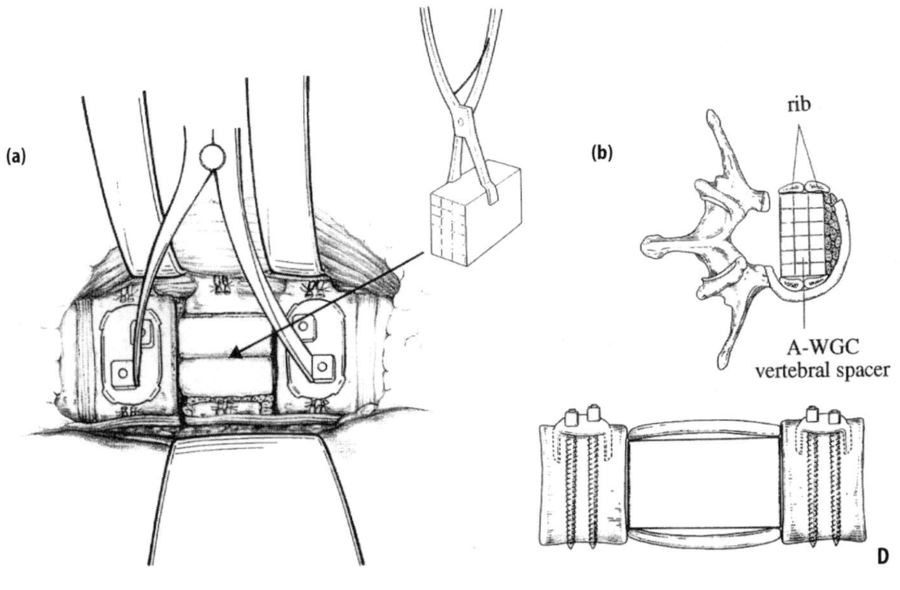

Fig. 16.1. **C** Placement of vertebral staples and screws. **a** A vertebral plate is properly placed at the lateral aspect of vertebral body. The spikes of the plate must be placed parallel to the intervertebral space and not penetrating into the disc spaces. **b** Posterior vertebral screws must be inserted 10°–15° anteriorly so as not to penetrate into the spinal canal. The screw tips must penetrate the opposite cortex to achieve bicortal screw purchase. The screw tip is blunt to avoid additional tissue damage. *Ao.*, aorta; *V.C.*, vena cava. **D** Placement of an A-W glass ceramic (A-WGC) vertebral spacer. **a** After correcting regional kyphotic deformity, autogenous rib graft and an A-WGC vertebral spacer of an appropriate length are inserted. **b** Autogenous rib graft at both sides of the A-WGC vertebral spacer and chip bone graft taken from the rib or healthy part of the vertebral body must be added. (*continued next page*)

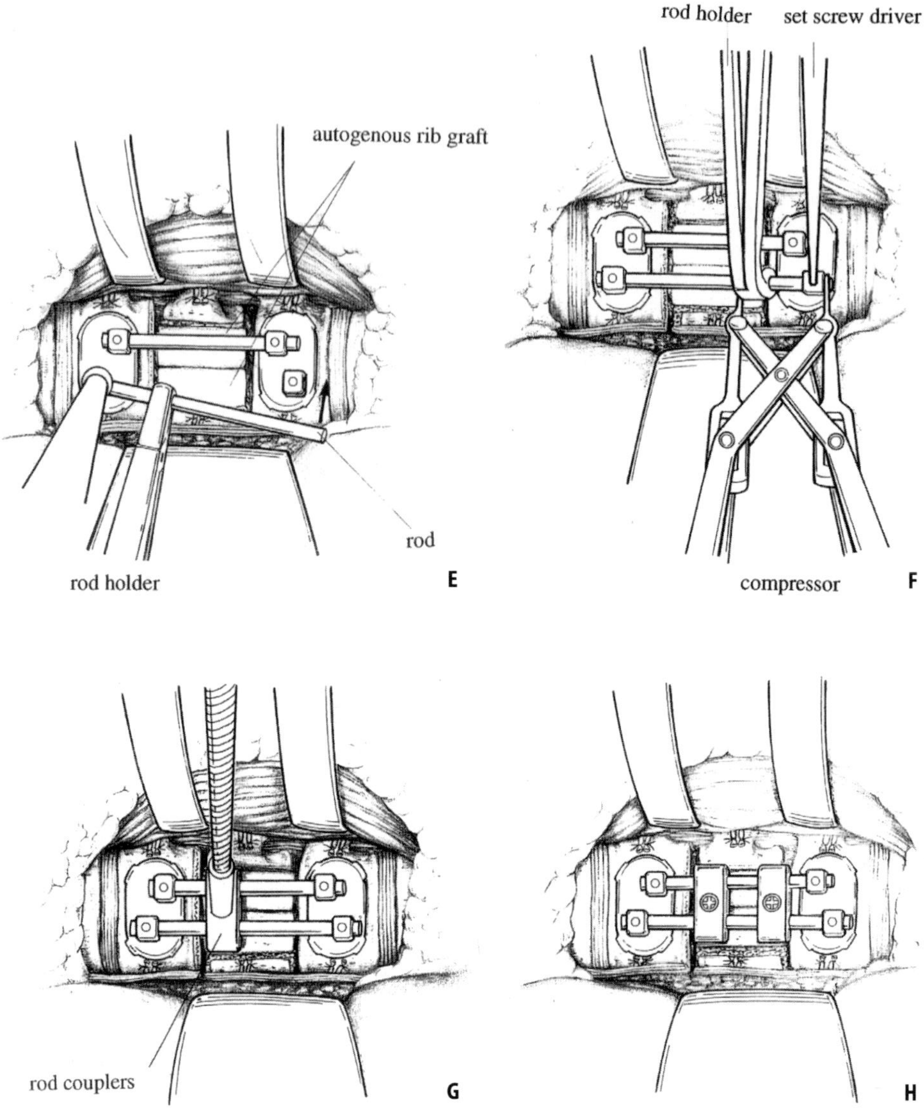

Fig. 16.1. **E** Placement of rod. By slightly rotating the screw head, it becomes easier to insert the rod into the screw hole. **F** Application of compression force to the construct. After firmly tightening the set screw over the screw head, compression force must be applied and the opposite screw tightened. **G** Placement of rod couplers. Two appropriate-sized rod couplers must be placed. **H** Completion of the Kaneda-SR system. (*continued next page*)

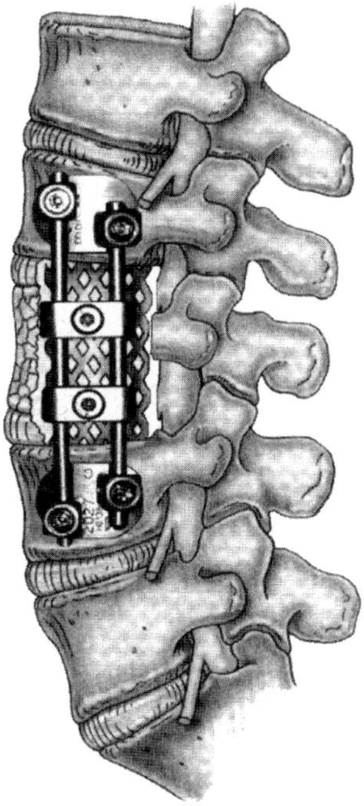

Fig. 16.1. I Placement of titanium mesh cage (Harms cage) and the Kaneda-SR system.

Surgical exposure of the thoracolumbar spine was via the extrapleural and retroperitoneal approach from the left side. Since osteoporotic/post-traumatic vertebral collapse usually occurs below T11, exposure of the surgical portion of the thoracolumbar spine can be achieved without thoracotomy (Fig. 16.1A). After exposing the vertebrae above and below the collapsed vertebra(e), the segmental vessels are ligated and cut. Discectomy is conducted above and below the collapsed vertebra to be resected. The resection is conducted using sharp osteotomes, chisels, curetts and Kerison rongeurs. During anterior spinal canal decompression, the posterior longitudinal ligament is left intact, which means detaching the retropulsed posterior part of the collapsed vertebra from the posterior longitudinal ligament. This is important to reduce bleeding from the epidural vein. It is not necessary to remove that ligament for neural decompression (Fig. 16.1B).

Following anterior spinal canal decompression by resection of the retropulsed bony mass compressing the neural tissue, application of Kaneda-SR anterior instrumentation is started. At first the vertebral staples are placed properly and fixed with screws as shown on the figure. The screw tip must penetrate the opposite cortex for stable fixation (Fig. 16.1C). Following insertion of the screws, the kyphosis is corrected by pushing the apex of the kyphosis with an assistant's palm and applying the spreader to the front screw heads. In keeping with the correction of kyphosis, one or two pieces of rib strut graft are placed as shown on the figure and the proper size of bioactive ceramic (A-W glass ceramic) [10] vertebral spacer (Fig. 16.1D), or a titanium cage with bone chip packing inside (Fig. 16.1I), is inserted tightly. The spreader is removed after checking the stability of the inserted spacer. Rib graft is placed on the spacer also. (Fig. 16.1D). The precut rods are inserted at the posterior screws first and tightened using the compressor. The anterior rod is set also (Fig. 16.1E). Compression force is applied to the inserted spacer by using the compressor between the rod holder and the screw head (Fig. 16.1F, I). Finally the two rod-couplers are applied for completion of Kaneda anterior instrumentation (Fig. 16.1G, H). Anterior column reconstruction using the titanium cage and Kaneda-SR is shown in Fig. 16.1I).

Within 3–5 days after surgery, patients were encouraged to start walking with TLSO. The brace is worn for about 6 months.

Results

Operating time was 228 min on average. Blood loss was 588 ml on the average. Blood transfusion was done in 47 of the 92 patients; 45 patients (49%) did not receive a blood transfusion. Postoperative follow-up period was 62 months on average (range 30–147 months).

Histological findings of the resected collapsed vertebrae were typical avascular necrosis without any vessels or blood cells in the collapsed portion.

Preoperatively, 76 (83%) of 92 patients suffered from devastating neurological damage due to late post-traumatic vertebral collapse. Nine had pure conus medullaris syndrome. Sixty-five (97%) of 67 patients (9 patients with pure conus syndrome were excluded from the 76 patients with neurological damage) showed a remarkable neurological recovery in Frankel grading (improvement of one or more Frankel grades). Of 45 patients with preoperative bladder–bowel disturbance, complete recovery occurred in 30 (67%); the others showed mild (incomplete) recovery. All 2 patients who did not show any neurological recovery in motor function in the lower extremities and/or in bladder–bowel function have had satisfactory pain relief with correction of increasing kyphosis. These 2 patients kept their paralytic status with increasing kyphosis for over 1 year without spinal canal decompression.

In terms of radiographic evaluation, stable fusion was gained in 72 (89%) of 81 patients treated by single anterior surgery and in all 11 patients (100%) treated by the scheduled combined anterior and posterior surgeries. Salvage posterior reinforcement following the anterior surgery was conducted in 9 patients; all were stabilized successfully. Correction of kyphotic deformity was from 33.2° preoperatively to 16.6° postoperatively and 20.2° at the survey. Existence of a "clear zone" at the border between the vertebral bone and A-W glass ceramic spacer was diminished with time. Though 67% of patients showed clear zone (0–2 mm) at 6 months postoperatively, this decreased to 45% at 18 months after operation. At 5 years after operation, most patients did not have a definite clear zone. Bone formation (consolidation) around the ceramic spacer became noticeable with time. All the patients showed moderate to marked bone consolidation at 5 years after surgery.

Subsequent compression fractures at levels other than the reconstructed site occurred in 33 patients during follow-up. There was no fracture at the fused vertebrae (just above and below the vertebral spacer, with the vertebral staple and screws inserted). It was not necessary to repair the subsequent compression fractures except in one patient of severe rheumatoid arthritis treated with steroid hormone.

Complications were pseudarthrosis in 9 patients (who were reinforced successfully by posterior instrumentation with fusion), migration of the vertebral spacer in 14 (15%) and dislodgment of the hooks of posterior instrumentation in 1. Nine of these were included in the pseudarthrosis group. There was no major complication (neurological, respiratory or circulatory). Death during follow-up occurred in 11 patients. One died at 4 months postoperatively from pneumonia. Of the remaining 10 patients, 3 died within 1–2 years, 2 in 2–5 years and 1 in over 5 years. All deaths seemed not to be related to surgery.

Case Reports

Case 1 (Fig. 16.2A–G)

This 62-year-old man suffered from alcoholism and secondary osteoporosis due to malnutrition. A T12 mild compression fracture occurred after a fall (Fig. 16.2A) and had been treated conservatively by another doctor. The patient noticed difficulty in walking due to muscle weakness of the lower extremities 4 months after injury and was referred to us with diagnosis of severe collapse of the T12 vertebral body (Fig. 16.2B). Myelotomography and MRI revealed the retropulsed-collapsed vertebral fragments compressing the spinal cord with unstable kyphosis (Fig. 16.2C, D). Anterior spinal canal decompression by vertebrectomy and anterior spinal reconstruction with A-W glass ceramic vertebral spacer, autogenous rib bones and Kaneda-SR was conducted. Complete neural recovery occurred after surgery. Four years postoperatively the spinal column was successfully reconstructed with complete bonding between the ceramic spacer and the vertebral bone. Bone union between autogenous rib graft and vertebral bodies was completed (Fig. 16.2E, F, G-tomogram).

Case 2 (Fig. 16.3A–E)

This 82-year-old woman suffered L1 and L2 compression fracture as a result of mild trauma and had been treated by bracing. The two vertebrae with compression fracture gradually collapsed with progression of unstable kyphosis. When she noticed urinary disturbance and difficulty in walking at 8 months after injury, her doctor found osteoporotic/post-traumatic vertebral collapse at L1 and L2 (Fig. 16.3A–C). Myelography showed severe compression of the dural tube by a retropulsed bony fragment at L1/2. Kyphosis between L1 and L2 was 48°. After anterior decompression and stabilization with correction of kyphosis using a Harms titanium cage and Kaneda-SR with rib graft, urinary function recovered and motor weakness in the lower extremities disappeared. At 2 years after surgery, the reconstructed portion of the spine was stable and neural function was maintained (Fig. 16.3D, E).

Discussion

In our series, vertebral collapse after osteoporotic compression fracture of the thoracic and lumbar spine occurred within 3 months in 41% of patients and within 6 months in 63%. Eleven per cent occurred over 1 year after fracture. The levels of vertebral collapse are concentrated at T12 and L1. Therefore, osteoporotic compression fractures, especially at T12 and L1, should be followed up carefully for at least 1 year after the fracture.

Causes of late vertebral collapse after osteoporotic compression fracture are unknown. From our surgical findings, the collapsed vertebra was ischemic and fragile, and the resection of the collapsed vertebra could be conducted easily because of reduced bleeding due to avascular necrosis. Histological study of the resected

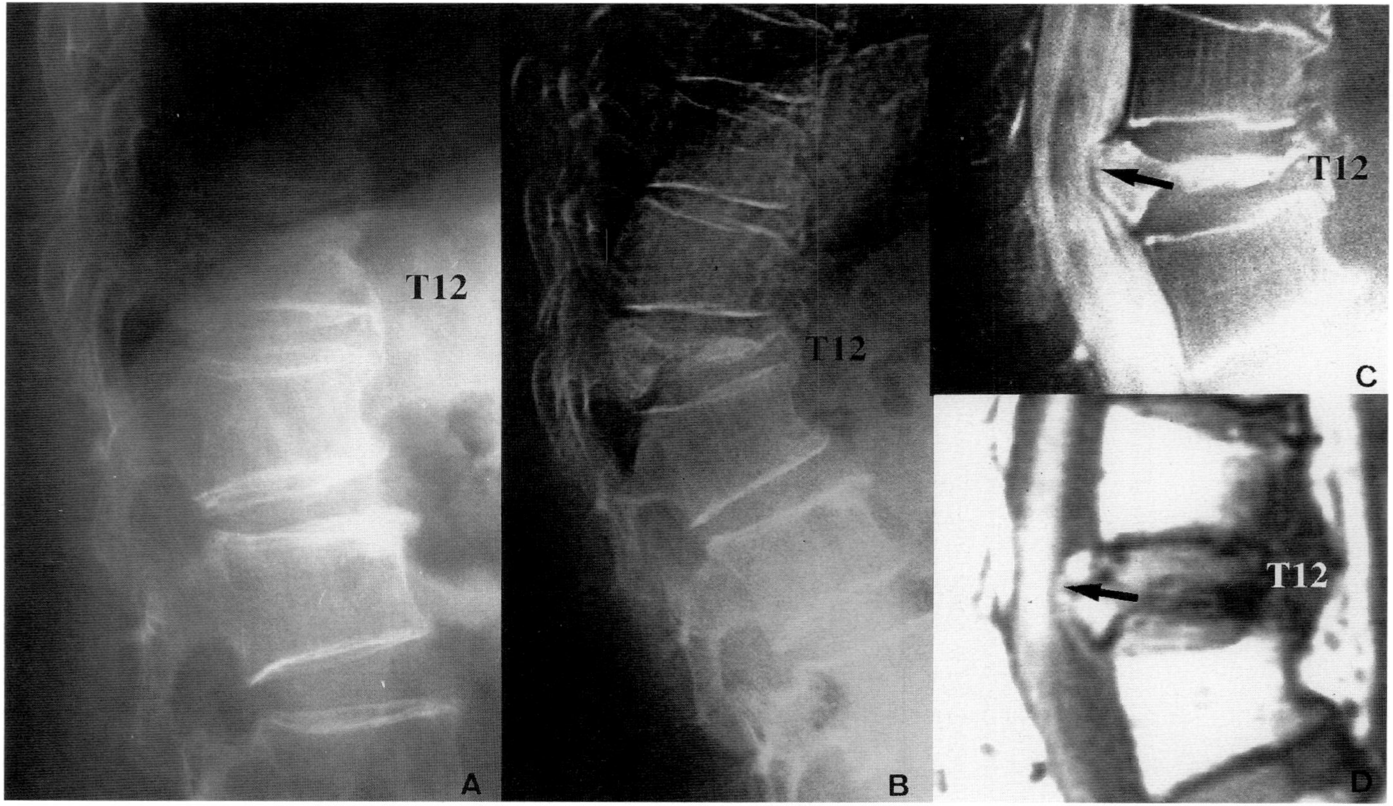

Fig. 16.2. **A–G** Case 1. A 62 year-old man with osteoporotic post-traumatic vertebral collapse of T12. **A** T12 mild compression fracture occurred after falling. **B** At 4 months after the initial injury, severe collapse of T12 vertebral body caused neurological problems. **C** Myelotomogram showed the retropulsed vertebral fragments compressing the spinal cord (*arrow*). **D** T1-weighted MR image. (*continued next page*)

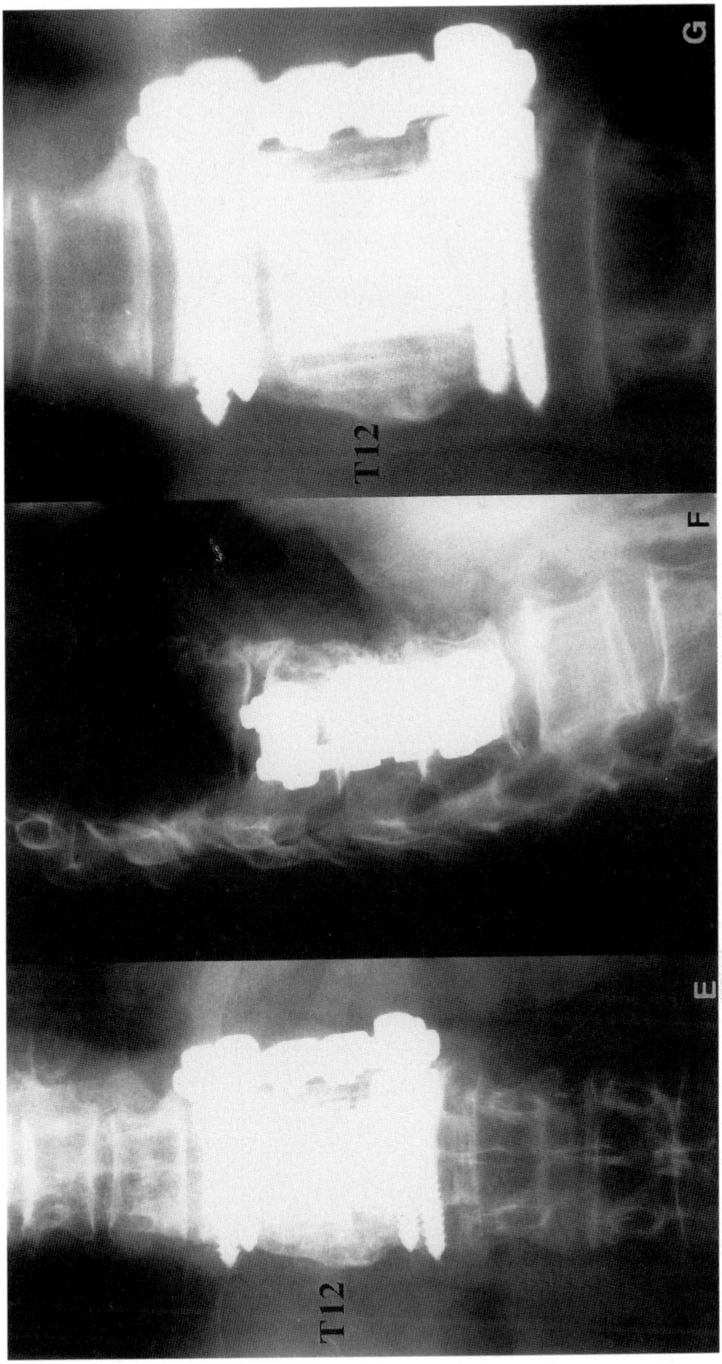

Fig. 16.2. **E,F** Radiographs at 4 years after surgery. Good spinal alignment was achieved. **G** Tomogram showed complete bone union between autogenous rib graft and vertebral bodies.

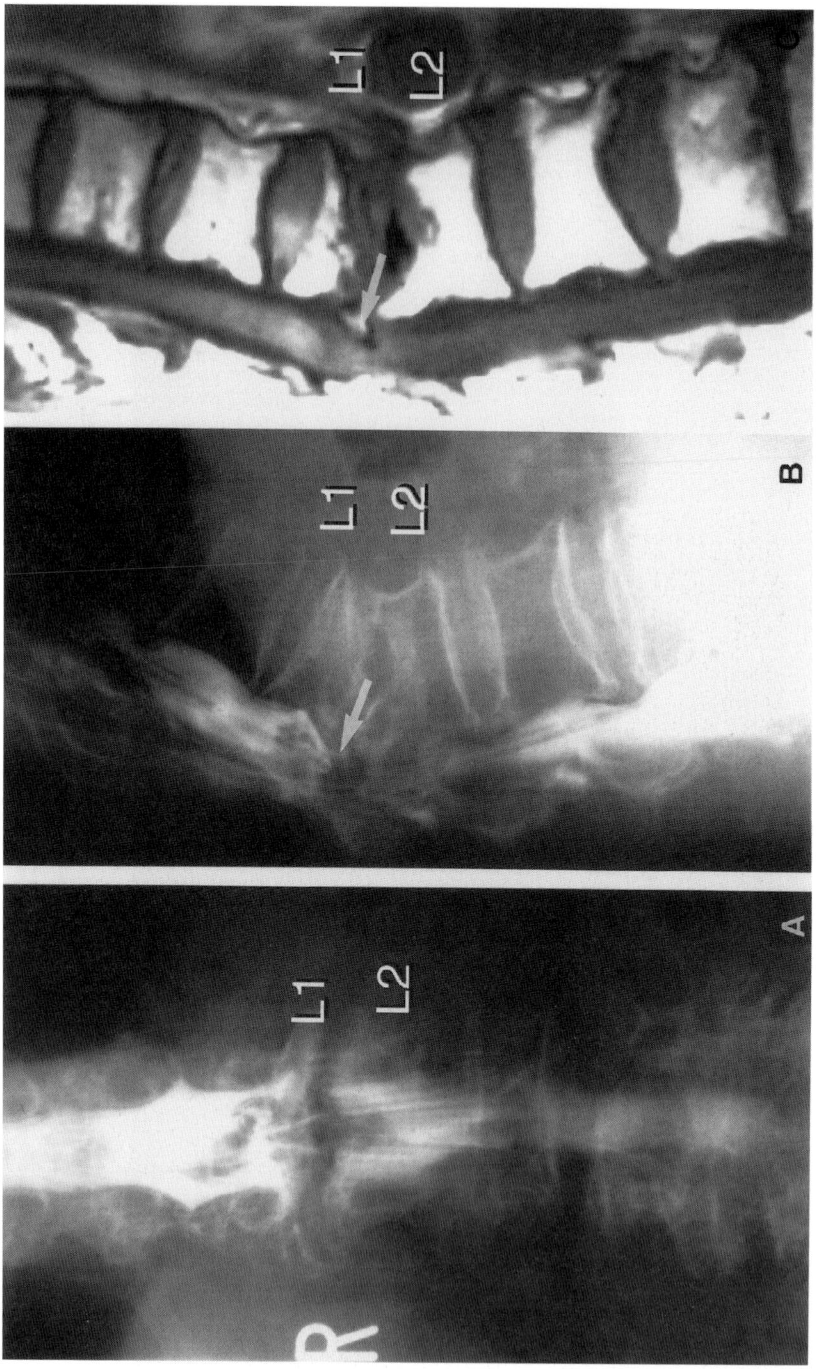

Fig. 16.3. **A–C.** Case 2. An 82-year-old woman with osteoporotic post-traumatic vertebral collapse of L1 and L2. **A,B** Myelogram showed severe compression of the dural tube by retropulsed bony fragments at L1/2 (*arrow*). **C** TI-weighted MR image. (*continued next page*)

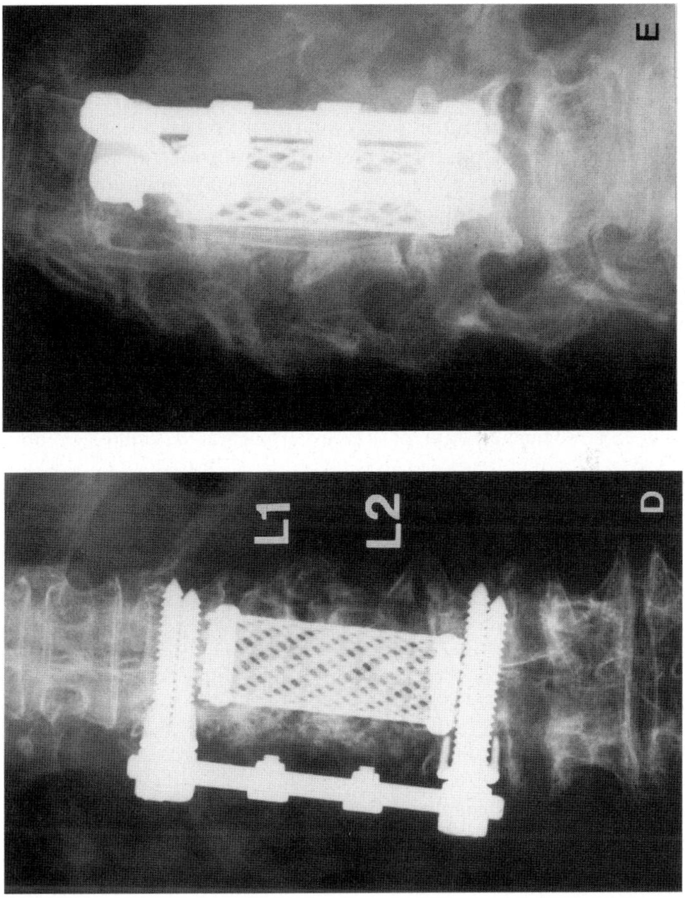

Fig. 16.3. **D,E** Radiographs showed that good spinal alignment was maintained at 2 years after surgery.

collapsed vertebra revealed necrotic tissue, which might be the result of secondary bone ischemia. The normal fracture healing process of the osteoporotic trabeculae would be disturbed due to the fragility of the osteoporotic bone. As a result, osteoporotic fractured trabeculae underwent fibrous union, which would have disturbed the blood circulation in the vertebral body.

There are several reports of posterior reconstruction with instrumentation for treatment of this disease [11]. Posterior reconstruction procedures have the following disadvantages: (1) indirect neural decompression, (2) destruction of intact posterior elements, (3) difficulty in reconstruction of anterior column support and (4) prolonged levels of instrumentation. The pathology of the devastating neural damage and progressively unstable kyphosis is located in the anterior pillar of the spinal column. The neural lesion is brought about by impingement on the neural tissue in the spinal canal by the retropulsed bony mass. Therefore, anterior spinal canal decompression by resection of the retropulsed bony fragment and the reconstruction of the stable anterior column support should be reasonable. This concept is supported in our series and satisfactory results have been gained without severe complications even in the very elderly. Our results showed that for this pathology an anterior procedure is indicated for treatment of "Osteoporotic/post-traumatic vertebral collapse with or without neurological deficit of the thoracolumbar spine".

In conclusion, late devastating neurological complications can be brought about by osteoporotic/post-traumatic vertebral collapse of the thoracolumbar spine. The cause of this pathology will be ischemic necrosis of vertebral bone, caused by secondary circulatory disturbance resulting from fibrous union of the fractured trabeculae. The principle of treatment should be anterior spinal canal decompression and reconstruction of the anterior spinal column using anterior instrumentation and a vertebral spacer.

References

1 Arciero, RA, Leung, KYK, Pierce, JH. Spontaneous unstable burst fracture of the thoracolumbar spine in osteoporosis. Spine 1989;14:114–117.

2 Golimbu, C, Firooznia, H, Rafii, M. The intravertebral vaccuum sign. Spine 1986; 11: 1040–1043

3 Kaneda, K et al. The treatment of osteoporotic/post-traumatic vertebral collapse using the Kaneda device and a bioactive ceramic vertebral prosthesis. Spine 1992;17: S295–S303.

4 Kaplan, PA et al. Osteoporosis with vertebral compression fractures, retropulsed fragments, and neurological compromise. Radiology 1987;165:533–535.

5 Maruo, S, Takekawa, F, Nakano, K. Paraplegia caused by vertebral compression fractures in senile osteoporosis. Z. Orthop 1987;3:125–320.

6 Salomon, C et al. Spinal cord compression; an exceptional complication of spinal osteoporosis. Spine 1988;13:222–224.

7 Lafforgue, P, Chagnaud, C, et al. The intravertebral vacuum phenomenon ("vertebral osteonecrosis") migration of intradiscal gas in a fractured vertebral body? Spine 1997; 22:1885–1891.

8 Ryan, P, Fogelman, I. Osteoporotic vertebral fractures: diagnosis with radiography and bone scintigraphy. Radiology 1994;190:669–672.

9 Kaneda, K. Anterior approach and Kaneda instrumentation for lesions of the thoracic and lumbar spine. In: Bridwell KH, Dewald RL, editors. Text book of spinal surgery. Philadelphia: Lippincott 1991:959–990.

10 Yamamuro, T. Reconstruction of the lumbar vertebrae of sheep with ceramic prosthesis. J Bone Joint Surg Br 1990;72:889–893.
11 Shikata, J et al. Surgical treatment for paraplegia resulting from vertebral fractures in senile osteoporosis. Spine 1990;15:485–489.

17 Fractures of the Proximal Humerus

P. Vienne and C. Gerber

Introduction

Fractures of the proximal humerus represent about 5% of all fractures of the human skeleton and correspond to approximately 45% of all fractures of the humerus. Together with femoral neck fractures, fractures of the spine and fractures of the distal radius, they mainly affect postmenopausal women suffering from osteoporosis. In this population, 75% of all fractures of the humerus concern its proximal end. They mostly occur after minor, low-energy trauma and present with varying degrees of diagnostic and therapeutic difficulties according to the exact type of fracture and patient. It is estimated that 80% of these fractures do well with conservative treatment but approximately 20% are sufficiently displaced and/or unstable that the natural history appears unacceptable and requires surgical correction for improvement of outcome.

Although classical techniques of internal fixation often allow anatomical reduction with restoration of nearly normal function in young patients, experience with these same classical techniques is much less favorable in elderly patients with compromised bone quality. Not only has stable open reduction and internal fixation not fulfilled expectations in elderly patients but also less invasive techniques such as closed reduction and percutaneous pinning can no longer be recommended in the presence of poor bone quality because insufficient fixation too frequently leads to loss of reduction and migration of the pins.

Failure to obtain anatomical reduction, secondary displacement, avascular necrosis and nonunion are frequent complications and require re-evaluation of the concepts of surgical treatment of these fractures. The challenge for the orthopaedic surgeon is to choose the best therapeutic option according to the type of fracture, the quality of the bone and the patient's compliance. There is currently no commonly recognized, optimal surgical way to avoid these complications and the success of treatment depends largely on the ability of the surgeon to deal with the problem of the osteoporotic bone. If internal fixation is needed, particular techniques including retention of the fragments without stable fixation and the use of cement and bone grafting to obtain stability will have to be considered. If internal fixation appears impossible because of poor bone quality, arthroplasty may be the only alternative. This option is often preferred for older patients, but it is neither associated with universally successful results nor devoid of complications. In the present chapter we will try to provide a better understanding of the approach and treatment of fractures of the proximal humerus in severely osteoporotic bone.

Etiology and Clinical Presentation

Fractures of the proximal humerus in osteoporotic patients are sustained through a low-energy accident, mainly by a direct fall on the shoulder or on the outstretched, abducted arm with the forearm pronated – a position which limits external rotation of the shoulder and produces great shear forces at the proximal humerus. Kiaer [1] has reported that the incidence of this type of fracture is 22 times higher for patients over the age of 65 years with a clear predominance of women and that there is a strong annual increase of the incidence of proximal fractures of the humerus after the age of 50 years [2–5].

Direct injury of the proximal part of the humerus and/or traction on the rotator cuff and thereby on the tuberosities causes the important displacement of the fragments. Patients affected by such fractures report acute pain in the shoulder and a nearly total loss of function. They present with the arm at the side supported by the opposite arm because passive and/or active mobilization are painful. Neurological deficits or vascular injuries are rare but have to be carefully sought as especially axillary nerve injuries compromise the final outcome substantially.

The diagnosis is confirmed by standard radiographs of the shoulder (anteroposterior view in neutral to internal rotation, scapular lateral (Neer or Y view) and axillary lateral views). These radiographs serve to assess the exact localization of the fracture, the displacement of the fragments and the bone quality. These three factors, combined with the general health of the patient, will be used for treatment selection.

Classification of the Fractures of the Proximal Humerus

The main goal of the different systems of classification of fractures of the proximal humerus is to define the "severity" of the condition by analyzing the exact morphology and predicting the biological implications of the fracture. The classification should allow a prognosis of the natural history and thereby assist in the selection of treatment.

The currently most widely recognized and used classification is the one presented by Neer in 1970 (Fig. 17.1) [6]. On the basis of the concept of the four fragments (head segment, greater tuberosity, lesser tuberosity, shaft) developed by Codman in 1934 [7], Neer redefined a classification system emphasizing the importance of the displacement of the fragments and the consequent risk of avascular necrosis of the cephalic segment. In his classification, Neer introduced a parameter of presumably great prognostic value, namely the amount of displacement of the four segments. He arbitrarily determined that displacements were only considered to be present if the distance between two fragments is at least 1 cm or if there is an angulation of at least 45° as determined radiographically. Any fracture with a displacement smaller than these two values is considered an undisplaced fracture. Undisplaced fractures can be distinguished from two-part fractures (anatomical neck, surgical neck, greater tuberosity, lesser tuberosity), three-part fractures and four-part fractures (all four segments displaced more than 1 cm or 45°) [8]. The

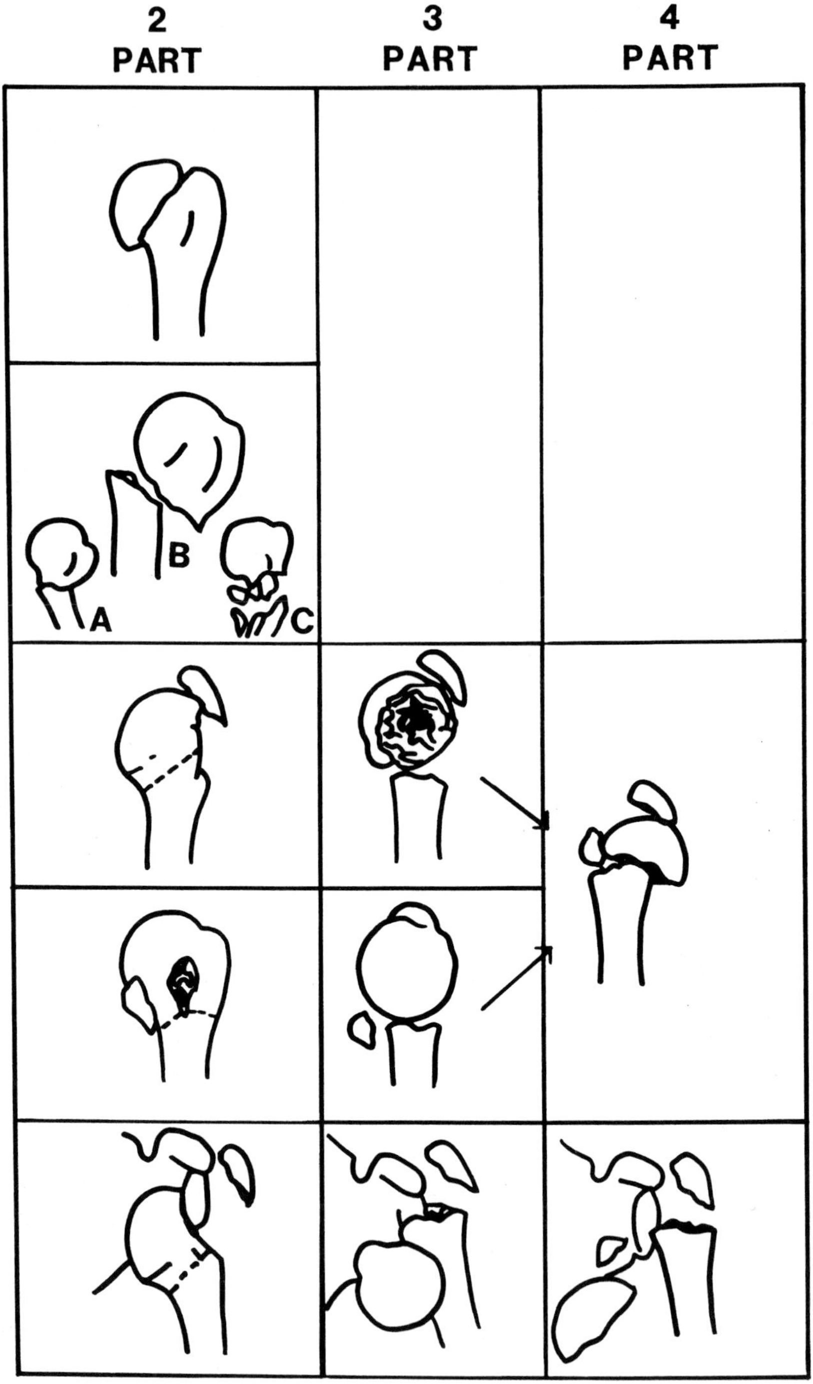

Figure 17.1. Neer's classification.

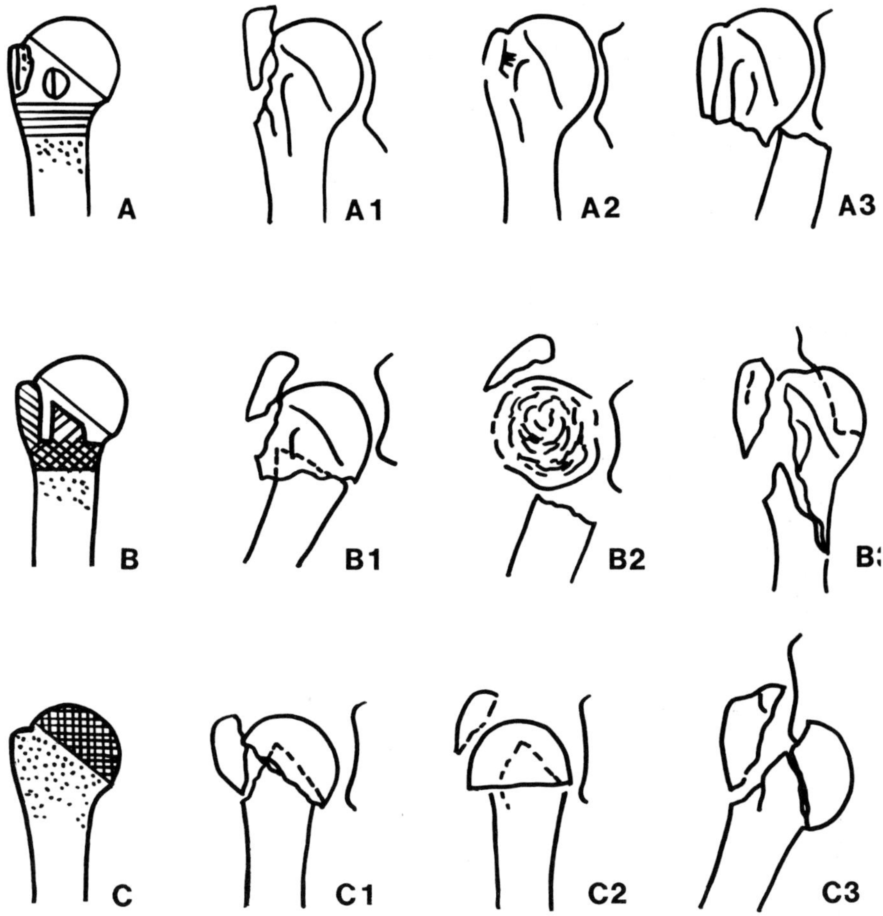

Figure 17.2. AO/ASIF classification.

Neer classification is conceptually simple and clear; its reproducibility, however, like that of so many other radiological classification systems, is relatively poor, so that the analysis and comparison of data from different sources is scientifically dubious [9].

Another system of classification which is often used in the literature was proposed in 1987 by the AO/ASIF group (Arbeitsgemeinschaft für Osteosynthese). This system is based on the retrospective analysis of 730 fractures of the proximal humerus submitted to surgical treatment [10]. The alphanumeric system common to the AO classification of all fractures attempts to represent the variety of fracture patterns observed (Fig. 17.2). The affected bone (proximal humerus) is coded as No. 11 and the individual fracture is then described as a fracture type (A, B or C) which is subdivided into three groups (A1, A2, A3, B1, B2, B3, C1, C2, C3), each group being then further subdivided into three subgroups. Type A corresponds to extra-articular unifocal fractures, type B consists of extra-articular, bifocal fractures and type C of intra-articular fractures. This system also allows for classification of the frequent (but in the Neer system hardly classifiable) valgus-impacted fracture of the proximal humerus (C1 or C2 fracture) [11].

The AO as well as the Neer classification suffers from imperfections regarding interobserver reliability and intraobserver repeatability [12–20]. This problem can not be solved by using more sophisticated imaging techniques such as routine CT scanning [21]. In practice, the Neer classification is used with the known reservation concerning reproducibility and treatment is selected on the basis of both the Neer type and the quality of the bone, which unfortunately is not included in the classification systems. The surgeon also considers the age, expectations and ability of the patient to cooperate when selecting the treatment.

Treatment Options and Final Outcome

The goal of treatment is optimal function and freedom from pain and the form of treatment selected and the quality of its execution will influence the likelihood of obtaining the desired result.

Nondisplaced, Stable Fractures, Good Quality Bone or Osteoporotic Bone

Conservative Treatment

Undisplaced fractures (which may be impacted) represent about 80% of all proximal humeral fractures. Conservative treatment will generally give good results without impairment of function and without residual pain [22–25]. The arm is immobilized in a sling and swathe and after about 10 days passive and assisted active exercises (pendulum exercises) are begun. After 3 weeks active mobility is resumed and elevation of the arm is started. Healing of the fracture is expected to be obtained by 6 weeks and functional recovery by 3 months. It is not our experience that early, aggressive range of motion exercises are beneficial. Overly aggressive early management leads to secondary displacement with compromised outcome. In contrast to many other authors we therefore think that protection of the arm in the first 3 weeks is crucial. In conservatively treated cases this does not lead to intractable stiffness. If the patient is young, range of motion exercises are commenced somewhat earlier but the arm is protected sufficiently to prevent secondary displacement of the segments.

Complications

The most common complication of conservative treatment of an undisplaced fracture is secondary displacement of the fracture fragments. This happens when mobilization of the arm is too intensive in the early rehabilitation period or when the bone is particularly osteopenic. In this case, the surgeon has to decide between neglect in elderly debilitated patients who do not depend on the function of the affected arm, surgical treatment by open reduction and internal fixation in cases of moderate osteoporosis but a definitely vital head segment, or hemiarthroplasty in cases of interrupted blood supply to the humeral head or very severe osteopenia which will probably not allow satisfactory internal fixation.

Complex Fractures, Good-Quality Bone

Complex fractures, with major dislocation of the fragments and important comminution, are treated surgically provided the patient has functional demands justifying an intervention. In cases with good-quality bone, no particular method of treatment can be preferred statistically. The aim of treatment is to obtain and maintain an anatomical reduction of the fracture until healing. This treatment goal is valid for closed reduction and percutaneous pinning [26,27], for open reduction and minimal internal fixation [28] or other fixation techniques [29–34]. In very general terms it can be said that the danger of open reduction and stable fixation using plate and screws is failing to achieve anatomical reduction. The danger of closed reduction and minimal internal fixation is secondary displacement. Each form of treatment has the additional potential of devascularization of the head segment and should be chosen accordingly. For young patients, we prefer open or closed reduction with minimal internal fixation to preserve vascularity of the head and cause as little soft tissue damage as possible. We do not, however, accept any displacement of more than 1 cm or 45° on the postoperative radiographs but attempt to obtain as anatomical a reduction as possible [28]. This because we have been able to show that even the development of avascular necrosis does not necessarily imply a poor clinical result if the necrosis developed after restoration of the anatomy of the proximal humerus [28,35–37]. Hemiarthroplasty is avoided in young patients except in rare cases of splitting of the humeral head. Hemiarthroplasty has so far been associated with a relatively poor functional outcome and a high complication rate [28].

Complex Fractures, Osteoporotic Bone

In severely osteoporotic bone the treatment is often different and does not correspond to generally accepted standards of internal fixation of fractures. The challenge for the surgeon is to find a solution to retain a near-anatomical reduction with little and soft bone to work with and a patient who may not be able to cooperate in the postoperative situation [38].

Open Reduction and Internal Fixation (ORIF)

The commonest fractures in osteoporotic patients are two- and three-part part fractures with displacement or dislocation of the head segment and an associated displacement of one (usually the greater) tuberosity. As opposed to fractures in the young, which are often characterized by impaction and stability, fractures in the elderly are often displaced and unstable. In addition the head may be split, and thereby partially devascularized and not suitable for internal fixation.

If, in such unstable situations, closed reduction is attempted, percutaneous pinning is at very high risk of secondary failure with migration of the pins and secondary displacement of the fracture fragments (Fig. 17.3). Open reduction with internal fixation using bone graft, cement or tension band wiring with suture material are therefore considered. If augmentation is used it should compensate the bone defect in the zone of comminution, provide intrinsic stability for the fracture and improve the holding characteristics of the implants. Clearly unconventional techniques and implants may be successful [31,38–40].

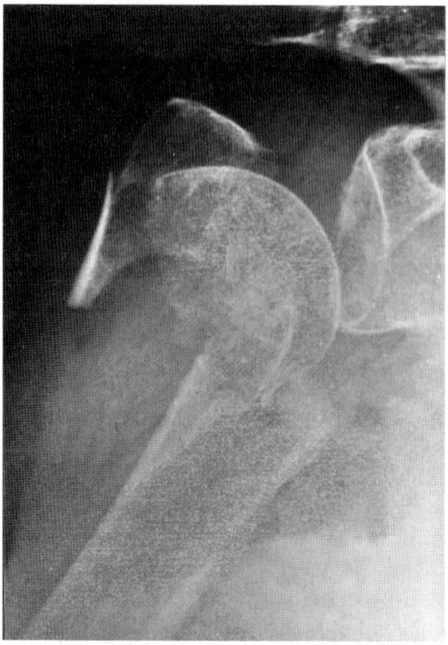

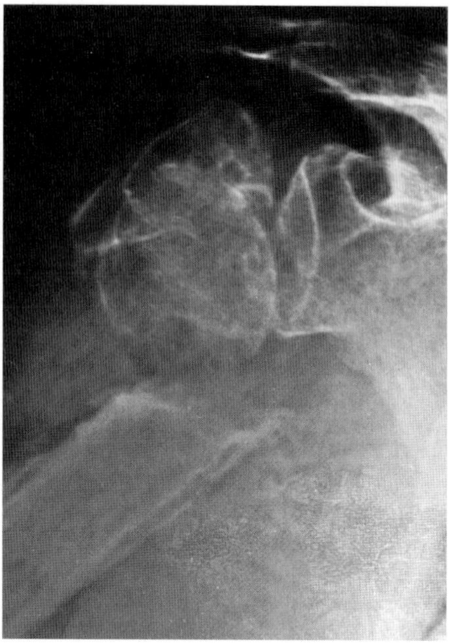

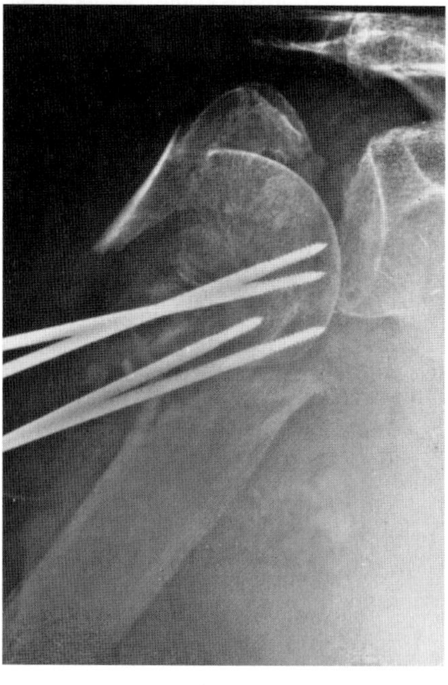

Figure 17.3. A 78-year-old woman with a four-part fracture. There is secondary displacement resulting from treatment with closed reduction and percutaneous pinning.

Surgical Technique: Open Reduction, Internal Fixation with Bone and Cement Augmentation. The patient is installed in a beach-chair position under general anesthesia and/or interscalenic bloc. The shoulder to be operated on should be well exposed and at the lateral rim of the operating table. Intravenous antiobiotic prophylaxis with a second-generation cephalosporin is administered 10 min before skin incision. The shoulder and the ipsilateral iliac crest are draped. A deltopectoral approach is used. The cephalic vein is identified and protected laterally against the deltoid muscle. The dissection goes further between the deltoid muscle laterally and the conjoined tendon medially, taking great care of the long biceps tendon. After incision of the clavipectoral fascia and excision of the subdeltoid bursa the fracture site is exposed. By preserving the soft tissue mantle around the fracture and after evacuation of the fracture hematoma, the fracture fragments are identified. The greater tuberosity is attached to the tendon of the supra-/infraspinatus tendon and forms a triangular bone fragment which is retracted dorsally and proximally. The lesser tuberosity is attached to the tendon of the subscapularis muscle and displaced medially. The fracture line invariably separates the two tuberosities lateral to the bicipital groove. The humeral head is generally displaced dorsally or impacted in a valgus position against the humeral shaft. By axial traction and internal rotation of the arm, the head segment can be exposed and reduction can be obtained with disimpaction of the head.

This maneuver leaves an important bony defect between the two tuberosities. The humeral head is checked for vascularity by drilling a hole into the cartilage. If the head is well vascularized, internal fixation is achieved by bone grafting the defect and anatomical reduction of the tuberosities using suture fixation. If the humeral head does not bleed, hemiarthroplasty should be preferred at this point. The two tuberosities can be sutured to the shaft and to each other using #5 or at least #3 nonabsorbable sutures. The head segment is stabilized by the bone graft and the tuberosities; occasionally screws or pins may serve as an internal splint for the head. If the fracture is lower, e.g. at the level of the surgical neck, plate fixation may be possible and two plates (1/3 tube), one on the internal side medial to the bicipital groove and one on the external side at the level of the greater tuberosity, are preferred. In very osteoporotic bone, the use of bone cement (polymethylmethacrylate) will secure the fixation of the screws and improve the stability of the fixation. It should be understood that a screw is not a suitable implant for fixation in soft bone and this should be avoided. The quality of the reduction is checked with anteroposterior and axillary lateral radiographs and the stability is checked intraoperatively together with range of motion. This serves to guide postoperative management. After abundant rinsing, the wound is closed over two suction drains.

Alternative surgical techniques have to be considered, especially in salvage situations. The goal is then to provide nothing more than a nondisplaced fracture which can be treated conservatively. This is only possible with nonrigid fixations. The proximal fragments are grasped with heavy sutures and a tension band principle is then used to fix the proximal fragments to the shaft, possibly by tying the sutures to a screw in the metadiaphysis which serves as a post. If vascularity is preserved and the relation of the tuberosities to the head is maintained, this technique may be much more successful than rigid fixation (Fig. 17.4).

Postoperative Rehabilitation

The postoperative rehabilitation depends greatly on the stability of the reduction and the internal fixation. In general terms it is the same as the treatment of an undisplaced fracture. The arm is protected in a sling for the first 3–5 days and depending on the stability of the fixation and the compliance of the patient passive

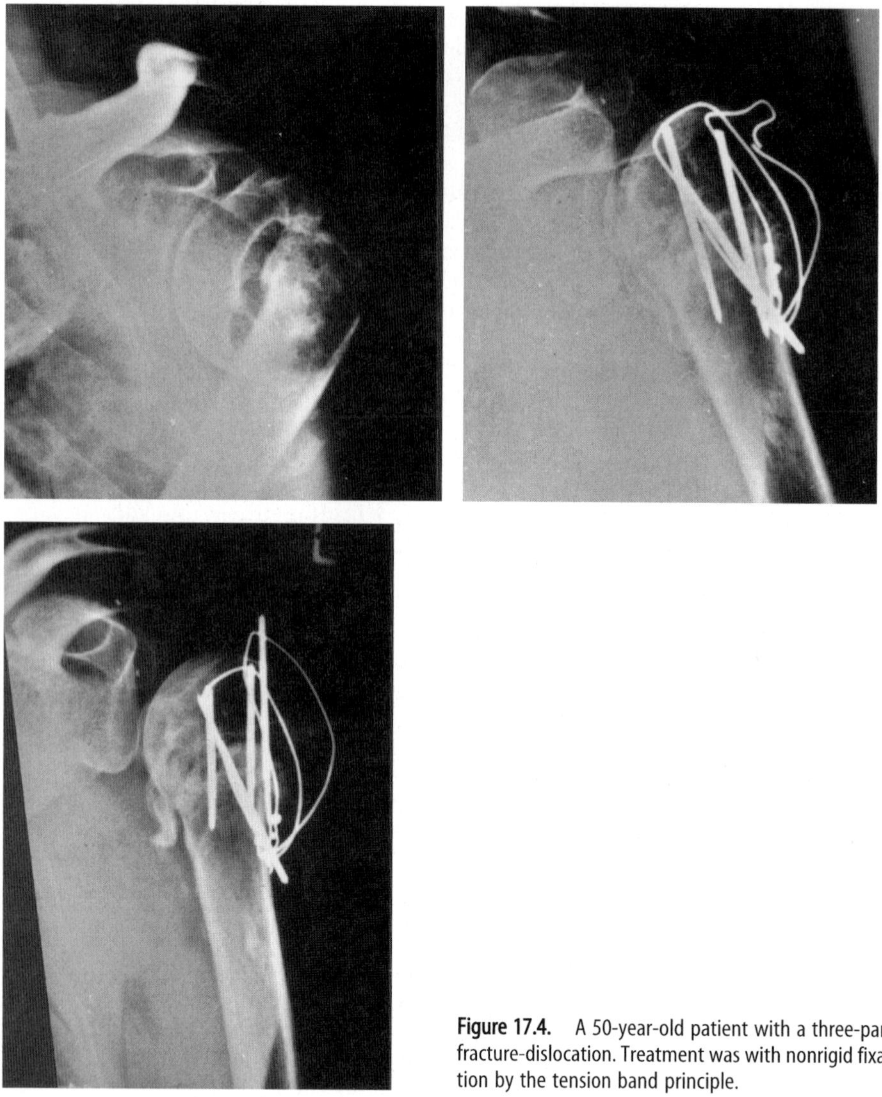

Figure 17.4. A 50-year-old patient with a three-part fracture-dislocation. Treatment was with nonrigid fixation by the tension band principle.

range of motion is progressively increased in physiotherapy. We avoid all active motion until healing of the fracture, which is generally obtained after 6 weeks.

Complications

The most frequent complications of open reduction and internal fixation are nonunion and malunion of the fracture [26,31,39–41]. They are due either to insufficient primary reduction or to secondary displacement because of insufficient stabilization (Fig. 17.5).

In three- or four-part fractures with important displacement of the head fragment, the rate of avascular necrosis is high (more than 50% in some studies) and

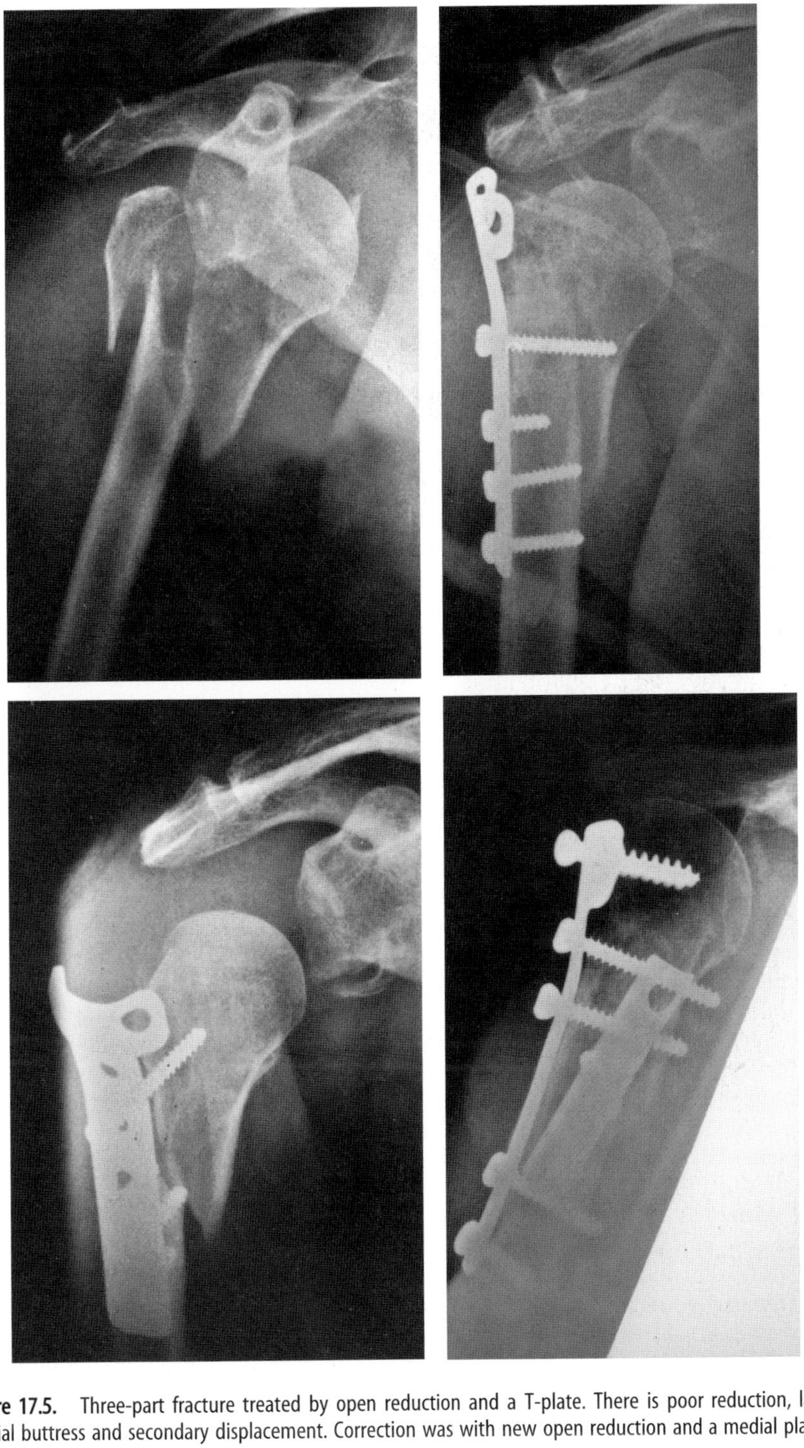

Figure 17.5. Three-part fracture treated by open reduction and a T-plate. There is poor reduction, lack of medial buttress and secondary displacement. Correction was with new open reduction and a medial plate.

its onset can greatly compromise the final outcome, especially if the reduction of the fracture is not anatomical. In the advent of nonunion/malunion and avascular necrosis, chronic pain and substantial limitation of function are consistently present. In such cases, implantation of a hemiprosthesis becomes the only treatment option. The procedure is difficult because of scarring, lack of anatomical references and joint stiffness, and the final outcome is not spectacular [28,41].

Hemiarthroplasty

The treatment of complex proximal humeral fractures by an open reduction and internal fixation technique in the presence of poor bone quality remains a difficult challenge for the orthopaedic surgeon. The complications are frequent and the outcome is often unsatisfactory. One should therefore consider the possibility of hemiarthroplasty in such cases [44]. It is the authors' conviction that osteoporosis is the most important indication for hemiarthroplasty – more important than the exact fracture type according to the various classification systems. Unfortunately even treatment with hemiarthroplasty, which is described in detail in many other texts, does not yield universally satisfactory results, mostly due to secondary displacement of the greater and/or lesser tuberosity and possibly also because these fractures are often treated by surgeons who do not have sufficient experience of these difficult situations [45–51].

Surgical Technique: Hemiarthroplasty

A crucial step in the success of hemiarthroplasty is preoperative planification. In the presence of marked shortening or comminution, the contralateral side may be taken to plan the exact height of the prosthesis. Usually, however, this is not necessary because the greater tuberosity fragment is triangular and can be identified exactly. Also its counterpart on the shaft can be exactly defined. The distance of the tip of this triangular fragment to the insertion of the supraspinatus is then measured on the inside of the greater tuberosity fragment. This distance is then measured from the tip of the triangular fracture site on the shaft proximally. At the level of the insertion of the cuff or exactly the length of the fragment above the tip of the triangular defect in the shaft is the level of the head of the humerus. Retrotorsion of the humeral head can usually not be assessed and the differences between right and left are so important that verifying on the opposite shoulder is not warranted. We use the mean usual retrotorsion of 20° with respect to the axis of the epicondyles of the distal humerus or roughly 30° to the 90° flexed forearm. Inclination of the prosthesis is usually 130°.

The patient is installed in a beach-chair position under general anesthesia or interscalenic block. Preoperative antibiotic prophylaxis with cephazolin is used 10 min before skin incision. After usual disinfection and sterile draping a deltopectoral approach is used. The proximal part of the humerus is reached between the deltoid muscle and the conjoined tendon, taking care to identify the long head of biceps. After incision of the deltopectoral fascia and excision of the subdeltoid bursa the fracture is exposed. Both tuberosities and their respective tendon attachment are identified and preserved to be reinserted after setting of the prosthesis. The isolated head fragment is excised. In the presence of important comminution of

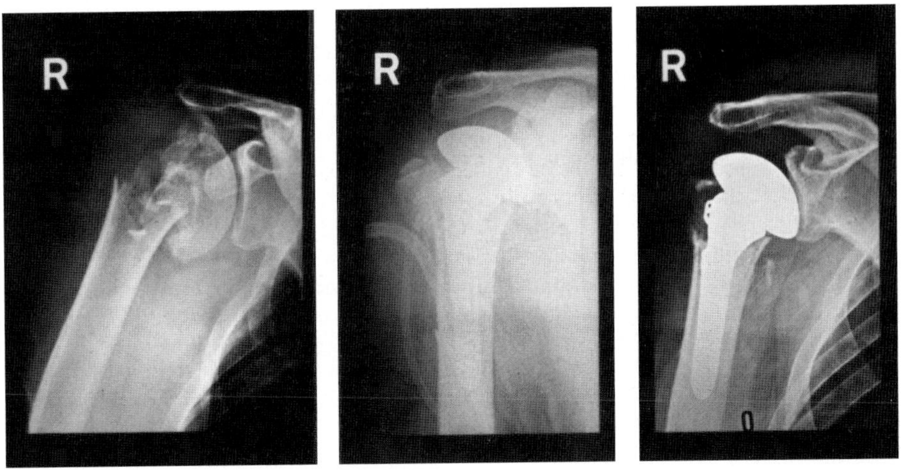

Figure 17.6. A 65-year-old patient with a four-part fracture. Treatment was with a primary hemiarthroplasty. Note the displacement of the lesser tuberosity at follow-up.

the proximal humerus, the anatomical position of the two tuberosities can be difficult to identify and the length is defined by the length of the greater tuberosity fragment as described above.

We use a third-generation prosthesis (Anatomica, Sulzer Medica, Winterthur, Switzerland) which allows the original retrotorsion, inclination, offset and head size to be reproduced as exactly as possible.

The stem is always cemented and the two tuberosities are reattached to the humeral shaft and to the prosthesis using osteosutures (Ethibond #3, or preferably #5). The biceps is usually released at the supraglenoid tubercle and tenodesed in the region of the groove. The wound is closed over two suction drains.

Postoperative Rehabilitation

The arm of the patient is held in a sling and early passive mobilization is begun 48 h after the operation after removing the drains. The intensity of mobilization depends greatly on the stability of the fixation of the two tuberosities. We usually begin with gentle, pendular exercises and progressively increase the amplitude of passive range of motion in flexion, abduction, internal and external rotation. The aim of the rehabilitation is to reach a normal passive range of motion after 6 weeks. The rehabilitation goes on with progressive active assisted mobilization and strengthening until 12 weeks postoperatively. At this time the patient should have reached a functional range of motion and satisfactory strength.

Complications

Hemiarthroplasty for complex proximal humeral fractures in osteoporotic bone is not a common procedure. The risks of complication are important and the surgeon should be experienced enough to treat them. Intraoperatively, because of the poor bone quality, the risk of periprosthetic fracture exists. Great care should be taken when preparing the humeral shaft with the different reamers. Complications such as hematoma, iatrogenic nerve lesions or infections can occur but are rather rare (1–2%). Nonunions or malunions of the tuberosities are common complications (Fig. 17.6). A secondary displacement of the tuberosities will cause an important limitation of function and persistent pain [28]. To avoid this complication, it is important to reduce the tuberosities anatomically and to improve the quality of the fixation by securing the sutures with very strong sutures in the cement mantle. When a nonunion or a malunion of the tuberosities occurs, a surgical revision with reduction and refixation may be necessary to reduce pain and improve function. Most of the time this revision, however, will produce only a minor improvement of function.

Conclusions

Fractures of the proximal humerus are frequent in elderly patients and particularly in those with severely osteoporotic bone. Though 80% of these fractures are simple and can be treated conservatively with good results, the remaining 20% are more complicated fractures with major displacement of the fragments and need open reduction and internal fixation to improve the outcome. In these situations, because of the very poor quality of bone and the lack of compliance of these patients, the surgeon has to use some special techniques to achieve either an optimal reduction and fixation of the fracture or an optimal implantation of a hemiprosthesis. Using open reduction and internal fixation, some unconventional techniques must be chosen to improve the quality of the fixation, such as use of cement or bone grafting. With hemiarthroplasty, the exact reduction and fixation of the two tuberosities and the exact reconstruction of the proximal humerus in height and retrotorsion are very important factors in achieving satisfactory results. An analysis of the current literature clearly shows that the results of treatment of acute fractures using hemiarthroplasty are better than those for chronic fractures. The surgeon's experience, although difficult to account for, may often be decisive. Postoperative rehabilitation should be more careful than previously recommended and the fragments need to be protected until healing and to avoid secondary displacement. This rehabilitation should be adapted to the quality of the internal fixation and to the abilities of the patient.

References

1. Kiaer T. Proximal fractures of the humerus. An epidemiological and descriptive study of fractures. Ugeskrift for Laeger 1986;148:1894–1897.
2. Bengner U, Johnell O, Redlund-Johnell I. Changes in the incidence of fracture of the upper end of the humerus during a 30-year period. Clin Orthop 1988;231:179–182.
3. Kuner EH, Schaefer DJ. Epidemiologie und Behandlung von Frakturen im hohen Alter. Orthopäde 1994;23:21–31.
4. Horak J, Nilsson BE. Epidemiology of fracture of the upper end of the humerus. Clin Orthop 1975;112:250–253.
5. Rose SH, Melton LJ, Morrey BF, Ilstrup DM, Riggs BL. Epidemiologic features of humeral fractures. Clin Orthop 1982;168:24–30.

6. Neer CS II. Displaced proximal humeral fractures. Part I: classification and evaluation. J Bone Joint Surg Am 1970;52:1077–1089.
7. Codman EA. Fractures in relation to the subacromial bursa. In: The shoulder: rupture of supraspinatus tendon and other lesions in or about the subacromial bursa. Miller, Brooklin, 1934.
8. Neer CS II. Displaced proximal humeral fractures. Part II: treatment of three-part and four-part displacement. J Bone Joint Surg Am 1970;52:1090–1103.
9. Brien H, Notfall F, MacMaster S, Cummings T, Landells C, Rockwood P. Neer's classification system: a critical appraisal. J Trauma 1995;38:257–260.
10. Müller ME, Allgöwer M, Schneider R, Willenegger H. Manual der Osteosynthese. AO-Technik. Berlin Heidelberg New York: Springer, 1992.
11. Jakob RP, Miniaci A, Anson PS, Jaberg H, Osterwalder A, Ganz R. Four-part valgus impacted fractures of the proximal humerus. J Bone Joint Surg Br 1991;73:295–298.
12. Bernstein J. Fracture classification systems: do they work and are they useful? J Bone Joint Surg Am 1994;76:792–793.
13. Bigliani LU. Fracture classification systems: do they work and are they useful? J Bone Joint Surg Am 1994;76:790–792.
14. Burstein AH. Fracture classification systems: do they work and are they useful? J Bone Joint Surg Am 1993;75:1743–1744.
15. Cuomo F. Fracture classification systems: do they work and are they useful? J Bone Joint Surg Am 1994;76:792.
16. Kristiansen B. The Neer classification of fractures of the proximal humerus. An assessment of intraobserver variation. Skel Radiol 1988;17:420–422.
17. Neer CS II. Fracture classification systems: do they work and are they useful? J Bone Joint Surg Am 1994;76:789–790.
18. Rockwood CA Jr. Fracture classification systems: do they work and are they useful ? J Bone Joint Surg Am 1994;76:790.
19. Sidor ML, Zuckermann JD, Lyon T, Koval K, Cuomo F, Schoenberg N. The Neer classification system for proximal humeral fractures. An assessment of interobserver reliability and intraobserver reproducibility. J Bone Joint Surg Am 1993;75:1745–1750.
20. Siebenrock KA, Gerber C. Frakturklassifikation und Problematik bei proximalen Humerusfrakturen. Orthopäde 1992;21:98–105.
21. Sallay PI, Pedowitz RA, Mallon WJ, Vandemark RM, Dalton JD, Speer KP. Reliability and reproducibility of radiographic interpretation of proximal humeral fracture pathoanatomy. J Elbow Shoulder Surg 1997;6:60–69.
22. Zyto K, Ahrengart L, Sperber A, Törnkvist H. Treatment of displaced proximal humeral fractures in elderly patients. J Bone Joint Surg Br 1997;79:412–417.
23. Rommens P, Heywaert G. Conservative treatment of subcapital humerus fractures. A comparative study of the classical Desault bandage and the new Gilchrist bandage. Unfallchirurgie 1993;19:114–118.
24. Wiedemann E, Schweiberer L. Closed treatment of fractures of the humeral head. Indications, technique, limits. Orthopäde 1992;21:106–114.
25. Towfigh H, Buhl W, Obertacke U. Results ot treatment after conservative and surgical management of proximal humerus fractures. Aktuelle Traumatol 1993;23:354–360.
26. Jaberg H, Warner JP, Jakob RP. Percutaneous stabilization of unstable fractures of the humerus. J Bone Joint Surg Am 1992;74:508–515.
27. Kocialkowski A, Wallace A. Closed percutaneous K-wire stabilization for displaced fractures of the surgical neck ot the humerus. Injury 1990;21:209–212.
28. Vienne P, Gerber C. Les fractures complexes de l'humérus proximal chez l'adulte. A propos du traitement par réduction chirurgicale et ostéosynthèse à minima. MD thesis, University of Zurich, 1997.
29. Gautier E, Slongo T, Jakob RP. Die Behandlung der subkapitalen Humerusfraktur mit dem Prevot-Nagel. Z Unfallchir Vers Med 1992;85:145–155.

30. Geneste R, Durandeau A, Gauzere JM, Roy J. Traitement de la fracture-luxation de la tête humérale parenclouage percutané. Rev Chir Orthop Rep App Moteur 1980;66:383–386.
31. Kohler A, Simmen HP, Duff C, Käch K, Trentz O. Osteosynthese subkapitaler Humerusfrakturen mit unkonventionell applizierten Implantaten. Swiss Surg 1995;2:114–117.
32. Mestdagh H, Butruille Y, Tillie B, Bocquet F. Résultats du traitement des fractures proximales de l'humérus par enclouage percutané. A propos de 142 cas. Ann Chir 1984;38:5–13.
33. Mouradian WA. Displaced proximal humeral fractures. Seven years' experience with a modified zickel supracondylar device. Clin Orthop 1986;212:209–218.
34. Zifko B, Poigenfürst J, Pezzei C. Die Marknagelung unstabiler proximaler Humerusfrakturen. Orthopäde 1992;21:115–120.
35. Gerber C, Hersche O, Berberat C. The clinical relevance of posttraumatic avascular necrosis of the humeral head. J Shoulder Elbow Surg 1998;7:586–590.
36. Resch H. Reconstruction of the valgus-impacted humeral head fracture. J Shoulder Elbow Surg 1995;4:73–80.
37. Schai P, Imhoff A, Preiss S. Comminuted humeral head fractures: a multicenter analysis. J Shoulder Elbow Surg 1995;4:319–330.
38. Hertel R, Aebi M, Ganz R. Osteosynthese bei hochgradiger Osteoporose. Unfallchirurg 1990;93:479–484.
39. Hawkins RJ, Kiefer GN. Internal fixation for proximal humeral fractures. Clin Orthop 1987;223:77–85.
40. Koval KJ, Blair B, Takei R, Kummer FJ, Zuckermann JD. Surgical neck fractures of the proximal humerus: a laboratory evaluation of ten fixation techniques. J Trauma 1996;40:778–783.
41. Speck M, Lang FJH, Regazzoni P. Proximale Humerusmehrfragmentfrakturen. Misserfolge nach T-Platten-Osteosyntheses. Swiss Surg 1996;2:51–56.
42. Resch H, Thöni H. Luxationsfrakturen der Schulter. Sonderstellung und Therapiekonzepte. Orthopäde 1992;21:131–139.
43. Norris TR, Green A, Mc Guigan FX. Late prosthetic shoulder arthroplasty for displaced proximal humerus fractures. J Shoulder Elbow Surg 1995;4:271–280.
44. Neer CS II. Articular replacement of the humeral head. J Bone Joint Surg Am 1955;37:215–228.
45. Bosch U, Fremerey RW, Skutek M, Lobenhoffer P, Tscherne H. Die Hemiarthroplastik: Primär- oder Sekundärmassnahmen für 3- und 4-Fragment-Frakturen des proximalen Humerus beim älteren Menschen? Unfallchirurg 1996;99:656–664.
46. Hawkins RJ, Switlyk P. Acute prosthetic replacement for severe fractures of the proximal humerus. Clin Orthop 1993;289:156–160.
47. Kraulis J, Hunter G. The results of prothetic replacement in fracture-dislocations of the upper end of the humerus. Injury 1977;8:129–131.
48. Compito CA, Self EB, Bigliani LU. Arthroplasty and acute shoulder trauma. Reasons for success and failure. Clin Orthop 1994;307:27–36.
49. Moeckel BH, Dines DM, Warren RF, Altchek DW. Modular hemiarthroplasty for fractures of the proximal part of the humerus. J Bone Joint Surg Am 1992;74:884–889.
50. Neumann K, Muhr G, Breitfuss H. Die Endoprothese bei Oberarmkopftrümmerbrüchen. Eine ermutigende Alternative. Unfallchirurg 1988;91:451–458.
51. Pietu G, Deluzarches P, Gouin F, Letenneur J. Traumatismes complexes de l'extrémité supérieure de l'humérus traités par prothèse céphalique. A propos de 21 cas revus avec un recul moyen de 4 ans. Acta Orthop Belg 1992;58:159–169.

18 Fractures of the Distal Humerus

H. Hastings II and M. R. Robichaux

Introduction

As our population ages fractures of the distal humerus will become increasingly common, with a nearly threefold increase projected by the year 2030 [1]. The major determinant in this expected rise in fracture rates is a corresponding increase in the number of patients with osteoporosis. The treatment of the osteoporotic distal humerus fracture has traditionally posed great difficulty and surgical results have often been disappointing [2–6]. However, with the advent of newer fixation techniques and evolving treatment modalities, the initial despair with which these injuries were viewed has given way to a more optimistic outlook. Significant osteoporosis is no longer considered a contraindication to aggressive surgical stabilization and good results can be obtained even in the severely osteopenic patient [7–14]. The liberal use of bone graft, multiple plate and screw fixation techniques, and the use of methylmethacrylate for enhanced screw fixation have all been important developments in the treatment of these fractures. Furthermore, total elbow arthroplasty provides us with a salvage procedure for those rare injuries that are not amenable to operative reconstruction. It is imperative that the treating physician has a thorough understanding of modern surgical principles and techniques in order to treat fractures of the osteoporotic distal humerus effectively.

Anatomy and Biomechanics

The elbow is classified as a trochoginglymoid joint allowing for flexion and extension in the sagittal plane as well as rotation about a central axis. This motion occurs through the interactions of three distinct articulations. The ulnohumeral joint provides for flexion and extension while the proximal radioulnar joint and radiohumeral joints allow for rotation. Because of the proximity of these articulations, injuries to any one of the joints can result in a "spillover effect" to the others [15]. Therefore, inadequate restoration of one articulation may predispose an adjacent articulation to abnormal wear and early degenerative changes.

Elbow flexion and extension occurs at the ulnohumeral articulation between the semilunar notch of the olecranon and the trochlea. This articulation is highly constrained, with the prominent medial and lateral ridges of the "spool-like" trochlea

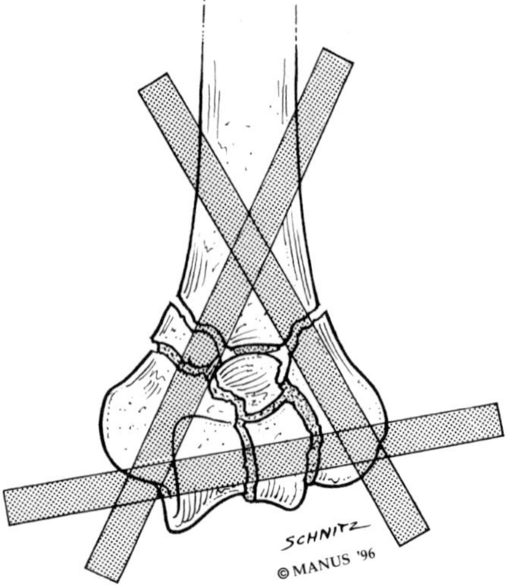

Figure 18.1. The distal humerus triangle composed of a lateral column, medial column and distal articular platform. Stable reconstruction requires securing all three of these osseous elements.

contributing greatly to the intrinsic stability of the elbow [11,16]. It is, therefore, imperative that the trochlea be anatomically reconstructed when treating fractures of the distal humerus. Special surgical attention should be given to avoiding iatrogenic narrowing of the trochlea which could prevent its normal seating within the semilunar notch. Anatomically, the trochlea projects more distally than the capitellum in the coronal plane and a resulting valgus posture is imparted to the extended elbow. Thus, the extended elbow has a carrying angle ranging from 11° to 17° [17–19]. The capitellum also projects further anteriorly than the trochlea with a resulting varus posture being assumed by the elbow in flexion.

In structural terms the distal humerus can be thought of as an equilateral triangle with its sides being formed by the medial and lateral columns of the distal humerus and its base by the trochlea (Fig. 18.1). The capitellum is part of the lateral column and represents its distal anterior extension. The medial and lateral columns diverge from the humeral shaft at 45° and 20° respectively, and are separated by the coronoid fossa anteriorly and the olecranon fossa posteriorly. These columns are composed of triangular-shaped cortical bone which provides for adequate screw purchase even in the presence of significant osteoporosis [11]. The goal of surgery should be to reconstruct all three arms of the triangle in a manner sufficiently stable to support early postoperative mobilization. Instability of any one arm will affect the integrity of the entire construct, resulting in its failure to withstand the rigors and stresses of early motion. Because additional elbow stability is imparted by the radiocapitellar joint, its reconstruction is also important for optimal long-term functional recovery [20].

A detailed understanding of the normal architecture of the distal humerus is required if complex fractures are to be reconstructed, especially if gaps have been created by bone loss or fragment impaction. The articular surface is tilted 30° anteriorly with respect to the humeral shaft such that the axis of the trochlea is in line with the anterior cortex of the humerus. The articular condyles are also rotated

Table 18.1. Classification of distal humeral fractures

I.	Intraarticular fractures			
	A.	Single-column fractures		
		1.	Medial	
			a.	High
			b.	Low
		2.	Lateral	
			a.	High
			b.	Low
	B.	Bicolumn fractures		
		1.	T pattern	
			a.	High
			b.	Low
		2.	Y pattern	
		3.	H pattern	
		4.	Lambda pattern	
			a.	Medial
			b.	Lateral
		5.	Multiplane pattern	
	C.	Capitellum fractures		
	D.	Trochlear fractures		
II.	Extra-articular intracapsular fractures			
	A.	Transcolumn fractures		
		1.	High	
			a.	Extension
			b.	Flexion
			c.	Abduction
			d.	Adduction
		2.	Low	
			a.	Extension
			b.	Flexion
III.	Extracapsular fractures			
		A.	Medial epicondyle	
		B.	Lateral epicondyle	

Reprinted with permission from McKee et al. [22].

internally 3°–8° relative to a line drawn from the medial to lateral epicondyles. The distal articular surface is in approximately 6° of valgus. Recognition of these seemingly minor anatomical facts enables the surgeon accurately to reconstruct potentially devastating distal humerus fractures [21].

Fracture Classification

Historically, numerous fracture classification systems have been developed for the distal humerus. The system proposed by McKee et al. [22] is preferred by the authors (Table 18.1). In this system fractures are separated based upon the column involved as well as whether there is intra-articular, intracapsular or extracapsular involvement. Elements of older classification systems are incorporated in this newer system. Milch [23] has previously described single-column intra-articular fractures as being high or low depending upon how proximal the fracture started before travelling obliquely across the trochlea (Fig. 18.2). These fractures represent a continuum in

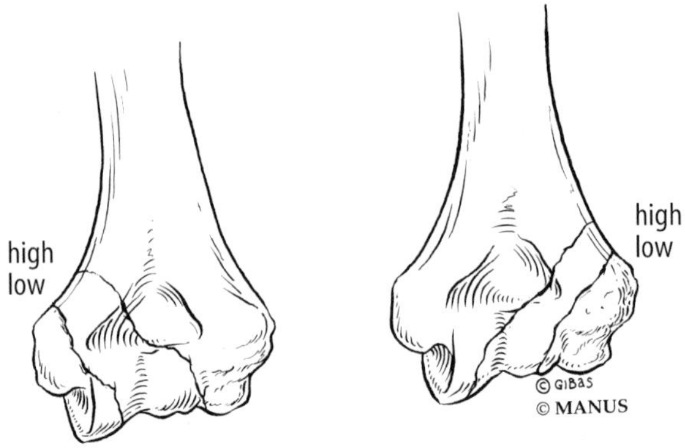

Figure 18.2. Milch classification of single-column fractures including high and low variants of the medial and lateral columns.

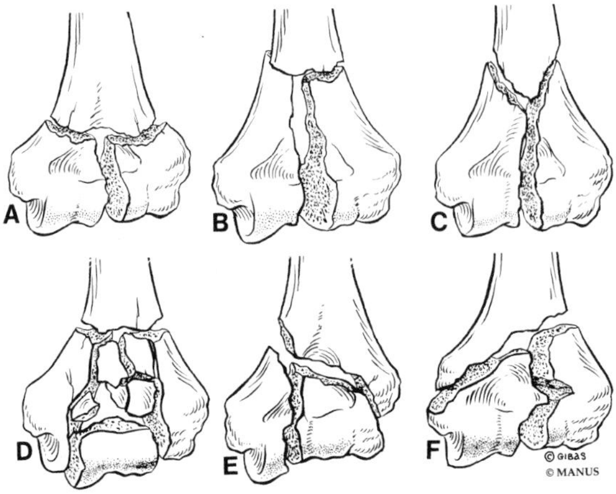

Figure 18.3A-F. Classification of osteochondral bicolumnar fracture variants of the distal humerus. **A** Low T bicolumnar fracture. **B** High T bicolumnar fracture. **C** Y bicolumnar fracture. **D** H bicolumnar fracture. **E** Medial lambda fracture. **F** Lateral lambda fracture.

which high fractures involve a majority of the trochlea and are inherently unstable while low fractures involve little or none of the trochlea and tend to be stable. Divergent single-column fractures occur in adolescents through an impaction injury in which the olecranon is driven proximally, splitting off the medial or lateral condyle in a divergent fashion [24].

Bicolumn fractures have garnered multiple descriptive labels and include T fractures, Y patterns, H variants, medial and lateral Lambda fractures and the more complex multiplane fractures (Fig. 18.3) [22,25]. Isolated capitellar and trochlea fractures represent the last two subsets of intra-articular fractures. These distal osteochondral fractures have been further divided into subsets by Bryan and Morrey (Fig. 18.4) [26]. Type I fractures (Hahn–Steinthal fracture) are simple capitellar fractures involving a substantial portion of cancellous bone. Type II

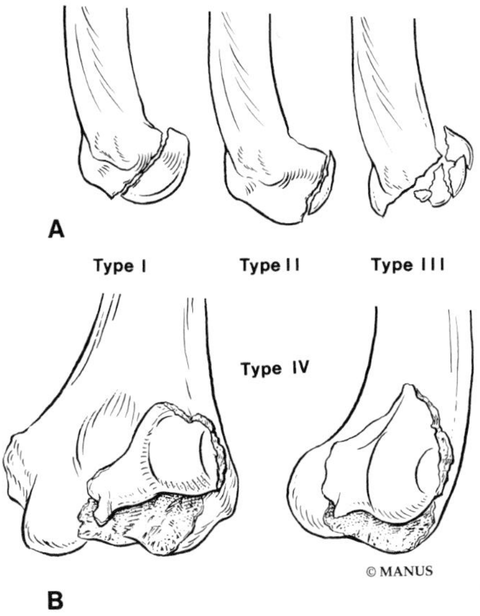

Figure 18.4A,B. The four types of osteochondral injuries. Adapted with permission from Jupiter [12].

fractures (Kocher–Lorenz fracture) are superficial lesions involving only the anterior cartilage of the capitellum and a thin layer of subchondral bone. Type III fractures represent comminuted osteochondral fractures of the capitellum. The final subset, type IV fractures, includes the coronal shear fractures described by McKee and associates [27]. As the name suggests, these fractures involve a shearing injury to the distal humerus in which the capitellum and a major portion of the trochlea are sheared off as a single fragment. The extra-articular intracapsular fractures are the next group, coming in both high and low transcolumn variants. These fractures are described mechanistically as flexion, extension, abduction or adduction types. Finally, extracapsular fractures are divided into those involving either the medial or lateral epicondyle.

The AO classification provides us with another useful method to precisely group the myriad fracture patterns seen in the distal humerus. While this system is complex it is extremely helpful in comparing results among different investigators. The system divides fractures into three main groups based upon fracture location (Fig. 18.5). Type A fractures are extra-articular. Type B fractures are partial articular fractures meaning that at least a part of the distal articular surface remains attached to the proximal humerus. Type C fractures are complete articular fractures involving complete disruption of the distal articular surface from the more proximal supporting osseous structures. Each type of fracture is further subclassified based upon the location of the major fracture lines and the degree of comminution [28]. This system is particularly useful in predicting those fractures which pose reconstructive difficulties and are prone to postoperative complications.

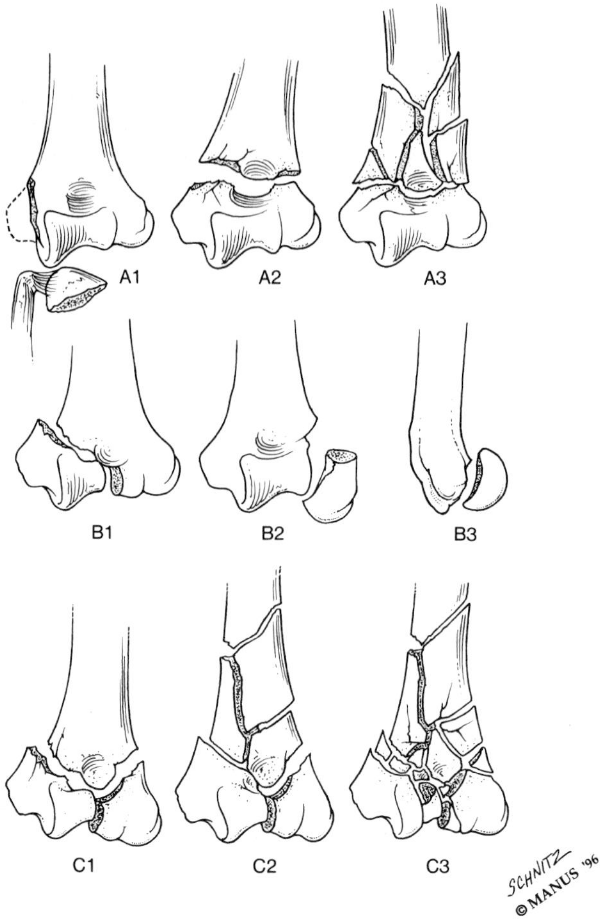

Figure 18.5. AO classification of distal humerus fractures.

Preoperative Evaluation

History

A thorough medical history provides the foundation for any treatment that is contemplated in the trauma setting. A complete analysis of all pre-existing medical conditions is imperative, especially in elderly patients. Those patients with metabolic bone diseases such as osteoporosis will often reveal a history of multiple low-energy fractures. Such a patient's long-term functional outlook may depend greatly upon a thorough metabolic investigation and the institution of appropriate medical management.

Careful questioning regarding the mechanism of injury is essential. The position of the arm at the time of injury, the direction of the applied force and the estimated energy absorbed at impact are all important historical considerations. This information allows an assessment of the complexity of the trauma to the elbow as well as of the likelihood of associated injuries.

An appreciation of the patient's overall medical condition and pre-injury functional level is vital in determining appropriate treatment. The physician should always inquire into any previous elbow injuries or surgery. Pre-existing elbow arthritis, instability or limitations in motion can alter the treatment plan dramatically. Finally, associated symptoms of weakness and paresthesias are always sought as they may portend possible neurovascular compromise.

Physical Examination

The examination of the extremity begins with a complete neurovascular evaluation. Appropriate motor and sensory function of the median, ulnar, anterior interosseous, posterior interosseous and radial nerves should be documented. Vascular status is assessed through the palpation of peripheral pulses and capillary refill. A Doppler examination is employed in equivocal cases, with arteriography indicated only in those rare circumstances in which the site and/or nature of vascular compromise are not apparent.

Further examination of the extremity involves careful inspection, palpation and range of motion evaluation of the wrist, elbow and shoulder. Gross deformity or crepitus at the elbow may necessitate that radiographic studies proceed before a more thorough examination is performed. The soft tissue envelope must always be fully assessed with special attention directed toward skin integrity and the possibility of open fractures. While documentation of ligamentous stability is also important it is usually impossible to delineate its presence in the face of unstable fractures. Therefore, coexisting ligamentous instability is not typically appreciated until the osseous components of the instability are repaired.

Radiographic Examination

Initial radiographic evaluation should include an anteroposterior (AP) and lateral view of the distal humerus. The AP view should be obtained with the beam directed perpendicular to the distal humerus with the elbow flexed approximately 40°. This disengages the olecranon from its fossa permitting better visualization of the distal humerus. The lateral view is taken with the shoulder abducted and the elbow flexed 90° and resting on the cassette. The beam is directed parallel to the elbow axis of rotation such that the humeral condyles are superimposed on the film. An additional AP view of the proximal radius and ulna can be obtained with the beam orthogonal to the antebrachial region yielding better images of this area.

Additional views are also available to evaluate specific areas of the elbow more fully. Oblique radiographs can be helpful in assessing the extent of medial and lateral column comminution. The radial head–capitellum view is a lateral view of the elbow taken with the beam canted 45° toward the ipsilateral shoulder joint with the forearm fully supinated. This view provides a magnified image of the radial head without the overlap of the proximal ulna [29–32]. The coronoid view is a reverse of the radial–capitellum view, with the beam directed at the lateral elbow canted 45° away from the ipsilateral shoulder. It provides excellent definition of the coronoid process.

Traction views of the distal humerus are often extremely helpful in assessing complex fracture patterns. Distortion caused by fragment overlap and rotation due to unopposed muscle pull is minimized. Fragment size can be more clearly defined and previously hidden fracture lines and segmental bone loss can be visualized. Fragments can also be traced accurately for templating future reconstructive procedures.

CT provides an excellent method of further elucidating anatomical detail in the injured elbow. Fracture fragment size and displacement are well visualized using 2 mm or smaller axial and coronal cuts. Axial images are especially helpful in assessing the degree of comminution of the capitellum, trochlea and radial head as well as the presence of pre-existing arthritic changes. Sagittal CT views usually require reconstructed images and are highly dependent upon the thickness of the initial sequences. They may not be reliable in assessing articular incongruity.

Nonoperative Treatment

Nonoperative treatment has a limited role in the management of distal humerus fractures in adults. This is because of the inability to correct intra-articular displacement as well as the severe fibrosis and ankylosis that often follows prolonged immobilization. The conservative treatment modalities currently in use include splint immobilization, closed reduction and cast immobilization, traction, and the "bag of bones" technique.

We use a long arm posterior splint at 90° for the rare nondisplaced fracture of the distal humerus. Initial weekly radiographic follow-up allows for assessment of possible displacement. Early active motion is begun at between 2 and 3 weeks. While loss of complete extension is common, it is rarely functionally significant.

Closed reduction and immobilization has been described for both flexion- and extension-type transcondylar fractures. All closed reduction attempts performed on adults should be done under general anesthesia. Soltanpur [33] has successfully treated flexion-type transcondylar fractures using a reduction maneuver in which following gentle traction the elbow is brought into flexion and the condylar fragments are pushed posteriorly through the axis of the fully supinated forearm. The elbow is immobilized by starting with a circular cast around the upper arm which is then used as a buttress onto which the final fracture reduction is completed. The plaster is then extended into a long arm cast. Despite 6 weeks of immobilization, Soltanpur reports near complete restoration of elbow motion [33]. Closed reduction of extension-type transcondylar fractures has also been described using techniques similar to those used in the pediatric population [34,35]. We have limited experience with both these techniques in adults as these transcondylar fractures are usually unstable and often require prolonged immobilization to maintain their reduction. While we prefer surgical stabilization in most cases, closed treatment remains a viable option in those patients whose overall medical condition may prohibit operative reconstruction.

The use of olecranon pin traction has historically been important in the treatment of distal humerus fractures [36,37]. Overhead skeletal traction allows for early elbow motion and facilitates edema control. Its use today has largely been supplanted by open reduction and internal fixation. However, traction remains a useful temporizing measure in those cases where definitive surgical treatment must be deferred while more pressing medical problems are addressed.

The "bag of bones" technique described by Eastwood [38] in the 1930s continues to be a useful treatment option for those elderly patients whose confounding medical conditions prohibit surgery. This technique involves placing the arm in a collar and cuff with the elbow initially in maximal flexion. The elbow hangs free allowing gravity to aid in reducing the fragments into a more anatomical alignment. As the pain and swelling resolve the elbow is gradually allowed to extend and at 6 weeks the fracture is typically healed allowing the discontinuation of the sling. In cooperative patients therapy can be continued for an additional 3–4 months resulting in an average arc of motion of 70° [38].

Operative Treatment

Surgical Exposure

Several methods of exposing the distal humerus have been described in the literature. The most commonly used technique is a straight posterior approach combined with an olecranon osteotomy. However, familiarity with the Bryan–Morrey triceps-sparing approach and the extended Kocher approach is necessary if distal humerus fractures are to be optimally treated in elderly patients [39,40].

It is our practice to position the patient in the lateral decubitus position with a sterile arm-holder under the brachium (Fig. 18.6). This provides excellent exposure of the posterior elbow and allows the arm to be rotated freely through the shoulder. This position also allows easy access to the ipsilateral iliac crest, which is always prepared and draped in the event that bone grafting proves necessary.

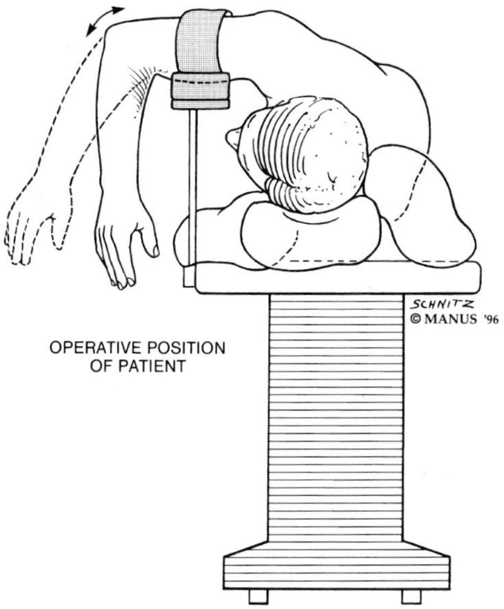

Figure 18.6. Lateral decubitus positioning for approaching the distal humerus.

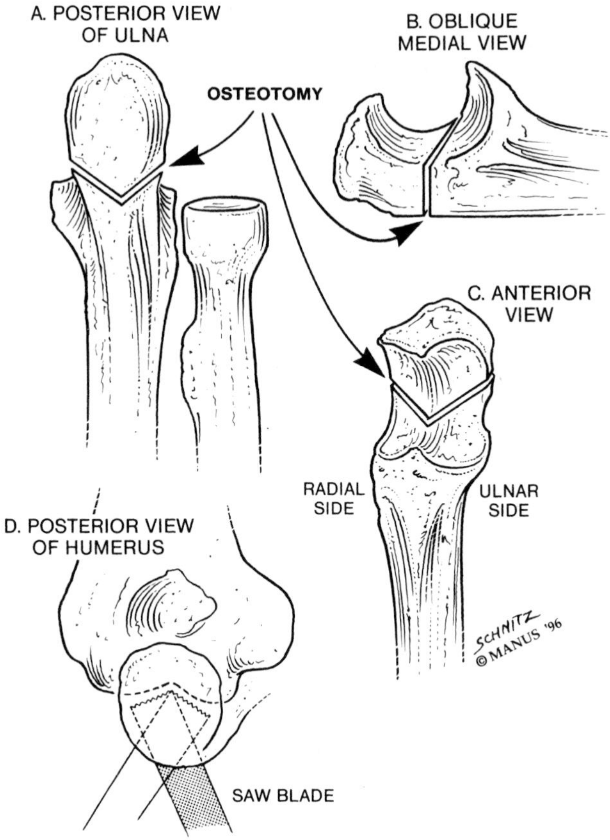

Figure 18.7A-D. Proper orientation of olecranon osteotomy cuts.

We typically use a straight midline posterior approach, curving our incision slightly either medially or laterally over the apex of the olecranon in order to prevent scar sensitivity. After the ulnar nerve is exposed, a chevron-type olecranon osteotomy is performed (Fig. 18.7). The osteotomy is started using a thin-bladed sagittal saw with the cuts converging just distal to the midportion of the semilunar notch. This places the osteotomy within the bare area of the semilunar notch where the synovial membrane inserts and the least amount of articular cartilage is found. A sponge is placed from medial to lateral under the olecranon to protect the distal humerus and to provide countertraction while the osteotomy is completed using a thin osteotome. An osteotome is used so as to avoid the articular distortion that results from the kerf of a saw blade. This approach allows excellent visualization of the intra-articular components of the elbow joint. The triceps and proximal olecranon can be reflected proximally allowing exposure of the distal 7 cm of the humerus before the radial nerve is jeopardized [11]. It is our practice to repair the osteotomy with the AO tension-band wire technique using 0.045 inch Kirschner (K) wires [15,41]. The tension band is then applied proximally by passing a 16-gauge needle under the triceps and against the periosteal surface. The wire transverse passage hole of the distal wire is drilled at a point where the osteotomy will be equidistant from the proximal and distal transverse wire sites. A double twist is performed to ensure symmetric compression across the osteotomy. Care must be taken to bend and impact the proximal ends of the K wires into bone in order to prevent migration.

The triceps-sparing approach described by Bryan and Morrey [39] is our approach of choice in simple type I and II fractures. The need for retraction of the reflected triceps with resultant untoward torque on columnar fragments makes this a less suitable approach for more complex distal humerus fractures. However, if there is a possibility that a fracture is beyond reconstruction and a total elbow arthroplasty may be necessary, the triceps-sparing approach is preferred.

An extended Kocher approach provides excellent exposure of most of the distal humerus especially the capitellum and lateral trochlea. We use this exposure for treatment of isolated distal osteochondral fractures (types I–IV). The extensive stripping of the soft tissue attachments along the lateral column prohibits its use in other fractures. Our incision is made along the supracondylar ridge extending distally along the interval between the extensor carpi ulnaris and anconeus. The interval between the triceps, posteriorly, and the brachioradialis and ECRL, anteriorly, is developed. The anconeus and triceps are then elevated as a continuous flap off the proximal ulna. The brachioradialis and extensor carpi radialis longus are elevated anteriorly with subperiosteal release continuing distally elevating the common extensor origin and the lateral collateral/annular ligament complex off the lateral epicondyle. After release of the anterior capsule, the elbow joint can be dislocated through a varus stress providing generous exposure of the distal humerus. Upon completion of the procedure the triceps are repaired back to the olecranon through drill holes using #5 braided nylon suture. A similar repair of the common extensor origin and lateral collateral/annular ligament complex is carried out to the lateral epicondyle.

Handling of Ulnar Nerve

It is imperative that the ulnar nerve always be identified and protected during surgery on the distal humerus. Ulnar neuritis is a well-recognized and potentially disabling complication of distal humerus fractures and their treatment. Factors related to ulnar neuritis include operative manipulation of the nerve, inadequate release of Osborne's fascia (fascia overlying the two heads of the flexor carpi ulnaris) or the medial intermuscular septum, and postoperative immobilization. The authors recommend simple decompression of the ulnar nerve in surgical exposure of all distal humerus fractures. This is accomplished through its complete release in the retrocondylar groove and beneath Osborne's fascia in the cubical tunnel.

Transposition of the nerve is indicated in three situations [15]. The first is when plate and screw purchase around the medial epicondyle is necessary for fracture fixation. In this instance the hardware would interfere with the nerve unless it is transposed. Second, if the nerve is felt to be unstable with flexion and extension of the elbow after fracture fixation, it is best transposed. Lastly, patients with prior symptomatology consistent with ulnar nerve irritation at the elbow also warrant transposition. When performing a transposition, Osborne's fascia should be released completely with care taken to preserve the motor branches to the flexor pronator muscles. Likewise, excision of the distal extent of the medial intermuscular septum in the arm will also prevent postoperative nerve constriction.

Fracture Reconstruction

Reconstruction of distal humerus fractures begins with the provisional reconstitution of the trochlea and the distal articular surface of the humerus. The reconstructed articular unit is then reduced and stabilized to the largest and least comminuted column. This is followed by fixation of the remaining column to the construct. The construct is only considered rigid if the articular surface is stabilized to both the medial and lateral columns. When only one column is stabilized to the articular unit, the stability is insufficient for early postoperative mobilization and the risk of hardware failure and nonunion is great. Supplemental cast immobilization in this setting is notoriously disappointing.

Reconstruction of the trochlea can often be challenging especially when severe comminution and segmental bone loss exists. It is important to avoid narrowing the normal articular contour of the trochlea. Areas of comminution and segmental bone loss are replaced with cancellous and corticocancellous bone grafts so as to maintain the proper breadth of the trochlea. Bone grafts used to bridge central trochlea defects are most easily placed at the end of the reconstructive effort, after the articular platform has been stabilized to both columns.

The typical distal humerus reconstruction involves the following steps. The trochlea fragments are reduced and provisionally stabilized with K wires or cannulated screw guide pins. Definitive stabilization of the trochlea is accomplished most easily using one or two cannulated 3.5 mm screws (AO/Synthes, Paoli, PA) (Fig. 18.8). These cannulated screws make impingement with previously placed K wires less likely. The generous use of washers is helpful especially in osteoporotic bone. Alternatively, a lag screw can be used in noncomminuted fractures in those patients with strong compression-resistant bone stock. This is unfortunately not typically the case in elderly patients with pre-existing osteoporosis. More commonly, a nonlagged neutralization screw technique is used. Most small fragment sets (i.e., AO/Synthes, Paoli, PA) contain 3.5 mm and partially threaded 4.0 mm screws only up to 50 mm in length. Fully threaded 4 mm screws are provided in lengths up to 60 mm. When the articular platform width exceeds these dimensions, longer 3.5 mm screws are available in the pelvic implant set (AO/Synthes, Paoli, PA). While these transversely oriented screws are used to stabilize fractures in the sagittal plane, articular fragments displaced in the coronal plane can best be stabilized with Herbert screws buried under the articular cartilage. Two alternative fixation methods used for very small fragments include buried fine-threaded K wires and buried bioabsorbable pins.

After the articular platform has been reconstructed, the least comminuted column is then stabilized to it. This is followed by the fixation of the more severely involved column. A dual-plate construct is usually needed with one plate placed medially on the medial column and a second plate posteriorly on the lateral column (Fig. 18.9). This orthogonal plate arrangement imparts increased mechanical stability [42]. The medial plate can be contoured to bend around the medial epicondyle and to cradle it. This allows the distal screws to be directed at near right angles, producing a mechanical interlocking construct. The lateral plate is placed as far distally as possible abutting the posterior border of the capitellar cartilage. The distal screw is again directed proximally providing an interlocking construct [22]. In severely comminuted bone the plates are contoured so as to buttress and support the bone fragments in their anatomical position [43]. The "Du Pont" precontoured plate is available for these situations [22].

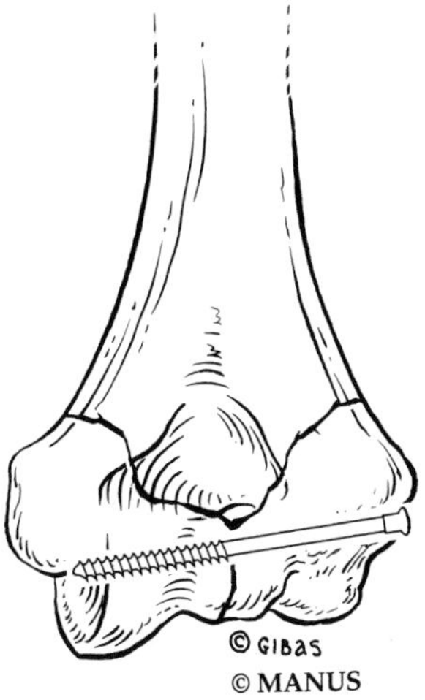

Figure 18.8. Stabilization of the trochlea with a cannulated screw.

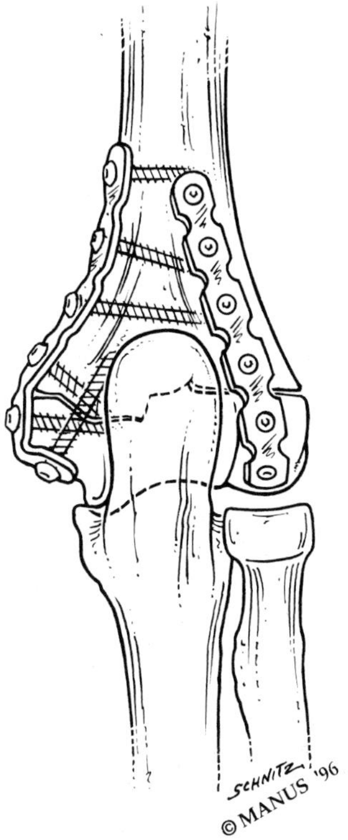

Figure 18.9. Orthogonal plate fixation.

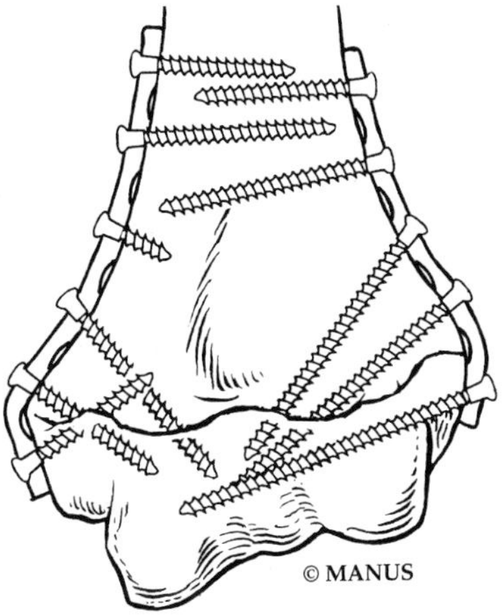

Figure 18.10. Medial and lateral plating technique to optimize the number of screws in the distal fracture fragment.

Recent data detailing the stability of different plate configurations against varying loads indicate that an orthogonally arranged medial 3.5 mm reconstructive plate and a lateral 3.5 mm dynamic compression plate provide the greatest stability (Scott Jacobson, MD, personal communication, 1997). Other authors have found that a third contoured plate along the lateral aspect of the lateral column is useful especially in elderly patients in need of supplemental distal fixation [11]. This plate is also used to provide an additional buttress in severely comminuted intra-articular fractures. The origin of the brachioradialis and extensor carpi radialis longus are elevated in these cases and their suture repair at the completion of the reconstruction is required. It is extremely important to pay special attention to the number of screws inserted into the distal fragments as this is usually the weakest link of the construct. In very low fractures we have found the use of isolated medial and lateral plates helpful to optimize the number of screws in the distal fragments (Fig. 18.10). Care should always be taken to avoid violating articular surfaces and anatomical fossae with screws during plate application. Rather, the screws should be directed so as to engage the substantial triangular cortical bone of the columns where reproducible and reliable purchase can be obtained.

Enhanced Fixation Techniques

Liberal use of bone graft to fill defects, enhance stability and augment bone healing is a mainstay of the treatment of distal humerus fractures in the elderly. If stable fixation of both columns to the trochlea proves impossible due to segmental comminution, contoured corticocancellous bone graft can be used to bridge the involved area (Fig. 18.11). Similar bridging grafts may be required to reconstruct the trochlea in a way that preserves its normal dimensions (Fig. 18.12). Methods of stabilizing interpositional grafts are similar to those used in fracture reconstruction, with the grafts being positioned last and stabilized through multiple screw or plate constructs. Placement of bone graft should not obstruct the coronoid, olecranon or radial fossae, as a block to elbow flexion and extension will result. Finally, any small fracture gaps or crevices are filled and impacted with generous cancellous bone graft.

Because adequate screw purchase can prove difficult in osteopenic bone, supplemental fixation methods are often required. The use of polymethylmethacrylate provides a useful way of enhancing screw fixation in these patients. The method described by Jupiter [11] involves pouring the methylmethacrylate while in its liquid phase into a straight-tipped 12 mm syringe. The tip is placed into those previously identified screw holes that require enhanced fixation and the cement is injected. Screws are then reinserted and remain in place until the cement begins to harden, at which time the final one or two turns are made. Cement extravasation into the fracture site is to be avoided.

Total Elbow Arthroplasty

The use of joint arthroplasty in the trauma setting is well established in the treatment of severe fractures involving the hip and shoulder. With the advent of newer total elbow arthroplasty systems, this has also become a viable treatment alternative in those elderly patients with severely comminuted distal humerus fractures. While some authors maintain that elderly patients all have adequate bone stock to obtain stable fixation [11,44], this becomes a much more challenging prospect with increasing fracture comminution and coexisting osteopenia. We consider patients older than 65 years of age with severe osteopenia and severely comminuted intercondylar fractures to be candidates for immediate elbow arthroplasty (Fig. 18.13). Advanced pre-existing rheumatoid arthritis with elbow involvement may be an additional indication. While long-term follow-up is not available, short-term results using the modified Coonrad–Morrey total elbow implant compare favorably with open reduction and internal fixation in carefully selected patients. A retrospective

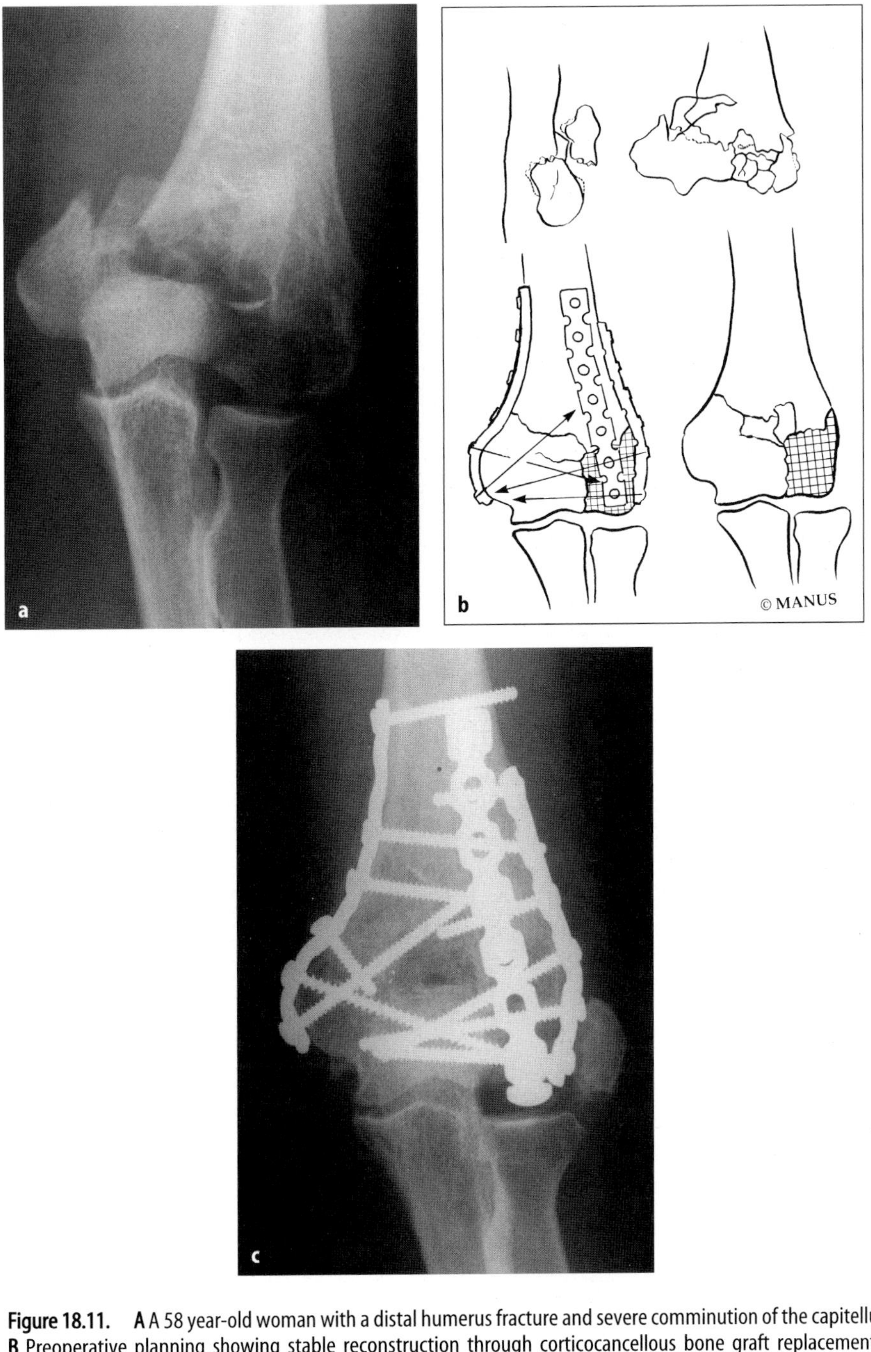

Figure 18.11. **A** A 58 year-old woman with a distal humerus fracture and severe comminution of the capitellum. **B** Preoperative planning showing stable reconstruction through corticocancellous bone graft replacement of the comminuted capitellum. **C** Final radiograph with stable fixation of the lateral column to the trochlea through bone grafting and triple-plating.

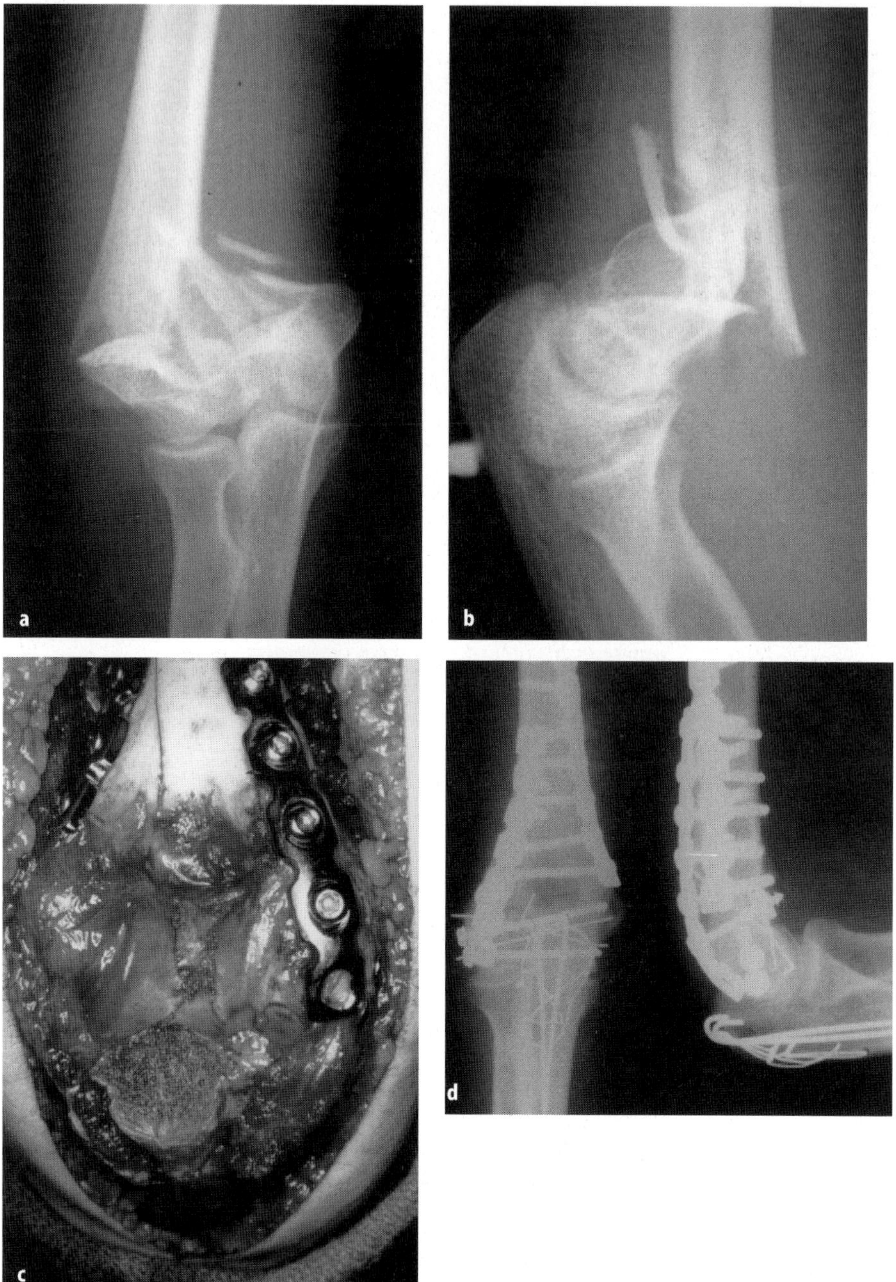

Figure 18.12. **A**, anteroposterior (AP) and **B**, lateral radiographs of comminuted AO C–3 distal humerus fracture. **C**, Central trochlear comminution is replaced by corticocancellous bone graft and stabilized by orthogonal plating. **D**, Final AP and lateral radiographs.

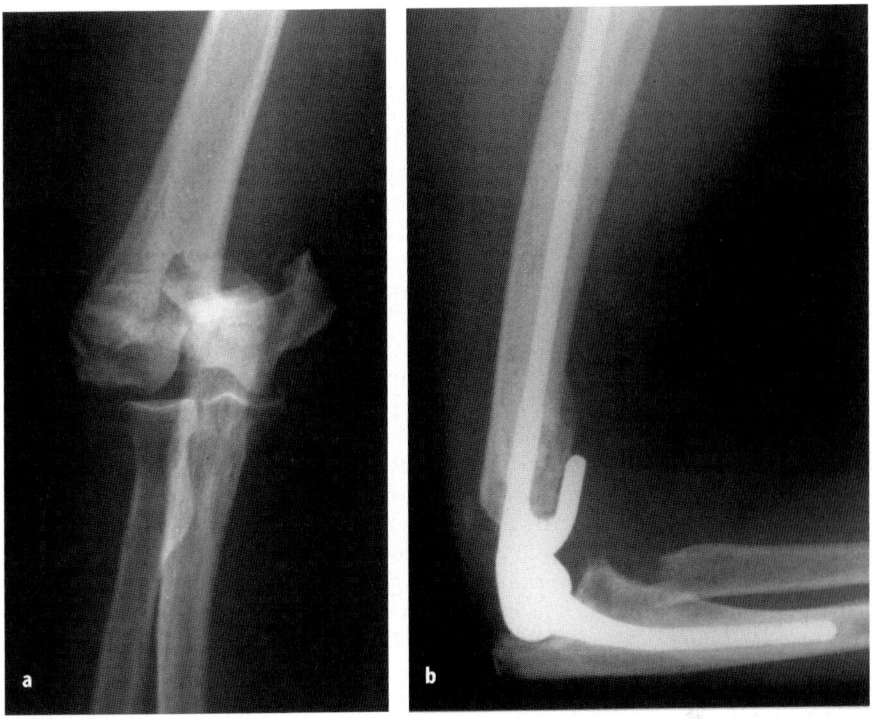

Figure 18.13A,B. A comminuted distal humerus fracture in an elderly female with osteoporosis. Because of the severe comminution an elbow arthroplasy was performed. **A**, Preoperative radiographs. **B**, Postoperative view of the total elbow arthroplasty.

study looking at 20 elbows with a minimum 2 year follow-up found a mean arc of motion from 25° to 130° with 100% good or excellent functional results [45]. Complications such as nonunion, malunion and avascular necrosis are avoided. It is worth emphasizing that immediate elbow arthroplasty should be performed only in those few elderly patients in whom no suitable alternative is available. It is not a treatment option in younger patients nor in those patients who have high functional demands placed upon their elbows.

Based on our preoperative planning, we use the surgical approach described by Bryan and Morrey [39] in any patient who we feel may require a total elbow replacement. An alternative approach maintaining the triceps attachment and exposing the elbow through combined medial and lateral dissection around the triceps can also be used [46]. This allows for adequate exposure and provides the advantage of allowing unrestricted active elbow extension in the immediate postoperative period. After the fracture is exposed the soft tissue attachments to the distal humerus are released and all bone fragments are excised. The remaining operative technique is well described and is similar to that used in elbow arthroplasty for other indications. Experience with total elbow arthroplasty is a prerequisite for performing this operation.

Rehabilitation

Our postoperative rehabilitation proceeds through one of two possible paths depending upon the stability of our fixation. The senior author has classified fracture fixation as being either rigid or stable [15]. Rigid fixation is present when the operative construct has excellent bone apposition, all plates are well contoured, screws have adequate purchase to resist pull-out and multiple K wires are not required to supplement fixation. Stable fixation involves small fracture gaps, tenuous screw purchase and the need for enhanced fixation techniques. It is imperative that an honest assessment of fixation be made in each case in order to prevent early hardware failure and nonunion.

Rigidly stabilized fractures done through a posterior approach can be mobilized at 3 days postoperatively with both active and passive measures being instituted. We have also found immediate continuous passive motion to be helpful in these patients. On the other hand, while stable fracture constructs will withstand active motion they are at risk of failure with unabated passive motion. As a result, active motion only is begun at 3 days and passive motion is withheld for 6 weeks. Those patients undergoing a Bryan–Morrey approach must avoid active extension for the first 6 weeks. Extension is achieved through a supervised program of gravity-assisted extension with the arm kept at the patient's side, as well as through gentle passive assisted exercises. Close supervision by a properly trained therapist and frequent postoperative follow-up is necessary in all cases for optimal results.

Complications

Complications associated with the care of distal humerus fractures are frequent. Joint stiffness, nonunion and malunion, ulnar neuritis, heterotopic ossification and wound problems are most commonly encountered. Each of these represents a serious challenge for the treating physician.

Significant joint stiffness is usually a function of inadequate fixation and the resulting prolonged immobilization needed to ensure fracture healing. Early active range of motion is paramount if a full functional arc is to be restored. If stiffness is a problem a static progressive range of motion splint can be instituted as soon as fracture healing has occurred. These splints can result in improved motion up to 6 months after surgery [47,48]. If a functional range of motion continues to be elusive, open release of the offending area of fibrosis is indicated.

The combination of an insufficiently stable surgical construct and poor osteogenic potential will lead to fracture nonunion. This has become less of a problem with the advent of the liberal use of bone graft and newer fixation techniques. However, special attention with respect to the quantity and quality of screw purchase in the distal fragments continues to be important in avoiding this complication. Nonunion is typically a disabling problem because of the associated pain, loss of motion and ulnar nerve irritation[11,49–52]. Its treatment involves either repeat open reduction and internal fixation (ORIF) with bone grafting or a semiconstrained total elbow arthroplasty. We prefer to perform repeat ORIF with bone grafting in patients younger than 65 years old and in those patients older than 65 years old who have high functional demands and adequate bone stock. Total elbow arthroplasty is performed on those elderly patients who place low functional demands on their elbow. Favorable results can be obtained with each of these methods[51,53–56].

Similar treatment options and considerations are given to those patients with symptomatic malunions.

The ulnar nerve is predisposed to injury with complex distal humerus fractures. The fracture deformity may place stretch on the nerve, swelling may lead to compression of the nerve, and bony fragments or hardware may impinge on or damage the nerve. In nearly all distal humerus fractures simple decompression of the nerve is advised through release of Osborne's ligament. Postoperative transient neuritis should be observed for at least 6 weeks. If symptoms do not improve over time, formal decompression of the nerve and anterior transposition is advised. In most instances it is recommended that the nerve be placed subcutaneously so as not to impede recovery of joint range of motion. Only in late established severe cases is a submuscular position preferred.

Ectopic calcification frequently follows trauma to the elbow but rarely leads to significant impairment of function. Ectopic ossification (heterotopic ossification) is uncommon but may lead to severe disturbance of range of motion. Risk factors include severe open injury, fracture-dislocations, high-energy trauma, multiple surgical procedures, head injury and repeat surgical intervention within 3 months of injury. In most instances problematic ectopic ossification can be seen within 2–6 weeks of injury on the radiographs. The limits of bone involvement are usually well established by 12 weeks after injury. Operative excision is recommended when a functional range of motion can not be restored by therapy within 3–6 months of injury. An operative excision can safely be performed when soft tissue homeostasis is apparent and the bone is approaching clear definition and maturity by radiography.

Infection rates vary from 0 to 6% in the literature [57,58]. Grade 3 open fractures associated with high-energy trauma pose the greatest risk. Deep infections are treated with appropriate intravenous antibiotics, aggressive irrigation and debridement, and soft tissue coverage as needed. If the hardware is securely fixed, it should be left in place until union has occurred. If the hardware is loose it should be removed and treatment of the nonunion is deferred until the infection has been eradicated.

Conclusion

Reconstruction of an osteoporotic distal humerus fracture is immensely challenging, especially when severe comminution or segmental bone loss is present. Success requires thoughtful preoperative planning, extensive surgical exposure, and skillful reduction and fixation techniques. The liberal use of bone graft and enhanced fixation methods such as methylmethacrylate supplementation are often necessary. The goal is to obtain rigid fixation of each of the three osseous arms of the distal humerus allowing for early unrestricted motion. A thorough understanding of the normal distal humerus anatomy and of modern fixation principles is a prerequisite for success. Despite the difficulties and potential complications, aggressive surgical stabilization is the preferred method of treating these fractures and good functional results can be obtained. The rare fracture in the elderly patient that is not amenable to surgical reconstruction can be treated effectively with immediate total elbow arthroplasty.

References

1. Palvanen M, Kannus P, Niemi S, Parkkari J. Secular trends in the osteoporotic fractures of the distal humerus in elderly women. Eur J Epidemiol 1998;14:159–164.
2. Brown RF, Morgan RG. Intercondylar T-shaped fractures of the humerus. Results in ten cases treated by early mobilisation. J Bone and Joint Surg Br 1971;53:425–428.
3. Evans EM. Supracondylar Y fractures of the humerus. J Bone Joint Surg Br 1953; 35:381–385.
4. Keon-Cohen BT. Fractures at the elbow. J Bone Joint Surgery Am 1966;48:1623–1639.
5. Miller WE. Comminuted fractures of the distal end of the humerus. J Bone Joint Surg Am 1964;46:644–656.
6. Riseborough EJ, Radin EL. Intercondylar T fractures of the humerus in the adult. A comparison of operative and nonoperative treatment in twenty-nine cases. J Bone Joint Surg Am 1969;51:130–141.
7. Jupiter JB, Neff U, Holzach P, Allgower M. Intercondylar fractures of the humerus. An operative approach. J Bone Joint Surg Am 1985;67:226–239.
8. Gabel GT, Hanson G, Bennett JB, Noble PC, Tullos HS. Intra-articular fractures of the distal humerus in the adult. Clin Orthop 1987;216:99–108.
9. Aitken GK, Rorabeck CH. Distal humeral fractures in the adult. Clin Orthop 1986;207:191–197.
10. Holdsworth BJ, Mossad MM. Fractures of the adult distal humerus. Elbow function after internal fixation. J Bone Joint Surg Br 1990;72:362–365.
11. Jupiter JB. Complex fractures of the distal part of the humerus and associated complications. Instr Course Lect 1995;44:187–198.
12. Kundel K, Braun W, Wieberneit J, Ruter A. Intra-articular distal humerus fractures. Factors affecting functional outcome. Clin Orthop 1996;332:200–208.
13. Zagorski JB, Jennings JJ, Burkhalter WE, Uribe JW. Comminuted intra-articular fractures of the distal humeral condyles. Surgical vs nonsurgical treatment. Clin Orthop 1986;202:197–204.
14. Hubert J, Rosso R, Neff U, Bodoky A, Regazzoni P, Harder F. Operative treatment of distal humeral fractures in the elderly. J Bone Joint Surg Br 1994;76:793–796.
15. Hastings H, II, Engles DR. Fixation of complex elbow fractures, Part I. General overview and distal humerus fractures. Hand Clin 1997;13:703–719.
16. Morrey BF. Post-traumatic stiffness: distraction arthroplasty. In: Morrey BF, editor. The elbow and its disorders, 2nd ed. Philadelphia: Saunders, 1993:476–491.
17. Atkinson WB, Elftman H. The carrying angle of the human arm as a secondary symptom character. Anat Rec 1945;91:49.
18. Keats TE, Teeslink R, Diamond AE, et al. Normal axial relationships of the major joints. Radiology 1966;87:904.
19. Beals RK. The normal carrying angle of the elbow: a radiographic study of 422 patients. Clin Orthop 1976;119:194.
20. Halls AA, Travill A. Transmission of pressures across the elbow joint. Anat Rec 1964;150:243.
21. Morrey BF. Anatomy of the elbow joint. In: Morrey BF, editor. The elbow and its disorders, 2nd ed. Philadelphia: Saunders, 1993:16.
22. McKee MD, Mehne DK, Jupiter JB. Trauma to the adult elbow and fractures of the distal humerus. II. Fractures of the distal humerus. In: Browner BD, Jupiter JB, Levine AM, Trafton PG, editors. Skeletal Trauma. 2nd ed. Philadelphia: Saunders, 1998:1488.
23. Milch H. Fractures and fracture-dislocations of the humeral condyles. J Trauma 1964;4:592–607.
24. Kuhn JE, Louis DS, Loder RT. Divergent single-column fractures of the distal part of the humerus. J Bone Joint Surg Am 1995;77:538–542.
25. Jupiter JB, Barnes KA, Goodman LJ, Saldana AE. Multiplane fracture of the distal humerus. J Orthop Trauma 1993;7:216–220.

26. Bryan RS, Morrey BF. Fractures of the distal humerus. In: Morrey BF, editor. The elbow and its disorders. Philadelphia: Saunders, 1985:302–339.
27. McKee MD, Jupiter JB, Bamberger HB. Coronal shear fractures of the distal end of the humerus [see comments]. J Bone Joint Surg Am 1996;78:49–54.
28. Muller ME, Nazarian S, Koch P. AO Classification of fractures. Berlin Heidelberg New York: Springer, 1987.
29. Greenspan A, Norman A. Radial head-capitellum view: an expanded imaging approach to elbow injury. Radiology 1987;164:272.
30. Greenspan A, Norman A, Rosen H. Radial head-capitellum view in elbow trauma: clinical application and radiographic-anatomic correlation. AJR 1984;143:355.
31. Greenspan A. The radial head–capitellum view: another example of its usefulness [letter]. AJR 1982;139:193.
32. Head RW. Radial head–capitellum view in elbow trauma. AJR 1983;140:1273.
33. Sultanpur A. Anterior supracondylar fracture of the humerus (flexion type): a simple technique for closed reduction and fixation in adults and the aged. J Bone Joint Surg Br 1978;60:383–386.
34. Hotchkiss RN. Fractures and dislocations of the elbow. In: Rockwood CA Jr, Green DP, Bucholz RW, Heckman JD, editors. Fracturs in adults, 4th ed. Philadelphia: Lippincott-Raven, 1996:937–939.
35. Bohler L. The treatment of fractures. Philadelphia: Grune & Stratton, 1956.
36. Smith FM. Surgery of the elbow, 2nd ed. Philadelphia: Saunders, 1972.
37. Conn J, Wade PA. Injuries of the elbow (a ten-year review). J. Trauma 1961;1:248–268.
38. Eastwood WJ. The T-shaped fracture of the lower end of the humerus. J Bone Joint Surg 1937;19:364–369.
39. Bryan RS, Morrey BF. Extensile posterior exposure of the elbow: a triceps-sparing approach. Clin Orthop 1982;166:188.
40. Morrey BF. Surgical exposures of the elbow. In: Morrey BF, editor. The elbow and its disorders, 2nd ed. Philadelphia: Saunders, 1993:139–167.
41. Weber B, Vasey H. Osteosynthese bei Olecranon Fraktur. A Unfallmed Berufskr 1963;2:90.
42. Helfet DL, Hotchkiss RN. Internal fixation of the distal humerus: a biomechanical comparison of methods. J Orthop Trauma 1990;4:260–264.
43. Waddell JP, Hatch J, Richards R. Supracondylar fractures of the humerus: results of surgical treatment. J Trauma 1988;28:1615–1621.
44. Jupiter JB, Morrey BF. Fractures of the distal humerus in the adult. In: Morrey BF, editor. The elbow and its disorders, 2nd ed. Philadelphia: Saunders, 1993:328–366.
45. Cobb TK, Morrey BF. Total elbow arthroplasty as primary treatment for distal humeral fractures in elderly patients. J Bone Joint Surg Am 1997;79:826–832.
46. Morrey BF, Adams RA. Semiconstrained elbow replacement for distal humeral nonunion [see comments]. J Bone Joint Surg Br 1995;77:67–72.
47. Conney WP. Contractures of the elbow. In: Morrey BF, editor. The elbow and its disorders, 2nd ed. Philadelphia: Saunders, 1993:466.
48. Morrey BF. Post-traumatic contracture of the elbow. Operative treatment, including distraction arthroplasty. J Bone Joint Surg 1990;61:601.
49. Sim FH, Morrey BF. Nonunion and delayed union of distal humeral fractures. In: Morrey BF, editor. The elbow and its disorders, 2nd ed. Philadelphia: Saunders, 1993:367–382.
50. Ackerman G, Jupiter JB. Non-union of fractures of the distal end of the humerus. J Bone Joint Surg 1988;70:75–83.
51. Figgie MP, Inglis AE, Mow CS, Figgie HE. Salvage of non-union of supracondylar fracture of the humerus by total elbow arthroplasty. J Bone Joint Surg 1989;71:1058–1065.
52. Mitsunaga MM, Bryan RS, Linscheid RL. Condylar nonunions of the elbow. J Trauma 1982;22:787–791.

53. Jupiter JB, Goodman LF. The management of complex distal humerus nonunions in the elderly by elbow capsulotomy, triple plating, and ulnar nerve neurolysis. J Shoulder Elbow 1992;1:37–46.
54. McKee M, Jupiter J, Toh CL, Wilson L, Colton C, Karras KK. Reconstruction after malunion and nonunion of intra-articular fractures of the distal humerus. Methods and results in 13 adults. J Bone Joint Surg Br 1994;76:614–621.
55. Morrey BF, Adams RA. Total replacement for post-traumatic arthritis of the elbow. J Bone Joint Surg Br 1991;73:607.
56. Cobb TK, Linscheid RL. Late correction of malunited intercondylar humeral fractures. J Bone Joint Surg Br 1994;76:622.
57. Lecestre R. Round table on fractures of the lower end of the humerus. Societe Francaise de Chirurgie Orthopedique et Traumatolgie. Orthop Trans 1980;4:123.
58. Groh GI, Bennett JB. Fractures of the elbow region. In: Peimer CA, editor. Surgery of the hand and upper extremity. New York: McGraw-Hill, 1996:425–448.

19 Acetabular Fractures

P. M. Rommens and M. H. Hessmann

Introduction

Compared with surgery for fractures in other regions of the body, the operative treatment of acetabulum fractures is a recent development. This is so for several reasons: acetabulum fractures are rare, their analysis is complex and the surgery is difficult. In young people acetabulum fractures are caused by high-energy trauma. The early operative treatment of this fracture has the same advantage as the osteosynthesis of long bone fractures in the severely injured: fracture fixation permits early mobilization of the patient and prevents the complications of prolonged bed rest [1,2]. In addition, since acetabular fractures are articular fractures, the goal of treatment should be the same as for other joint injuries: the anatomical and stable reduction of the joint surfaces [3].

This chapter reviews the place of early surgery for acetabulum fractures in the elderly. To determine whether or not the same advantages of anatomical reduction and stable fixation occur in the older age group, an analysis of the specific situation of the elderly patient with an acetabulum fracture was undertaken.

Hip Fractures in the Elderly

Before dealing with acetabular trauma, it makes sense to review the treatment of hip fractures in the elderly. For these fractures, be they intracapsular, extracapsular or subtrochanteric, conservative management is not an acceptable treatment alternative. It is well known that nonoperative treatment has high morbidity, with a high mortality [4]. Prolonged and painful immobilization results in specific complications such as pneumonia, urinary infection, decubitus, cachexia and, not least, mental deterioration. An unacceptable number of fractures develop nonunion, delayed union or malunion, which makes functional rehabilitation difficult or impossible.

Although technical solutions for these fractures are numerous and different, their common aim is to make early out-of-bed-mobilization of the elderly possible. To achieve this goal the restoration of anatomy is not as important as the creation of functional stability, which allows early active mobilization. Total hip arthroplasty and hemiarthroplasty create an immediate weightbearing stability; femoral neck screws, extramedullary and intramedullary hip screws create a controlled instability, which allows impaction of the fracture fragments.

It is also accepted that hip fractures in elderly patients should be operated on as early as possible. In many of these patients primary surgery is not feasible due to the suboptimal condition in which the patient is admitted and the hospital's logistics. A high number of elderly patients will have associated diseases such as hypertonia, cardiac failure, atherosclerosis, limited pulmonary function, diabetes, Alzheimer's disease and risk factors such as anemia and hypothermia. In order to minimize dangers of anesthesia and surgery, a short but intensive preparation time is necessary. Nevertheless, all patients should be operated upon within the first 48 h after admission.

Acetabular Fractures in the Elderly

Why do acetabular fractures differ from hip fractures? In comparison with the thousands of articles that have been written about the operative treatment of hip fractures in the elderly, there is a paucity of literature about acetabular fractures in old people. There are at least two explanations for this difference: there are many fewer acetabular fractures than hip fractures, and there are no current valid guidelines for the treatment of acetabular fractures in the elderly.

The acetabulum is part of the solid three-dimensional construct of the innominate bone and since it is situated deep in the pelvic region, it is protected by several layers of soft tissue. As a consequence, acetabular fractures are not typical lesions of poor quality bone such as humeral head and neck fractures, femoral neck fractures and distal radius fractures. The acetabulum typically needs much more energy to be broken: the fracture usually occurs in a younger, more active and better risk-adapted population. The acetabular fracture of the elderly patient is the result of a different, lower-energy trauma compared with the fracture of younger patients. High-velocity traffic accidents will be less frequent than falls from a bicycle, pedestrian accidents or injuries in the home. While the type of fracture is dependent on the position of the femoral head and neck at the time of accident, fracture types in the elderly population will also be different. Whereas posterior wall fractures, transverse fractures and transverse with posterior wall fractures are common lesions in the younger population, anterior wall and column fractures are more frequent lesions in the elderly (Fig. 19.1). In motor vehicle accidents, the hip joint of the victim is flexed and the force comes from the front or the side. The energy applied on the acetabulum is transmitted through the femoral neck and head and directed in an upper and posterior direction to produce fractures involving the posterior wall and column. In falls either as pedestrians or in the home, the leg will be in a more extended position. The anteversion of the femoral neck will guide the forces coming from the trochanteric region in a more anterior direction, producing fractures involving the anterior wall and anterior column. In the series of 900 acetabular fractures, presented by Letournel [5], 65% of 129 patients older than 65 years had anterior column involvement. In a series of 25 patients, treated conservatively by Spencer [6], 76% had anterior column involvement. All 19 acetabular fractures in patients older than 60 years, operated on by Helfet et al. [7] had fracture types with involvement of the anterior column.

Treatment alternatives of acetabular fractures in the elderly range from bed rest with or without skeletal traction, to open reduction and internal fixation, and

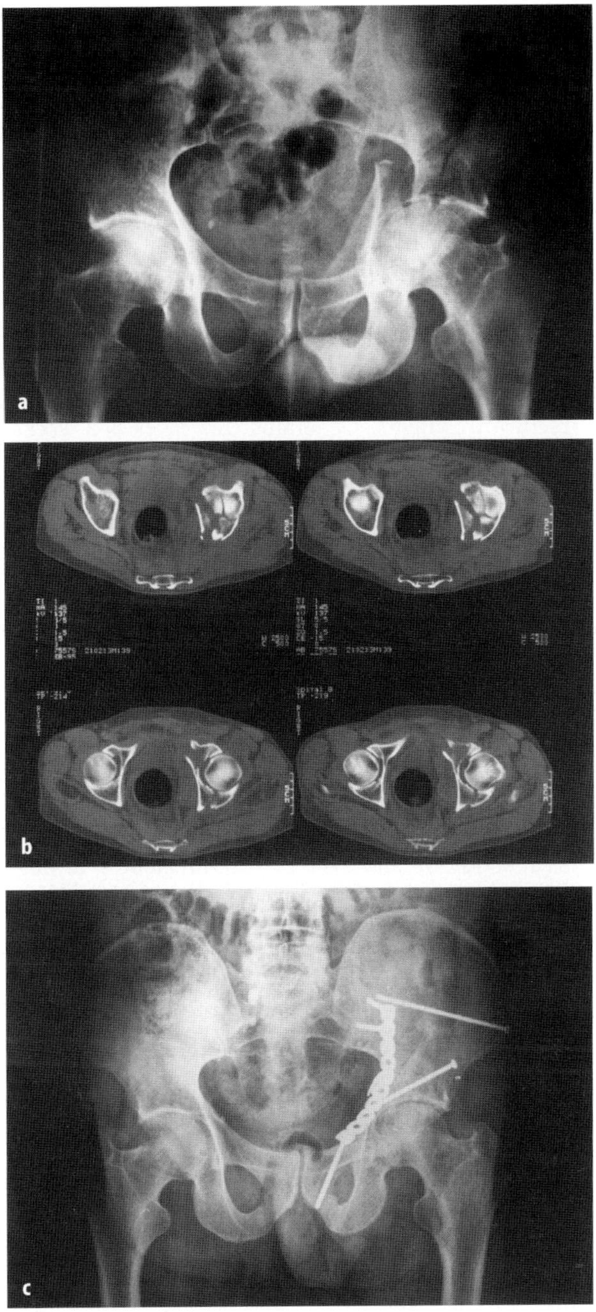

Figure 19.1. **a** Anterior column and posterior hemitransverse fracture of the left acetabulum after a fall in a 74-year-old male. **b** CT scans through the acetabular roof give an impression of its fragmentation. **c** Internal stabilization via the ilioinguinal approach. An additional spring plate is implanted for reposition of the posterior hemitransverse fracture part. An excellent functional and radiological result is achieved.

primary and secondary total hip arthroplasty. None of these regimens is generally accepted because they all have significant dangers and disadvantages. On the other hand, there is a great variety of fracture types of the acetabulum and pre-existing quality of the hip joint. Therefore, there cannot be a unique treatment regimen for all acetabular fractures in all elderly people. Advantages, limitations and dangers of each method have to be balanced against the personality of the patient with the acetabular fracture and the complexity of the fracture situation itself.

Conservative Treatment

Conservative treatment is certainly the oldest and, until now, most common method of treatment. The patient is placed in the supine position in bed and often put in femoral traction which is maintained as long as needed for early, incomplete bone union between fracture fragments. Generally, this takes 6–8 weeks. In this time, mobilization of the hip joint in traction and general rehabilitation measures are started. A period of out-of-bed mobilization with partial and gradually increasing weightbearing follows. Full weightbearing and good range of motion of the hip joint with independent walking is not reached before 4–6 months, if it can be obtained at all [6].

This type of treatment is all but equivalent to doing nothing. Long-term bed rest with prolonged skeletal traction represents a significant physical and mental burden for the patient. As conservative treatment demands motivation and cooperation, it is contraindicated in patients with severe mental illness. Moreover, long hospitalization in an unknown environment, chronic pain and discomfort can cause mental deterioration in old healthy patients, which makes the outcome of conservative treatment uncertain. Prolonged bed rest with traction is also associated with many medical problems. Sacral decubitus and ischemic heel ulcers have to be prevented actively and continuously. Urinary and/or pulmonary infections can deteriorate the patient's physical condition and even be life-threatening through sepsis. Their first clinical signs can be nonspecific: they have to be looked for regularly and treated aggressively. Deep venous thrombosis and pulmonary embolism are feared complications in all patients with prolonged immobilization. Food intake and nitrogen balance must be controlled in this older population; sometimes supplemental intravenous feeding will be necessary. Other consequences of prolonged immobilization are muscle wasting, disuse osteoporosis, joint contracture and stiffness.

Last but not least, it is not likely that closed reduction and skeletal traction will bring an anatomical position of the fracture fragments in most fracture types. A discongruence between the femoral head and the acetabular roof will remain visible. An exception is the double-column fracture, in which secondary congruence of the fracture fragments around the femoral head is possible [5]. If the patient survives without major medical problems but with articular discongruence, rehabilitation will be difficult and the patient's quality of life will be diminished due to limited hip mobility, limited walking capacity and chronic pain. In the literature there are only a few series of conservatively treated acetabular fractures in elderly patients. Spencer [6] found 30% unacceptable functional results in a group of 25 patients, of whom 68% initially had limited fracture displacement.

Conservative therapy is the treatment of choice only in minimally displaced fractures, in small posterior wall fractures after a posterior dislocation without hip instability, and in patients with clear contraindications for operative treatment due to their extremely precarious preoperative physical condition. Poor mental condition is more a contraindication than an indication for conservative treatment.

Operative Stabilization

If the operative management of hip fractures in the elderly is generally accepted, this is not so for acetabular fractures. Many surgeons are reluctant to perform or are even against internal fixation due to the complexity of the fracture and the difficulty of the surgery. They fear implant loosening and suboptimal reduction due to the low holding power of the screws. They also argue that most elderly patients are not able to walk with partial weightbearing postoperatively, which is of major importance for uneventful fracture healing. The long, difficult and risky surgical procedure and the uncertain prognosis of the hip joint thereafter make the risk-benefit analysis of operative stabilization seem unfavorable.

However, surgeons who are familiar with acetabular surgery in a younger population, have a different opinion. Since they are aware of the poor results of conservative treatment and primary hip arthroplasty, they promote open reduction and internal fixation [7–10]. Their arguments are as follows: each fracture and each patient has to be regarded individually; the great majority of fractures can be stabilized through one approach; primary hip arthroplasty is at least as difficult and risky as open reduction and internal fixation; and long-term results are as gratifying as in the younger population if good reduction and fixation is achieved.

All fractures displaced more than 2 mm, fractures running through the acetabular roof, as well as fractures with intra-articular fragments and residual instability after hip reduction, with the exception of osteoarthritic hips, should be considered for internal stabilization [11]. They have to be analyzed before a therapeutic decision is made just as acetabular fractures in younger patients are studied. Anteroposterior, ala and obturator oblique pelvic radiographs are taken, and the fracture is identified in accordance with the classification system of Letournel and Judet [5]. CT examination is mandatory; three-dimensional reconstructions may be helpful for better evaluation of the damage to the acetabular roof and its cartilage. Different methods of fracture reduction, fracture stabilization and alternative operative approaches are considered. Fractures with major involvement of the posterior column can be operated on through the Kocher-Langenbeck approach, fractures with major involvement of the anterior column through the ilioinguinal approach. The use of extensile approaches is avoided because of the duration of the operative procedure, and the higher risk of intrinsic problems such as massive blood loss, infection, damage to the sciatic nerve, heterotopic ossification and abductor weakness.

Each patient has to be evaluated preoperatively as well. The following questions have to be answered before a decision is taken:

- What is the biological age of the patient?
- What are his or her concomitant medical problems?
- Can the patient's medical condition be stabilized or improved in a few days before surgery?
- Will the patient be able to cooperate with the surgeon postoperatively?
- What is the patient's motivation for rehabilitation?

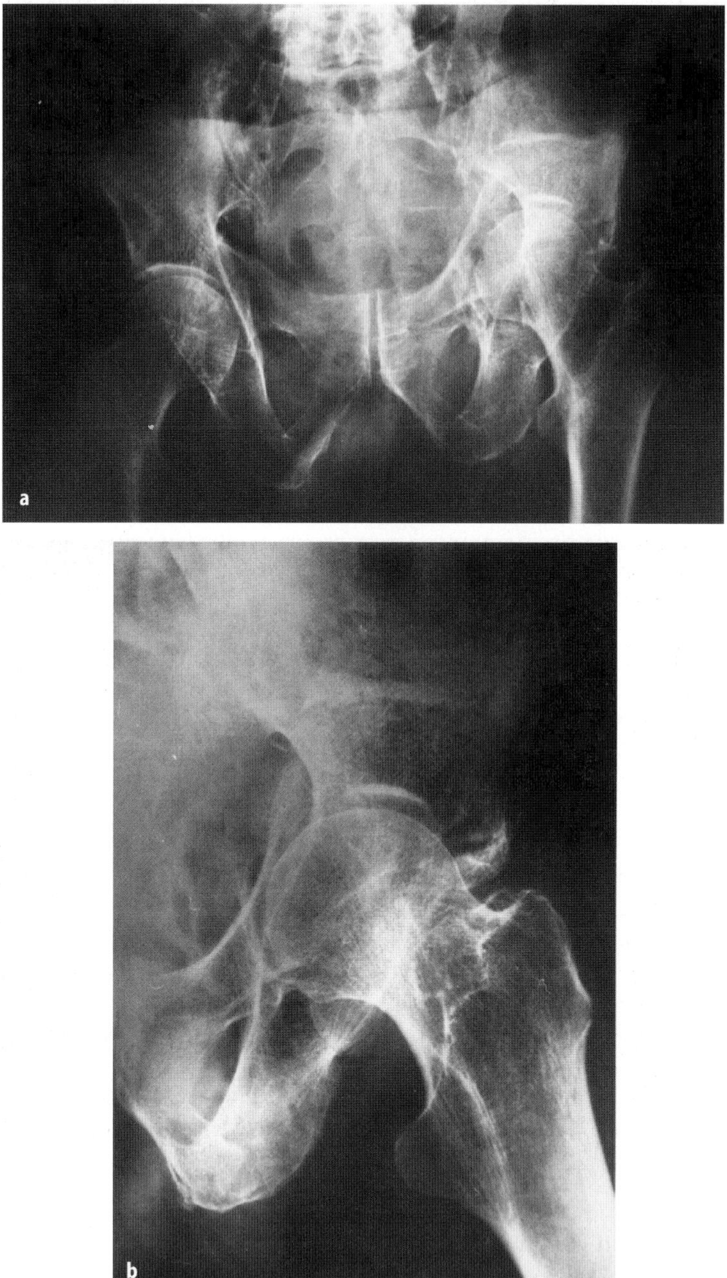

Figure 19.2. **a** Anterior column and posterior hemitransverse fracture of the left acetabulum after a fall at home in an 83-year-old healthy man. **b** The ala view shows the protrusion of the femoral head proximally and medially. (*continued on facing page*)

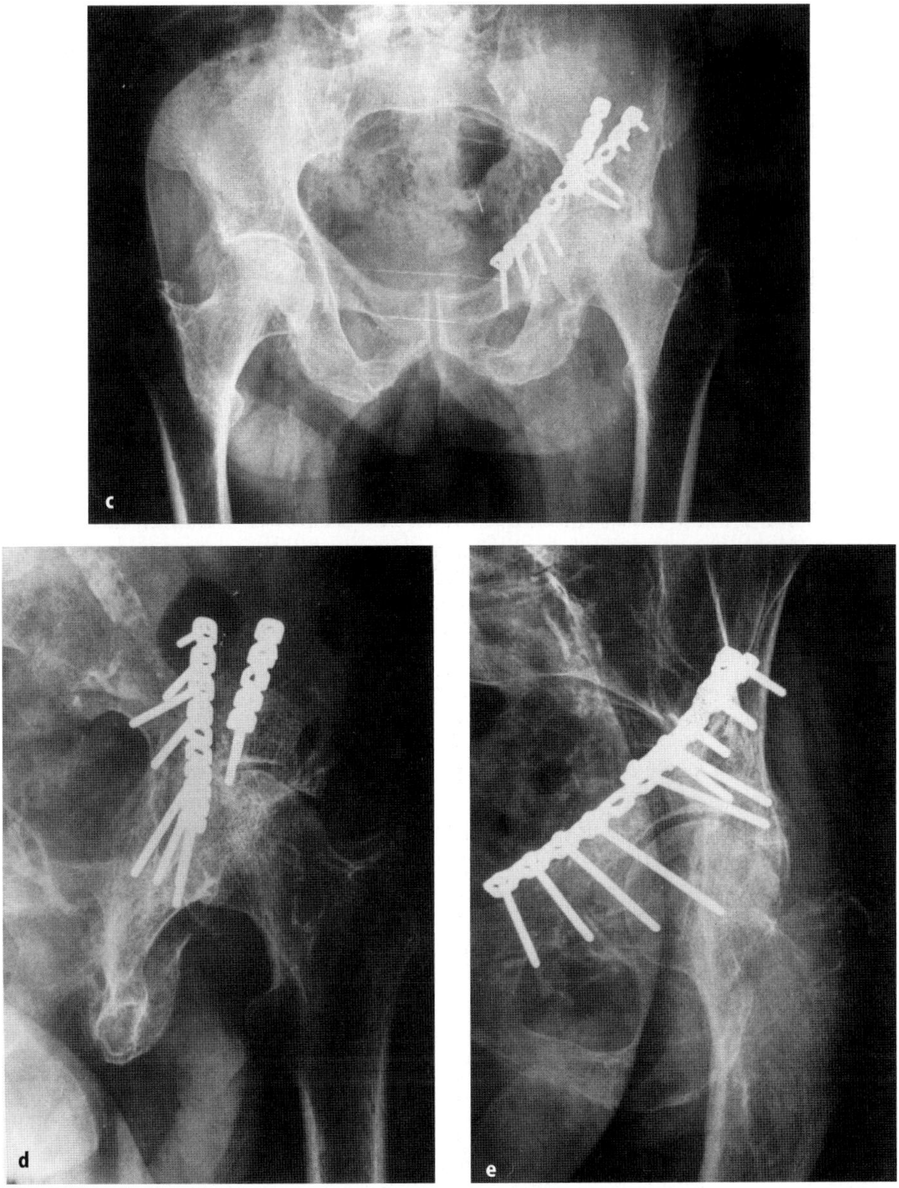

Figure 19.2. (*continued*) **c** Pelvic overview 6 months after internal stabilization. A slight protrusion of the femoral head is still visible. The fracture is healed. **d** Ala view after 6 months. **e** Obturator view after 6 months. The patient is able to walk shorter distances than before, but without any pain.

Patients who have an acceptable medical and mental condition are good candidates for open reduction and internal fixation. However, patients who are almost bedridden or have a poor mental condition must be considered for internal stabilization. In this patient group, the primary goal is not to obtain an anatomical reconstruction but to create a stable hip joint. This will certainly make mobilization and nursing easier. Consequently, the overall prognosis for survival might be better than if nonoperative treatment was selected. As with hip fractures, patients have to be prepared quickly but intensively for operation. The risk of anesthesia for these patients is no higher than for patients with an unstable hip fracture or for patients with acetabular fractures treated by primary total hip arthroplasty if the surgery can be done without major blood loss within 90 min to 2 h of operating time. Typically, the operation is performed at the end of the first or the beginning of the second week after trauma.

As mentioned in the introduction, most fractures will involve the anterior column and can be stabilized through the ilioinguinal approach [12]. This is certainly the most anatomical and the less aggressive approach to the acetabulum. The structures at highest risk are the lateral femoral cutaneous nerve and the external iliac vessels. The surgeon exposes and reduces the fracture fragments through three surgical windows. The lateral window exposes the internal iliac fossa from the sacroiliac joint to the pectinate eminence. The middle window shows the lower part of the anterior column from the pectinate eminence to the pubic tubercle and the quadrilateral surface, which corresponds to the inner surface of the acetabulum. The medial window gives access to the symphysis pubis and the retropubic space from the symphysis to the obturator foramen. In the case of a low fracture pattern of the anterior column, the approach can be limited to the middle and medial windows [13].

With one long reconstruction plate on the anterior side of the pelvic brim, if necessary combined with additional shorter plates at the acetabular roof and the inner pelvic fossa or with one or several very long lag screws, a stable and anatomical fixation can be obtained (Fig. 19.2). It is very important to obtain good holding power at the proximal and distal ends of the plate, at a distance from the fracture. It is advisable to choose long pathways for the small fragments screws in order to obtain maximal bony anchorage and holding power for each screw. When the posterior column is involved as well, it must be reduced indirectly through the middle window and fixed with long lag screws, coming from the front. Alternative fixation techniques are the spring plate and cerclage wires [13] (see also Fig. 19.1). The extended Pfannenstiel approach promoted by Cole and Bolhofner [15] and the median retroperitoneal approach described by Biert and Goris (4) are other less invasive approaches to the inner side of the small pelvis. The reconstruction plate is placed at the inner side of the innominate bone and pushes the quadrilateral surface laterally against the direction of the forces coming from the femoral neck and head. In fractures with exclusive posterior wall or column involvement, the Kocher-Langenbeck approach is chosen. In our experience, stable internal fixation can be obtained in nearly all cases, including double-column fractures. Also Helfet et al. [7] obtained stable fixation without secondary dislocation in all but one of 18 fractures . Thanks to the excellent perfusion of the pelvic bone, healing of the fracture can be expected between 8 and 12 weeks.

Healthy patients will have the same postoperative rehabilitation schedule as younger patients who underwent the same operation. Patients with mental illness or those who are not able to ambulate are mobilized out of bed and set in a chair.

Weightbearing is prevented as much as possible. Although only small experience is available, we are persuaded that open reduction and internal fixation is the best treatment for the great majority of the biologically and/or mentally older patients, provided that intensive medical stabilization and thorough diagnostics and planning are performed preoperatively and that the surgeon is familiar with acetabular surgery.

Primary Total Hip Arthroplasty

The idea of primary total hip arthroplasty (PTHA) in older patients with acetabular fractures is not new. Although the literature on PTHA is more extensive than that on open reduction and internal fixation, all series are small and little is known about long-term results. PTHA has to be differentiated from secondary THA (STHA). PTHA is defined as the placement of a total hip prosthesis as primary treatment for acute acetabular fractures. STHA can be defined as the placement of a total hip prosthesis in patients with an old acetabular fracture treated primarily with skeletal extension, with open reduction and internal fixation or with primary reconstruction of the acetabular roof in order to create a stable and vital foundation for insertion and fixation of the acetabular component of the total hip prosthesis. Proponents of PTHA argue that open reduction and stable internal fixation mostly will not be possible due to the comminution of the fracture, the destruction of the cartilage of the acetabular roof and the poor holding power of the screws in the osteoporotic bone. For these authors, the best candidates for PTHA are patients with pre-existing osteoarthritis, severe cartilage damage to the acetabulum and/or the femoral head and concomitant fractures of the femoral head and neck [16–18].

Although different approaches and techniques of implantation are described, the same therapeutic goals can be defined for all of them. To achieve a stable fixation of the cup component of the total hip prosthesis to the pelvic ring, both columns of the acetabulum have to be fixed together to make a stable construct. For this, rigid fixation is more important than restoration of anatomy. This can be achieved with a reconstruction plate and/or lag screws. Both columns can best be visualized after removal of the femoral head and neck. Furthermore, bony defects in the acetabular roof must be filled with spongious bone from the femoral head combined with corticocancellous bone blocks from the iliac wing. The polyethylene cup, which is cemented, is fixed in a metal ring which fits in the reconstructed acetabulum and is held with several cancellous screws (Fig. 19.3). The shaft component of the prosthesis is fixed as a cemented or noncemented implant, depending on the bone quality of the proximal femur. The aftertreatment is similar to that of THA in osteoarthritis. Partial weightbearing is recommended for several weeks, if possible; otherwise full weightbearing is allowed after wound healing. Only in patients with a posterior dislocation of the hip combined with a smaller posterior wall or column fracture is reconstruction of the acetabular roof neither necessary nor quick and easy (Fig. 19.4).

Also for this type of surgery, the patient has to be prepared intensively. Due to the acetabular reconstruction the duration of the operative procedure and the amount of blood loss will be much higher than in THA for osteoarthritis. In cases of complex acetabular fractures, the whole procedure may be more demanding for both patient and surgeon than internal stabilization.

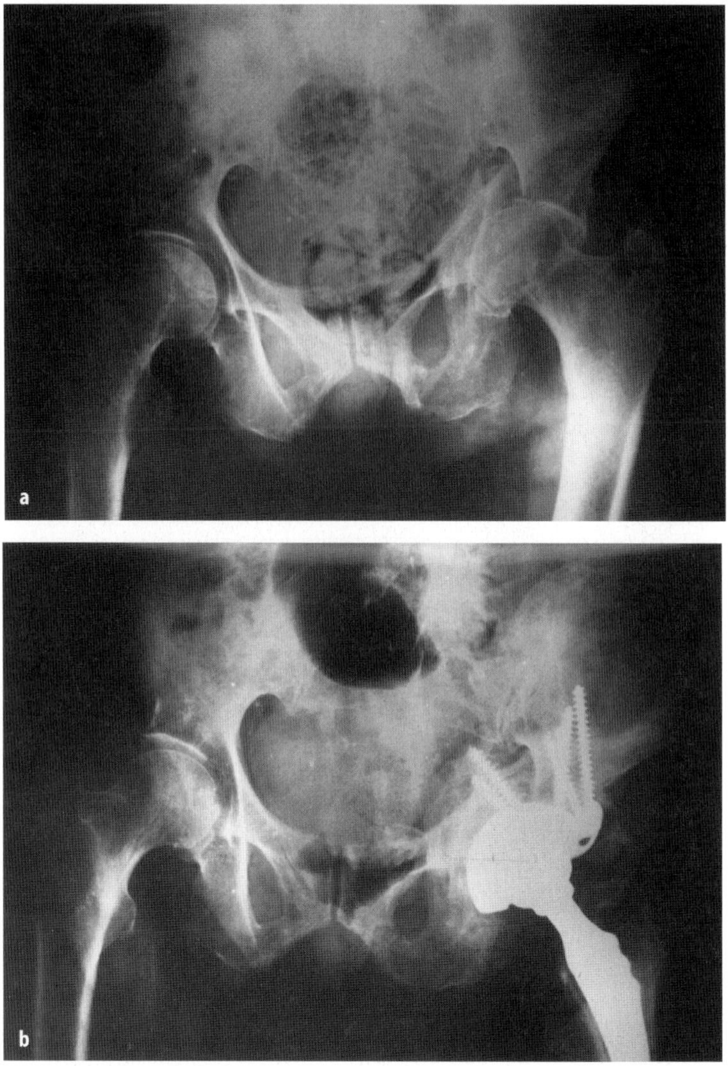

Figure 19.3. **a** Both-column fracture of the left acetabulum in an 89-year old woman after a fall at home. **b** Primary total hip arthroplasty with metal reinforcement ring, cemented polyethylene cup and cemented shaft component. The position of the new acetabulum is clearly medialized, the metal cup is attached with four cancellous screws to the acetabular roof and with two additional screws to loose fracture fragments.The stability of the whole construct is questionable. Survival time of the patient was only 6 months.

Although perioperative mortality in the series described in literature is comparable to series of femoral neck fractures treated with THA, morbidity is higher. But no series contains more than 26 patients and the limited follow-up time varies between 6 and 38 months, which certainly limits the validity of the conclusions [19–21]. The most important local problems described in the follow-up are the formation of massive periarticular ossifications, hip dislocation, infection and loosening of the acetabular component of the prosthesis. The advanced age of the

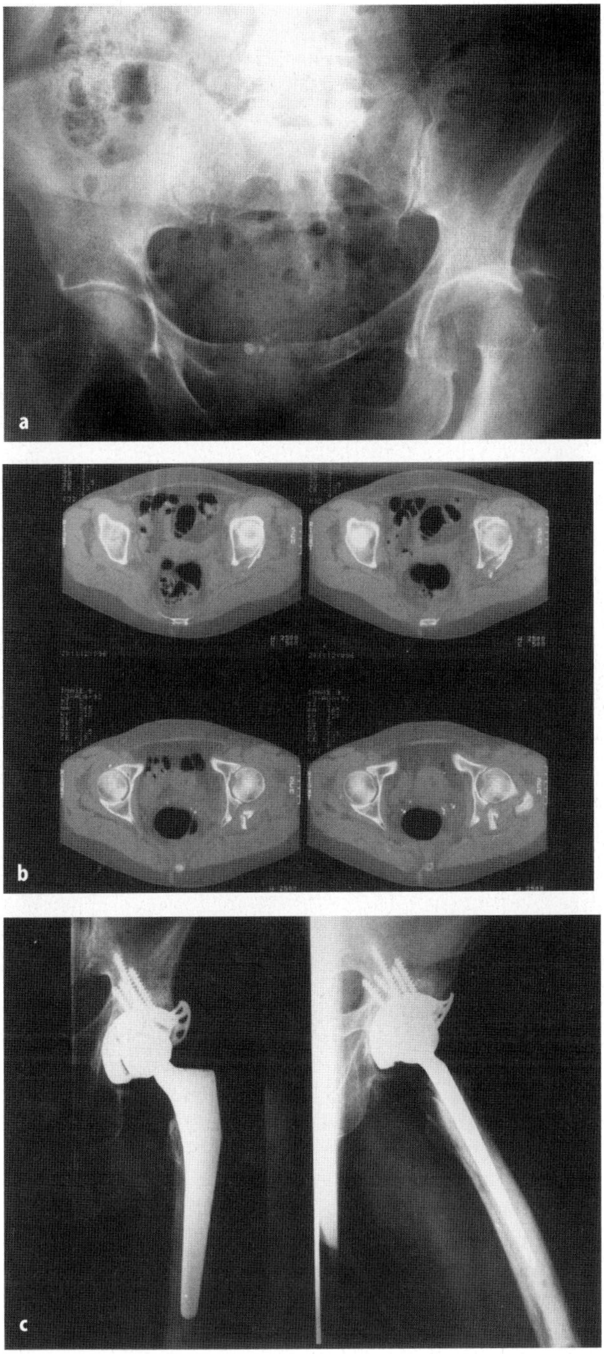

Figure 19.4. **a** Posterior hip dislocation and posterior wall fracture of the left acetabulum in a 72-year-old woman. **b** CT scans through the acetabular roof reveal a good bone socket for cup implantation. **c** Primary total hip arthroplasty with reinforcement ring. There is an excellent functional end-result.

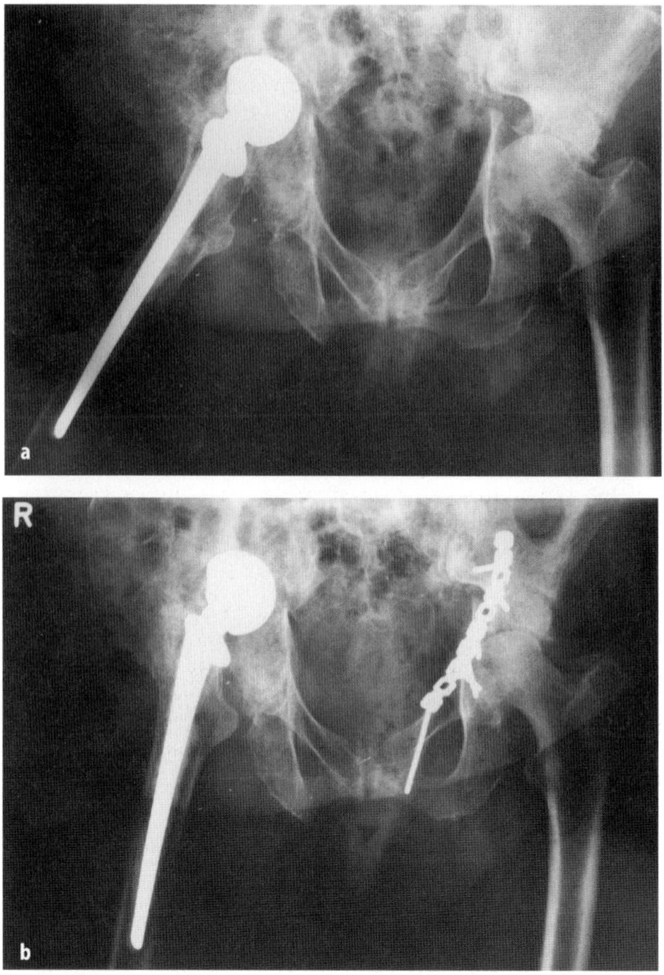

Figure 19.5. **a** A 78-year-old woman with an acute transverse fracture of the left acetabulum and older transverse fracture of the right acetabulum. The right side was treated with primary bipolar hemiarthroplasty. No stabilization of the acetabulum or reconstruction of its roof was performed. There is massive protrusion of the prosthetic head through the fracture. Before the second accident, the patient was able to stand on the right leg, but range of motion was minimal. **b** Primary internal stabilization on the left side through the ilioinguinal approach: anteroposterior view. The functional outcome is acceptable.

patient, the altered anatomy, the manipulation of the soft tissues around the hip joint, the difficult fixation of the cup to the acetabular roof and the duration of surgery seem to be responsible for the higher complication rate. Although only a small proportion of the patients operated on could be reviewed, functional results were acceptable. As in patients treated for femoral neck fractures, only a few regain the same functional level they had before surgery.

Secondary Total Hip Arthroplasty

In the older English literature, acceptable results have been published with primary skeletal traction until fracture healing, followed by STHA. Nevertheless, in the only long-term follow-up study of a larger patient group treated with STHA, revision for loosening of the acetabular component of the prosthesis was 4 to 5 times higher than in THA for osteoarthritis [21]. As mentioned above (see Conservative Treatment), the acetabulum mostly will heal in a nonanatomical position. At the level of the acetabular roof, important bony defects may result, which make safe fixation of the acetabular component of the prosthesis difficult. As in PTHA, the creation of a stable, vital acetabular roof without bony defects is mandatory. STHA therefore does not avoid the risks of major primary surgery. During the period of conservative treatment before surgery, the condition of the patient may deteriorate mentally as well as physically. If the patient survives the period of skeletal traction without major medical problems, one risks operating on a patient with disuse osteoporosis, hip contracture, muscle weakness and latent, subclinical infection. For these reasons, STHA following conservative treatment is no longer recommendable. It unnecessarily prolongs the period of treatment and endangers the whole outcome of the patient.

In some patients with acetabular fractures combined with pre-existing osteoarthritis, femoral head damage or bony defects at the acetabular roof, the complex problem of instability must be solved in several operative sessions. In a first operative procedure, the acetabular fracture is stabilized through an ilioinguinal or a Kocher-Langenbeck approach. The patient is stabilized after this surgery and, in an early second procedure, a total hip prosthesis is implanted [23]. With this staged reconstruction, a long surgical procedure with manipulation and mobilization of the gluteal muscles proximal to the acetabulum is prevented. The formation of periarticular ossifications is also prevented. Marchesi and Ganz [23], Baumgärtel et al. [19] and Pohlemann and Baumgärtel [13] report good to acceptable results in small series.

Conclusion

Acetabular fractures in the elderly are infrequent lesions, but constitute a real problem for the patient and a challenge for the surgeon. Whereas operative treatment of hip fractures in the elderly is generally accepted, therapeutic options for acetabular fractures range from conservative treatment to primary total hip arthroplasty. The problem created by the fracture has to be analyzed individually. For the classification of the injury, the descriptive system of Letournel and Judet [5] is as valid as it is in a younger population. Due to different trauma mechanisms, more fractures with involvement of the anterior column are seen. The medical and mental status of the patient has to be evaluated before a decision on the therapeutic strategy is taken.

Conservative management includes long-time bed rest with skeletal traction and is associated with a large number of complications. Moreover, the fracture usually will not heal in an anatomical position, which makes rehabilitation difficult and overall functional outcome fair to poor. Internal fixation should be performed by surgeons who are familiar with acetabular surgery.

Preoperative planning and decision making on the approach are similar in older patients and in younger patients. To reduce operation time and/or to enhance fracture stability, limited approaches and different implants such as spring plates or cerclage wires may be used. The best candidates for open reduction and internal fixation are healthy, active people who are able to cooperate postoperatively and who have a high motivation for rehabilitation. Also patients, who are nearly bedridden or with a limited mental or physical state can be treated with osteosynthesis. Primary total hip arthroplasty requires good bone stock for fixation of the prosthesis (Fig. 19.5). This may include osteosynthesis of the acetabular roof and insertion of corticocancellous grafts in bony defects. The cup usually is inserted in a metal ring, which is attached to the pelvic ring with several long cancellous screws. The whole procedure is longer than THA in osteoarthritis or femoral neck fractures and associated with a higher ratio of dislocation, periarticular ossification, early cup loosening and infection. Therefore, it should be performed by an experienced hip surgeon. STHA prolongs the duration of treatment and may compromise the mental and physical condition of the patient before surgery. As in PTHA, the acetabular roof must be prepared for optimal attachment of the cup. It is no longer accepted as a standard therapy. In some patients, early STHA is preferred after primary acetabular stabilization. This procedure has the advantage of dividing one long procedure into two consecutive, less aggressive operations. In the first procedure, the acetabular roof is repaired so that a sufficient bone stock is available for the THA, which is performed soon thereafter.

References

1. Rommens PM, Hessmann MH. Early versus delayed surgery for musculoskeletal trauma in polytraumatized patients. Curr Opin Crit Care 1998;4:424–428.
2. Tscherne H, Regel G, Pape HC, Pohlemann T, Krettek C. Internal fixation of multiple fractures in patients with polytrauma. Clin Orthop 1998;347:62–78.
3. Matta J, M. Surgical treatment of acetabular fractures. In: Browner BD, Jupiter JB, Levine AM, Trafton PG, editors. Skeletal trauma. Philadelphia: Saunders, 1992:899–912.
4. Stappaerts KH, Deldycke J, Broos PLO, Staes FFGM, Rommens PM, Claes P. Treatment of unstable peritrochanteric fractures in elderly patients with a compression hip screw or with the Vandeputte (VDP) endoprothesis: a prospective randomized study. J Orthop Trauma 1995;9:292–297.
5. Letournel E, Judet R. Fractures of the acetabulum, 2nd ed. Berlin Heidelberg New York: Springer, 1993.
6. Spencer RF. Acetabular fractures in older patients. J Bone Joint Surg Br 1989;71: 774–776.
7. Helfet DL, Borrelli J, DiPasquale T, Sanders RW. Stabilization of acetabular fractures in elderly patients, J Bone Joint Surg Am 1992;74:753–765.
8. Borrelli J Jr, Koval KJ, Helfet DL. Pelvis and acetabulum. In: Koval J, Zuckermann JD, editors. Fractures in the elderly. Philadelphia: Lippincott-Raven, 1998:159–174.
9. Rommens PM. Azetabulumfrakturen: Diagnostik, Therapie, Ergebnisse. Chir Praxis 1995/1996;50:685–710.
10. Rommens PM, Van den Bossche M, Fevery S, Blum J. Bilaterale Azetabulumfrakturen der vorderen Pfeiler- und Wirbelkörperfraktur nach alkoholinduziertem Krampfanfall. Unfallchirurg 1996;99:704–707.
11. Rommens PM, Vanderschot P, Broos PL. Vorbereitung und Technik der operativen Behandlung von 225 Azetabulumfrakturen. Zweijahresergebnisse in 175 Fällen. Unfallchirurg 1997;100:338–348.

12. Rommens PM, Hessmann M. The ilioinguinal approach. Osteo Int 1999;7:74–83.
13. Pohlemann T, Baumgärtel F. Azetabulumfrakturen im Alter. In: Tscherne H, Pohlemann T, editors. Tscherne Unfallchirurgie. Becken und Acetabulum. Berlin Heidelberg New York: Springer, 1998:446–455.
14. Cole J, Bolhofner B. Extended Pfannenstil approach for intrapelvic fixation of acetabular fractures. Proceedings of the first international symposium on surgical treatment of acetabular fractures, Paris, 10–11 May 1993.
15. Biert J, Goris RJA. The median extra peritoneal approach to the pelvic ring in perspective. Indications and limitations. Osteo Int 1999;7:45–47.
16. Boardman KP, Charnley J. Low-friction arthroplasty after fracture-dislocations of the hip. J Bone Joint Surg Br 1978;60:495–497.
17. Coventry MB. The treatment of fracture-dislocation of the hip by total hip arthroplasty J Bone Joint Surg Am 1974;56:1128–1134.
18. Palin HC, Richmond A. Dislocation of the hip with fracture of the femoral head. A report of 3 cases. J Bone Joint Surg Br 1954;36:442–445.
19. Baumgärtel F, Feld C, Bohnen L, Gotzen L. Azetabulumfrakturen im höheren Lebensalter. In: Ramanzadeh R, Meissner A, Würtenberger C, editors. Unfall- und Wiederherstellungschirurgie des proximalen Femurs und des Beckengürtels. Einhorn: Schwäbisch Gmünd, 1994:98–100.
20. Berner M, Ulrich C. Die primäre endoprothetische Versorgung von Azetabulumfrakturen. Osteo Int 1999;7:93–100.
21. Hoellen IP, Mentzel M, Bischoff M, Kinzl L. Azetabulumfrakturen beim alten Menschen. Primäre endoprothetische Versorgung. Orthopäde 1997;26:348–353.
22. Romness DW, Lewallen DG. Total hip arthroplasty after fracture of the acetabulum. Long-term results. J Bone Joint Surg Br 1990;72:761–764.
23. Marchesi DG, Ganz R. Totalendoprothesenimplantation mit zusätzlicher Beckenosteosynthese. Orthopäde 1989;18:483–488.

20 Fractures of the Distal Femur

P. L. O. Broos and F. M. A. Robijns

Introduction

Supracondylar and intercondylar fractures of the femur are relatively uncommon, representing only 4–6% of all femoral fractures [1,2].During the past decades the term "supracondylar" has included fractures of the distal 15 cm, the distal 9 cm and the distal 7.5 cm [3–6]. The AO classification was born when Müller et al. [7,8] defined supracondylar–intercondylar lesions as fractures whose center lies within a square of which the side length is determined by the width of the condyles. Most recent studies use this classification.

The management of distal femoral fractures is particularly difficult because they are often associated with other injuries in younger persons and achieving rigid fixation can be difficult in the elderly, due to osteoporotic bone. Regaining full knee motion and function may be difficult, because of the proximity of these fractures to the knee joint. No single method of management has overcome all problems associated with these fractures. Before 1970, the majority of supracondylar fractures were treated nonoperatively. Nowadays, the goal of treatment for these fractures in the elderly is similar to that of hip fractures: early mobilization. Operative reduction and stabilization are necessary to obtain early mobilization in patients with fractures of the distal femur. The benefit of operative treatment has recently also been shown in aged patients [9,10].

Etiology

The mechanism of injury in most supracondylar–intercondylar fractures is thought to be axial loading with varus-valgus or rotational forces. In younger patients, the injury typically occurs after high-energy trauma (motor vehicle or motorcycle accidents). In such patients there may be considerable fracture displacement, open fractures and associated injuries. In a study by Siliski and co-workers [11] 19% of the patients had craniofacial lesions, 12% thoracic trauma and 73% other fractures of the extremities.

In elderly patients, fractures frequently occur after a fall at home on a flexed knee (Table 20.1). Despite the low-energy trauma, the fall often leads to comminuted fractures through osteoporotic cortical bone. Pritchett et al. [12] reviewed 23

Table 20.1. Mean age of patients and number of fractures caused by simple falls in different studies

Author	n	Mean age (years)	Simple fall
Shahcheraghi [2]	51	34	5 (20%)
Lucas [14]	24	39	4 (17%)
Siliski [11]	51	42.9	11 (22%)
Ostrum [15]	30	48.4	–
Zehntner [1]	59	51.9	8 (14%)
Pritchett [12]	23	66	11 (48%)
Shewring [13]	19	62.8	10 (53%)
Janzing [9]	25	74	16 (64%)

fractures of the distal femur. The median age of the patients was 66 years; 11 fractures resulted from a fall from sitting or standing position. There was radiographic evidence of advanced osteoporosis in 12 patients.

In elderly patients, associated injuries are few. Janzing et al. [9] reported about 25 supracondylar fractures in elderly patients, mean age 74 years. In 17 patients the distal femoral fracture was an isolated injury; in 16 cases the fracture was caused by a simple fall. Siliski et al. [11] reviewed the records of 52 supracondylar–intercondylar fractures of the femur. The age of the patients ranged from 15 to 92 years with an average of 47 years. In 22% of the patients (all of them older than 50 years), the fracture was caused by a fall.

Classification of the Distal Femur Fractures

During the past decades the term "supracondylar" has included fractures of the distal 15 cm, the distal 9 cm and the distal 7.5 cm [3–6]. Müller et al. [7,8]defined supracondylar–intercondylar lesions as fractures whose center lies within a square of which the side length is determined by the width of the condyles. Most recent studies use this definition. There is no universally accepted method of classification for supracondylar fractures of the femur. Many systems of classification have been used, all of which distinguish between extra-articular, intra-articular and isolated condylar lesions. Fractures are further subdivided according to the degree and direction of displacement, the amount of comminution and the involvement of the joint surface. In the past decades the following classification systems have been used: the classification of Neer and associates, Stewart et al., Schatzker, Seinsheimer and Müller et al. [3,6–8,16]. The last is undoubtedly widely accepted and is used by most of the latest studies. Although this ASIF-AO classification is solely based on the radiographic appearance of the fracture, it correlates well with its complexity and with the surgical techniques needed for adequate stabilization. Siliski et al. [11] advocate this classification because of its simplicity and believes that it is as accurate in predicting outcome as more complex systems based on the pattern of the fracture and on associated injuries of the ligaments, patella and soft tissue. Obviously, some fractures do not neatly fit into any classification. This emphasizes the fact that each case must be evaluated individually.

The classification of Müller is based on the location and pattern of the fracture and considers all fractures within the transepicondylar width of the knee

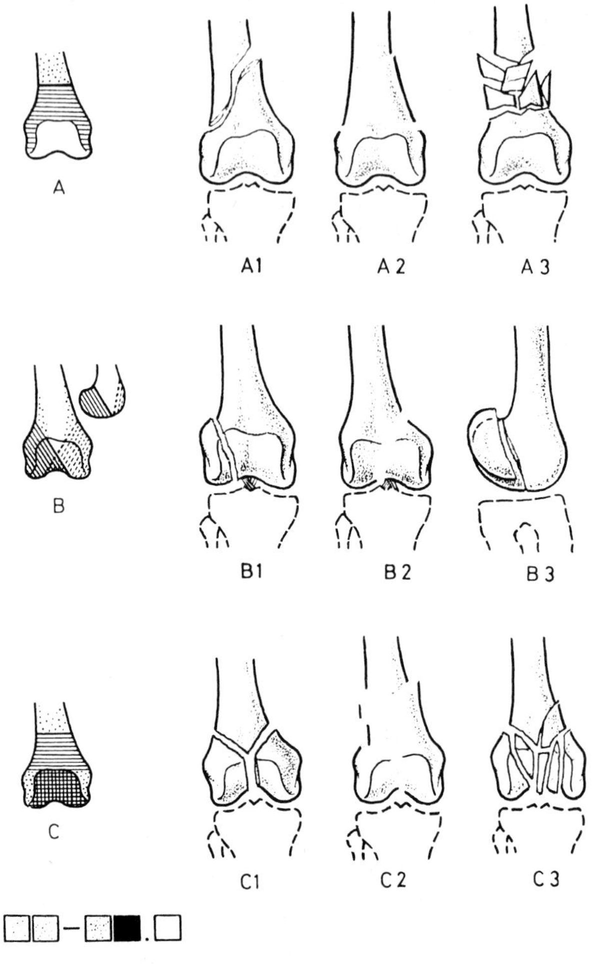

Figure 20.1. Main parts of the distal femur.

(Fig. 20.1). Type A fractures involve the distal shaft of the femur with varying degrees of comminution. Type B fractures are unicondylar fractures; type B1 is a sagittal split of the lateral condyle, type B2 is a sagittal split of the medial condyle and type B3 is a coronal plane fracture. Type C fractures are T- and Y-shaped condylar fractures; type C1 fractures have no comminution, C2 fractures have a comminuted shaft fracture with two principal articular fragments and type C3 fractures have intra-articular comminution.

Associated Injuries

Supracondylar–intercondylar fractures of the femur are complex lesions which are often associated with other injuries about the knee. Ligamentous injuries (cruciate ligaments, collateral ligaments), fractures (patella, tibial plateau), lesions of the articular cartilage and neurovascular injuries are mentioned in literature. These injuries are closely related to the fracture itself and they are therefore also seen in elderly patients. Siliski et al. [11] found 8 tears of the anterior cruciate ligament, 1 of the posterior cruciate ligament and 1 of the collateral ligament in the 52 patients he reviewed. There were ten ipsilateral patellar fractures and one tibial plateau fracture.

On the other hand, there are fractures related to the energy of the trauma: thoracic lesions, craniofacial lesions and fractures of the other extremities. Taking the injury mechanism into account, these lesions are rather seldom seen in elderly patients [2].

Ligamentous Injuries

Ligamentous injuries are rarely diagnosed preoperatively because of the close proximity to the fracture site. The most commonly injured ligament is the anterior cruciate. In supracondylar fractures with significant comminution of the articular surface, the anterior cruciate ligament can be detached with one of the fracture fragments. It is recommended that this injury is repaired at the time of fixation of the fracture. Midsubstance tears of the anterior cruciate ligament should initially be treated nonoperatively.

Vascular Injuries

The incidence of vascular injury accompanying supracondylar femur fracture is estimated to be only 2–3% [1, 2]. Injuries to the superficial or profound femoral arteries often occur after fractures of the femoral shaft and injuries of the popliteal artery occur after proximal tibia fractures. Vessel injuries can be caused by direct laceration or contusion of the artery or vein by fracture fragments or indirectly by stretching. In supracondylar fractures, however, the incidence of popliteal artery injury is low. Clinical examination of the leg for signs of ischemia is essential. If any doubt exists about the integrity of the vessels, it is wise to proceed with an angiogram to rule out an occult vascular injury. Doppler ultrasound cannot rule out initial tear and is therefore not recommended.

Pre-existing Hip Pathology

Moran et al. [10] identified 5 of their 24 patients as having either osteoarthritis or previous hip fracture which reduced hip mobility. This obviously occurred in elderly patients. Therefore, the status of the ipsilateral hip joint must be assessed by preoperative radiographs. Perioperative complications can be minimized by modification of patient positioning during osteosynthesis (intramedullary nailing) of the femur.

Rating Systems

The comparison of published series of fractures is often difficult because of the use of different systems for rating the results of treatment: the rating systems of Neer et al., Pritchett, Schatzker and Lambert [3,6,12]. We often see a discrepancy between alignment, pain, function and results according to different rating systems [1]. This stresses the need for future standardized reporting and classification of rating. Laros [17] grouped the "excellent" category of Neer et al. and the "excellent–good–fair" category of Schatzker and Lambert because of similar requirements to compare different series. We advocate the use of the rating system of Neer et al. because it emphasizes the functional results and because of its simplicity. The Neer score is rather forgiving and classifies more cases in the excellent range, whereas the Schatzker score almost requires a preinjury status. Considering the fractures included, the study of Neer et al. included the distal 7.5 cm of the femur, which most closely approximates the AO classification; Schatzker and Lambert included the distal 15 cm of the femur, which represents another category of fractures. Obviously, alignment and knee function must be analyzed more critically for these more proximal lesions. Zehntner et al. [1] concluded, however, that some revision of the Neer score is necessary, because it tends to overrate the final scores.

Since many aged patients already have impaired function before the injury, Janzing et al. [9] created "a relative score of Neer": 100 − (pretrauma score − final score) = relative score of Neer. This is a good adaptation, though it is not always easy to determine the pretrauma range of motion of the knee joint, e.g., after the accident has happened.

Treatment of Distal Femoral Fractures

Closed or Operative Treatment?

In the 1960s, before the development of reliable surgical techniques and implants, nonoperative treatment methods produced better results than operative treatment of supracondylar fractures of the femur. Early attempts at internal fixation of these fractures were often associated with malunion, nonunion, severe knee stiffness and infection. Stewart et al. [16], who popularized the two-pin method of skeletal traction retrospectively, reviewed 213 supracondylar fractures [16]. Results were satisfactory in 67% of fractures treated nonoperatively and in 54% of those treated operatively. Neer et al. [6] also compared operative with nonoperative treatment in 77 supracondylar femoral fractures. In patients treated with nonoperative methods, 84% had satisfactory results, while satisfactory results were obtained in only 52% of the patients operatively treated. Other possible complications related to skeletal traction and cast bracing are urinary tract infection, deep-vein thrombosis, pulmonary lung embolism and pressure sores. These methods also require confinement to bed, are time-consuming, expensive and not indicated in elderly people.

In the 1970s, the combination of properly designed implants, a better understanding of soft tissue handling, perioperative antibiotics and improved anesthetic methods made internal fixation safe and practical [18]. Improved results were reported after open reduction and internal fixation and surgery gained widespread acceptance as the treatment of choice of fractures of the distal part of the femur.

In the 1990s, the management of elderly patients with displaced supracondylar femoral fractures still poses a challenge. In 1996, Butt et al. [19] performed a prospective randomized trial of operative versus nonoperative treatment of 42 displaced fractures of the distal femur in elderly patients. There were 20 patients with a mean age of 77.6 years in the operatively treated group. The fractures were fixed with a dynamic condylar screw and knee mobilization was started 24 h postoperatively. Good results were achieved in 53% of this group. In the nonoperative group, 22 patients were included (mean age 80.6 years) with a good result in 31%. Skeletal traction was applied in a Thomas splint and Pearson knee attachment and exercises started 3–4 weeks after injury. In the latter group, there were more complications and the time to discharge was considerably longer.

With the development of improved internal fixation devices by the AO group, treatment recommendations began to change. Rigid internal fixation has enabled earlier range of motion exercises and weightbearing, which help to prevent some of the serious complications attributed to prolonged bed rest and traction. This surgery has gained widespread acceptance as the treatment of choice for fractures of the distal part of the femur with exception of simple, nondisplaced fractures.

Halpenny and Rorabeck [20] retrospectively reviewed 61 fractures of the distal femur. These fractures were treated nonoperatively or with internal fixation using a blade plate. In extra-articular fractures, results were better with operative treatment. Intra-articular fractures had less satisfactory results and the results of operative and nonoperative treatment were equal. Healy and Brooker [21] compared operative treatment (mainly with a plate and screw device) with nonoperative treatment in fractures of the distal femur and found good functional results in 81% of fractures treated surgically, compared with only 35% of those treated by closed methods.

In young patients, the goal of treatment for this fracture is restoration of length and axial alignment with stable fixation. In elderly people, emphasis is on early mobilization. Impaction of metaphyseal fragments with small amounts of shortening or malalignment may therefore be a reasonable technique for rapid fracture union in osteoporotic patients [11,15,22].

Operative Treatment

When treating complex fractures of the distal femur the choice is between plate fixation and intramedullary nailing. Both techniques have their own advantages and complications. Devascularization of the fragments and, in elderly people, advanced osteoporosis may compromise the stability of the fixation and the bone healing. To solve these problems some authors advise the use of bone grafts and bone cement [1,11,23–26].

Implants

Two major types of internal fixation devices are widely used in the management of supracondylar femur fractures: condylar plates and screws, and intramedullary nails.

1. "Lateral Fixation Devices"

Blade Plate. The blade plate was one of the first plate and screw devices to gain wide acceptance in the treatment of these fractures and it remains a useful implant. The placement of the 95° blade plate is technically demanding because the surgeon is required to place the blade simultaneously in three planes. When used by an experienced surgeon, this device restores alignment and provides stable fixation [20].

Mize reported good or excellent results in 76% of 68 fractures treated with this technique [23,24]. Siliski et al. [11] evaluated 52 fractures treated with a blade plate. Good or excellent results were obtained in 81% of fractures and range of motion averaged 107° [11]. The use of the 95° blade plate in elderly patients with variable degrees of osteoporosis must, however, be individualized.

Dynamic Condylar Screw. The dynamic condylar screw (DCS) is a less technically demanding alternative to the blade plate. This device consists of a 95° compression screw and a sideplate. The implant shares many of the features of a compression hip screw, making it familiar to most surgeons and therefore easier to manage. A minimum of 4 cm of uncomminuted bone in the femoral condyles above the intercondylar notch is necessary for successful fixation. While the blade plate requires accurate insertion in three planes simultaneously, the DCS allows a degree of freedom in the sagittal plane. Other advantages are its ability to apply interfragmentary compression across the femoral condyles and better purchase in osteoporotic bone [19].

The major disadvantage with the DCS is that insertion of the condylar lag screw requires removal of a large amount of bone to ensure a low-profile fit. The "shoulder" of this device is more prominent compared with the 95° blade plate and this often causes knee syndromes as the iliotibial band slides over the edge of the implant. In our opinion, the DCS shows no advantages compared with the blade plate for experienced surgeons.

Condylar Buttress Plate. The condylar buttress plate is a one-piece device, specifically designed for the distal femur. It is a broad dynamic compression plate with a cloverleaf-shaped distal portion designed to accommodate up to six cancellous screws. The condylar buttress plate does not provide such rigid fixation as a blade plate or DCS, so should not be used as a substitute for these two preferred implants. We prefer the buttress plate to the blade plate and the DCS only for fractures with less than 3–4 cm of intact femoral condylar bone, fractures with a large amount of articular comminution and in cases where the lateral femur condyle is comminuted. Additionally, the condylar buttress plate is used to salvage delayed unions and nonunions after the use of a 95° blade plate or a DCS.

The major disadvantage of this device is that the screws passing through the distal holes do not have a fixed relationship to the plate so that they may shift relative to the plate, especially in osteoporotic bone. Improved systems such as the Less Invasive Stabilization System (LISS) for the distal femur have been developed, providing fixation of the screws into the plate and less soft tissue damage as the implant can mostly be fixed percutaneously.

Double Condylar Buttress Plate. A second medial plate is often indicated to prevent varus deformities in cases with extensive medial comminution [27]. Chapman and Henley [28] reported on an inverted large-fragment T-plate inserted through a separate medial subvastus incision.

Isolated Screw Fixation. In cases of condylar fractures type B1 and B2 according the AO classification, percutaneous cannulated screw fixation can be considered. However, when the articular incongruity is more than 2 mm in elderly patients, a buttress plate should be applied.

2. Intramedullary Nails

Firstly, supracondylar fractures tend to collapse into varus. When using a lateral fixation device, the shaft of the femur is often pulled laterally. This creates a rotational moment arm at the fracture site causing the distal fragment to displace into varus or leading to fatigue fracture of the device. Obviously, an intramedullary nail reduces this tendency.

Secondly, fixation in osteoporotic bone frequently leads to failure with screws and plates cutting out of the soft bone. As the bending moment of an intramedullary device is reduced, failure of fixation in osteoporotic bone should be less likely.

Flexible Intramedullary Implants. The Ender nail, the Rush rod and the Zickel supracondylar device have been used with some success to treat distal femoral fractures. Since the development of more rigid plate and screw devices and interlocking intramedullary nails, the indications for their use are, however, limited.

In 1970, Zickel et al. [29,30] developed a nail especially for the distal femur. This has a flexible stem and a rigid, curved condylar end allowing it to be anchored into the femoral condyles by transfixing screws. The Zickel nail was designed to be inserted by an open method, but closed nailing is possible. The most important disadvantage of this device is that it cannot prevent shortening. The use of the Zickel nail should therefore be restricted to elderly patients in whom impaction and shortening at the fracture site can be accepted. Other candidates are frail patients with concurrent medical problems who are poor candidates for a more open procedure. Marks et al. [31] reported 33 cases of distal femoral fractures in such debilitated patients (with a mean age of 79 years) and achieved excellent results in terms of pain relief, movement and function.

Supracondylar Femoral Nail. A retrograde intramedullary nail specifically for supracondylar/intracondylar femoral fractures has been developed. The implant is a fully cannulated, single-piece stainless steel nail with an 8° apex anterior bend near the distal end to accommodate the geometry of the posterior aspect of the femoral condyles. The nail has a wall of 2 mm and there are multiple holes along its length for percutaneous placement of 5 mm locking screws. The portal of entry for the nail is in the intracondylar notch just anterior to the femoral attachment of the posterior cruciate ligament. In patients with intra-articular extension, careful reconstruction of the joint surface is essential before nail passage. Intrafragmentary screws must be placed quite anteriorly or posteriorly so as not to impede nail passage. Additionally, the nail must be countersunk several millimeters so as not to interfere with the patellofemoral articulation.

This device obtains more "biological" fixation than plates because they are load-sharing rather than load-sparing plates and it has the potential to stabilize complex fractures with less soft-tissue dissection [32–36]. The retrograde nailing of extra-articular distal femoral fractures is a fast procedure which can be performed through a small incision and with minimal blood loss. Finally, in patients with ipsilateral hip and distal femoral fractures, both fractures can be stabilized independently and securely [9,14,35,37].

The design of the retrograde supracondylar nail is associated with potential disadvantages as well. The intra-articular entry portal can potentially lead to knee stiffness and sepsis, synovial metallosis and patellofemoral degeneration. Biomechanical testing has shown that retrograde supracondylar nails do not provide such rigid fixation as a 95° blade plate and sideplate devices. In a synthetic bone osteotomy model, Firoozbakhsh et al. [38] found the latter devices stiffer in valgus bending and torsion compared with the former. However, the clinical relevance of these biomechanical studies is unclear.

Early studies of this device reported a relatively high incidence of implant failure. The interlocking screws were changed from 6.4 to 5.0 mm in diameter. The diameter of the screw holes was decreased and the diameter of the nails augmented from 11 to 13 mm. This greatly decreased the incidence of implant failure. Lucas et al. [14] and Iannacone et al. [35]reported good results using the supracondylar retrograde femoral nail for supracondylar fractures of the femur.

Janzing et al. [9] reported the results of 26 supracondylar nailings in 25 patients with a mean age of 74 years. They counted 92% excellent and good results using the Neer score. In osteoporotic bone, the locking bolts often had a very poor grip, and in 5 patients bone cement was used to fix the distal screws. Only one implant failure was described: breakage of a distal locking screw with protrusion of the nail into the knee [9].

Helfet et al. [34] concluded that the intramedullary nail is a reasonable option in the treatment of most type A and some specific type C (especially the Y-shaped fractures) supracondylar fractures.

3. Use of Cement

Pritchett, Ostrum, Zehnter and Struhl advocated the use of cemented internal fixation to improve screw fixation in these fractures in osteoporotic patients [1,12,15,25,26]. On the other hand, Siliski et al. [11] did not use bone cement in his study and elderly patients did not have a poorer outcome. Distal locking screw purchase can be compromised by osteoporotic bone in the distal femoral metaphysis. Janzing et al. [9] therefore used cement in osteoporotic patients treated for a distal femoral fracture with a retrograde intramedullary supracondylar nail.

In our own department, we use a self-developed "cement screw". The fixation in the epimetaphyseal area in patients with severe osteoporosis is supplemented with low-viscosity radio-opaque bone cement (Palacos E Flow), injected through a specially designed 7.3 mm cannulated screw (Fig. 20.2). The "cement screw" is a partially cannulated, self-drilling and self-tapping 7.3 mm screw at the top closed by the insertion of a press-fit metal plug. In the threaded portion, two side holes of 2 mm have been drilled. Through these holes, the injected cement can flow sideways into the cancellous bone.

In normal cases of osteoporosis, one central "cement screw" surrounded by solid 6.5 mm cancellous bone screws are used. These screws are embedded in low-viscosity bone cement. The injection of this bone cement is monitored by an image intensifier (Fig. 20.3). The latter is important to prevent forceful injection into the joint. No more than 4 cm^3 of bone cement per screw is needed, which is injected using an ordinary plastic syringe without the need for a special adapter.

4. Use of Bone Grafting

In the past, comminution of the medial cortex and fractures in osteoporotic bone were an absolute indication for bone grafting. Schatzker et al. even recommended bone grafting for all comminuted supracondylar fractures [3,4]. The most common donor site is the ipsilateral iliac crest; alternative sites are the greater trochanter

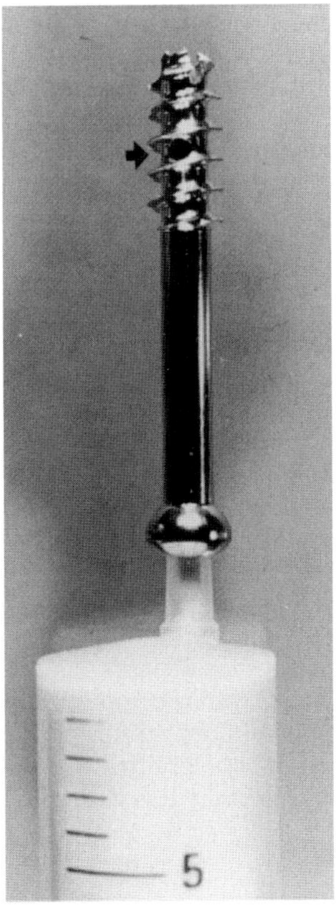

Figure 20.2. "Cement screw" with side hole.

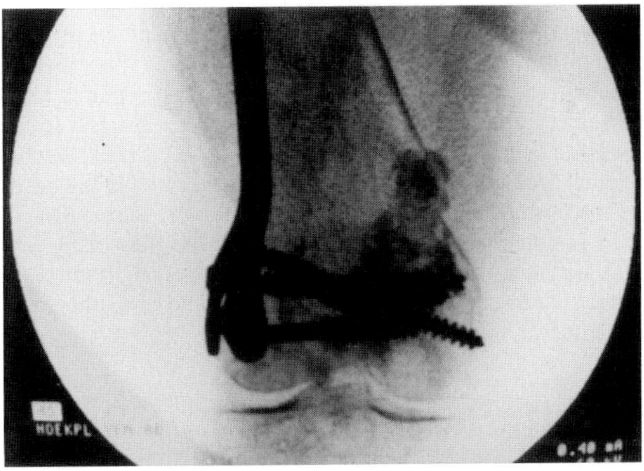

Figure 20.3. Monitoring of injection of bone cement by an image intensifier.

and proximal tibia. In osteoporotic patients who have little usable bone, cancellous chips from a bone bank are indicated.

Current methods of fixation with the use of indirect reduction techniques and soft tissue preservation have decreased the need for bone grafting. This may be attributed to the decreased periosteal stripping of the fracture and the intramedullary reams which serve as a bone graft. Fractures with major bone loss still remain a strong indication for the use of bone grafts. Relative indications still include selected A3, C2 and C3 fracture patterns, as well as many severe open fractures treated on a delayed basis to prevent nonunion.

In the study by Ostrum and Geel [15], supracondylar fractures of the distal femur were treated in a prospective series using an indirect reduction technique with femoral distractors or external fixators. Patients who entered the protocol had undergone fixation with a DCS without stripping of the medial soft tissues and without bone grafting. Using the Neer score, 86.6% excellent and satisfactory results were achieved. This result compares favorably with other reports in literature. The nonunion rate in this study compares as well with the recent literature on surgical treatment of these fractures.

Younger and Chapman [39], reviewing 243 autogenous bone graft procedures, demonstrated that obtaining an iliac bone graft has a high associated morbidity. Major complications including infection, prolonged wound drainage, large hematoma, reoperation, pain for longer than 6 months and sensory loss were seen in 8.6% of cases. An incidence of 20.6% of minor complications including superficial infection, minor wound problems, temporary sensory loss and mild pain was also seen.

Thus, the role of supplemental bone grafting of supracondylar distal femur fractures after internal fixation has become less clear.

Postoperative Treatment

Apart from the usual problems of confining elderly patients to bed, conservative methods may at any age be complicated by knee stiffness, malunion and nonunion [6,16]. When stable internal fixation has been achieved, range of motion exercises for the knee and isometric hamstrings and quadriceps exercises can be started in the first days after operation with the assistance of a physical therapist [12]. A continuous passive motion (CPM) device is often used. The rationale for the use of CPM includes enhanced knee motion, decreased limb swelling and a lower incidence of quadriceps adhesions. A mobilization with only toe touch and partial weightbearing on the operated extremity is encouraged with full weightbearing when clinical and radiographic evidence of healing is present [14]. The use of a functional brace is recommended to protect the repair of associated disruptions of ligaments and in patients who cannot comply with weightbearing limitations (e.g., elderly patients). Either a cast brace or a removable dorsal splint is used. Shewring et al. [13] maintained functional bracing for all patients until there was clinical and radiological evidence of union.

Treatment Strategy in Leuven

All elderly people with a fracture of the distal femur are treated operatively in our department. The operation is performed as soon as possible, but never as a night-

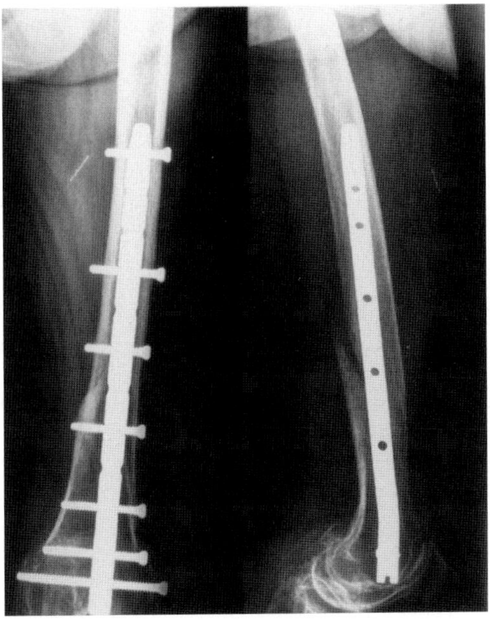

Figure 20.4. Type A fracture healed with intramedullary nailing.

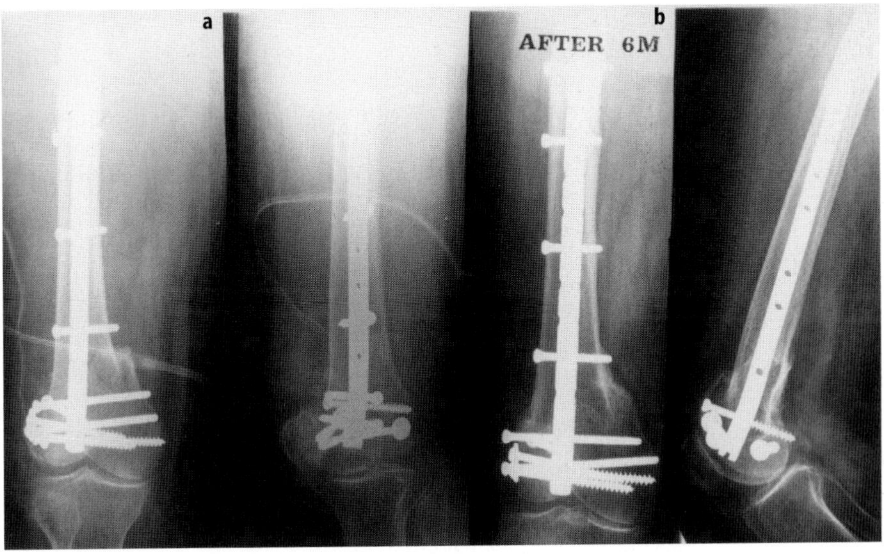

Figure 20.5. **a** Type C fracture treated with intramedullary nail and separate cannulated cement screws. **b** Status after 6 months.

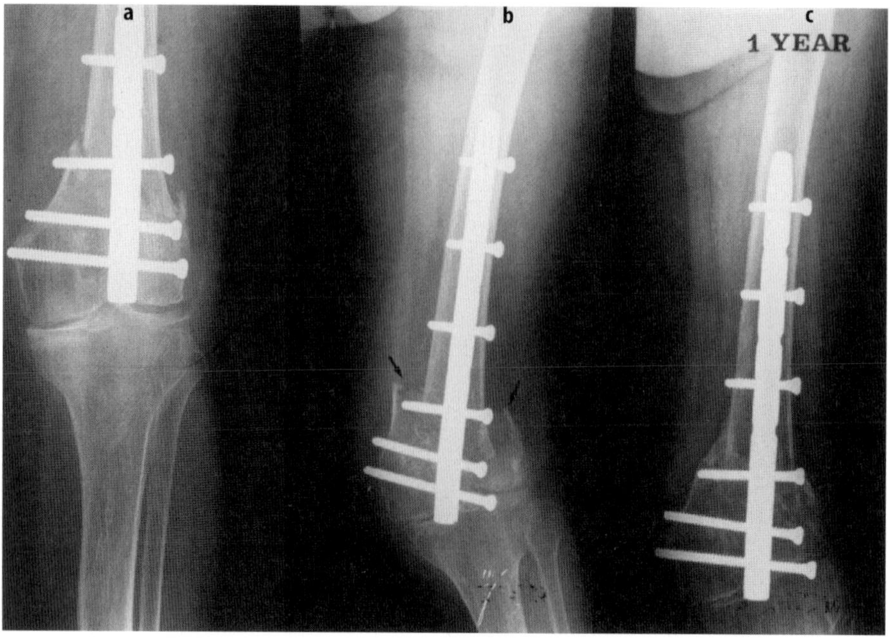

Figure 20.6. **a** Type A fracture treated with intramedullary nail. **b** Redislocation after 2 weeks. **c** Healing after 1 year.

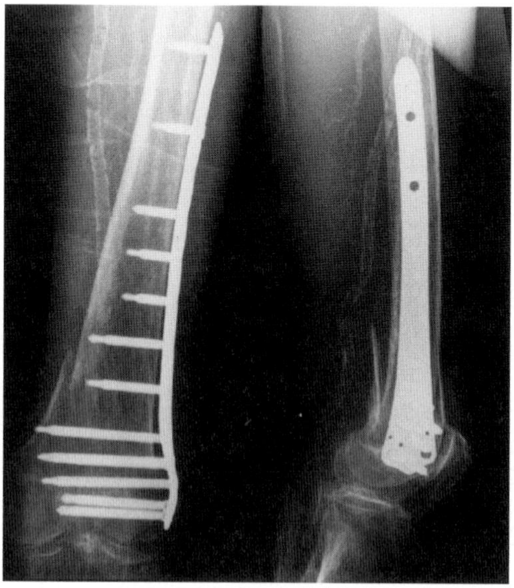

Figure 20.7. Type C fracture healed after use of the Less Invasive Stabilization System (LISS).

time emergency. If possible, an intramedullary fixation is chosen. In osteoporotic people, adjacent bone cement is used to fix the distal interlocking screws. As reported by Janzing et al. [9], this technique is associated with excellent results in type A fractures (Fig. 20.4). An intramedullary nail can also provide sufficient stability to make early motion possible for the great majority of type C fractures. In these cases, however, the introduction of the nail has to be preceded by the reconstruction of the condylar region with separate cannulated cement screws (Fig. 20.5). In elderly people an absolute anatomical reconstruction, although always desirable, does not have to be obtained at any price as they can carry on their activities of daily living even with some restriction of mobility of the knee joint. The risk of developing late degenerative osteoarthritis is also only a relative problem in the aged. Even redislocation is sometimes well tolerated and does not always need a reintervention (Fig. 20.6).

Our experiences with the LISS, which are still limited in the elderly, are encouraging (Fig. 20.7). The condylar buttress plate with cannulated cement screws still is an excellent implant for the very comminuted type C2–3 fractures. Nevertheless, this procedure has to be considered as a very severe one and has to be performed by the most experienced staff members. Early mobilization of the limb has to be possible, even after plate fixation. Nowadays, the CPM device is very useful. Full weightbearing can, however, only be allowed when the radiographs demonstrate the onset of callus formation, which does not occur earlier than 8 weeks after operation.

References

1. Zehntner MK, Marchesi DG, Burch H, Ganz R. Alignment of supracondylar–intercondylar fractures of the femur by internal fixation by AO/ASIF technique. J Orthop Trauma 1992;6:318–326.
2. Shahcheraghi GH, Doroodchi HR. Supracondylar fractures of the femur: closed or open reduction? J Trauma 1993;34:499–502.
3. Schatzker J, Lambert DC. Supracondylar fractures of the femur. Clin Orthop 1979; 138:77–83.
4. Seinsheimer F. Subtrochanteric fractures of the femur. J Bone Joint Surg Am 1978; 60:300.
5. Seinsheimer F. Fractures of the distal femur. Clin Orthop 1980;153:169–179.
6. Neer CS II, Grantham SA, Shelton ML. Supracondylar fracture of the adult femur. A study of one hundred and ten cases. J Bone Joint Surg Am 1967;49:591–613.
7. Müller ME, Nazarian S, Koch P, Schatzker J. The comprehensive classification of fractures of long bones. Berlin Heidelberg New York: Springer, 1990.
8. Müller ME, Allgöwer M, Schneider R, Willenegger H. Manual of internal fixation. Berlin Heidelberg New York: Springer, 1979.
9. Janzing HMJ, Vaes F, Broos PLO. Treatment of distal femoral fractures in the elderly. Unfallchirurgie 1998;24:55–59.
10. Moran C, Gibson M, Cross A. Intramedullary locking nails for femoral shaft fractures in elderly patients. J Bone Joint Surg Br 1990;72:19–22.
11. Siliski JM, Mahring M, Hofer HP. Supracondylar-intercondylar fractures of the femur. J Bone Joint Surg Am 1989;71:95–104.
12. Pritchett JW. Supracondylar fractures of the femur. Clin Orthop 1984;184:173–177.
13. Shewring DJ, Meggitt BF. Fractures of the distal femur treated with the AO dynamic condylar screw. J Bone Joint Surg Br 1992;74:122–125.
14. Lucas SE, Seligson D, Henry SL. Intramedullary supracondylar nailing of femoral

fractures: a preliminary report of the GSH supracondylar nail. Clin Orthop 1993;296: 200–206.
15. Ostrum RF, Geel C. Indirect reduction and internal fixation of supracondylar femur fractures without bone graft. J Orthop Trauma 1995;9:278–284.
16. Stewart MJ, Sisk TD, Wallace SL Jr. Fractures of the distal third of the femur. J Bone Joint Surg Am 1966;48:784–807.
17. Laros GS. Supracondylar fractures of the femur: editorial comment and comparative results. Clin Orthop 1979;138:9–12.
18. Gustilo RB, Anderson JT. Prevention of infection in the treatment of one-thousand and twenty-five open fractures of long bones. Retrospective and prospective analysis J Bone Joint Surg 1976;58A:453–458.
19. Butt MS, Krikler SJ, Ali MS. Displaced fractures of the distal femur in elderly patients. Operative versus nonoperative treatment. J Bone Joint Surg Br 1996;78:110–114.
20. Halpenny J, Rorabeck CH. Supracondylar fractures of the femur: results of treatment in 61 patients. Can J Surg 1984;27:606–609.
21. Healy WL, Brooker AF Jr. Distal femoral fractures: comparison of open and closed methods of treatment. Clin Orthop 1983;174:166–171.
22. Mast J, Jakob RP, Ganz R. Planning and reduction technique in fracture surgery. Berlin Heidelberg New York: Springer, 1989.
23. Mize RD. Supracondylar and articular fractures of the distal femur. In: Chapman M, editor. Operative orthopedics. Philadelphia: Lippincott, 1988:401–412.
24. Mize RD, Bucholz RW, Grogan DP. Surgical treatment of displaced, comminuted fractures of the distal end of the femur. J Bone Joint Surg Am 1982;64:871–879.
25. Struhl S, Szporn MN, Cobelli NJ, Sadler AH. Cemented internal fixation for supracondylar femur fractures in osteoporotic patients. J Orthop Trauma 1990;4:151–157.
26. Benum P. The use of bone cement as an adjunct internal fixation of supracondylar fractures of osteoporotic femurs. Acta Orthop Scand 1977;48:52–56.
27. Sanders R, Swiontkowski M, Rosen H, Helfet D. Double plating of comminuted, unstable fractures of the distal part of the femur. J Bone Joint Surg Am 1991;73:341–346.
28. Chapman JR, Henley MB. Double plating of distal femur fractures: indications and techniques. Tech Orthop 1994;9:210–216.
29. Zickel RE, Fietti VG, Lawsing JF, Cochran GVB. A new intramedullary fixation device for the distal third of the femur. Clin Orthop 1977;125:185–191.
30. Zickel RE, Hobeika P, Robbins DS. Zickel supracondylar nails for fracture of the distal end of the femur. Clin Orthop 1986;212:79–88.
31. Marks DS, Isbister ES, Porter KM. Zickel supracondylar nailing for supracondylar femoral fractures in elderly or infirm patients. A review of 33 cases. J Bone Joint Surg Br 1994;76:596–601.
32. Brown A, D'Arcy JC. Internal fixation for supracondylar fractures of the femur in the elderly patients. J Bone Joint Surg Br1971;53:420–424.
33. Gellman RE, Paiement GD, Hillary DG, et al. Treatment of supracondylar femoral fractures with a retrograde inramedullary nail. Clin Orthop 1996;332:90–97.
34. Helfet DL, Lorich DG. Retrograde intramedullary nailing of supracondylar femoral fractures. Clin Orthop 1998;350:80–84.
35. Iannacone WM, Bennett FS, De Long WG Jr, et al. Initial experience with the treatment of supracondylar fractures using the supracondylar intramedullary nail: a preliminary report. J Orthop Trauma 1993;7:322–327.
36. Leung KS, Shen WY, So WS, et al. Interlocking intramedullary nailing for supracondylar and intercondylar fractures of the distal part of the femur. J Bone Joint Surg Am 1991;73:332–340.
37. Johnson EE, Marroquin CE, Kossosky N. Synovial metallosis resulting from intra-articular intramedullary nailing of distal femoral nonunion. J Orthop Trauma 1993;7: 320–324.

38. Firoozbakhsh K, Behzadi K, De Coster TA, et al. Mechanics of retrograde nail versus plate fixation for supracondylar femur fractures. J Orthop Trauma 1995;9:152–157.
39. Younger EM, Chapman MW. Morbidity at bone graft sites. J Orthop Trauma 1989;3:192–195.
40. Johnson KD, Hicken G. Distal femoral fractures. Orthop Clin North Am 1987;18:115–132.

21 Tibial Plateau Fractures

J. L. Marsh

Introduction

Decreased bone stock from osteoporosis or from osteopenia for other reasons, complicates the management of patients with fractures of the tibial plateau. There is an increased risk of fracture displacement after both conservative and operative management. When a tibial plateau fracture results from high-energy trauma in a patient with osteoporosis, greater comminution occurs than in a proximal tibia without osteoporosis. If an operative approach is chosen, implant fixation is less secure, decreasing the effectiveness of the device. Finally, patients with osteoporosis are frequently elderly and have poor tolerance for certain nonoperative treatment techniques, particularly traction, which requires prolonged bed rest.

Despite these difficulties, there are some factors that make management of tibial plateau fractures easier compared with other osteoporotic periarticular fractures in the lower extremity. Patients with a tibial plateau fracture can often be mobilized without surgical stabilization, unlike when similar fractures occur in the proximal or distal femur. When stabilization is chosen, the implant frequently needs to supply only a buttressing effect and does not need to withstand the bending forces that occur in the proximal and distal femur. In addition, function is often good after tibial plateau fractures despite significant joint disruption, and articular depression. Although radiographic signs of post-traumatic degenerative arthritis are not uncommon, they do not always cause patient symptoms and decreased function. Because of these reasons, the surgeon can often avoid complex difficult surgery or can use surgeries to maintain alignment of the limb without precise articular reconstruction, and still obtain a satisfactory result with a relatively low complication rate.

Deciding among treatment options for patients with osteoporotic tibial plateau fractures is complicated by the fact that there are few data in the literature that specifically relate to these patients. The majority of studies on tibial plateau fractures do not identify a subset of patients with osteoporosis and there is no study particularly focused on this patient cohort. There are some data on the affect of patient age, which has some relevance since many elderly patients will have osteoporosis.

Incidence and Prevalence

Fractures of the proximal tibia involving the articular surface occur throughout the full span of life: in young patients who sustain intra-articular physeal injuries and in very elderly patients. The highest incidence of tibial plateau fractures in several studies has been in the fifth decade, closely followed by the fourth and sixth decades [1,2].

There is a gender difference in age occurrence of tibial plateau fractures, which resembles the distribution of any osteoporotic fracture. Men have a higher incidence in the second, third and fourth decades when fractures secondary to high-energy mechanisms are most common. Women have an increasing incidence with age, not peaking until the sixth or seventh decade [2]. Most of these fractures in older women are in osteoporotic proximal tibias.

The exact incidence of osteoporosis complicating tibial plateau fractures is unknown but, particularly in women, it is very common. In studies of tibial plateau fractures where a radiographic assessment of osteoporosis has been made, it has been noted to be present in approximately 30–40% of all cases [2,3]. In these studies osteoporosis has been assessed only on plain radiographs taken at the time of injury. More accurate techniques for assessing for osteoporosis would most likely find a higher incidence.

Classification

Tibial plateau fractures represent a diverse group of injuries. Fractures from totally different mechanisms, with different prognosis requiring different evaluation and treatment techniques, are all included under the broad heading of tibial plateau fractures. These injuries span the spectrum from low-energy valgus loading fractures to high-energy knee dislocations with rim avulsions and bumper injuries with proximal metaphyseal disruption and proximal fracture lines extending into the joint. Numerous fracture classifications have been proposed to help categorize and stratify these diverse injuries. Currently, the two most commonly used classifications are that of Schatzker et al. [3] and the AO comprehensive classification [4]. Despite the wide general acceptance of the AO classification in many anatomical regions, for fractures of the tibial plateau the Schatzker classification continues to be the most commonly used. The six subtypes are a manageable number of subgroups to remember and span the spectrum of tibial plateau fractures. These groups are as follows: type I, pure cleavage fracture without local compression; type II, the classic split depression fracture; type III, local compression without a split fracture; type IV, medial condyle fracture often involving the intercondylar eminence; type V, bicondylar fracture with the intercondylar eminence intact with the shaft; type VI, a metaphyseal/diaphyseal disruption fracture where the diaphysis is broken separately from the condyles with associated intra-articular fracture lines [3].

All the subtypes of the Schatzker classification occur in elderly and osteoporotic patients; however, there are significant shifts in relative incidence compared with tibial plateau fractures in patients with normal bone stock. The Schatzker II split depression fracture is more common in patients with osteoporosis [5]. A mild valgus load in patients with good bone stock may produce a hemorrhage or bruise within the bone, but the bone resists structural failure, leading to a medial collateral and/or anterior cruciate ligament injury. In the patient with decreased bone strength from osteoporosis, a split depression fracture occurs. The Schatzker type I fracture is much less common in patients with osteoporosis. This type of pure cleavage fracture occurs in good structural bone that can withstand the local compression forces, developing only the split. Bicondylar fractures can occur in elderly patients from relatively lower-energy mechanisms. The high-energy fractures such as Schatzker type VI are less common in the elderly because these patients are less likely to be involved in the type of high-speed activities which result in these fractures [6]. However, when they do occur, if there is osteoporosis, comminution and small fragments close to the joint result, which present significant problems for management.

Evaluation

Tibial plateau fractures may be associated with open wounds, compartment syndrome, vascular injuries and other system injuries. These problems are all most common when tibial plateau fractures are sustained from a high-energy mechanism. Although these associated injuries are less common in patients with osteoporosis, they should still be considered and ruled out.

Knee ligament injuries may be associated with tibial plateau fractures. The classic association is a medial collateral ligament injury with a split depression or a local compression fracture of the lateral tibial plateau. This association has been reported to occur in up to 20–25% of lateral tibial plateau fractures; however, in elderly patients early failure of the lateral tibial plateau prevents the medial collateral ligament injury, and in one series in elderly patients the association was only seen in 3.2% of cases [5]. Osteoporotic bone tends to be protective of the ligaments and decreases the incidence of medial collateral ligament injuries.

On physical examination, besides a detailed neurovascular examination, the stability of the knee should be tested. Achieving perfect articular congruity is less important in patients with significant osteoporosis, but achieving a reasonably stable knee and satisfactory angular alignment should be considered an important goal [1]. In deciding among treatment options, an initial assessment of knee stability is therefore important. Usually in the acute phase this assessment can be made without an anesthetic by gentle valgus testing of the injured knee in slight flexion.

The soft tissues around the proximal tibia should be carefully assessed. The low-energy mechanisms that create most osteoporotic fractures do not create a severe soft tissue injury. However, elderly patients with osteoporosis may have very thin, relatively poorly perfused skin that will tolerate less than the skin in younger patients.

The imaging for patients with tibial plateau fractures is the same regardless of the presence or absence of osteoporosis. An anteroposterior, lateral and 10° caudal view radiographs of the proximal tibia are required. For significantly displaced fractures where surgery is being contemplated an axial CT scan with 2 mm cuts is a very useful adjunct for preoperative planning. A CT scan should not be used to decide on surgical indications, particularly in patients with osteoporosis. Significant comminution may be appreciated that was not noted on plain films, and this might lean the surgeon towards a surgical indication. However, if there is satisfactory limb alignment as determined on initial radiographs and preoperative physical examination, an excellent result may be achieved from conservative treatment.

In cases where surgery is indicated a CT scan helps in planning incisions, implants and reduction maneuvers.

Treatment Concepts

Factors That Relate to Outcome

In assessing outcomes and treatment priorities in elderly patients and patients with osteoporosis several facts should be considered. First, patients with decreased bone stock are more likely to have low demands and a shorter life expectancy, and have somewhat decreased expectations. Second, complications, while always problematic, are particularly bad in elderly and infirm patients.

It is clear from the literature that there are a variety of techniques which can achieve satisfactory outcomes after tibial plateau fractures in both young patients and elderly patients with osteoporosis. Indeed it is hard to find reports of techniques that do not result in satisfactory knee function in the vast majority of patients. In considering treatment for the difficult group with osteoporosis, some comfort can be taken from this information.

In deciding among the treatment options, the surgeon should consider the factors that predict favorable versus nonfavorable outcomes. There are abundant data in the literature that define these factors. Angular alignment is an important determinant of outcome after a tibial plateau fracture. If, after treatment of a tibial plateau, the limb is accurately aligned, most patients generally have a favorable prognosis [7]. Significant angular malalignment, particularly greater than 10°, tends to alter the weightbearing forces over the injured plateau, and predisposes to poor outcomes. Although elderly patients with osteoporosis may be more tolerant of malalignment, achieving accurate limb alignment remains an important goal of treatment.

Closely related to angular alignment is knee stability. When healing results in significant angular malalignment, this will result in coronal plane instability. The converse is also true: if the knee is well aligned, severe coronal instability is rarely a problem. Particularly in osteoporotic patients, in whom collateral ligament injuries are unusual, good limb alignment usually results in adequate knee stability.

The data on whether millimeters of articular displacement is an important factor to consider in deciding on treatment are controversial. Unreduced articular displacement has been considered by some authors to lead to poor outcomes and to be an absolute indication for anatomical surgical restoration [8]. Others feel that treatment based on restoring angular alignment without regard to the exact amount of articular depression leads to excellent results in the majority of patients [1,7]. Treatment based on restoring alignment will generally lead to less surgery and less aggressive operations when surgery is chosen. In elderly patients with osteoporosis, surgery based on millimeters of displacement of the articular surface is not required or sensible. These patients are unlikely to put the type of demands on the knee that will lead to symptomatic degenerative arthritis. Rather the goal should be to obtain reasonably accurate angular alignment.

If an open operative approach is chosen, the menisci should be preserved. In studies where this variable has been assessed, meniscal excision leads to poor outcomes. Indeed, nonoperative treatment is better than surgical treatment where the meniscus is sacrificed [9].

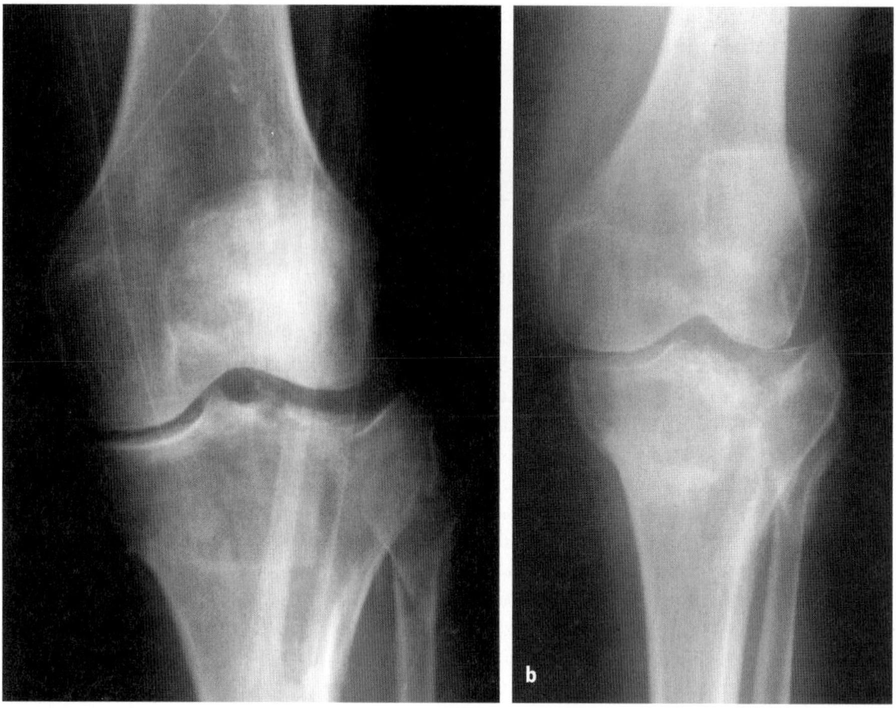

Figure 21.1. **a** An anteroposterior (AP) radiograph of a split depression fracture in a 78-year-old woman with osteoporosis. Note the calcified popliteal artery. **b** One year after treatment in a cast brace an AP radiograph shows healing of the fracture. There is some increased displacement but the coronal alignment is good. The patient has a 115° arc of knee motion and minimal discomfort.

Early joint mobility has generally been considered to be important after any articular fracture. For tibial plateau fractures the data suggest that early motion is most important after aggressive surgical approaches. In these knees early joint motion leads to better results. There is considerable evidence that tibial plateau fractures that are not treated surgically tolerate 4–6 weeks of immobilization very well [6,10].

One thing that is abundantly clear from the literature is that complications of treatment must at all costs be avoided. These include problems such as infection, wound breakdown, missed compartment syndrome, and the development of peroneal nerve palsy. These things are more likely than any other single factor to lead to poor patient outcome. These complications occur most frequently in high-energy fractures [11].

Nonoperative Treatment Techniques

The majority of tibial plateau fractures with associated osteoporosis carry the option to be treated conservatively. Unlike in fractures of the hip or distal femur, prolonged bed rest or traction is not necessary. In most cases nonoperative treatment can be expected to provide a satisfactory outcome for the knee. This fact, coupled with the increased difficulties of operatively fixing tibial plateau fractures with poor bone stock, increases the indications for nonoperative treatment when a patient has osteoporosis.

Many split depression fractures with only a few millimeters of displacement and without significant valgus instability on examination, can be treated with a lightweight brace and protected weightbearing. Early joint movements through hinges at the knee are indicated. Progression to full weightbearing will almost always be safe at 6 weeks. Symptoms should recede and there should be a full return to function within a few months of injury.

If there is concern for increased displacement, either because of the fracture pattern or because of uncontrolled weightbearing in an elderly patient, or if the initial examination shows valgus instability, a formal cast brace can be applied (Fig. 21.1). The hinges should be set to prevent valgus displacement at the knee. Free motion is allowed. These heavier molded cast braces provide greater protection against valgus displacement. Segal et al. [12] have shown that weightbearing in a cast brace can be allowed with an expectation of no greater than 2 mm of increased displacement. The treatment of bicondylar fractures by early application of a cast brace leads to less satisfactory results [13].

In bicondylar fractures, fractures with a high degree of valgus instability (greater than 10°), cases with an associated fibular head fracture or other cases where satisfactory alignment cannot be obtained, traction can be considered [14]. However, elderly patients and patients with osteoporosis may not tolerate the prolonged immobility required, and in these circumstances operative intervention may be preferable.

Operative Treatment Techniques

Before choosing operative intervention, the surgeon should consider several factors. In case series on the results of reduction and internal fixation of tibial plateau fractures using AO techniques, patients with significant osteoporosis consistently have poorer outcomes than those without osteoporosis [3]. There is a high risk of postoperative collapse of the reduced plateau. In addition there is decreased holding strength of the applied implant. Despite operative fixation the patient may still have poor mobility secondary to general debility and associated medical problems.

Despite these warnings some patients with tibial plateau fractures and associated osteoporosis will benefit from carefully planned surgical intervention. The exact indications must be individualized based on the fracture, the quality of the bone and the patient's expectations and demands. Nonoperative treatment that results in significant coronal malalignment will often lead to pain and decreased function, and subsequent reconstruction by knee arthroplasty will be more difficult. The degree of instability on initial examination combined with the radiographic features of the fracture provide clues to when this result is likely. Split lateral depression fractures with 1 cm or greater depression of a large portion of the lateral plateau, or certain bicondylar fractures with large depressions or those with medial tilting, are at high risk for malalignment and poor results [13].

Split Depression Lateral Plateau

Since the split depression lateral plateau fracture is the most common type of fracture in patients with osteoporosis, and since it may lead to unacceptable valgus

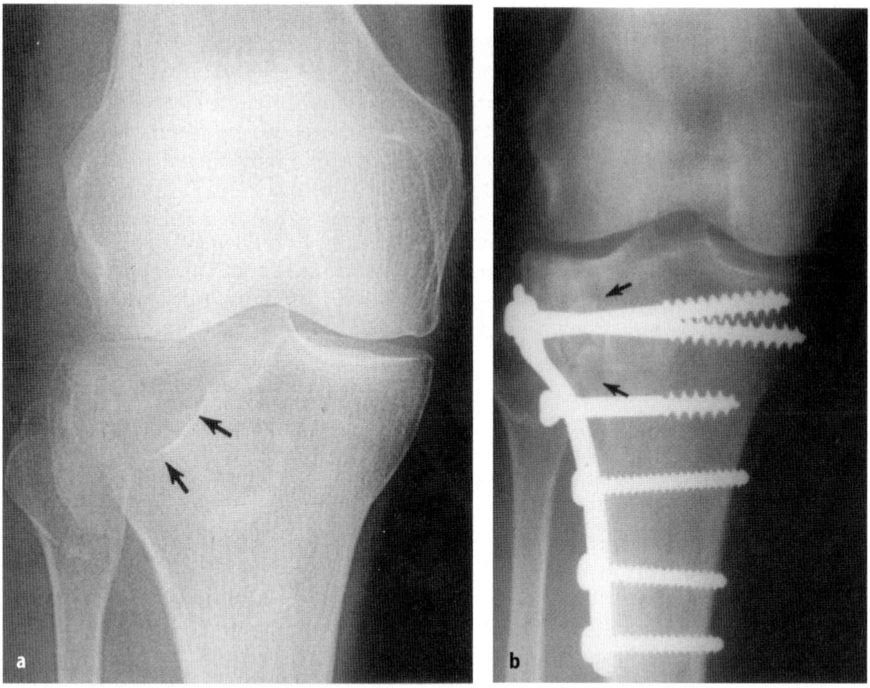

Figure 21.2. **a** A split depression lateral plateau fracture in a patient with osteoporosis. **b** A postoperative AP radiograph shows reduction and internal fixation. The *arrows* point to corticocancellous grafts. Bone graft substitutes and the use of more proximally placed small fragment plates and screws would be satisfactory alternatives.

alignment, surgery will sometimes be contemplated for this fracture pattern. A preoperative CT scan is a help in surgical planning. This will demonstrate the exact location of the split fracture line as it exits anteriorly and the location in the lateral joint of the depressed fragments.

The surgical approaches for reducing, and the techniques for evaluating the reduction are similar to those utilized in patients with normal bone, except that direct joint visualization by arthrotomy or arthroscopy is rarely considered necessary in elderly patients with osteoporosis. Indirect reduction and evaluation techniques are always preferred. An incision is made over the anterior fracture line of the split fragment. The joint surface is reduced through this fracture line from below using awls and elevators. The joint is not directly visualized; rather the reduction is evaluated fluoroscopically. The lateral plateau should be elevated to the anatomical level above the medial plateau and evaluated fluoroscopically on the lateral and caudal view.

In the elderly patient with a valgus split depression fracture, the elevated fragments will leave a cavity which will almost always have to be filled to support the reduction and minimize the amount of redisplacement. Structural support is required since the problem is not with fracture healing, but with fracture redisplacement. This support has traditionally been supplied by blocks of cortical cancellous bone harvested from the iliac crest and placed underneath the reduced articular surface prior to returning the split fragment into position (Fig. 21.2). Blocks of interporous hydroxyapatite have been shown to provide equivalent support for the lateral tibial plateau to autogenous grafts [15]. Newer bone graft substitutes have phase changing characteristics where pastes set into cement, which has higher compressive strength than cancellous bone [16]. These osteoconductive agents will soon have a role in the treatment of osteoporotic lateral tibial plateau fractures by providing structural support without the morbidity of an iliac graft [17].

Osteoporotic split depression tibial plateau fractures require buttress plate fixation. Unlike in young patients, where in some cases cancellous screws placed through the split fragment provide enough stability, in patients with osteoporosis, the buttressing effect of the split fragment should always be augmented by plate fixation. Traditional plate fixation has been with large-fragment T and L buttress plates, but recently better fixation has been found with multiple small-fragment screws placed close to the subchondral area in conjunction with slightly smaller plates [18].

Schatzker V or VI Bicondylar or Metaphyseal/Diaphyseal Disruption Fractures

These difficult fracture patterns most commonly occur in young patients from high-energy mechanisms, but may be seen in elderly patients with osteoporosis. When they occur there is often severe metaphyseal and sometimes intra-articular comminution, making management difficult. Associated injuries to the soft tissues are common. There are no data in the literature on the treatment of these specific fracture types in elderly or osteoporotic patients, so all recommendations must be based on experience and general wisdom.

Treatment of these injuries leads to more complications than treatment of lower-energy tibial plateau fractures. The difficulties are compounded when there is poor bone stock. The treatment options include traction, medial and lateral plating, external fixation or combinations of these methods. Traction is rarely utilized in elderly patients with tibial plateau fractures.

The complications of medial and lateral plating have decreased the popularity of this method and its use is mostly limited to lower-energy bicondylar fractures [11]. In these cases the use of an external fixator can be avoided. The bone quality must be reasonable and there should not be a severe injury to the soft tissues. When the medial plateau is not comminuted and not widely displaced, it is stabilized with a small fragment implant placed in the interval between the pes tendons and the medial head of the gastrocnemius. The posterior medial plate is applied with little stripping under good soft tissue cover. This converts a bicondylar fracture to a standard split lateral depression. A standard approach through an anterolateral incision, widely spaced from the posteromedial incision, can then be made for the split lateral depression portion of the bicondylar fracture [19].

External fixation techniques have become popular and the results of several series have been reported in the literature [6, 20–23]. These techniques have decreased the complications when compared with extensile approaches with medial and lateral plating. However, there are no data specific to the use of external fixation for the tibial plateau in patients with osteoporosis (Fig. 21.3).

Reductions can often be achieved percutaneously with the assistance of reduction forceps and intraoperative distraction. When the major metaphyseal disruption is not too close to the joint, excellent fixation can be obtained percutaneously with either pin or wire fixators. Primary attention should be directed to alignment of the limb, and the metaphyseal area should not be disturbed. High healing rates without bone grafts have been reported.

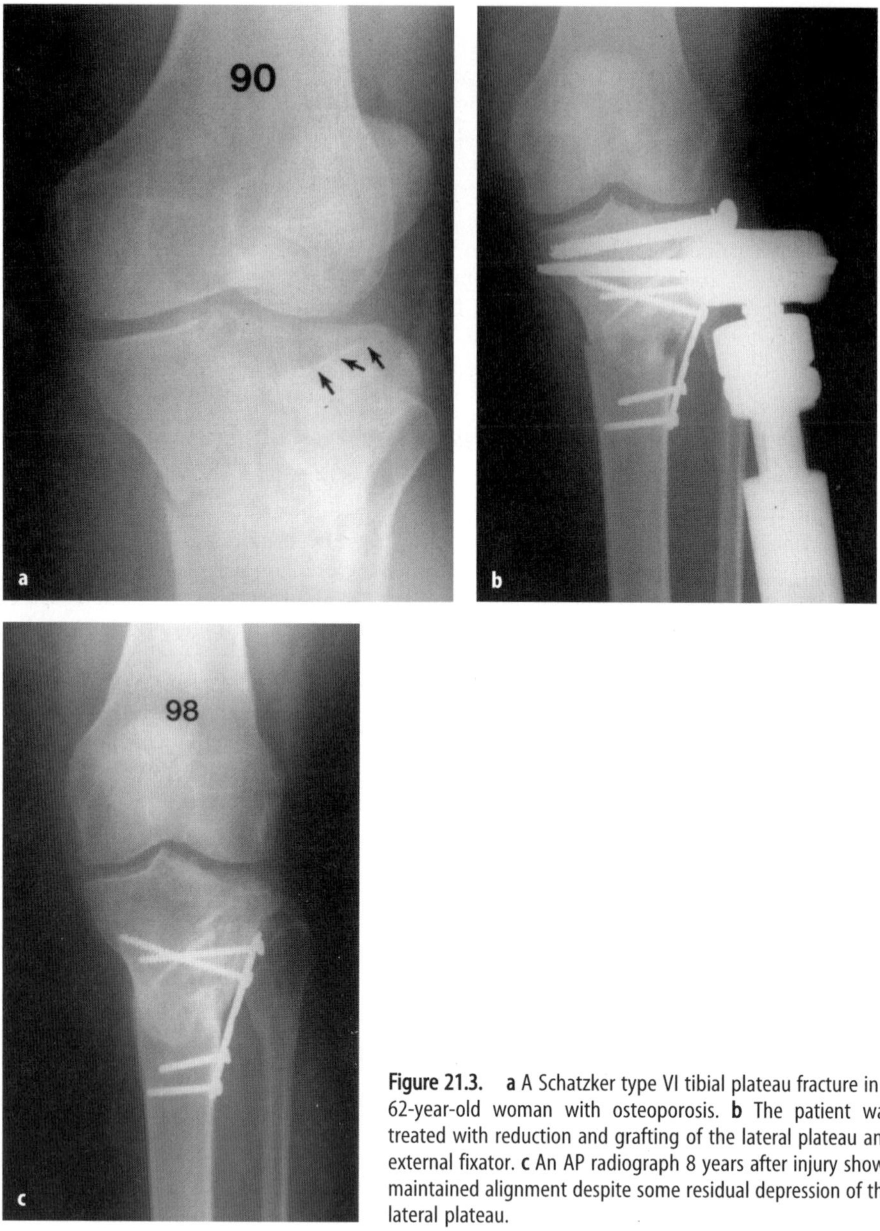

Figure 21.3. **a** A Schatzker type VI tibial plateau fracture in a 62-year-old woman with osteoporosis. **b** The patient was treated with reduction and grafting of the lateral plateau and external fixator. **c** An AP radiograph 8 years after injury shows maintained alignment despite some residual depression of the lateral plateau.

When the fracture is close to the joint and comminution in the proximal tibia increases, fixation becomes increasingly difficult. This can be a particular problem when there is significant osteoporosis. In these cases, fracture instability despite external fixation leads to pin or wire sepsis close to the knee which may lead to septic arthritis [6,20]. In these cases, the judicious use of a period of spanning external fixation can decrease the rate of this significant complication. The fixator

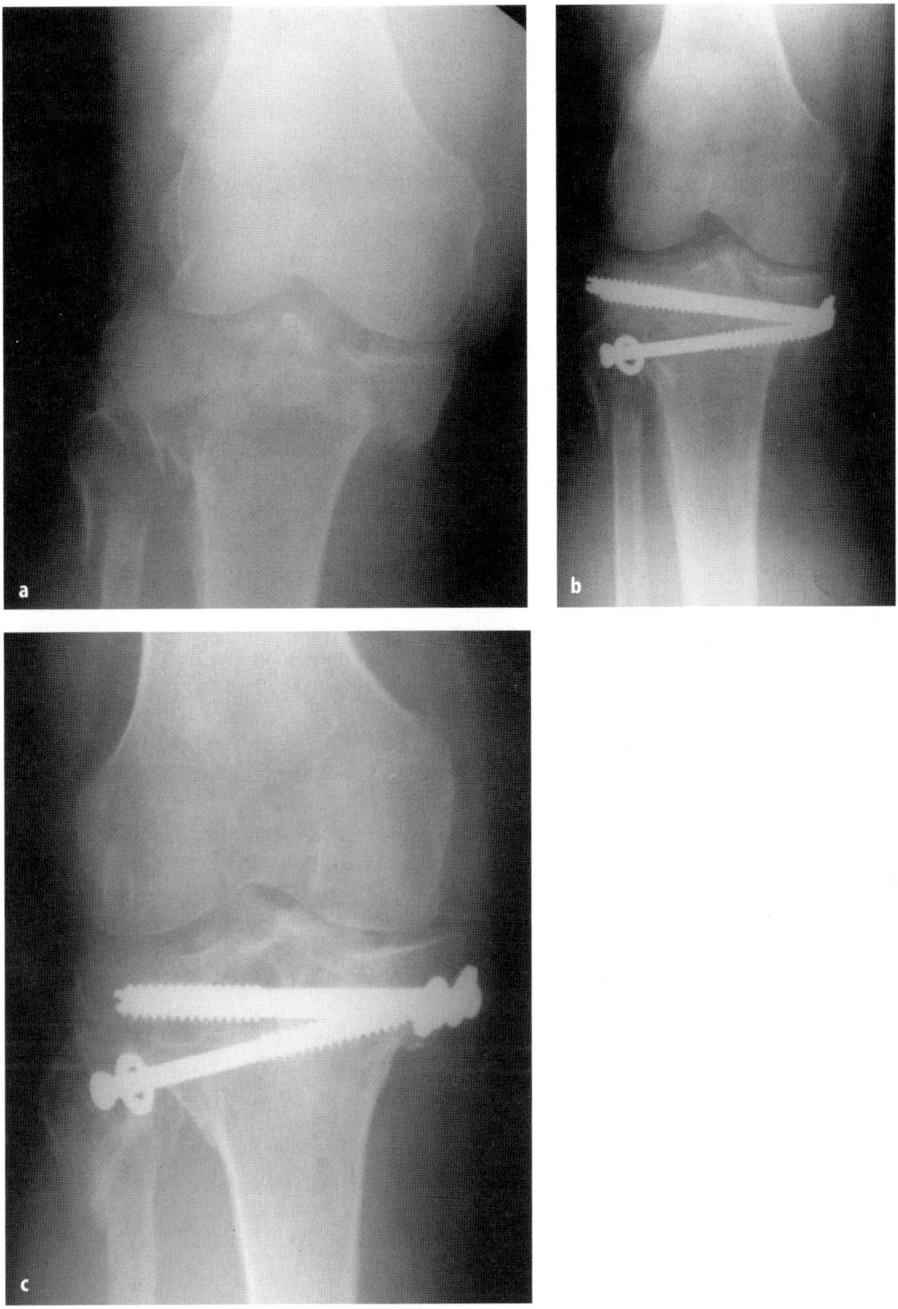

Figure 21.4. **a** A comminuted bicondylar fracture in a 79-year-old woman. **b** Treatment was by percutaneous screw fixation and cast bracing. **c** Eighteen months after injury the patient is healed and her alignment is satisfactory despite some residual displacement. She has good function with a 105° arc of motion.

pins or wires are not placed in the area of the proximal tibia, but instead span from the mid-femur to distal femur down to the mid-tibia. This technique requires a period of knee joint immobility, which is well tolerated in the majority of patients, and knee mobility rapidly recovers [6]. The timing of across-knee frame removal and conversion to a cast brace, or alternatively change to a below-knee fixator, depends on the particular fracture pattern and the condition of the soft tissues.

Results

Redisplacement after operatively treated tibial plateau fractures is common and can be expected to be more of a problem in osteoporotic fractures. In 3 of 5 cases studied by radiographic stereophotogrammetric analysis, displacement of the reduced fragment averaged 2.8 mm [24]. Further displacement after initial conservative treatment is also expected, particularly in osteoporotic proximal tibias.

Although redisplacement is a cause for significant concern and all efforts should be made to minimize its occurrence, several studies have shown that there is little correlation between the radiographic and functional results. Rasmussen [1] could find no correlation between radiographs and function, and Honoken and Järvinen [25] found no correlation of results with the amount of articular step-off. Instead, results correlated with the tilt of the plateaus or angular malalignment. Lansinger et al. [7] found 90% good and excellent results 20 years after the treatment of tibial plateau fractures where the only criterion for operative intervention was 10° of instability in full extension. All other fractures were treated in a cast.

There are few data in the literature on the results of treatment specifically in elderly or osteoporotic patients. One study noted that there was no correlation between the appearance of the knee on radiographs and the clinical outcome, in a group of operatively treated patients greater than 65 years of age [5]. Twenty-three of 32 patients studied had good or excellent results after open reduction and internal fixation. There were no serious complications. An additional series of patients treated operatively showed no significant difference in results by age [26]. However, another study showed that both nonoperatively and operatively treated patients with tibial plateau fractures had worse results when significant osteoporosis was present on radiographs [3].

In reviewing these reported results it is clear that, particularly in elderly and osteoporotic patients, there is at best only a loose association between radiographs and functional outcome. The surgeon can make an argument to pay close attention to the radiographic results in young patients, by hypothesizing that radiographic results may lead to functional differences long after the fracture has healed. In elderly patients, such as those who have significant osteoporosis, this argument is clearly not valid. For this reason, obtaining reasonable angular alignment, avoiding complications and generally choosing simpler interventions should be the guiding principles (Fig. 21.4).

Conclusion

Osteoporosis complicates over one-third of tibial plateau fractures. It is found more frequently in women in the fifth, sixth and seventh decades. The most common fracture pattern is a split depression fracture of the lateral plateau. Pure split fractures are uncommon.

There are more options for treating osteoporotic tibial plateau fractures than equivalent fractures of the proximal or distal femur. In many cases conservative treatment can be expected to lead to a reasonable functional result. The surgeon should be aware that redisplacement of a fragment or increased displacement beyond that measured on initial radiographs is more common in osteoporotic patients than in patients with good bone stock.

When operative approaches are chosen, they should be based on obtaining satisfactory limb alignment rather than on achieving exact reduction of the articular surface. In addition to plate fixation, either structural grafts or other bone substitutes are required to support the lateral plateau. When high-energy fractures occur in patients with decreased bone stock, the complications of management are increased, and the surgeon should follow a plan that minimizes these adverse outcomes.

References

1. Rasmussen PS. Tibial condylar fractures. J Bone Joint Surg Am 1973;55:1331–1350.
2. Honkonen SE. Indications for surgical treatment of tibial condyle fractures. Clin Orthop Rel Res 1994;302:199–205.
3. Schatzker J, McBroom R, Bruce D. The tibial plateau fracture: the Toronto experience. Clin Orthop 1979;138:94–104.
4. Müller ME, Nazarian S, Koch P, Schatzker J. The comprehensive classification of fractures of long bones. Berlin Heidelberg New York: Springer, 1990.
5. Biyani A, Reddy NS, Chaudhury J, Simison AJM, Klenerman L. The results of surgical management of displaced tibial plateau fractures in the elderly. Injury 1995;26:291–297.
6. Marsh JL, Smith ST, Do TT. External fixation and limited internal fixation for complex fractures of the tibial plateau. J Bone Joint Surg Am 1995;77:661–673.
7. Lansinger O, Bergman B, Korner L, Anderson G. Tibial condylar fractures: a 20 year follow up. J Bone Joint Surg Am 1986;68:13–19.
8. Burri C, Bartzke G, Coldewey J Muggler E. Fractures of the tibial plateau. Clin Orthop 1979;138:84–93.
9. Jensen D. Tibial plateau fractures: a comparison of conservative and surgical treatment. J. Bone Joint Surg Br 1990;72:49–52.
10. Gausewitz S, Hohl M. The significance of early motion in the treatment of tibial plateau fractures. Clin Orthop 1986;202:135–138.
11. Young MJ, Barrack RL. Complications of internal fixation of tibial plateau fractures. Orthop Rev 1994;23:149–154.
12. Segal D, Mallik AR, Wetzler MJ, Franchi AV, Whitelaw GP. Early weightbearing of lateral tibial plateau fractures. Clin Orthop 1993;294:232–237.
13. DeCoster TA, Nepola JV, El-Khoury GY. Cast brace treatment of proximal tibial fractures: a ten-year follow-up study. Clin Orthop 1988;231:196–204.
14. Apley A. Fractures of the lateral tibial condyle treated by skeletal traction and early mobilisation. A review of sixty cases with special reference to the long-term results. J Bone Joint Surg Br 1956;38:699–708.
15. Bucholz RW, Carlton A, Holmes R. Interporous hydroxyapatite as a bone graft substitute in tibial plateau fractures. Clin Orthop 1989;240:53–62.
16. Goodman S, Bauer T, Carter D, Casteleyn P, Goldstein S, Kyle R, Larsson, et al. Norian SRS cement augmentation in hip fracture treatment. Clin Orthop 1998;348:42–50.
17. Yetkinler D, McClellan T, Reindal E, Carter D, Poser R. Biomechanical evaluation of the fracture stability between ORIF and cement augmentation with proper void

preparation in a central depressed tibial plateau fracture. Presented at the Orthopaedic Trauma Association Annual Meeting, Vancouver, British Columbia, Canada, 8–10 October 1998.
18. Herriott G, Hubbard D. Low-profile fixation of tibial plateau fractures. Presented at the Orthopaedic Trauma Association Annual Meeting, Vancouver, British Columbia, Canada, 8–10 October 1998.
19. Georgiadis GM. Combined anterior and posterior approaches for complex tibial plateau fractures. J Bone Joint Surg Br 1994;76:285–289.
20. Weiner LS, Kelley M, Yang E, Steuer J, Watnick N, Evans M, et al. The use of combination internal fixation and hybrid external fixation in severe proximal tibia fractures. J Orthop Trauma 1995;9:244–250.
21. Gaudinez RF, Mallik AR, and Szporn M. Hybrid external fixation of comminuted tibial plateau fractures. Clin Orthop 1996;328:203–210.
22. Stamer DT, Schenk R, Staggers B, Aurori K, Aurori B, Behrens F F. Bicondylar tibial plateau fractures treated with a hybrid ring external fixator: a preliminary study. J Orthop Trauma 1994;8:455–461.
23. Dendrinos GK, Kontos S, Katsenis D, Dalas A. Treatment of high-energy tibial plateau fractures by the Ilizarov circular fixator. J Bone Joint Surg Br 1996;78:710–717.
24. Ryd L, Toksvig-Larsen S. Stability of the elevated fragment in tibial plateau fractures. Int Orthop 1994;18:131–134.
25. Honkonen SE, Järvinen MJ. Classification of fractures of the tibial condyles. J Bone Joint Surg Br 1992;74:840–104.
26. Lachiewicz PF, Funik T. Factors influencing the results of open reduction and internal fixation of tibial plateau fractures. Clin Orthop 1990;259:210–215.

22 Ankle Fractures

J. Karlsson, S. Brandsson and M. Möller

Introduction

The ankle is a complex hinge joint, in which the skeletal structures and the ligaments play an important role in terms of function, movement and stability. Normal function of the ankle is dependent on the precise structural integrity. Not only the ligaments but also the tight fit between the talus and the malleoli in the ankle mortise play an important stabilizing role. During weightbearing, the ankle is exposed to forces of between 1.2 and 5.5 times the weight of the body. This load increases the inherent stability of the joint [1].

Ankle fractures are the most common lower extremity fractures. Current treatment protocols appear to produce better results than older alternatives, especially in terms of fewer and less severe complications and more rapid rehabilitation, and there has been a general trend toward surgical treatment, especially in the case of more severe injuries. In recent studies there appears to be an increase in the prevalence of ankle fractures, as well as an increase in the severity of the fractures in the elderly population with severely osteoporotic bone. Most ankle fractures involve the lateral or medial malleolus and are produced through indirect trauma, by shearing forces directed through the talus. The management of ankle fractures requires a thorough assessment of the anatomical structures involved, not only the bone but also ligaments and tendons crossing the joint. There is substantial evidence that reduced vascular flow in the lower extremities is associated with an increased rate of bone loss, at both the hip and the foot [2].

Although the treatment of ankle fractures is well described, there is still some controversy, due in part to recent advances in the understanding of the biomechanics of the ankle, and these areas of controversy mainly relate to the indications for surgical treatment and postoperative rehabilitation. The question whether isolated lateral malleolar fractures should be operated on or not is therefore under discussion; the operative treatment and postoperative management of syndesmotic injuries have been questioned and the length of the postoperative immobilization has also been debated. Even though there is general agreement that surgical treatment of ankle fractures produces better clinical results, this has not been effectively demonstrated in well-conducted comparative studies [3]. Surgical treatment should be undertaken in patients in whom exact reductions in the joint surface fragments can be expected to produce better results than nonsurgical treatment. Regretfully, relatively little is known about the treatment of ankle fractures in severely osteoporotic bone and the optimal treatment for these patients has not as yet been established.

The incidence of osteoporotic fractures (also known as fragility fractures) increases with age, is higher in overall terms in women than men and in most cases these fractures are correlated with only minimal trauma. These fractures, including ankle fractures, are expensive and can lead to major morbidity, requiring repeated surgery and prolonged immobilization. To be able to deal with these areas of controversy, a sound knowledge of functional anatomy and ankle biomechanics is therefore necessary.

Anatomical Considerations

The ankle joint is composed of three bones: the articular surfaces of the distal tibia, the distal part of the fibula and the talus. These three bones form a highly congruent saddle-shaped joint surface. During weightbearing, most of the load is transmitted via the tibial joint surface to the talar dome. With varus or valgus stress, the load can shift to either the medial or the lateral facet of the talus. Almost one-fifth of the load is transmitted through the proximal fibula via the syndesmosis and the interosseous membrane [1].

The distal parts of the tibia and fibula are closely connected by the ligaments of the syndesmosis. These are the anterior and posterior tibiofibular ligaments and, between them, the interosseous ligament extending into the interosseous membrane more proximally. Laterally, the fibula is attached to the talus and calcaneus by three ligaments. These ligaments are anatomically weak and are often damaged. Of these, the calcaneofibular ligament is located deep in relation to the peroneal tendons, which serve as major dynamic stabilizing structures of the lateral aspect of the ankle. The function of the interosseous membrane is not fully understood. The medial side of the ankle is stabilized by the deltoid ligament, which is composed of two layers: one deep and one superficial. The deltoid ligament is stronger and is more seldom damaged than the lateral ligaments. Isolated deltoid ligament injuries are infrequent. The talus and the fibula move synchronously; in other words, as the dorsiflexion of the ankle increases, the fibula moves posteriorly and laterally and rotates externally. The primary movement of the skeletal structures in cases of fracture of the lateral malleolus is external rotation of the talus. The primary stabilizing structures of the ankle are on the medial side, i.e., the medial malleolus and the deltoid ligament [1].

Classification of Ankle Fractures

Every classification system for ankle fractures is designed to help the surgeon decide on appropriate treatment and assess the prognosis. Two main classification systems are in use: those of Lauge-Hansen and Danis-Weber (AO). Neither of these systems has been shown to be prognostic, but both can be used to guide the treatment.

The Lauge-Hansen system was created in 1942 and was the first modern classification system for fractures related to the ankle [4]. This system is based on the reproduction of experimentally produced fractures in cadavers and is a further development of a previous classification system, published by Ashurst and Bromer in 1922 [5]. The following groups of ankle fractures were established: supination-adduction, supination-eversion, pronation-abduction, pronation-eversion and pronation-dorsiflexion. The main groups can then be divided into subgroups (stages), depending on the severity of the trauma. The first description denotes the position of the foot at the time of the injury and the second the direction of the force applied. Supination of the foot places the lateral structures under stress and pronation places the medial structures under stress. The Lauge–Hansen classification was originally designed to guide the surgeon in the closed treatment of ankle fractures. It was thought that by reversing the injury mechanism, manipulative treatment was facilitated and optimal results could be achieved. The Lauge–Hansen system is not easy to apply and one major disadvantage is that it is not prognostic. Yde [6] demonstrated that the Lauge–Hansen classification provided a very precise description of all ankle fractures. In his study, only 1.2% of the fractures could not be classified using this system and this is the major advantage of the stystem. Yde [6] added the isolated fracture of the posterior tibial margin as a special type of ankle fracture.

At the present time, modern treatment protocols consisting of surgical methods, based on open reduction and rigid internal fixation which can permit early mobilization and weightbearing, are preferred. A second and simpler classification system, more suitable for application to surgical treatment, was first introduced by Danis in 1949, subsequently modified by Weber and has predominantly been used by the AO group [7]. The AO system is based on dividing ankle fractures into three major groups – A, B and C – according to the height of the fibular fracture in relation to the syndesmotic joint and the tibiotalar joint space. This system is simpler and is more suited to surgical rather than nonsurgical treatment and is easier to use [8].

Each system has its advantages and disadvantages and it has been suggested that they could be merged into one system involving three basic patterns [9]. It has been questioned whether reliance on the localization of the fibular fracture is warranted, as the fibular fracture configuration does not correlate well with ankle stability. However, the classical supination-external rotation type of fracture is not produced by a pure supination and external rotation mechanism but also includes doriflexion movement and a talofibular force that is laterally directed. The relationship of radiologically occult injuries in a classical supination-external rotation type of fracture is not always based on the fracture pattern which is observed.

Both classification systems have their inherent disadvantages but can be used in elderly patients with ankle fractures. Neither of these systems has proved reliable. The interobserver reliability of both systems is at best fair and agreement between observers (not dependent on their experience) of less than 60% has been reported. The use of two (lateral and true anteroposterior radiograph of the ankle) or three (anteroposterior, lateral and mortise) radiographic projections is also discussed. There appears to be a strong economic argument in favor of the routine use of only two radiographs [10,11].

Epidemiology of Ankle Fractures

There are several studies which focus on the epidemiology of ankle fractures. Most of them are retrospective. It appears that the epidemiology of ankle fractures is changing and this might be due to increasing longevity [12]. Fewer data can be found when it comes to the epidemiology of peripheral fractures, such as the ankle, compared with hip fractures. Before the age of 70–75, ankle fractures are more common than fractures of the hip. There is also a more pronounced age-related increase in the risk of fracture when it comes to proximal (hip) limb fractures than distal ones (e.g., the ankle) [13–15].

Bengner and coworkers [16] reported on the increasing incidence of ankle fractures in Sweden between the 1950s (65 per 100 000 persons a year) and the 1980s (107 per 100 000 persons a year) and Kannus and coworkers [17] demonstrated a similar trend in Finland between 1970 (66 per 100 000 persons a year) and 1994 (162 per 100 000 persons per year). These authors stated that the increasing rate of ankle fractures could not be explained by demographic changes alone and that vigorous preventive measures should be implemented to reduce this increasing problem. Daly and coworkers [18] determined an incidence of 184 fractures per 100 000 persons a year in the USA.

Below the age of 50 years, ankle fractures are most common in men, but after that age there is a female predominance, probably due to reduced bone quality in postmenopausal women. Court-Brown and coworkers [19] found that the incidence of ankle fractures was highest in women aged between 75 and 84 years in a survey of 1500 fractures. There is some evidence that ankle fractures should not be characterized as fragility fractures because compared, for instance, with the continued increase in well-known fragility fractures, such as hip fractures, the incidence of ankle fractures has been shown in some studies to decrease after the age of 60–70 years. Baron and coworkers [20,21] did not find any difference in the incidence of ankle fractures beween men and women over the age of 65 years. This was in contrast to the increased risk in women of this age sustaining fractures of the hip, distal forearm and proximal humerus. Jensen and coworkers [22] studied the epidemiology in Denmark in a prospective population-based study. The overall incidence was 107 fractures per 100 000 individuals a year. Their findings indicated that most of the fractures were caused by large-scale trauma during physical activity; the main cause was a fall, on the ground, stairs or from a height, in 87% of the patients. Osteoporosis thus did not appear to have any major effect on the incidence of ankle fractures.

Lauritzen and Lund [23] found that the relative risk of subsequent hip fracture was 4.8 after lumbar spine fracture, 4.1 after olecranon fracture, 3.5 after knee fracture, but only 1.5 after ankle fracture. Bengner and coworkers [16], on the other hand, stated that bi- and trimalleolar, but not unimalleolar fractures could be regarded as fragility fractures, due to the marked increase in incidence with age. This could have specific implications in terms of the choice of treatment. Gunnes and coworkers [24] investigated the effect of a previous fracture on the risk of a new fracture in a population-based study of postmenopausal women. They found that it might be possible to select women for intervention against osteoporosis by the information obtained about fragility fractures earlier in life. The occurrence of a fracture 5–10 years before answering the questionnaire increased the risk (measured as the odds ratio) of having sustained a hip fracture to 3.5 times for a previous humerus fracture and 1.6 for a previous ankle fracture. In a similar population-based study, Honkanen and coworkers [25] studied 12 192 perimenopausal women. They found that the menopause was significantly related to an increase in incidence of wrist fractures but not of ankle fractures. However, an increase (1 SD) in body mass index increased the relative risk of ankle fracture by 24%. Contrary to this, an increase in body mass index reduced the relative risk of wrist fracture. Smoking was also related to an increased risk of sustaining an ankle fracture, as opposed to a wrist fracture.

The profiles of risk factors for ankle and foot fractures are not entirely known and the question of whether low bone mass is the most important risk factor is being discussed. The risk factors for ankle and foot fractures were analyzed by Seeley and coworkers [26] in 9704 women aged 65 years and over. The questionnaire included lifestyle factors and functional impairment and the objective investigation included assessments of bone mineral density (BMD) and neuromuscular performance tests. The relative risks (RR) of ankle and foot fractures were estimated during a 6-year follow-up. During this period, 191 women sustained an ankle fracture. Factors associated with ankle fractures were an increased tendency to fall during the year preceding baseline (RR 1.5), vigorous physical activity (RR 1.2 for twice a week), weight gain since the age of 25 years (RR 1.4 for a 20% gain), osteoarthritis (RR 0.5) and a sister's history of hip fracture after the age of 50 years (RR 1.7). The relative risk associated with low distal radius BMD was 1.2 for −0.1 g/cm^2. The conclusion of this study was that the risk factors for ankle fracture were largely independent of low bone mass and that ankle fractures should therefore not be classified as fragility fractures.

One known risk factor for sustaining a fragility fracture is a nonosteoporotic fracture earlier in life. In a retrospective study, Karlsson and coworkers [27] followed 767 patients who had sustained a tibial shaft fracture and 786 patients who had sustained an ankle fracture. It was shown that these individuals who had sustained previous tibial or ankle fractures ran an increased risk of fragility fractures later in life, without any difference in the localization of the fracture or a difference between men and women. Thus, the occurrence of a fracture earlier in life might serve as a predictor of subsequent fragility fractures and this might have implications for future treatment, especially in terms of the prevention of osteoporosis.

Management of Ankle Fractures

Adequate care of ankle fractures can often prevent permanent disability. The main priorities are (a) an evaluation of peripheral circulation; (b) acute reduction of any major deformity, e.g., dislocation; (c) wound care, e.g., open fracture; (d) during operations, the exact reduction of any skeletal deformity and maintenance of stable reduction throughout the healing period; (e) repair of associated injuries; (f) rehabilitation including early range of motion training and early weightbearing, if possible, and (h) adequate identification and treatment of secondary problems and complications [28] (Fig. 22.1).

It is well known that the best results after treating unstable ankle fractures follow accurate reduction and internal fixation of the fragments. Experience in elderly patients, however, indicates that the results are less satisfactory when osteoporosis prevents secure internal fixation. In a prospective study of unstable fracture-subluxations of the ankle in patients over the age of 65 years, Litchfield [29] found satisfactory results in only 58% of his patients. No specific risk factors associated with inferior results were reported. Beauchamp and coworkers [30] also reported a high incidence of complications in elderly patients following the open reduction and internal fixation of ankle fractures. Fernandez [31] described a simple technique for the internal fixation of the common Danis–Weber type B fracture of the

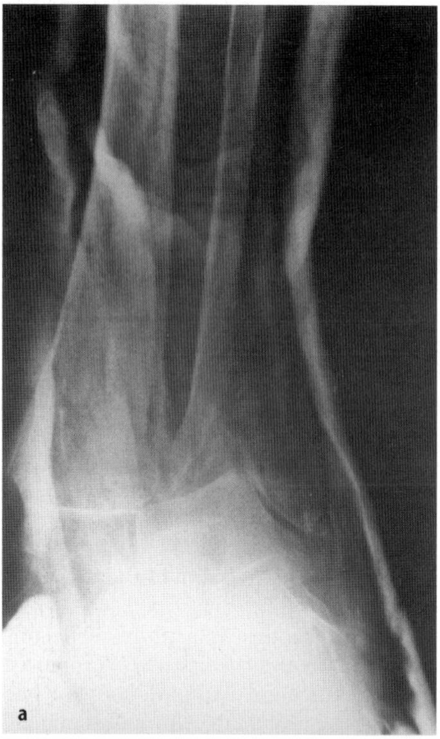

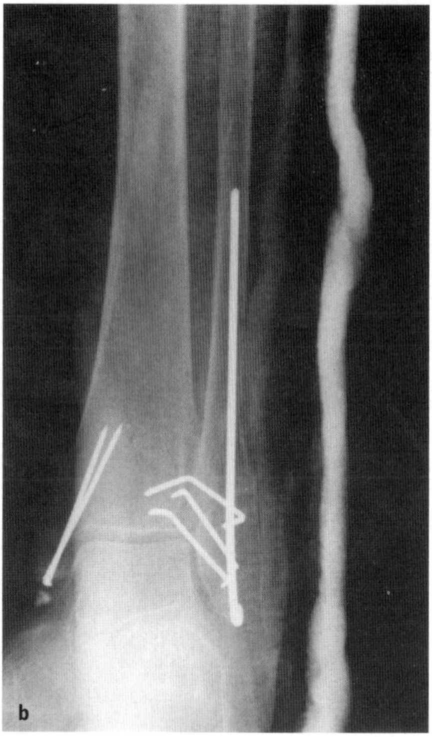

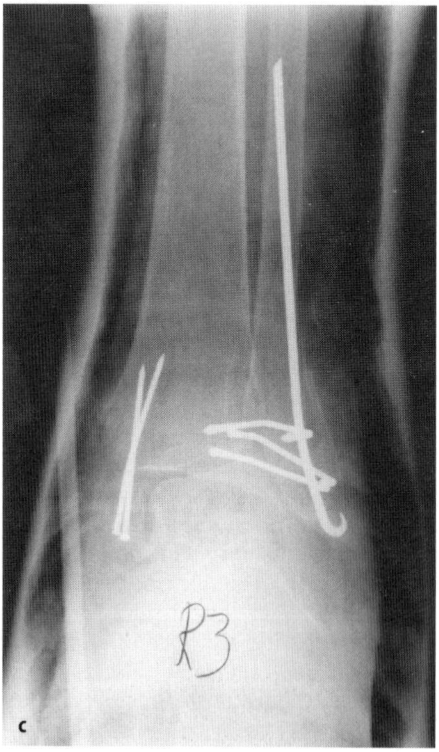

Fig. 22.1. **a** An 85-year-old woman who fell while walking on uneven ground. She sustained an open trimalleolar ankle fracture with major dislocation. There was disruption of the skin on the medial side of the ankle and loss of bone from the medial malleolus. **b** The patient was operated on within 24 h with semi-rigid osteosynthesis. The wound on the medial side was left open. An adequate reduction of the fragments was achieved. During the operation it was noted that the bone was very soft (osteoporotic) and the patient was recommended no weightbearing postoperatively. **c**, **d**, Radiographs 1 week later showed a redislocation of the fragments and there was a partial breakdown of the wound on the medial side with marginal necrosis. (*continued*)

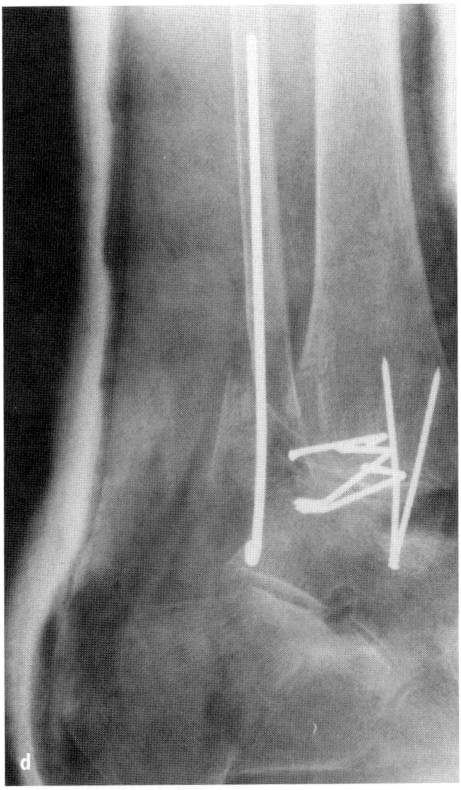

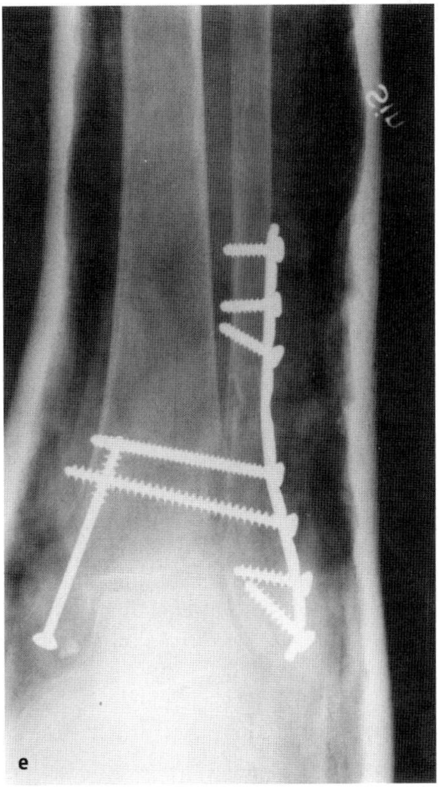

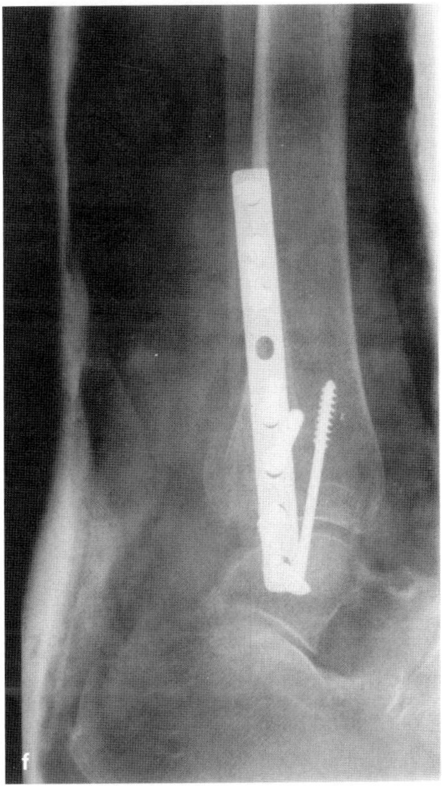

Fig. 22.1. (*continued*) **e, f,** The fracture was reoperated on 10 days after the initial trauma, in order to reduce the risk of further skin necrosis and to improve the reduction of the fragments. Using an AO plate and screws, stable internal fixation was achieved in spite of inferior bone quality.

lateral malleolus in elderly osteoporotic patients. This study, however, included only a limited number of patients.

In spite of less satisfactory overall results in the elderly population after the surgical treatment of ankle fractures, it is widely accepted that these patients should be treated as a medical emergency, i.e., on the day of the injury. Elderly patients are also best treated by definitive fracture care, permitting early mobilization, including weightbearing. Surgical treatment in unstable, displaced fractures should therefore be directed at obtaining exact reduction and stable fracture fixation, as this can facilitate an early functional return. In the case of ankle fractures, this particularly involves early weightbearing. In intra-articular fractures with displacement of the fragments, anatomical reduction is especially important. The need for internal fixation to secure fracture reduction must be weighed against the risk of operating on osteoporotic bone which lacks the strength to hold screws and plates. The failure of internal fixation can therefore be due to the low internal strength of the bone rather than an implant failure. The choice of implant for ankle fractures in osteoporotic bone is thus crucial. Implants that minimize stress shielding should be chosen to reduce the risk of further skeletal damage.

Complications of ankle injuries, including fractures, are infection, soft tissue problems, malunion and osteoarthritis. Malunion can be caused by inadequate reduction or loss of reduction due to inferior bone quality.

References

1 Michelson JD. Fractures about the ankle. Current concepts review. J Bone Joint Surg AM 1995;77:142–152.
2 Vogt MT, Cauley JA, Kuller LH, Nevitt MC. Bone mineral density and blood flow to the lower extremities: The study of osteoporotic fractures. J Bone Miner Res 1997;12: 283–289.
3 Bauer M, Bengner U, Johnell O, Redlund-Johnell I. Supination-eversion fractures of the ankle joint: Changes in incidence over 30 years. Foot Ankle 1987;8:26–28.
4 Hansen LN. Fractures of the ankle. II. Combined experimental-surgical and experimental-roentgenologic investigations. Arch Surg 1950;60:957–985.
5 Ashurst A, Bromer R. Classification and mechanism of fractures of the leg involving the ankle. Arch Surg 1922;4:51.
6 Yde J. The Lauge Hansen classification of malleolar fractures. Acta Orthop Scand 1980; 51:181–192.
7 Weber BG. Die Verletzungen des oberen Sprunggelenkes, 2nd ed. 1972; Bern: Hans Huber.
8 Lindsjö U. Classification of ankle fractures: the Lauge–Hansen or AO system. Clin Orthop 1985;199:12–16.
9 Harper MC. Ankle fracture classification systems: a case for integration of the Lauge–Hansen and AO–Danis–Weber schemes. Foot Ankle 1992;13:404–407.
10 Michelson J, Solocoff D, Waldman B, Kendall K, Ahn U. Ankle fractures. The Lauge–Hansen classification revisited. Clin Orthop 1997;345:198–205.
11 Nilsson BER. Age and sex incidence of ankle fractures. Acta Orthop Scand 1969; 40: 122–129.
12 Johnell O, Nilsson B, Obrant K, Sernbo I. Age and sex patterns of hip fracture-changes in 30 years. Acta Orthop Scand 1984;55:290–292.
13 Nguyen T, Sambrook P, Kelly P, Jones G, Lord S, Freund J, Eisman J. Prediction of osteoporotic fractures by postural instability and bone density. BMJ 1993;307:1111–1115.

14 Singer BR, McLauchlan GJ, Robinson CM, Christie J. Epidemiology of fractures in 15,000 adults. The influence of age and gender. J Bone Joint Surg Br 1998;80:243–248.
15 Jones G, Nguyen T, Sambrook PN, Kelly PJ, Gilbert C, Eisman JA Symptomatic fracture incidence in elderly men and women: the Dubbo Osteoporosis Epidemiology Study (DOES). Osteoporos Int 1994;4:277–282.
16 Bengner U, Johnell O, Redlund-Johnell I. Epidemiology of ankle fractures 1950 and 1980. Increasing incidence in elderly women. Acta Orthop Scand 1986;57:35–37.
17 Kannus P, Parkkari J, Niemi S, Palvanen M. Epidemiology of osteoporotic ankle fractures in elderly patients in Finland. Ann Intern Med 1996;125:975–978.
18 Daly PJ, Fitzgerald RH, Melton LJ, Ilstrup DM. Epidemiology of ankle fractures in Rochester, Minnesota. Acta Orthop Scand 1987;58:539–544.
19 Court-Brown CM, McBirnie J, Wilson G. Adult ankle fractures: an increasing problem? Acta Orthop Scand 1988;69:43–47.
20 Baron JA, Barrett J, Malenka D, Fisher E, Kniffin W, Bubolz T, Tosteson T. Racial differences in fracture risk. Epidemiology 1994;5:42–47.
21 Baron JA, Barrett JA, Karagas MR. The epidemiology of peripheral fracture. Bone 1996; 18 (Suppl): 209S–231S.
22 Jensen SL, Andresen BK, Mencke S, Nielsen PT. Epidemiology of ankle fractures. A prospective population-based study of 212 cases in Aalborg, Denmark. Acta Orthop Scand 1988;69:48–50.
23 Lauritzen JB, Lund B. Risk of hip fracture after osteoporosis fractures: 451 women with fracture of lumbar spine, olecranon, knee or ankle. Acta Orthop Scand 1993;64: 297–300.
24 Gunnes M, Mellström D, Johnell O. How well can a previous fracture indicate a new fracture? A questionnaire study of 29,802 postmenopausal women. Acta Orthop Scand 1998;69:508–512.
25 Honkanen R, Tuppurainen M, Kroger H, Alhava E, Saarikoski S. Relationships between risk factors and fractures differ by type of fracture: a population-based study of 12 192 perimenopausal women. Osteoporos Int 1998;8:25–31.
26 Seeley DG, Kelsey J, Jergas M, Nevitt MC. Predictors of ankle and foot fractures in older woman. The Study of Osteoporotic Fractures Research Group. J Bone Miner Res 1996;11:1347–1355.
27 Karlsson MK, Hasserius R, Obrant K. Individuals who sustain nonosteoporotic fractures continue to also sustain fragility fractures. Calcif Tissue Int 1993;53:229–231.
28 Bauer M, Bergström B, Hemborg A, Sandegård J. Malleolar fractures: nonoperative versus operative treatment. A controlled study. Clin Orthop 1987;199:17–27.
29 Litchfield JC. The treatment of unstable fractures of the ankle in the elderly. Injury 1987;18:128–132.
30 Beauchamp CG, Clay NR, Thaxton PW, Displaced ankle fractures in patients over 50 years of age. J Bone Joint Surg Br 1983;65:329–332.
31 Fernandez GN. Internal fixation of the oblique, osteoporotic fracture of the lateral malleolus. Injury 1988;19:257–258.

23 Periprosthetic Fractures after Total Hip and Knee Replacements in Patients with Osteoporosis

Å. Carlsson and L. Sanzén

Introduction

Are there periprosthetic fractures directly related to osteoporosis and occurring after only minor trauma? The answer is yes but more often so after knee replacement than after hip replacement.

In osteoporotic patients fractures close to intact acetabular prostheses are mostly cracks through the inferior part of the acetabulum which can be treated conservatively. In the femur minor trauma may cause a fracture of the greater trochanter but provided the stem prosthesis is stable, comminuted fractures at the level of the middle or distal part of the stem prosthesis are uncommon. Most fractures at the latter levels are a result of loss of cortical bone secondary to stem loosening or localized osteolysis, caused either by fragmented bone cement or polyethylene wear particles generated in the bearing. These latter complications are discussed in Ch. 40.

Total knee arthroplasty is mainly performed in old persons, patients being on average about 10 years older than for hip arthroplasty. The most common periprosthetic fractures after total knee replacement occur in the supracondylar part of the distal femur and are particularly seen in severely osteoporotic bone. The tibial component, whatever the construction and fixation principle, may tilt or subside, but fractures of the proximal tibia below this component are relatively seldom seen, either in normal or in osteoporotic bone.

If a periprosthetic fracture occurs in a very osteoporotic skeleton, which is common notably in the knee, the situation is delicate. It is of course the patient who is to be treated, not only the fracture. This implies that less traditional methods are sometimes required; for example, the best surgical treatment for a person with preserved walking ability may not be appropriate for a person confined to bed or a wheelchair. Irrespective of the cause of osteoporosis and type of fracture, the goal of the treatment must be to stabilize the fracture in such a way that at least sitting in a chair is possible. This can be achieved by conservative methods but more easily after successful surgical fixation. If sitting is not possible there is a great risk of pressure sores and pneumonia.

Table 23.1. Proportion of satisfactory results following different treatment methods for femoral fractures after total hip arthroplasty according to Mont and Maar [3]

Treatment	Type of fracture			
	Periprosthetic	Around tip	Distal to stem	Comminuted
Traction and/or cast	26/46	25/58	59/77	1/3
Cerclage	15/15	14/15	9/16	1/1
Screw plate	7/15	12/25	28/57	0/1
Long stem revision	29/36	26/32	37/50	11/14

Figures (n/n) show number of satisfactory results/ number of cases treated.

Periprosthetic Fractures after Hip Replacement

Fractures of the Pelvic Ring

Isolated fractures of the pubic bone can be treated conservatively, as in any patient without a hip implant. Fractures at the bottom of the acetabulum can also be treated conservatively in patients with a total hip arthroplasty, but in patients with a hemi-arthroplasty one should be more cautious, allowing only ambulation without weightbearing or sitting for about 6 weeks.

Fractures of the Femur

Bethea at al. [1] introduced a commonly applied system for classification of periprosthetic femoral fractures after hip replacement, which is similar to that of Johansson et al. [2]. An extended classification was described by Mont and Maar [3]. Duncan et al. [4] suggested a less stringent system, also taking into consideration whether the stem prosthesis is loose or not.

Femoral fracture after hip arthroplasty was the reason for revision with implant exchange in 1% of 4858 hips in the Swedish Hip Arthroplasty Register [5]. Only a small number of cases treated for this complication have been published and no comparative studies have been performed. In 1994, Mont and Maar [3] published a review of the literature up to 1991 including 487 fractures in 26 studies. In Table 23.1 we have summarized data from this review regarding the most common types of fracture and treatment. Interpretation of these figures should be done with care and it should be noted that satisfactory results apply to fracture healing, and not to a long-term well-fixed prosthesis. Improvements and new methods for treatment were introduced in clinical practice during the 1990s.

Factors predisposing to fracture in addition to osteoporosis are perforations or windows in the femur and localized osteolytic lesions. The goals of treatment should be early mobilization and functional recovery, fracture healing in an anatomical position and retained prosthetic fixation.

Fractures of the Greater and Lesser Trochanter

Fractures through the greater or lesser trochanter (type A(g) and A(l) according to the classification by Duncan et al. [4], dislocated or not, can be treated

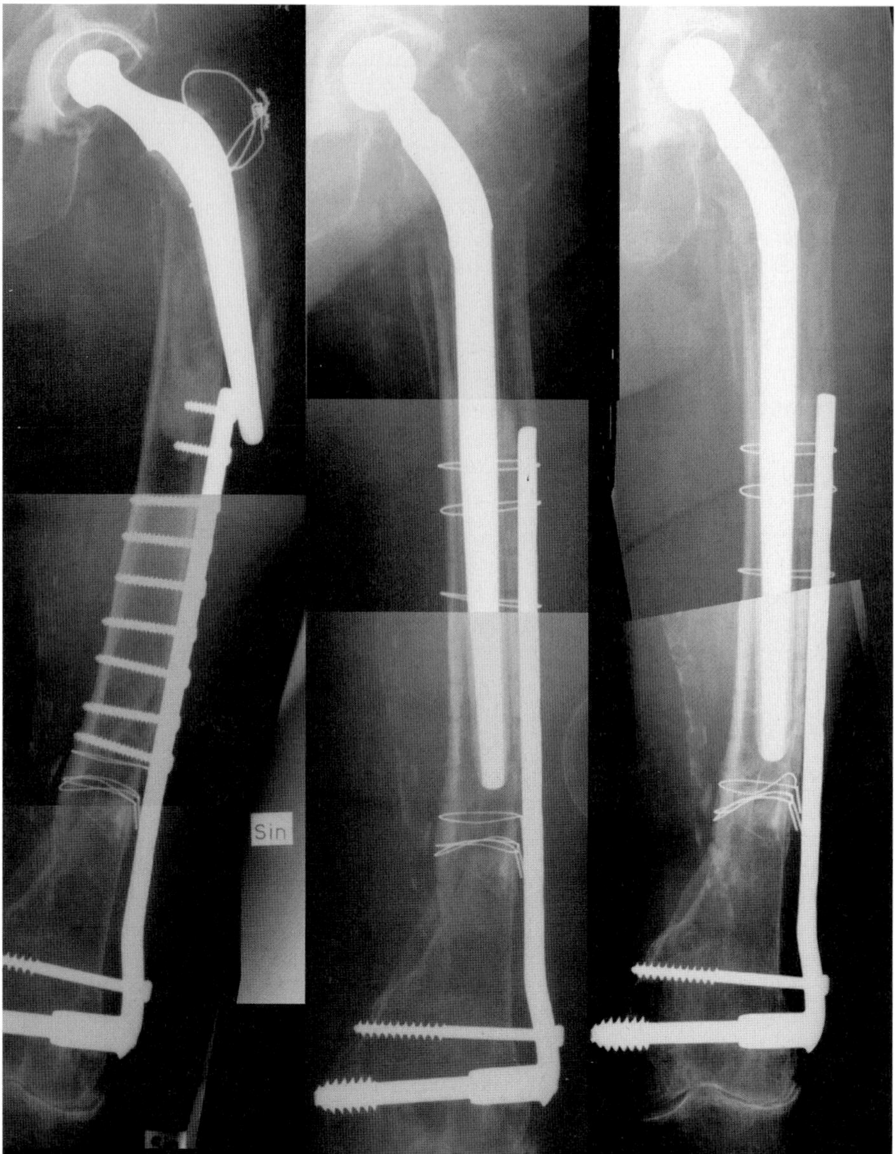

Figure 23.1. A 92-year-old woman, previously operated on due to a supracondylar femoral fracture, sustained a periprosthetic fracture at the upper end of the femur (*left*). The screws fixating the fracture device were replaced by cerclage wires. Thereafter the Charnley stem and the surrounding bone cement were removed and a 265 mm long uncemented Wagner stem introduced. Although the acetabular prosthesis was stable it was also replaced to allow for a 28 mm femoral head (*middle*). After 6 months the fracture had healed (*right*).

conservatively. Reinsertion of an osteoporotic greater trochanter is hazardous and will not essentially improve the final function.

Comminuted Fractures of the Femoral Shaft

Comminuted fractures engaging the upper third of the femur, above the tip of the stem prosthesis (Bethea type C and Duncan type B3), are, as previously mentioned, most common after major trauma or when the stem has loosened and caused thinning of the cortical bone. However, patients with osteoporosis and a hip replaced due to femoral neck fracture or rheumatic disease may also suffer a major trauma. In such a relatively infrequent but difficult situation, there are in principle only two treatment alternatives –neither of them ideal. One is conservative and implies traction in bed for several months. When the fracture has stabilized the stem will be loose and the patient cannot expect a future ambulatory life. A more attractive alternative is to extract the stem prosthesis and any bone cement, relying on distal fixation of a new uncemented implant in spite of the poor bone quality. In Europe the Wagner self-locking revision stem (Sulzer, Baar, Switzerland) or the MP-reconstruction prosthesis (W. Link, Hamburg, Germany) are the most commonly used designs (Fig. 23.1). Kolstad [6] presented 9 cases successfully treated with the Wagner stem. The experience with long femoral stems, distally fixed with screws through holes in the stem, is at present limited.

Spiral and Long Oblique Fractures

Spiral and long oblique fracture at the mid-stem level and at the tip of the prosthesis (Bethea type A and B) can be treated in several ways. We prefer open reduction and some kind of internal fixation to allow the patient to ambulate as quickly as possible. The following techniques are available (not in rank order):

1. Fixation with cerclage wires or, preferably, multistrand steel wires, the ends of which are clamped together by a special locking device. A graded tensioner may be used to prevent overtightening of the wires. These devices and instruments are supplied by different companies and could also be combined with a metal plate. Nylon-strap cerclages, so-called Partridge bands, are less suitable as they do not offer rigid fixation and notably because in our experience and that of others they cause local bone resorption [7,8].
2. Plating. When the plate is fixated by screws it is unusual to be able to pass screws through all holes and it is therefore often necessary also to use multistrand wires, as described in the previous paragraph (Fig. 23.2). A small series with fracture healing in 9 of 10 cases only using screws was presented by Serocki et al. [9]. Specially constructed devices, such as the "Mennen clamp-on plate" (C.H. Medical, UK) which clamps the fragments together, resulted in healing within 4 months in 11 cases of a series of 12. Nonunion occurred in one case and the plate broke twice [10]. In our experience the Mennen plate does not give a fixation stable enough to prevent angulation, and was only successful in undisplaced fractures in a series of 14 cases, presented by Otremski et al. [11].
3. Removal of the stem prosthesis and any cement, reduction of the fracture and fixation according to either of the two methods described above, and insertion of a new cemented or uncemented stem. The latter principle for fixation is theoretically the most attractive but the former has to be accepted in osteoporotic and debilitated patients. Cement fixation after fracture reduction and

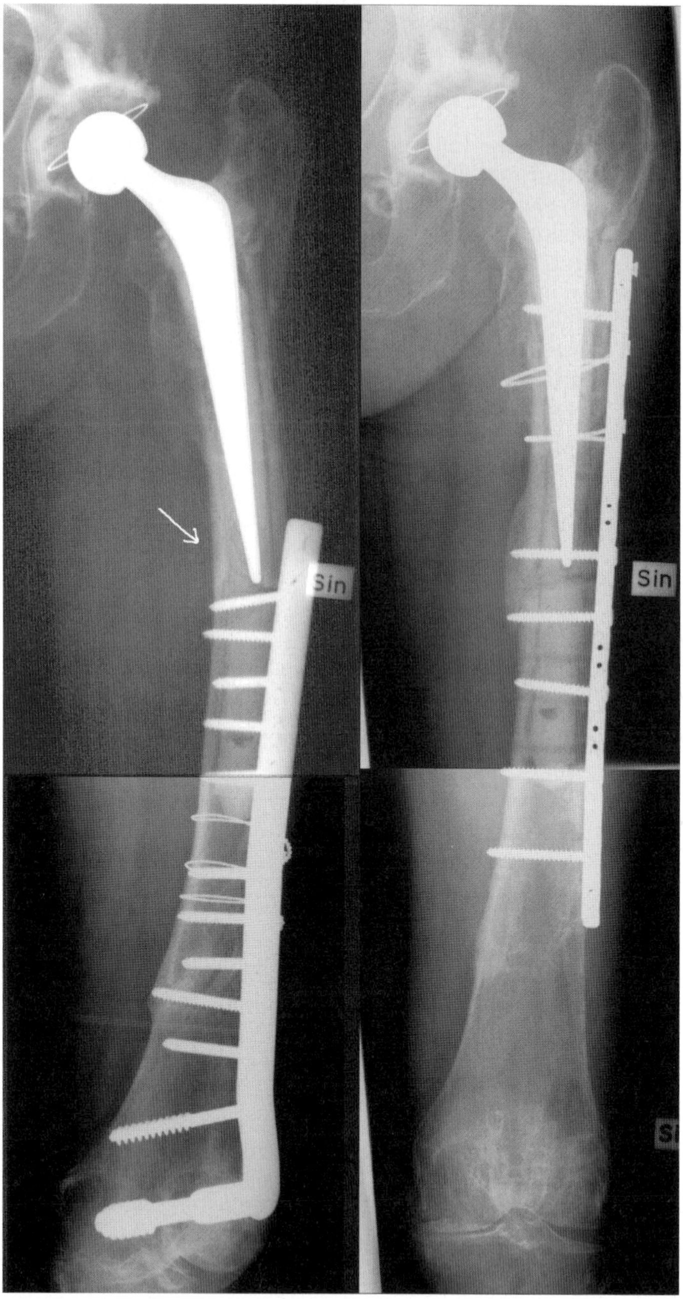

Figure 23.2. An 81-year-old woman, previously treated due to a high supracondylar femoral fracture. She sustained a short oblique fracture at the tip of her cemented Exeter prosthesis (*left*). The fracture device was removed, whereafter the fracture was aligned and fixated with a plate, screws and wires, leaving the prosthetic components in place. Autologous bone was used at the fracture site. After 3 months (*right*) the fracture had healed.

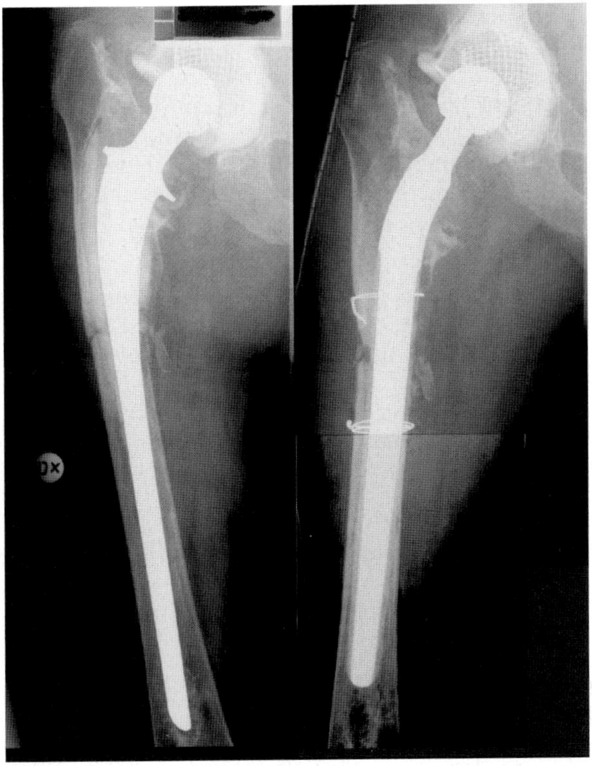

Figure 23.3. A 66-year-old woman with rheumatoid arthritis who sustained a transverse fracture at the upper part of the femur. The long cemented hip prosthesis had subsided. The loose stem and the surrounding bone cement were removed and an uncemented 265 mm long Wagner stem subsequently inserted.

impaction grafting might promote fracture healing in selected cases. As seen in Table 23.1 bypassing the fracture by a long stem prosthesis was satisfactory in about 75% of the cases.

4. If the fracture do not extend too far distally and the cortical bone of the distal fragment is not too fragile, insertion of an uncemented Wagner or Link stem without extra wires or plates may be considered. These prosthesis are not dependant on an exact and stable reduction of the fracture (Fig. 23.3).

Fractures At or Just Below the Tip of the Stem

The following treatment options may be considered:

1. These fractures are typically square or of the short oblique type (Bethea type A). The ideal treatment of this type of fracture is removal of the old stem prosthesis, loose or not, and insertion of a new uncemented stem. We prefer the Wagner type of stem. This type of fracture should be grafted with autogenous cancellous bone to enhance healing.
2. Open reduction and fixation with plate and screws is a less reliable method and should be reserved for patients too medically debilitated to tolerate stem

exchange. However, with a well-fixed prosthesis, reasonably good bone quality and a modern plate which can be used with multistrand wires, the results can be expected to improve. Bone grafting the fracture site seems advantageous.
3. Conservative treatment implies a very long time in traction and a high risk of a painful nonunion and should therefore be avoided.
4. In a patient who was nonambulatory before the fracture, extraction of the prosthesis and fixation of the fracture by an intramedullary nail may be considered.

Fractures Distal to the Prosthesis

In fractures distal to the prosthesis, the prosthesis is unaffected by the fracture and should usually be retained. Since proximally inserted locked nails cannot be used, other less ideal methods must be used. Retrograde intramedullary nails inserted from the knee as in supracondylar femoral fractures could be used (see below). Plates with screws and wires can offer good fixation in healthy bone. In osteoporotic bone intramedullary semiflexible rods give a less stable fixation and might necessitate a supplementary external support such as a splint or a period of traction.

Periprosthetic Fractures after Total Knee Replacement

Supracondylar Fractures

Typically fractures after total knee replacement occur in the supracondylar region in osteoporotic patients and as the result of only minimal trauma. Fortunately, these supracondylar fractures are not common: a prevalence of 0.15% was reported by Ritter et al. [12], 0.54% by Merkel and Johnson [13] and 1.8% by Figgie et al. [14]. The risk of sustaining such a fracture increases if an osteoporotic femur is also notched at its anterior femoral cortex at the index operation [13,15,16]. Although Ritter et al. [12] only found 2 fractures in 180 "notched" total knees, one should be particularly careful to avoid notching in osteroporotic knees. Also, manipulation of a stiff total knee under anesthetic implies a risk of sustaining a fracture in the supracondylar region. The risk factors are summarized in Table 23.2.

Supracondylar fractures after total knee replacement were first reported in the early 1980s [17–19], and since that time about 250 such fractures have been presented in a number of case reports [13–16,19–29] (Table 23.3). In the 1990s, with the introduction of anatomically formed condylar plates and notably locked intramedullary rods, the treatment possibilities of these challenging fractures dramatically improved. The indication for surgical treatment of displaced fractures will therefore presumably increase. Excellent and updated reviews have been presented by Ayers [30] and Dennis [31].

Table 23.2. Risk factors for supracondylar periprostetic fracture

Osteoporosis
Neurological disorders
Anterior notching of the femur
Manipulation of stiff knees under anaesthetic
Revision arthroplasty

Table 23.3. Major clinical reports on the treatment of supracondylar femoral fracture after knee replacement

Author	No.of cases	Treatment			
		Conservative	Operative	Locked intramedullary rod	External fixation[a]
Sisto and Insall 1985 [19]	15	12	3		
Cain et al.1986 [15]	14	10	4		
Merkel and Johnson 1986 [13]	36	26	7		3
Culp et al. 1987 [16]	61	30	31		
Cordeiro et al. 1990 [20]	10	2	8 (including 5 long stem revisions)		
Figgie et al. 1990 [14]	24	10	14		
Healy et al. 1993 [21]	20		20		
McLaren et al. 1994 [22]	7			7	
Jabczenski and Crawford 1995 [23]	4			4	
Ritter et al. 1995 [24]	22		22 Rush rods		
Murrel and Nunley 1995 [25]	3			3	
Rolston et al. 1995 [26]	4			4	
Moran et al. 1996 [27]	29	14	15		
Smith et al. 1996 [28]	1			1	
Total number	250				

[a]This treatment is contraindicated [29].

The goal of treatment is to achieve healing within about 3 months retaining the mechanical axis of the leg. Also, the range of knee motion should ideally not decrease more than 10°. This goal may be met by conservative or surgical methods depending on the type of fracture and whether the femoral component is loose or not.

The treatment of choice for stable and aligned fractures without loosening of the femoral component has for long been closed treatment. After initial treatment in a cast for 3–4 weeks, a brace is applied and flexion exercises begun. However, in old debilitated persons this regimen is in practice very difficult to accomplish. Internal fixation is therefore being performed more often in stable fractures also.

Skeletal traction in bed as the only treatment for unstable fractures, is no longer a current treatment option. In an old patient population, often with concurrent diseases, traction in bed implies a great risk of pressure sores, pulmonary complications, etc. Early surgical attempts to overcome this problem included semiflexible rods and blade plates. We advise against the use of Rush rods and lockable Zickel supracondylar rods, which in our experience give a less rigid fixation, notably in osteoporotic bone. However, Ritter et al. [24] reported good results in 20 of 22 cases and Nielsen et al. [32] found it useful in displaced fractures.

Increased knowledge of this type of fracture and development of fixation devices for use in the presence of total knee prostheses has obviously improved the results.

Antegrade intramedullary rods were recommended by Hanks et al. [33] for treatment of supracondylar fractures provided they were located at least 8 cm above the joint line. McLaren et al. [22] were the first to report on the use of locked *retrograde* intramedullary nails which allowed stable fixation also of the more difficult fractures close to the joint line. All their 7 cases healed. Three months postoperatively the loss of motion ranged from 0° to 20°. They reported the procedure to be fairly quick and straightforward and with minimal morbidity (Fig. 23.4). One drawback with this technique is that it cannot be used in cases with a posterior sacrificing

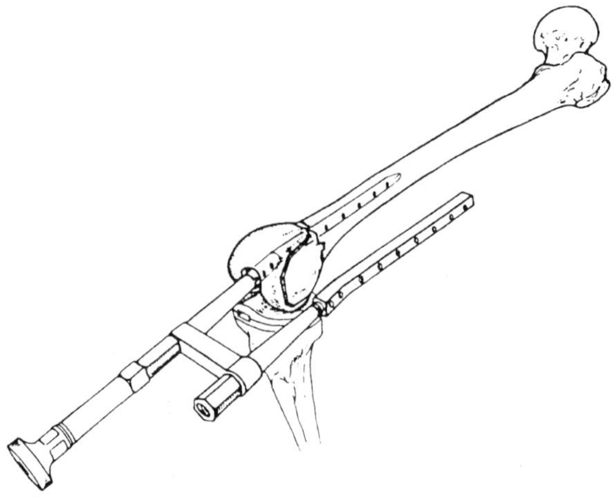

Figure 23.4. The technique for inserting a retrograde intramedullary nail in cases with a supracondylar femoral fracture and anterior cruciate retaining total knee prostheses. Reprinted with permission of Lippincott Williams & Wilkins.

prosthesis, in which the box prevents access to the femoral canal. Since the original report several authors have described the successful use of similar techniques [23,25,26,28] (Fig. 23.5).

In persons with very fragile bone the stability of the fracture may be augmented by bone cement [34]. Bone cement may also be the only way to accomplish a firm grip of screws in the fractured area. In very comminuted fractures the use of a structured distal femoral allograft in combination with a stemmed femoral component may be an option [35,36]. If the femoral component is loose, revision knee arthroplasty using a component with a long stem should be seriously considered irrespective of the type of fracture. Treatment of supracondylar femoral periprosthetic fractures by external fixation is always contraindicated [29].

Fractures of the Tibia

Postoperative periprosthetic fractures of the tibia have been less commonly reported than fractures in the distal femur. The reason may be that treatment is less controversial and less problematic. Of the four fracture types according to Felix et al. [37], type I, consisting of a depression or split of the tibial plateau, is the most common. This fracture mostly occurs without trauma and on the medial side in varus aligned knees. It has been most frequently observed in early prosthetic designs and where the tibial component has loosened. In the latter situation revision surgery is the treatment of choice [37,38]. The less common type II fractures are localized in the methaphysis and occur usually in modern designs after trauma. The tibial component is usually intact and the fracture could be treated in a cast and with partial weightbearing. Type II fractures may also occur in the proximal diaphysis in the case of a long-stemmed cemented component. Such prostheses, which regularly became loose and caused considerable bone loss, have not been used for a long time. Fractures of the tibial shaft and the tibial tubercle – type II and IV – are beyond the scope of this chapter.

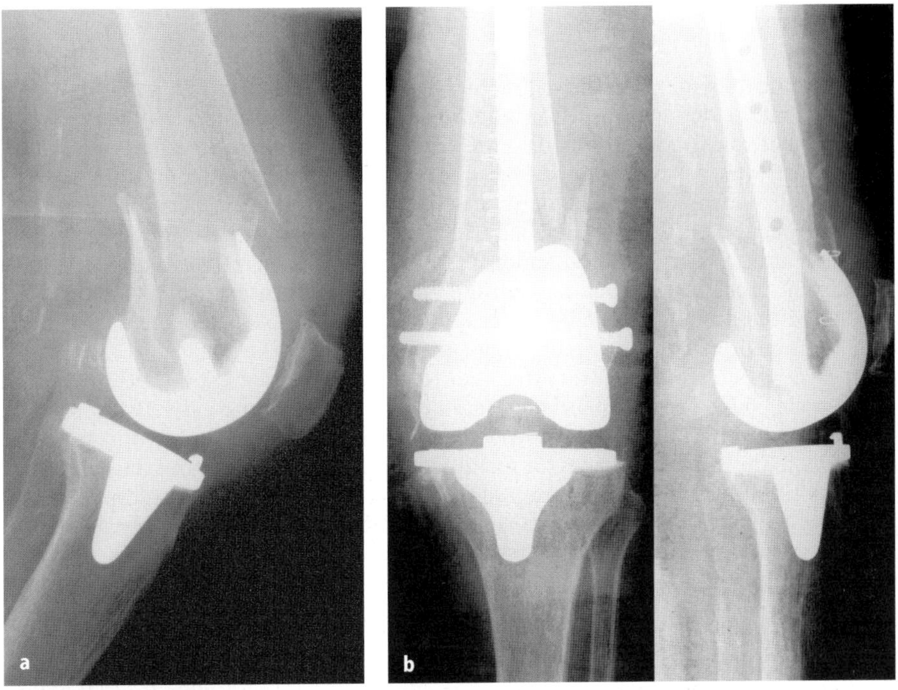

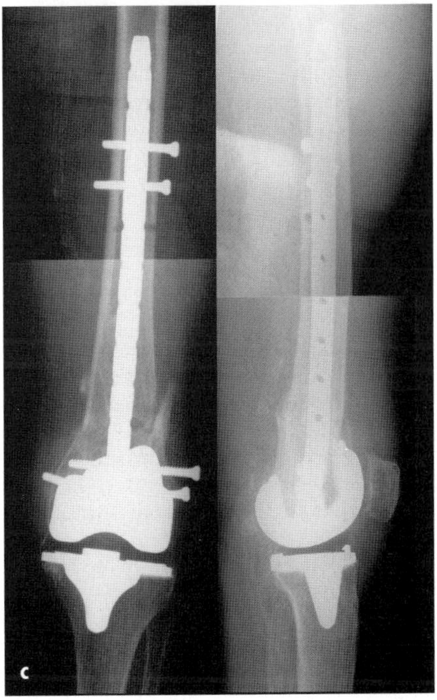

Figure 23.5. A 72-year-old woman who 1 year after total knee surgery sustained a distal ipsilateral supracondylar femoral fracture (**a**). The fracture was reduced and a retrograde intramedullary nail introduced. The nail was locked distally and proximally with screws (**b**). Motion exercises were started after 2 weeks and walking with partial weightbearing after 6 weeks. After 3 months the fracture had healed (**c**).

Summary

The treatment of periprosthetic fractures of the femur after hip and total knee replacements is demanding. If, in addition, the bone is of inferior quality due to osteoporosis, the situation is still more delicate. The optimal treatment obviously depends on whether the component is loose or not, cemented or not, the type and location of the fracture and the physical and mental condition of the patient.

Periacetabular fractures can usually be treated conservatively. A good functional outcome after a periprosthetic femoral fracture most often necessitates some kind of surgical procedure. Dependent on the type and localization of the fracture and quality of the bone, cerclage and wires, plates, revision to a long stem prosthesis and combinations of these methods are available.

Regarding periprosthetic fractures after total knee replacement the treatment has, from having been predominantly conservative in the 1970s and early 1980s, become increasingly active in order to allow early ambulation. This is also demonstrated in Table 23.3. The range of devices for fixation of periprosthetic fractures has increased. Notably the introduction of retrograde intramedullary rods for fixation of supracondylar femoral fractures, which can be introduced through a minimal incision without removing the knee prosthesis, seems to be a major step forwards, although clinical reports are still few.

References

1. Bethea JS, DeAndrade JR, Fleming LL, Lindenbaum SD, Welch RB. Proximal femoral fractures following total hip arthroplasty. Clin Orthop 1982;170:95–106.
2. Johansson JE, McBroom R, Barrington TW, Hunter GA. Fracture of the ipsilateral femur in patients with total hip replacement. J Bone Joint Surg Am 1981;63:1435–1442.
3. Mont MA, Maar DC. Fractures of the ipsilateral femur after hip arthroplasty. J Arthroplasty 1994;9:511–519.
4. Duncan CP, et al.. Fractures of the femur after hip replacement. Instr Course Lect 1995;44:293–304.
5. Malchau H, Herberts P, Ahnfelt L. Prognosis of total hip replacement in Sweden. Acta Orthop Scand 1993;64:497–506.
6. Kolstad K. Revision THR after periprosthetic femoral fractures. Acta Orthop Scand 1994;65:505–508.
7. Jones DG. Bone erosion beneath partridge bands. J Bone Joint Surg Br 1986;68:476–477.
8. Nafei A, Steinke NM, Saeter J, Thomsen PB. Complications after osteosynthesis using Partridge´s method in femoral fracture near the prosthesis. Ugeskr Laeger 1990;152: 1092–1094.
9. Serocki JH, Chandler RW, Dorr LD. Treatment of fractures about hip prostheses with compression plating. J Arthroplasty 1992;7:129–135.
10. Robinson AHN, Ayllon-Garcia A, Hallett JP, Meggitt BF. Periprosthetic fractures of the hip: the Mennen clasp plate. Hip Int 1995;5:20–24.
11. Otremski I, Nusam I, Glickman M, Newman RJ. Mennen paraskeletal plate fixation for fracture of the femoral shaft in association with ipsilateral hip arthroplasty. Injury 1998;29:421–423.
12. Ritter MA, Faris PM, Keating EM. Anterior femoral notching and ipsilateral supracondylar femur fracture in total knee arthroplasty. J Arthroplasty 1988;3:185–187.
13. Merkel KD, Johnson EW Jr. Supracondylar fracture of the femur after total knee arthroplasty. J Bone Joint Surg Am 1986;68:29–43.
14. Figgie MP, Goldberg VM, Figgie HE, Sobel M. The results of treatment of supracondylar

fracture above total knee arthroplasty. J Arthroplasty 1990;5:267–276.
15. Cain PR, Rubash HE, Wissinger HGA, McClain EJ. Periprosthetic femoral fractures following total knee arthroplasty. Clin Orthop 1986;208:205–214.
16. Culp RW, Schmidt RG, Hanks G, Mak A, Esterhai JL Jr, Heppenstall RB. Supracondylar fracture of the femur following prosthetic knee arthroplasty. Clin Orthop 1987;222: 212–222.
17. Hirsh DM, Bhalla S, Roffman M. Supracondylar fracture of the femur following total knee replacement. Report of four cases. J Bone Joint Surg Am 1981;63:162–163.
18. Short WH, Hootnick DR, Murray DG. Ipsilateral supracondylar femur fractures following knee arthroplasty. Clin Orthop 1981;158:111–116.
19. Sisto DJ, Lachiewicz PF, Insall JN. Treatment of supracondylar fractures following prosthetic arthroplasty of the knee. Clin Orthop 1985;196:265–272.
20. Cordeiro EN, Costa RC, Carazzato JG, Silva J dos S. Periprosthetic fractures in patients with total knee arthroplasties. Clin Orthop 1990;252:182–189.
21. Healy WL, Siliski JM, Incavo SJ. Operative treatment of distal femoral fractures proximal to total knee replacements. J Bone Joint Surg Am 1993;75:27–34.
22. McLaren AC, Dupont JA, Schroeber DC. Open reduction internal fixation of supracondylar fractures above total knee arthroplasties using the intramedullary supracondylar rod. Clin Orthop 1994;302:194–198.
23. Jabczenski FF, Crawford M. Retrograde intramedullary nailing of supracondylar femur fractures above total knee arthroplasty. J Arthroplasty 1995;10:95–101.
24. Ritter MA, Keating EM, Faris PM, Meding JB. Rush rod fixation of supracondylar fractures above total knee arthroplasties. J Arthroplasty 1995;10:213–216.
25. Murrell GA, Nunley JA. Interlocked supracondylar intramedullary nails for supracondylar fractures after total knee arthroplasty. A new treatment method. J Arthroplasty 1995;10:37–42.
26. Rolston LR, Christ DJ, Halpern A, O´Connor PL, Ryan TG, Uggen WM. Treatment of supracondylar fractures of the femur proximal to total knee arthroplasty. 1995;J Bone Joint Surg Am 77:924–931.
27. Moran MC, Brick GW, Sledge CB, Dysart SH, Chien EP. Supracondylar femoral fracture following total knee arthroplasty. Clin Orthop 1996;324:196–209.
28. Smith WJ, Martin SL, Mabrey JD. Use of a supracondylar nail for treatment of a supracondylar fracture of the femur following total knee arthroplasty. J Arthroplasty 1996; 11:210–213.
29. Engh GA, Ammeen DJ. Periprosthetic fractures adjacent to total knee implants: treatment and clinical results. Instr Course Lect 1998;47:437–448.
30. Ayers DC. Supracondylar fracture of the distal femur proximal to a total knee replacement. Instr Course Lect 1997;46:197–203.
31. Dennis DA. Periprosthetic fractures following total knee arthroplasty: the good, bad, & ugly. Orthopedics 1998;21:1048–1050.
32. Nielsen BF, Petersen VS, Varmarken JE. Fracture of the femur after knee arthroplasty. Acta Orthop Scand 1988;59:155–157.
33. Hanks GA, Mathews HH, Routson GW, Loughran TP. Supracondylar fracture of the femur following total knee arthroplasty. J Arthroplasty 1989;4:289–292.
34. Zehntner MK, Ganz R. Internal fixation of supracondylar fractures after condylar total knee arthroplasty. Clin Orthop 1993;293:219–224.
35. Gross AE. Revision total knee arthroplasty of bone grafts versus implant supplementation. Orthopedics 1997;20:843–844.
36. Ghazavi MT, Stockley I, Yee G, Davis A, Gross AK. Reconstruction of massive bone defects with allograft in revision total knee arthroplasty. J Bone Joint Surg Am 1997;79:17–25.
37. Felix NA, Stuart MJ, Hanssen AD. Periprosthetic fractures of the tibia associated with total knee arthroplasty. Clin Orthop 1997;345:113–124.
38. Rand JA, Coventry MB. Stress fractures after total knee arthroplasty. J Bone Joint Surg Am 1980;62:226–233.

Part IV

Nonpharmacological Prevention of Osteoporotic Fractures

24 Prevention of Falls

L. Wehren and J. Magaziner

Introduction

An important component of reducing disability among the elderly lies in fall prevention, and in prevention or amelioration of the injuries that occur as a consequence of falls. As the elderly and particularly the oldest of the old become a progressively larger segment of the population during the next 25 to 30 years, the personal and societal burdens of falling and its consequent morbidity and mortality will increase dramatically unless we develop effective means of managing risk factors for falls and injuries. Risk factors and management options differ somewhat for community-dwelling older persons and those who are in long-term care institutional settings, and throughout this chapter relevant differences will be indicated. Those who have fallen and sustained fractures comprise a population of special interest, because of their increased susceptibility to future adverse events.

Magnitude of the Problem

Prevalence

Approximately one-third of community-dwelling people aged 65 years and older and 50–60% of those in nursing homes and homes for the elderly fall each year [1–7]. The best estimates of rates of falling come from prospective studies. In a population-based study conducted in New Zealand among 684 persons aged 70 years and over, 507 falls occurred during 1 year of follow-up: 39.6% of women and 28.4% of men experienced at least one fall [4]. Similar findings have come from a study conducted in the United States among people aged 75 years or older [3], in which 34.6% of women and 29.1% of men fell at least once during the 12 months duration of the study. A survey conducted in Oxford, England found that, until about age 45 years, men experienced more falls than did women, but that the percentage of women falling increased sharply among those aged 50–54 years and this percentage remained higher than that reported by men for all older age groups [8]. Epidemiological studies have consistently shown higher rates of falling for women, in both community and institutional settings [1–4,6,7,9–24]. Similarly, some racial differences have been identified. Among Japanese men and women living in Hawaii, only 16.3% of women and 8.7% of men fell during 1 year of follow-up [13]. These rates are approximately half those seen among Caucasians of the same ages. Other studies also suggest that falling rates are lower for African-Americans than for Caucasian Americans [3, 19].

Consequences of Falls

Injury occurs in only a small percentage of falls, but fall-related injuries can be severe. Serious injuries (fractures, dislocations, head injuries or serious soft tissue damage) follow about 10–15% of falls among community-dwelling older persons [5,10,15,17,21,22,24–28]; about 15–20% of falls among institutionalized elderly result in serious injury [5,14,28]. Women are more likely than men to sustain serious injury, especially fractures, as a consequence of falling [10,15,17,22,27,29,30]. Fractures occur in from 3% to 12% of falls in the elderly; hip fractures follow about 1% of falls [10,13,14,17,19,26,30,31]. In many who fall, injuries such as hypothermia, pneumonia, dehydration and pressure injuries occur as a consequence of an inability to rise after falling [15,24]. Inability to rise without assistance has been reported in approximately 40–50% of falls in the elderly [32–34]. Minor injuries [abrasions, bruises, lacerations, or sprains] are seen in 40–50% of falls [26,35]. Falls are associated with a decline in functional status over the next 2–4 years [36,37], so the impact of the fall is not restricted to the event itself. The psychological impact of falling may also be clinically important. A substantial proportion of those who fall report a fear of falling again and may limit activities as a consequence, establishing a cycle of progressive functional impairment [3,15,26,38,39].

For those falls in which injury occurs, utilization of medical care is substantial: emergency rooms, physicians, hospitals and rehabilitation/extended care facilities are all involved in injury management. Approximately 70% of injuries among those 60 years of age or older who are treated at emergency departments have occurred as a consequence of falls, according to a study conducted in Sweden [40]. In the United States, it has been reported that over 40% of fall-related emergency department visits result in hospital admission [27]. Over 40% of persons who sustain injurious falls that require hospitalization are discharged to an extended care facility, and an additional 10% require assistance at home after discharge [26,33,41,42]. In the United States, falls account for the second greatest injury-related economic costs, and the lifetime costs of falls are greatest among the elderly [43].

Falling is an important cause of mortality among the elderly. According to the most current information available for the United States [44], unintentional injuries are the seventh most common cause of death among those aged 65 years and older, and falls are responsible for 23% of these injury deaths. Among persons aged 85 years and older, falls are responsible for 34% of all injury mortality. National Safety Council data for 1997 are shown in Fig. 24.1, from which the exponential increase in fall-related mortality with advancing age can clearly be seen, as can its contrast with that seen in other types of injury [45]. Despite the higher frequency of fall-related injury and fracture among women, men are more likely to die as a consequence of fall-related injury [17,27].

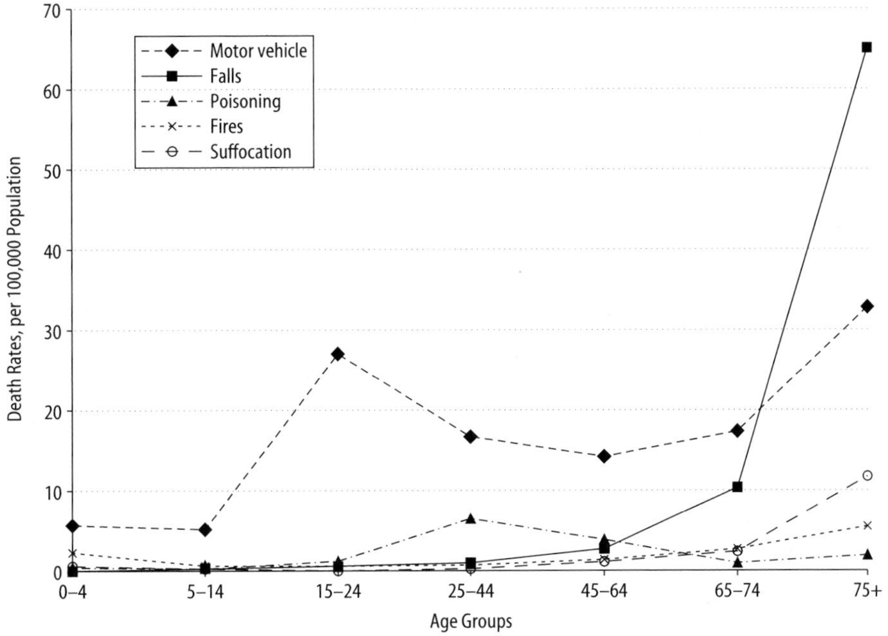

Figure 24.1. Death from unintentional injuries, United States, 1997. Data from the National Safety Council.

Risk Factors for Falls, Injuries and Fractures

Risk factors for falls and for fall-related injuries have been studied extensively. *Intrinsic risk factors* for falls (shown in Table 24.1) include older age, female gender, low body mass, medical comorbidities, musculoskeletal diseases, cognitive impairments, gait and balance disorders, sensory impairments, postural hypotension, having a history of previous falls, and use of certain medications, including long- and medium-acting benzodiazepines, sedative-hypnotic drugs, antidepressants, antihypertensive medications, anti-arrhythmic drugs, diuretics and antiseizure medications [1–4,6,10–12,16,19,20,22,30–32,46–49]. Postmenopausal status, independently of age, is also a risk factor for falls among women [50]. In addition, environmental hazards and the duration of exposure to them comprise *extrinsic risk factors* [1,10,15,17,26,35,51]. These include throw rugs, slippery and uneven floor surfaces, poor lighting, electrical cords that can be tripped over, footstools without handrails, slippery tub surfaces and unsuitable footwear. These extrinsic factors play a progressively smaller role in falls with advancing age, largely because intrinsic factors that affect the likelihood of falling assume a much more important role as the burden of chronic illness accumulates [7,20,52].

Risk factors for fracture and other fall-related injuries are similar to those for falling, but additionally include low bone mineral density and fall characteristics such as frequency, direction of the fall, and force of impact [29,30,32,53–56]. Risk factors for injury may differ among those who are independent and those who are

Table 24.1. Intrinsic risk factors for falling

Increasing age	
Female gender	
Decreasing body mass	
Postmenopausal status	
Medical comorbidities	
	Cardiovascular disease
	Diabetes mellitus
Musculoskeletal and neurological diseases	
	Arthritis
	Parkinson's disease
	Seizure disorder
Cognitive impairments	
	Dementia
	Alzheimer's disease
Gait and balance disorders	
Sensory impairments	
	Visual
	Auditory
	Vestibular
	Proprioceptive
Postural hypotension	
History of falling	
Medication effects	
	Long-acting benzodiazepines
	Medium-acting benzodiazepines
	Sedative-hypnotic drugs
	Anti-depressants
	Antihypertensives
	Anti-arrhythmics
	Diuretics
	Antiseizure drugs
Alcohol	

impaired in activities of daily living: risk factors for injury among the impaired have been shown to include not being married (unmarried, divorced, or widowed), a low body mass index, use of long-acting benzodiazepines, poor distant visual acuity and incomplete step continuity, whereas for those who were independent the presence of peripheral neuropathy and insomnia was important [57].

Prevention of Falls

The remainder of this chapter will address the currently available evidence about risk factors and interventions to reduce either the chance of falling or of experiencing adverse consequences. Relationships among the risk factors, falling, and fall consequences are complex, so that it may be difficult to reduce the risk of falling or the risk of injurious falls by modification of these factors. In addition, the effectiveness of many of the strategies discussed has not been demonstrated in randomized, controlled clinical trials nor have prospective studies, for the most part, provided follow-up for periods longer than 1 year, so inferences of effectiveness need to be made with caution. Still, many of the interventions appear to be beneficial, and in the absence of evidence that they could be harmful, warrant consideration.

Table 24.2. Environmental hazard modifications: Safety checklist for fall prevention in the home

Kitchen
Eliminate throw rugs
Use non-skid wax on floor
Keep frequently used items within easy reach
For items stored on high shelves, use assistive device or stepstool with handrail
Wipe up spills immediately
Bathroom
Eliminate throw rugs
Install night light
Use non-skid floor wax
Use rubber mat or adhesive non-slip pads in the tub or shower
Install grab rails at toilet, shower, and tub
Use shower stool
Keep bath/shower supplies (soap, shampoo washcloth) within easy reach
Consider installation of elevated toilet seat
Bedroom
Install night light
Be certain pathway to bedroom is unobstructed and well-lighted
Check height of bed for ease of transfer
Consider installation of bedrails
Use firm mattress
Consider bedside commode
Consider bedside telephone
Stairways
Be certain that stairs are well-lighted, especially at top and bottom
Be certain that handrails are sturdy and securely fastened
Be certain that steps are in good repair and have non-slip surfaces
Consider marking edges of steps, especially at top and bottom
If steps are carpeted, be sure this is well secured
General
Eliminate clutter, especially from floors
Keep traffic paths (hallways, within and between rooms) free of furniture
Install wall switches near doorways of all rooms
Keep floor surfaces between rooms even
Be sure carpeting is securely tacked down and has low pile
Have flashlights readily available in case of power failure
Be sure that electrical and telephone cords are well away from traffic paths
Use lightbulbs of adequate wattage in lighting fixtures
Consider use of assistive devices for walking and reaching
Clothing
Footwear should provide good traction and fit well
Avoid footwear with high heels or open backs or sides
Be sure that bedroom slippers fit well and stay securely on feet
Avoid floor-length robes
Wear clothing that is comfortable and allows easy movement
Outdoors
Keep walkways unobstructed and well-lighted
Clear snow and ice from walkways
Avoid soft or uneven surfaces when walking
Store lawn and garden tools and hoses when not in use
Eliminate gravel from driveway

Extrinsic Risk Factors

Environmental hazards are among the most straightforward to modify. While the effectiveness of these modifications has not been demonstrated in controlled trials, it seems reasonable to make the home environment as free as possible from elements that could lead to falls or increase fear of falling. Checklists of potential environmental hazards have been published [15,51,58–60], so that potentially dangerous elements can be identified readily by older persons, their families or health care providers. These alterations may enable the older person to be more independent within the home and to feel more secure in his or her home environment. A list of suggested modifications, compiled from the sources cited above, is shown in Table 24.2. Similar considerations for lighting, floor surfaces, clutter and grab-bars apply to long-term care facilities [61,62]. In addition, furniture, especially bedside tables and chairs, should be stable and not able to slip or roll. Handrails should line hallways and equipment should not obstruct access to these. Of course, nurse call-buttons must be easily accessible.

Studies of extrinsic risk factors have shown mixed results. A study of persons who sought medical care at hospitals as a consequence of fall-related injuries found no significant difference in environmental hazards among the cases and age- and gender- matched controls [63]. A trial of home hazard reduction that included home inspection, repair advice (but not the actual repairs) and four group meetings to address behavioral and physical aspects of fall risk, demonstrated only a minimal, nonsignificant decrease in falls in the intervention group [64]. On the other hand, a study of falling among community-dwelling elderly who agreed to have a free home safety inspection and simple home modifications (floor treatments and grab-rails) found over a 50% reduction in the number of falls sustained by participants during the 12 months after the modifications as compared with the preceding 12 months [65]. Home hazard reduction has been evaluated as part of a multifactorial intervention in the Frailty and Injuries: Cooperative Studies of Intervention Techniques (FICSIT) trial [66]. FICSIT is the largest trial of fall prevention conducted to date [67]. The multifactorial intervention, which also included medication adjustments and exercise programs, produced a significant decrease in falling after 1 year [68]. Because of the simultaneous alteration of several factors in this study, however, it is impossible to determine the relative contributions of individual modifications.

Medications

Considerable attention has been given to the use of specific medications that present risk to older persons. Medication use is very common among the elderly: in the United States approximately 30% of all prescriptions written are attributable to this 13% segment of the population [69]. The elderly experience a high risk of medication-related adverse events, the frequency of which increase with multiple drug use [69–72]. Although literature on the association of medication use and the risk of falling and injury is extensive, many studies were not designed specifically to address this question, and consequently have methodological limitations. Many studies failed to control for potential confounding by indication for use of the medication (if the disease itself affects the risk of falling), differential prescribing among those who have a history of falling, or duration of drug use or dosage. As a consequence, results have not been entirely consistent [73,74].

Psychoactive drug use has been associated with decreased tactile sensitivity, diminished dynamic balance, reduced quadriceps strength (in women) and increased postural sway on soft surfaces (in women) [47]. Weiner and colleagues [75] found that, even after adjusting for age, cognitive status, mobility status and depression, use of one such drug in elderly men was associated with a 50% increase in the likelihood of falling and use of two or more with over a twofold increase. Similarly, a study of community-dwelling elderly persons in Nottingham, England identified significant associations of falling with the use of sedative-hypnotic and antidepressant medications, although other medication use (including diuretics, antihypertensives and tranquilizers) was not a significant predictor of falls [12]. Cumming et al. [76] found that use of diuretics and diazepam was associated with the risk of multiple falls, after adjusting for potential confounders including medical conditions. Hale et al. [77] studied the prevalence of fainting, dizziness, and "blacking out" among community-dwelling elderly persons who used any of nine categories of antihypertensive medication, and found that women on these medications experienced significantly more of these central nervous system symptoms than did women who were not taking them.

In contrast, Nygaard [78], who studied long-term care residents in Norway, found no significant differences in drug use among fallers and non-fallers, although there was a tendency to increased falling among users of antipsychotic medications. Further, he found that among residents with restricted mobility who required a walking frame for ambulation or who were wheelchair users, use of hypnotics/anxiolytics was associated with a decreased risk of falling. As the author points out, depression and anxiety are themselves risk factors for falling, and amelioration of these conditions with medication may diminish the risk of falling to a greater extent than effects of the medication may increase it. This highlights the important question of whether a disease or the medication used for its treatment is the relevant risk factor for falling. Two studies conducted in long-term care facilities found an increased risk of falling among those who used certain drugs; this risk was more strongly associated with the drugs being used than with the diagnoses or with the degree of illness of the fallers [16,79].

Certain medications have also been shown to increase body sway, which is a measure of compensatory mechanisms used to maintain balance [80,81]. Thioridazine, a neuroleptic medication that is commonly used in nursing homes to manage dementia-related behavioral problems, has been shown to increase postural sway in both young (aged 20–42 years) and older (aged 70–76 years) men [80]. Diazepam, a long-acting benzodiazepine, has been shown to affect several components of the homeostatic balance mechanism in elderly persons. In addition to increasing postural sway, a single dose increases muscle latency in response to sudden perturbation and impairs neurocognitive performance [82].

A recent systematic review of English-language literature on drugs and risk of falling among the elderly provided evidence regarding psychotropic [83], cardiac and analgesic drugs [84]. Significant associations were reported for risk of falling with the use of any psychotropic medication, neuroleptics, sedative-hypnotics, antidepressants, short- and long-acting benzodiazepines, and the use of diuretics, type Ia antiarrhythmics and digoxin.

It is known that pharmacokinetics (how the body deals with a medication) are altered in the elderly, but changes in pharmacodynamics (drug actions) with aging are less well understood [85]. The processes by which drugs are metabolized, distributed and excreted change with advancing age because of changes in physiology.

It appears that even when controlling for pharmacokinetic changes, certain drugs, including benzodiazepines, opiates, anticholinergics, dopamine antagonists and antihypertensives, may have more potent effects in elderly persons [85]. Additionally, drug–drug interactions are common among medications utilized in older patients [70]. For all these reasons, it is essential to prescribe medications carefully and to monitor their effects closely in elderly patients.

The most carefully constructed recommendations for prescribing in the elderly have come from a group of experts in geriatrics from the United States and Canada [86]. Using a modified Delphi consensus approach, they compiled a detailed list of prescription medications that should be avoided in nursing home residents over the age of 65 years, among which are many that are associated with an increased risk of falling. These medications include certain sedative-hypnotics (diazepam, chlordiazepoxide, flurazepam, meprobamate, pentobarbital, secobarbital), the antidepressant amitriptyline, combination antidepressant and antipsychotic medications, propranolol, methyldopa, reserpine, and the anti-emetic trimethobenzamide. (Other medications were included on the list because of toxicities and lack of efficacy.) Wilcox and colleagues [87], using data collected from a nationally representative sample of 14 000 households in the United States (National Medical Expenditure Survey), estimated the prevalence of use of these medications and found that 23.5% of community-dwelling persons aged 65 years and older had received at least one of the non-recommended medications during 1987, and that use of potentially inappropriate medications was highest among those aged 80 to 84 years. Data from southern California showed that 20% of persons over age 65 years had used benzodiazepine medications at least twice during the preceding 12 months, and that 44% of those using benzodiazepine used long-acting forms, with diazepam the most commonly prescribed agent [88]. Benzodiazepine use was not, however, associated with falls during the preceding year.

Successful efforts have been made to modify prescribing behavior of physicians through educational programs designed to increase awareness of the hazards associated with medications [89]. Avorn et al. [90] conducted a randomized trial among nursing homes in which medical staff in some of the facilities received an educational intervention in which use of long-acting benzodiazepines, all antipsychotic medications, diphenhydramine, amitriptyline and doxepin was discouraged. After the 5 month intervention, use of these agents decreased approximately 27% in the intervention facilities, significantly more than was seen in the control facilities, and investigators found less deterioration in cognitive functioning, greater improvement in functional status, and no increase in disruptive behavior of residents in the intervention facilities. Falls were not explicitly measured as an outcome. Although medication adjustment has been a component of successful multifactorial fall reduction interventions [26,68], the importance of the medication element cannot be assessed.

Balance

Although balance may be considered a singular function, in reality it comprises several elements that interrelate in complex ways, so that disorders of balance are a heterogeneous group of dysfunctions involving one or more of the component systems [91–93]. It has been estimated that approximately 80% of falls among the elderly can be attributed to disorders of gait and balance [94], and studies have shown that postural instability is associated with an increased risk of falling and fracture [25,47,95]. The functions that regulate balance are under complex physiological control, involving sensory input, cerebral and cerebellar coordination, and neuromuscular function [96–98].

Postural Control

Postural control has been defined as "the maintenance of the body center of mass over its base of support or, more generally, within the limits of stability", in both static and dynamic situations [97]. The limits of stability depend on the biomechanics of the individual, the requirements of the task and the conditions of the support surface [97]. Changes in all functional realms occur with aging and with the development of chronic diseases associated with advancing age. Elderly women have demonstrated more pronounced impairment in postural control than men of comparable age, which plays an important role in their greater likelihood of falling [99].

Impairments in Visual Acuity and the Visual Field

Impairments in visual acuity and visual field develop progressively after age 50 years [100], and both falling and fall-related injury are associated with these decrements [48,101–103]. Impaired dark adaptation [104] and visual depth illusion (in which faulty visual fixation results in misperception of the distance of objects) [105] have also been associated with loss of balance and falling. There is also evidence to suggest that the elderly become progressively more dependent on visual stimuli to maintain postural control, so that deterioration in vision has an exaggerated influence [106,107].

Decline in Vestibular Function

Decline in vestibular function with advancing age and consequent vertigo produce increased postural sway and loss of balance [48,108], as do age- and disease-related alterations in somatosensory input [48,109]. Peripheral neuropathy that develops as a consequence of diabetes mellitus has been shown to affect postural control adversely [110]. Proprioceptive awareness of foot position declines with age, and can also be adversely affected by footwear [111], including soft, resilient soles [112,113] and high heels [114,115]. Impaired proprioception and vestibular function may force greater dependence on visual cues and increase the risk of falling.

Integration of Sensory Inputs

Integration of sensory inputs by the central nervous system becomes less efficient with advancing age, so that postural responses are slowed [116,117]. Dementia is also associated with postural instability [3]. Distractibility, or compromise of attention to standing or walking by addition of cognitive or manual tasks, has been shown to increase with aging and to increase postural instability [118,119]. The elderly are also susceptible to vertigo [120] and to defective blood pressure homeostasis, including both postprandial and orthostatic hypotension, both of which cause loss of balance [121,122].

Estrogen

Because of the well-documented increase in the risk of falling among women following menopause [8,50] and the greater degree of postural instability seen in women compared with men [99], a possible role for estrogen has been investigated. One study of women over the age of 65 years reported no difference between current users of estrogen and never users in reported falls or in measured gait speed, hip abductor strength, triceps extensor strength, or balance [123]. In contrast, Naessen et al. [124] compared long-term users of estradiol with non-users (mean age 68 years) and found significantly better postural balance among estrogen users. Similarly, Hammar et al. [125] studied the effect of estrogen replacement on balance in women of mean age 54 years. Balance perfomance was significantly improved on the two most difficult tests, in which sensory inputs were either cancelled or distorted, after only 4 weeks' use of estrogen. This improvement was maintained through 12 weeks of estrogen use and was not attenuated by the addition of progestin. The authors note that since baseline performance on the easier tests was well within normal limits, improvement could not be measured.

Gait

Gait disorders have been linked to risk of falling among both the community-dwelling elderly and nursing home residents [3,126–129]. Gait depends on multiple functions, including all those that contribute to balance, and both age- and disease-related changes are apparent in the gait of elderly persons. Older persons walk more slowly, take shorter steps, and spend a higher percentage of walking time with both feet on the ground than do younger persons [130–134]. In some elderly persons a shuffling "senile gait" develops, in which the feet are not lifted from the floor [135]. Muscular strength in the lower extremities is an important component of gait [136]: weakness of both quadriceps and ankle dorsiflexor muscles has been demonstrated in the elderly and has been shown to affect gait [129,137]. Muscle mass and strength are known to decline with age, with the decline beginning at an earlier age in women [138–141]. Symptoms of depression, especially psychomotor retardation, are also associated with gait impairment [142], although because persons with depression may be less active, falls may not be increased. A variety of tools have been developed to assess gait and balance in the elderly, using both functional and technology-based measures [127,143–147].

Exercise Interventions

It is difficult to separate effects of exercise on strength and balance, since interventions designed to affect either of these parameters have some effects on both, and it is likely that the combination of effects is important. Studies of postural sway and risk of falling have found only limited associations [148,149]. Hughes and associates [150] found no associations between measured postural sway and functional performance, suggesting that it is less a measure of functional status than of sensorimotor deficits. Tinetti and colleagues [3] found that although balance and gait were related to the risk of falling, cognitive impairment and medication use had stronger associations. Trials of interventions to improve balance have not consistently demonstrated substantial benefit. For example, regular brisk walking has been shown to be associated with greater postural stability in some studies [151], but a randomized intervention study of brisk walking found that falls were increased among members of the intervention group, although fracture injuries were not [152].

Balance Training

Earlier studies on balance training, in which falls were not assessed, reported some improvement in balance after interventions [153]. More recent studies, utilizing larger groups, have found that exercise interventions improved balance and decreased the risk of falling, with the greatest effect seen among those who were most compliant with the intervention [154,155]. In several recent studies, t'ai chi has been shown to be an effective intervention for balance training in the elderly. A study from Taiwan demonstrated that those who performed t'ai chi had less postural sway and better ankle dorsiflexor strength than did those with no t'ai chi experience [156], and regular practice of t'ai chi has also been shown to be associated with better preservation of cardiorespiratory function [157]. In a randomized trial of balance and strength training at the University of Connecticut FICSIT site, t'ai chi was used during a 26 week maintenance phase and was shown to sustain improvements throughout this period [158]. A more direct test of the effect of t'ai chi on falling was conducted at the Atlanta FICSIT site, in which it was found that although t'ai chi did not improve postural stability, fear of falling decreased and the risk of multiple falls declined by almost 50% in the intervention group [159–161].

Resistance Training

Resistance training has shown several benefits, including muscle hypertrophy, improved resistance to the development of disability, improved gait stability and increased functional capacity, even when subjects are frail, extremely elderly and residents in nursing homes [162–167]. Continued improvement with weight training has been shown for as long as 2 years [168]. Benefits of exercise have also been demonstrated in the early rehabilitation phase following hip fracture, as well as several months after the injury [169]. Reinsch and colleagues [170] failed to demonstrate a benefit from a combined program of exercise and cognitive-behavioral interventions, but their study population was relatively healthy and active and the exercise intervention was of low intensity. Another trial of a low-intensity exercise program combined with home safety assessment and behavioral risk modification demonstrated a small but significant reduction in the risk of falling [64]. At the Yale FICSIT site, a multifactorial intervention that included several types of exercise and balance training, as well as home hazard reduction, medication changes, and education demonstrated a 30% decrease in the odds of falling during 1 year of follow-up [68]. Rizzo and colleagues [26] demonstrated the cost-effectiveness of similar interventions in the community-dwelling elderly.

Modest, nonsignificant reductions in falls have been shown in nursing home residents after low-intensity physical rehabilitation [171]. Two FICSIT sites (San Antonio and Boston) conducted studies of more intense exercise, but were too short (16 weeks and 10 weeks, respectively) to demonstrate significant effects on falling [159]. Another strategy that has been tested in nursing home residents is the use of hip pads. Although these do not decrease the risk of falling, hip fracture occurrence is decreased among residents who wear these protective pads [172].

Compliance with use of pads has been problematic, however, especially among the cognitively impaired [173,174].

Mechanical Restraints

Many elderly residents of long-term care facilities in the United States are physically restrained at one time or another during their stay, with devices including Posey jackets, wrist and ankle restraints, lap belts, bedrails and restraining chairs. Although use of restraints has declined, the most common reasons given for use of restraints are prevention of wandering and prevention of fall-related injury [28,175]. Restraints are more commonly used in those who have cognitive impairments [175–177]. Risks associated with the use of restraints include accidental death from strangulation, impairment of circulation, nerve damage, increased agitation, skin injury, progressive muscle weakness and functional decline, incontinence, pressure ulcers and psychological sequelae [176]. Despite their use, there has been little evidence to document the effectiveness of restraints. As noted by Marks [176], the incidence of falls in acute care settings in England, where restraints are less commonly used than in the United States, is lower than that seen in the United States. Similarly, in a long-term care facility in England, falls were found to be most uncommon during the night, despite a prohibition on use of bed rails [178]. In a cohort of residents in skilled nursing care facilities who were unrestrained at baseline, and who subsequently became restrained, restraint use was independently associated with risk of serious fall-related injury relative to the unrestrained residents, even after controlling for other injury risk factors [28]. Several studies have now reported the consequences of efforts to reduce the use of restraints in both acute care and long-term care settings. Powell et al. [179] reported results from an acute care geriatric hospital in Winnipeg, Canada, in which restraint use application decreased from 52 per 1000 patient-days to 0.3 per 1000 patient-days, with a concomitant nonsignificant change in the incidence of falls. Bloom and Braun [180] found decreased agitation, fewer falls, improved sleep patterns, elimination of pressure ulcers, and an improved atmosphere of respect for the residents from the staff after elimination of restraints in almost all residents. Results from a study of restraint reduction in a group of seven nursing homes demonstrated a significant increase in the number of falls, but no increase in injurious falls [181]. Alternative strategies, including exercise, need to be implemented when restraint reduction is undertaken, because of the frailty of those residents and because many of the cognitively impaired are prone to "wander". Schnelle et al. [182] conducted a randomized controlled trial of an exercise protocol among physically restrained nursing home residents and found significant improvements in measures of injury risk and upper extremity strength. Several programs have been developed for management of wanderers without use of restraints [180,181,183].

Summary and Recommendations for the Orthopedist

Many of the risk factors associated with falling and injury are amenable to modification. Because of the prevalence of falls and serious fall-related injuries among the elderly, it is incumbent on medical professionals to minimize these occurrences by managing and modifying risk. Because previous falls are an independent risk factor for subsequent falls, it is especially important to investigate any individual who has fallen, particularly if injury has resulted, in order to determine the presence of any modifiable risk factors for that individual. This has been successfully utilized in PROFET [Prevention of Falls in the Elderly Trial], in which intervention decreased falls by 70% among patients who had presented to emergency departments with fall-related injuries [184]. The key elements of such programs of risk reduction are:

1. Individualized management, so that factors that are relevant to the individual are addressed;
2. Minimizing environmental hazards;
3. Reducing medication and multiple medication use;
4. Education of the individual in behavioral strategies to allow completion of tasks with minimal risk;
5. Education in techniques for rising from falls; and
6. Exercise programs to improve strength, balance and aerobic capacity.

Implementation of these strategies will not eliminate falls or fall-related injuries, but can result in substantial decreases in their incidence. The orthopedist, who is called upon to treat many such patients, is ideally placed to initiate and implement fall risk reduction programs.

Acknowledgement: The authors wish to acknowledge the sources of support for this project. These are the following grants: Training Grant NIA T32AG00262-01 and NIA R37 AG09901.

References

1. Prudham D, Evans JG. Factors associated with falls in the elderly: a community study. Age Ageing 1981;10:141–146.
2. Campbell AJ, Reinken J, Allan BC, Martinez GS. Falls in old age: a study of frequency and related clinical factors. Age Ageing 1981;10:264–270.
3. Tinetti ME, Speechley M, Ginter SF. Risk factors for falls among elderly persons living in the community. N Engl J Med 1988;319:1701–1707.
4. Campbell AJ, Borrie MJ, Spears GF. Risk factors for falls in a community-based prospective study of people 70 years and older. J Gerontol 1989;44:M112–M117.
5. Tinetti ME. Factors associated with serious injury during falls by ambulatory nursing home residents. J Am Geriatr Soc 1987;35:644–648.
6. Lipsitz LA, Jonnson PV, Kelley MM, Koestner JS. Causes and correlates of recurrent falls in ambulatory frail elderly. J Gerontol 1991;46:M114–M122.
7. Perry BC. Falls among the elderly: a review of the methods and conclusions of epidemiologic studies. J Am Geriatr Soc 1982;30:367–371.
8. Winner SJ, Morgan CA, Evans JG. Perimenopausal risk of falling and incidence of distal forearm fracture. BMJ 1989;298:1486–1488.
9. Stewart RB, Moore MT, May FE, Marks RG, Hale WE. Nocturia: a risk factor for falls in the elderly. J Am Geriatr Soc 1992;40:1217–1220.
10. Baker SP, Harvey AH. Fall injuries in the elderly. Clin Geriatr Med 1985;1:501–512.
11. Berg WP, Alessio HM, Mills EM, Tong C. Circumstances and consequences of falls in independent community-dwelling older adults. Age Ageing 1997;26:261–268.
12. Blake AJ, Morgan K, Bendall MJ, et al. Falls by elderly people at home: prevalence and associated factors. Age Ageing 1988;17:365–372.

13. Davis JW, Ross PD, Nevitt MC, Wasnich RD. Incidence rates of falls among Japanese men and women living in Hawaii. J Clin Epidemiol 1997;50:589–594.
14. Gryfe CI, Amies A, Ashley MJ. A longitudinal study of falls in an elderly population. I. Incidence and morbidity. Age Ageing 1977;6:201–210.
15. Kellogg International Work Group. The prevention of falls in later life: a report of the Kellogg International Work Group on the Prevention of Falls by the Elderly. Dan Med Bull 1987;34(Suppl 4):1–24.
16. Kerman M, Mulvihill M. The role of medication in falls among the elderly in a long-term care facility. Mount Sinai J Med 1990;57:343–347.
17. Lucht U. A prospective study of accidental falls and resulting injuries in the home among elderly people. Acta Soc Med Scand 1971;2:105–120.
18. Morris EV, Isaacs B. The prevention of falls in a geriatric hospital. Age Ageing 1980;9:181–185.
19. Nevitt MC, Cummings ST, Kidd S, Black D. Risk factors for nonsyncopal falls: a prospective study. JAMA 1989;261:2663–2668.
20. Nickens H. Intrinsic factors in falling among the elderly. Arch Intern Med 1985;145: 1089–1093.
21. Speechley M, Tinetti M. Falls and injuries in frail and vigorous community elderly persons. J Am Geriatr Soc 1991;39:46–52.
22. Tromp AM, Smit JH, Deeg DJH, Bouter LM, Lips P. Predictors for falls and fractures in the Longitudinal Aging Sudy Amsterdam. J Bone Miner Res 1998;13:1932–1939.
23. Wickham C, Cooper C, Margetts BM, Barker DJP. Muscle strength, activity, housing, and the risk of falls in elderly people. Age Ageing 1989;18:47–51.
24. Wild D, Nayak USL, Isaacs B. How dangerous are falls in old people at home? BMJ 1981;282:266–268.
25. Nguyen T, Sambrook P, Kelly P, et al. Prediction of osteoporotic fractures by postural instability and bone density. BMJ 1993;307:1111–1115.
26. Rizzo JA, Baker DI, McAvay G, Tinetti ME. The cost-effectiveness of a multifactorial targeted prevention program for falls among community elderly persons. Med Care 1996;34:954–969.
27. Sattin RW, Lambert-Huber DA, DeVito CA, et al. The incidence of fall injury events among the elderly in a defined population. Am J Epidemiol 1990;131:1028.
28. Tinetti ME, Liu W-L, Ginter SF. Mechanical restraint use and fall-related injuries among residents of skilled nursing facilities. Ann Intern Med 1992;116:369–374.
29. Melton LJI, Riggs BL. Risk factors for injury after a fall. Clin Geriatr Med 1985;1: 525–539.
30. Tinetti ME, Doucette J, Claus E, Marottoli R. Risk factors for serious injury during falls by older persons in the community. J Am Geriatr Soc 1995;43:1214–1221.
31. Grisso JA, Kelsey JL, Strom BL, et al. Risk factors for falls as a cause of hip fracture in women. N Engl J Med 1991;324:1326–1331.
32. Nevitt MC, Cummings SR, Hudes ES. Risk factors for injurious falls: a prospective study. J Gerontol 1991;46:M164–M170.
33. Grisso JA, Schwarz DF, Wolfson V, Polansky M, LaPann K. The impact of falls in an inner-city elderly African-American population. J Am Geriatr Soc 1992;40:673–678.
34. Tinetti ME, Liu W-L, Claus EB. Predictors and prognosis of inability to get up after falls among elderly persons. JAMA 1993;269:65–70.
35. King MB, Tinetti ME. Falls in community-dwelling older persons. J Am Geriatr Soc 1995;43:1146–1154.
36. Kiel DP, O'Sullivan P, Teno JM, Mor V. Health care utilization and functional status in the aged following a fall. Med Care 1991;29:221–228.
37. Wolinsky FD, Johnson RJ, Fitzgerald JF. Falling, health status, and the use of health services by older adults: a prospective study. Med Care 1992;30:587–597.
38. Tinetti ME, Richman D, Powell L. Falls efficacy as a measure of fear of falling. J Gerontol 1990;45:P239–P243.

39. Vellas BJ, Wayne SJ, Romero LJ, Baumgartner RN, Garry PJ. Fear of falling and restriction of mobility in elderly fallers. Age Ageing 1997;26:189–193.
40. Sjogren H, Bjornstig U. Unintentional injuries among elderly people: incidence, causes, severity, and costs. Accid Anal Prev 1989;21:233.
41. Alexander BH, Rivara FP, Wolf ME. The cost and frequency of hospitalization for fall-related injuries in older adults. Am J Public Health 1992;82:1020–1023.
42. Covington DL, Maxwell JG, Clancy TV. Hospital resources used to treat the injured elderly at North Carolina trauma centers. J Am Geriatr Soc 1993;41:847–852.
43. Rice DP, MacKenzie EJ, Associates. Cost of injury in the United States: a report to Congress. San Francisco: University of California, 1989.
44. Fingerhut LA, Warner M. Injury chartbook. Health, United States, 1996–97. Hyattsville, MD: National Center for Health Statistics, 1997.
45. National Safety Council. Accident facts 1998. Itasca, IL: National Safety Council, 1998.
46. Ashley MJ, Gryfe CI, Amies A. A longitudinal study of falls in an elderly population. II. some circumstances of falling. Age Ageing 1977;6:211–220.
47. Lord SR, Sambrook PN, Gilbert C, et al. Postural stability, falls, and fractures in the elderly: results from the Dubbo Osteoporosis Epidemiology Study. Med J Aust 1994; 160:684–691.
48. Manchester D, Woollacott M, Zederbauer-Hylton N, Marin O. Visual, vestibular and somatosensory contributions to balance control in the older adult. J Gerontol 1989;44: M118–M127.
49. Tideiksaar R. Preventing falls: how to identify risk factors, reduce complications. Geriatrics 1996;51:43–53.
50. Torgerson DJ, Garton MJ, Reid DM. Falling and perimenopausal women. Age Ageing 1993;22:59–64.
51. Josephson KR, Fabacher DA, Rubenstein LZ. Home safety and fall prevention. Clin Geriatr Med 1991;7:707–731.
52. Morfitt JM. Falls in old people at home: intrinsic versus environmental factors in causation. Public Health [Lond] 1983;97:115–120.
53. Nevitt MC, Cummings SR. Type of fall and risk of hip and wrist fractures: the study of osteoporotic fractures. J Am Geriatr Soc 1993;41:1226–1234.
54. Cummings SR, Nevitt MC. Non-skeletal determinants of fractures: the potential importance of the mechanics of falls. Osteoporos Int 1994;4(Suppl 1):S67–S70.
55. Greenspan SL, Myers ER, Maitland LA, Resnick NM, Hayes WC. Fall severity and bone mineral density as risk factors for hip fracture in ambulatory elderly. JAMA 1994; 271:128–133.
56. Tinetti ME, Doucette JT, Claus EB. The contribution of predisposing and situational risk factors to serious fall injuries. J Am Geriatr Soc 1995;43:1207–1213.
57. Koski K, Luukinen H, Laippala P, Kivela S-L. Risk factors for major injurious falls among the home-dwelling elderly by functional abilities: a prospective population-based study. Gerontology 1998;44:232–238.
58. Tideiksaar R. Preventing falls: home hazard checklists to help older patients protect themselves. Geriatrics 1986;41:26–28.
59. Tideiksaar R. Geriatric falls: assessing the cause, preventing recurrence. Geriatrics 1989;44:57–64.
60. Rhymes J, Jaeger R. Falls: prevention and management in the institutional setting. Clin Geriatr Med 1988;4:613–622.
61. Rubenstein LZ, Josephson KR, Osterweil D. Falls and fall prevention in the nursing home. Clin Geriatr Med 1996;12:881–902.
62. Connell BR. Role of the environment in falls prevention. Clin Geriatr Med 1996;12: 859–880.
63. Sattin RW, Rodriguez JG, DeVito CA, Wingo PA. Home environmental hazards and the risk of fall injury events among community-dwelling older persons. J Am Geriatr Soc 1998;46:669–676.
64. Hornbrook MC, Stevens VJ, Wingfield DJ, Hollis JF, Greenlick MR, Ory MG. Preventing

falls among community-dwelling older persons: results from a randomized trial. Gerontologist 1994;34:16–23.
65. Thompson PG. Preventing falls in the elderly at home: a community-based program. Med J Aust 1996;164:530–532.
66. Tinetti ME, Baker DI, Garnett PA, Gottschalk M, Koch ML, Horwitz RI. Yale FICSIT: risk factor abatement strategy for fall prevention. J Am Geriatr Soc 1993;41:315–320.
67. Ory MG, Schechtman KB, Miller JP, et al. Frailty and injuries in later life: the FICSIT trials. J Am Geriatr Soc 1993;41:283–296.
68. Tinetti ME, Baker DI, McAvay G, et al. A multifactorial intervention to reduce the risk of falling among elderly people living in the community. N Engl J Med 1994;331: 821–827.
69. Montamat SC, Cusack BJ, Vestal RE. Management of drug therapy in the elderly. N Engl J Med 1989;321:303–309.
70. Seymour RM, Routledge PA. Important drug-drug interactions in the elderly. Drugs and Aging 1998;12:485–494.
71. Cadieux RJ. Drug interactions in the elderly: how multiple drug use increases risk exponentially. Postgrad Med 1989;86:179–186.
72. Chrischilles EA, Segar ET, Wallace RB. Self-reported adverse drug reactions and related resource use: a study of community-dwelling persons 65 years of age and older. Ann Intern Med 1992;117:634–640.
73. Cumming RG. Epidemiology of medication-related falls and fractures in the elderly. Drugs Aging 1998;12:43–53.
74. Von Renteln-Kruse W. Falls in old age and drugs [German]. Z Gerontol Geriatr 1997;30:276–280.
75. Weiner DK, Hanlon JT, Studenski SA. Effects of central nervous system polypharmacy on falls liability in community-dwelling elderly. Gerontology 1998;44:217–221.
76. Cumming RG, Miller JP, Kelsey JL, et al. Medications and multiple falls in elderly people: the St. Louis OASIS study. Age Ageing 1991;20:455–461.
77. Hale WE, Stewart RB, Marks RG. Central nervous system symptoms of elderly subjects using antihypertensive drugs. J Am Geriatr Soc 1984;32:5–10.
78. Nygaard HA. Falls and psychotropic drug consumption in long-term care residents: is there an obvious association. Gerontology 1998;44:46–50.
79. Granek E, Baker SP, Abbey H, et al. Medications and diagnoses in relation to falls in a long-term care facility. J Am Geriatr Soc 1987;35:503–511.
80. Liu YJ, Stagni G, Walden JG, Shepherd AMM, Lichtenstein MJ. Thioridazine dose-related effects on biomechanical force platform measures of sway in young and old men. J Am Geriatr Soc 1998;46:431–437.
81. Macdonald JB. The role of drugs in falls in the elderly. Clin Geriatr Med 1985;1:621–632.
82. Cutson TM, Gray SL, Hughes MA, Carson SW, Hanlon JT. Effect of a single dose of diazepam on balance measures in older people. J Am Geriatr Soc 1997;45:435–440.
83. Leipzig RM, Cumming RG, Tinetti ME. Drugs and falls in older people: a systematic review and meta-analysis. I. Psychotropic drugs. J Am Geriatr Soc 1999;47:30–39.
84. Leipzig RM, Cumming RG, Tinetti ME. Drugs and falls in older people: a systematic review and meta-analysis: II. Cardiac and analgesic drugs. J Am Geriatr Soc 1999;47: 40–50.
85. Monane H, Avorn J. Medications and falls: causation, correlation, and prevention. Clin Geriatr Med 1996;12:847–858.
86. Beers MH, Ouslander JG, Rollingher I, Reuben DB, Brooks J, Beck JC. Explicit criteria for determining inappropriate medication use in nursing homes. Arch Intern Med 1991;151:1825–1832.
87. Wilcox SM, Himmelstein DU, Woolhandler S. Inappropriate drug prescribing for the community-dwelling elderly. JAMA 1994;272:292–295.
88. Mayer-Oakes SA, Kelman G, Beers MH, et al. Benzodiazepine use in older, community-dwelling southern Californians: prevalence and clinical correlates. Ann Pharmacother 1993;27:416–421.

89. Gurwitz JH, Soumerai SB, Avorn J. Improving medication prescribing and utilization in the nursing home. J Am Geriatr Soc 1990;38:542–552.
90. Avorn J, Soumerai SB, Everitt DE, et al. A randomized trial of a program to reduce the use of psychoactive drugs in nursing homes. N Engl J Med 1992;327:168–173.
91. Horak FB, Shupert CL, Mirka A. Components of postural dyscontrol in the elderly: a review. Neurobiol Aging 1989;10:727–738.
92. Rigler SK. Instability in the older adult. Compr Ther 1996;22:297–303.
93. Maki BE, McIlroy WE. Postural control in the older adult. Clin Geriatr Med 1996; 12:635–658.
94. Runge M. The multifactorial etiology of gait disorders, falls, and hip fractures in the elderly [German]. Z Gerontol Geriat 1997;30:267–275.
95. Maki BE, Holliday PJ, Topper AK. A prospective study of postural balance and risk of falling in an ambulatory and independent elderly population. J Gerontol 1994;49: M72–M84.
96. Leibowitz HW, Shupert CL. Spatial orientation mechanisms and their implications for falls. Clin Geriatr Med 1985;1:571–580.
97. Alexander NB. Postural control in older adults. J Am Geriatr Soc 1994;42:93–108.
98. Kuo AD, Speers RA, Peterka RJ, Horak FB. Effect of altered sensory conditions on multivariate descriptors of human postural sway. Exp Brain Res 1998;122:185–195.
99. Wolfson L, Whipple R, Derby CA, Amerman P, Nashner L. Gender differences in the balance of healthy elderly as demonstrated by dynamic posturography. J Gerontol 1994;49:M160–M167.
100. Maino JH. Visual deficits and mobility. Clin Geriatr Med 1996;12:803–823.
101. Tobis JS, Reinsch S, Swanson JM, Byrd M, Scharf T. Visual perception dominance of fallers among community-dwelling older adults. J Am Geriatr Soc 1985;33:330–333.
102. Simoneau GG, Cavanagh PR, Ulbrecht JS, Leibowitz HW, Tyrell RA. The influence of visual factors on fall-related kinematic variables during stair descent by older women. J Gerontol 1991;46:M188–M195.
103. Felson DT, Anderson JJ, Hannan MT, Milton RC, Wilson PWF, Kiel DP. Impaired vision and hip fracture: the Framingham study. J Am Geriatr Soc 1989;37:495–500.
104. McMurdo MET, Gaskell A. Dark adaptation and falls in the elderly. Gerontology 1991;37:221–224.
105. Cohn TE, Lasley DJ. Visual depth illusion and falls in the elderly. Clin Geriatr Med 1985;1:601–615.
106. Pyykko I, Jantti P, Aalto H. Postural control in elderly subjects. Age Ageing 1990; 19:215–221.
107. Hytonen M, Pyykko I, Aalto H, Starck J. Postural control and age. Acta Otolaryngol [Stockh] 1993;113:119–122.
108. Overstall PW, Hazell JWP, Johnson AL. Vertigo in the elderly. Age Ageing 1981; 10:105–109.
109. Kristinsdottir EK, Jarnlo G-B, Magnusson M. Aberrations in postural control, vibration sensation and some vestibular findings in healthy 64–92 year-old subjects. Scand J Rehabil Med 1997;29:257–265.
110. Uccioli L, Gaicomini PG, Pasqualetti P, et al. Contribution of central neuropathy to postural instability in IDDM patients with peripheral neuropathy. Diabetes Care 1997;20:929–934.
111. Robbins S, Waked E, McClaran J. Proprioception and stability: foot position awareness as a function of age and footwear. Age Ageing 1995;24:67–72.
112. Robbins S, Waked E. Balance and vertical impact in sports: role of shoe sole materials. Arch Phys Med Rehabil 1997;78:463–467.
113. Robbins S, Waked E, Krouglicof N. Improving balance. J Am Geriatr Soc 1998;46: 1363–1370.
114. Snow RE, Williams KR. High-heeled shoes: their effect on center of mass position, posture, three-dimensional kinematics, rearfoot motion, and ground reaction forces. Arch Phys Med Rehabil 1994;75:568–576.

115. Lord SR, Bashford GM. Shoe characteristics and balance in older women. J Am Geriatr Soc 1996;44:429–433.
116. Salthouse TA, Somberg BL. Time–accuracy relationships in young and old adults. J Gerontol 1982;37:349–353.
117. Stelmach GE, Phillips J, DiFabio RP, Teasdale N. Age, functional postural reflexes, and voluntary sway. J Gerontol 1989;44:B100–B106.
118. Barin K, Jefferson GD, Sparto PJ, Parnianpour M. Effect of aging on human postural control during cognitive tasks. Biomed Sci Instrum 1997;33:388–393.
119. Lundin-Olsson L, Nyberg L, Gustafson Y. Attention, frailty, and falls: the effect of a manual task on basic mobility. J Am Geriatr Soc 1998;46:758–761.
120. Froehling DA, Silverstein MD, Mohr DN, Beatty CW. Does this dizzy patient have a serious form of vertigo? JAMA 1994;271:385–388.
121. Lipsitz LA. Abnormalities in blood pressure homeostasis that contribute to falls in the elderly. Clin Geriatr Med 1985;1:637–645.
122. Aronow WS, Ahn C. Association of postprandial hypotension with incidence of falls, syncope, coronary events, stroke, and total mortality at 29-month follow-up in 499 older nursing home residents. J Am Geriatr Soc 1997;45:1051–1053.
123. Seeley DG, Cauley JA, Grady D, Browner WS, Nevitt MC, Cummings SR. Is postmenopausal estrogen therapy associated with neuromuscular function or falling in elderly women? Arch Intern Med 1995;155:293–299.
124. Naessen T, Lindmark B, Larsen H-C. Better postural balance in elderly women recceiving estrogens. Am J Obstet Gynecol 1997;177:412–416.
125. Hammar ML, Lindgren R, Berg GE, Moller CG, Niklasson MK. Effects of hormonal replacement therapy on the postural balance among postmenopausal women. Obstet Gynecol 1996;88:955–960.
126. Robbins AS, Rubinstein LZ, Josephson KR, Schulman BL, Osterweil D, Fine G. Predictors of falls among elderly people: results of two population-based studies. Arch Intern Med 1989;149:1628–1633.
127. Wolfson L, Whipple R, Amerman P, Tobin JN. Gait assessment in the elderly: a gait abnormality rating scale and its relation to falls. J Gerontol 1990;45:12–19.
128. Feltner ME, MacRae PG, McNitt-Gray JL. Quantitative gait assessment as a predictor of prospective and retrospective falls in community-dwelling older women. Arch Phys Medi Rehabil 1994;75:447–453.
129. Lord SR, Lloyd DG, Li SK. Sensori-motor function, gait patterns and falls in community-dwelling women. Age Ageing 1996;25:292–299.
130. Wolfson LI, Whipple R, Amerman P, Kaplan J, Kleinberg A. Gait and balance in the elderly: two functional capacities that link sensory and motor ability to falls. Clin Geriatr Med 1985;1:649–655.
131. Chen H-C, Ashton-Miller JA, Alexander NB, Schultz AB. Stepping over obstacles: gait patterns of healthy young and old adults. J Gerontol 1991;46:M196–M203.
132. Alexander NB. Differential diagnosis of gait disorders in older adults. Clin Geriatr Med 1996;12:689–703.
133. McIlroy WE, Maki BE. Age-related changes in compensatory stepping in response to unpredictable perturbations. J Gerontol 1996;51A:M289–M296.
134. Judge JO, Ounpuu S, Davis RBI. Effects of age on the biomechanics and physiology of gait. Clin Geriatr Med 1996;12:659–678.
135. Koller WC, Glatt SL, Fox JH. Senile gait: a distinct neurologic entity. Clin Geriatr Med 1985;1:661–668.
136. Wolfson L, Judge J, Whipple R, King M. Strength is a major factor in balance, gait, and the occurrence of falls. J Gerontol 1995;50A:64–67.
137. Judge JO, Davis RBI, Ounpuu S. Step length reductions in advanced age: the role of ankle and hip kinetics. J Gerontol 1996;51A:M303–M312.
138. Brown M, Sinacore DR, Host HH. The relationship of strength to function in the older adult. J Gerontol 1995;50A:55–59.

139. Hurley BF. Age, gender, and muscular strength. J Gerontol 1995;50A:41–44.
140. Marcus R. Relationship of age-related decreases in muscle mass and strength to skeletal status. J Gerontol 1995;50A:86–87.
141. Hurley MV, Rees J, Newham DJ. Quadriceps function, proprioceptive acuity and functional performance in healthy young, middle-aged and elderly subjects. Age Ageing 1998;27:55–62.
142. Buchner DM, Cress ME, Esselman PC, et al. Factors associated with changes in gait speed in older adults. J Gerontol 1996;51A:M297–M302.
143. Tinetti ME. Performance-oriented assessment of mobility problems in elderly patients. J Am Geriatr Soc 1986;34:119–126.
144. Tinetti ME, Ginter SF. Identifying mobility dysfunctions in elderly patients. JAMA 1988;259:1190–1193.
145. Trueblood PR, Rubenstein LZ. Assessment of instability and gait in elderly persons. Compr Ther 1991;17:20–29.
146. Alexander NB. Using technology-based techniques to assess postural control and gait in older adults. Clin Geriatr Med 1996;12:725–744.
147. Berg K, Norman KE. Functional assessment of balance and gait. Clin Geriatr Med 1996;12:705–723.
148. Fernie GR, Gryfe CI, Holliday PJ, Llewellyn A. The relationship of postural sway in standing to the incidence of falls in geriatric subjects. Age Ageing 1982;11:11–16.
149. Brocklehurst JC, Robertson D, James-Groom P. Clinical correlates of sway in old age – sensory modalities. Age Ageing 1982;11:1–10.
150. Hughes MA, Duncan PW, Rose DK, Chandler JM, Studenski SA. The relationship of postural sway to sensorimotor function, functional performance, and disablity. Arch Phys Med Rehabil 1996;77:567–572.
151. Brooke-Wavell K, Athersmith LE, Jones PRM, Masud T. Brisk walking and postural stability: a cross-sectional study in postmenopausal women. Gerontology 1998;44: 288–292.
152. Ebrahim S, Thompson PW, Baskaran V, Evans K. Randomized placebo-controlled trial of brisk walking in the prevention of postmenopausal osteoporosis. Age Ageing 1997;26: 253–260.
153. Buchner DM, Beresford SAA, Larson EB, LaCroix AZ, Wagner EH. Effects of physical activity on health status in older adults II: intervention studies. Ann Rev Public Health 1992;13:469–488.
154. Lord SR, Ward JA, Williams P, Strudwick M. The effect of a 12-month exercise trial on balance, strength, and falls in older women: a randomized controlled trial. J Am Geriatr Soc 1995;43:1198–1206.
155. Shumway-Cook A, Gruber W, Baldwin M, Liao S. The effect of multidimensional exercises on balance, mobility, and fall risk in community-dwelling older adults. Phys Ther 1997;77:46–57.
156. Lin PS, Tseng H-M. The effect of t'ai-chi-chuan on sensorimotor functions of the older people [abstract]. J Am Geriatr Soc 1997;45:S13.
157. Lai J-S, Lan C, Wong M-K, Teng S-H. Two-year trends in cardiorespiratory function among older t'ai chi chuan practitioners and sedentary subjects. J Am Geriatr Soc 1995;43:1222–1227.
158. Wolfson L, Whipple R, Derby C, et al. Balance and strength training in older adults: intervention gains and t'ai chi maintenance. J Am Geriatr Soc 1996;44:498–506.
159. Province MA, Hadley EC, Hornbrook MC, et al. The effects of exercise on falls in elderly patients: a preplanned meta-analysis of the FICSIT trials. JAMA 1995;273:1341–1347.
160. Wolf SL, Barnhart HX, Kutner NG, McNeely E, Coogler C, Xu T. Reducing frailty and falls in older persons: an investigation of t'ai chi and computerized balance training. J Am Geriatr Soc 1996;44:489–497.
161. Wolf SL, Barnhart HX, Ellison GL, Coogler CE. The effect of t'ai chi quan and computerized balance training on postural stability in older subjects. Phys Ther 1997;77: 371–381.

162. Fiatarone MA, Marks EC, Ryan ND, Meredith CN, Lipsitz LA, Evans WJ. High-intensity strength training in nonagenarians: effects on skeletal muscle. JAMA 1990;263: 3029–3034.
163. Charette SL, McEvoy L, Pyka G, et al. Muscle hypertrophy response to resistance training in older women. J Appl Physiol 1991;70:1912–1916.
164. Fiatarone MA, O'Neill EF, Ryan ND, et al. Exercise training and nutritional supplementation for physical frailty in very elderly people. N Engl J Med 1994;330:1769–1775.
165. Evans WJ. Effects of exercise on body composition and functional capacity of the elderly. J Gerontol 1995;50A(Special issue):147–150.
166. Tseng BS, Marsh DR, Hamilton MT, Booth FW. Strength and aerobic training attenuate muscle wasting and improve resistance to the development of disability with aging. J Gerontol 1995;50A(Special issue):113–119.
167. Krebs DE, Jette AM, Assmann SF. Moderate exercise improves gait stability in disabled elders. Arch Phys Med Rehabil 1998;79:1489–1495.
168. McCartney N, Hicks AL, Martin J, Webber CE. A longitudinal trial of weight training in the elderly: continued improvement in year 2. J Gerontol 1996;51A:B425–B433.
169. Sherrington C, Lord SR. Home exercise to improve strength and walking velocity after hip fracture: a randomized controlled trial. Arch Phys Med Rehabil 1997;78:208–212.
170. Reinsch S, MacRae P, Lachenbruch PA, Tobis JS. Attempts to prevent falls and injury: a prospective community study. Gerontologist 1992;32:450–456.
171. Mulrow CD, Gerety MB, Kanten D, et al. A randomized trial of physical rehabilitation for very frail nursing home residents. JAMA 1994;271:519–524.
172. Lauritzen JB, Petersen MM, Lund B. Effect of external hip protectors on hip fractures. Lancet 1993;341:11–13.
173. Ross JER, Maas ML, Huston JC, et al. Evaluation of two interventions to reduce falls and fall injuries: the challenge of hip pads and individualized elimination rounds. In: Funk SG, Tornquist EM, Champagne MT, Wiese RA, editors. Key aspects of elder care: managing falls, incontinence, and cognitive impairment. Berlin Heidelberg New York: Springer, 1992:97–103.
174. Wallace RB, Ross JE, Huston JC, Kundel C, Woodworth G. Iowa FICSIT trial: the feasibility of elderly wearing a hip joint protective garment to reduce hip fractures. J Am Geriatr Soc 1993;41:338–340.
175. Evans LK, Strumpf NE. Tying down the elderly: a review of the literature on physical restraint. J Am Geriatr Soc 1989;37:65–74.
176. Marks W. Physical restraints in the practice of medicine: current concepts. Arch Intern Med 1992;152:2203–2206.
177. DeSantis J, Engberg S, Rogers J. Geropsychiatric restraint use. J Am Geriatr Soc 1997; 45:1515–1518.
178. Morris EV, Isaacs B. The prevention of falls in a geriatric hospital. Age Ageing 1980; 9:181–185.
179. Powell C, Mitchell-Pedersen L, Fingerote E, Edmund L. Freedom from restraint: consequences of reducing physical restraints in the management of the elderly. Can Med Assoc J 1989;141:561–564.
180. Bloom C, Braun JV. Restraints in the 90s: success with wanderers. Geriatr Nursing 1991;Jan/Feb:20.
181. Ejaz FK, Jones JA, Rose MS. Falls among nursing home residents: an examination of incident reports before and after restraint reduction. J Am Geriatr Soc 1994;42:960–964.
182. Schnelle JF, MasRae PG, Giacobassi K, MacRae HSH, Simmons SF, Ouslander JG. Exercise with physically restrained nursing home residents: maximizing benefits of restraint reduction. J Am Geriatr Soc 1996;44:507–512.
183. Handysides S. Helping people with dementia feel at home. BMJ 1993;306:1115–1117.
184. Close J, Ellis M, Hooper R, Glucksman E, Jackson S, Swift C. Prevention of falls in the elderly trial (PROFET): a randomised controlled trial. Lancet 1999;353:93–97.

25 Hip Protectors

J. B. Lauritzen and W. C. Hayes

Introduction

Hip protectors used in prevention of hip fractures have been available in clinical practice for only a few years. Based on several recent clinical and biomechanical studies hip protection has been recommended by the European Commission in their 'Report on Osteoporosis in the European Community – Action for Prevention 1998': "Any bone will break if the force is strong enough, but reducing the impact of the force may prevent fracture. Hip protectors have been developed to reduce the impact of trauma and protect the bone when a fall occurs from a standing position. Studies have demonstrated the protective value of protectors worn by vulnerable older women and men who have already sustained a fracture, particularly those in nursing homes."

The following conditions have been considered important for a fall to cause hip fracture, impact near the hip, protective reflexes, local soft tissue energy absorption and bone strength [1]. More than 90% of hip fractures are related to direct impact on the hip [1–3], although only one-fourth of impacts to the hip in the elderly lead to a hip fracture [4]. Rarely does a hip fracture occur without direct trauma [5–7]. Moreover, falls directly on the hip raises the odds ratio for a hip fracture about 20-fold [8].

Occurrence of falls and hip fracture

For people living in the community the annual rate of falls is 28–35% among those older than 65 years of age [9–11], and 32–42% of subjects older than 75 years sustain at least one fall a year [12,13]. Among nursing home residents the occurrence of falls is 1.5 falls per resident per year, and more than 80% of nursing home residents experience at least one fall per year [4].

Most falls do not cause major injuries [14], but the risk of injuries after falls in the elderly is very high [15]. The annual incidence of falls on the hip among nursing home residents is 36 per 100 falls among women and 16 falls per 100 among men [4]. For cases of impact to the hip, the risk of fracture is 0.25 and 0.33 in women and men in nursing homes [4].

The incidence of hip fracture among nursing home residents is 6.8 and 5.3 per 100 per year among women and men respectively [4]. The incidence among frequent fallers is about 14%. The risk of hip fracture among recurrent fallers treated for fall-related trauma in the emergency room is 41% within the next year. Orthopedic inpatients older than 75 years of age have an annual risk of hip fracture of 4.1%, while those with dementia have a 6.5% risk. Those admitted due to fall have a risk of 5.6%, and those admitted with hip fracture a risk of an additional hip fracture of 4.7%. For those with a tendency to fall, the risk of a hip fracture is 6.6% per year and for those with visual impairment the risk is 6.2% per year [16].

Force and Energy in Falls on the Hip

A fall from standing height is associated with a potential energy that may be sufficient to produce hip fracture even in young, healthy subjects [17,18]. For 82 patients who sustained a hip fracture, the potential energy has been estimated to be 442 joules (J) [8]. However, this estimate may be too high based on data from unprotected falls performed by a stunt woman on a force platform. In this case the energy was only 113 J, corresponding to an effective load acting on the hip of 35% of the body weight [19], and a force of 3.5 kN. These results suggest that susceptible subjects are far more likely to suffer a hip fracture in case of impact to the hip.

Protective Responses

Elderly subjects experience far more trauma compared with young subjects. Reduced reaction time and degraded coordination are related to risk of fractures [20]. Many patients with hip fractures are admitted from nursing homes, and this group is characterized by disturbances in their neuromuscular functions [21].

Energy Absorption

Energy absorption in soft tissue may be a more important factor than bone strength in relation to hip fractures [17,22]. Experimental studies have shown that energy absorption in soft tissue may account for up to 75% of the energy available in a fall [23]. This may partially explain why being overweight protects against hip fractures.

Women with a hip fracture weigh on average 5 kg less than controls [24,25]. In addition, women with a hip fracture seem to possess less soft tissue covering their hips compared with controls, even after adjustment for body mass index [25]. It has been suggested that body mass index is a surrogate for measuring the thickness of trochanteric soft tissue thickness [26].

In one study about 42% of registered falls sustained within the home occurred in the bathroom [27]. However, impact attenuation of floor coverings has only a minor effect on the peak force from falls, even when one compares terrazzo with a carpet floor covering [28].

Bone Strength

The fracture threshold in the hip has been studied in cadavers and the results may differ according to set-up and loading velocity. The loading angle to the neck seems important [29]. Depending on density the breaking strength in elderly cadaveric bone ranges from 1000 N to 6000 N, with coefficients of determinations (r^2) between bone strength and density ranging from 0.7 to 0.9 [17,30]. Bone strength can thus be estimated from bone mineral density [30]. However, bone density on its own is not a good clinical predictor of a later hip fracture as indicated by the major overlap in bone density among elderly fallers between hip fracture patients and controls [31]. In fact, the impact direction and impact site may be stronger predictors of hip fracture risk than femoral bone density [32], whereas the potential energy available and the body mass index provide about the same level of predictability as density.

Hip Padding Systems

Various hip padding systems have emerged. There may be an energy shunting type (horse-shoe) [33] including the crash helmet type [34,35], an energy absorptive type[36–38] and an airbag type [39]. Laboratory experiments have suggested that some of the energy absorptive protectors may be insufficient to prevent hip fractures [40–42].

Clinical Studies

Nursing Homes

The effect of external hip protectors has been tested in four randomized controlled trials in nursing homes (Table 25.1), and two nonrandomized observational studies [36,43] (Table 25.2). The randomized studies showed a reduction in the rate of hip fractures between 0.0 to 0.44 [4,37,44,45] with a pooled average of 0.34. The two largest randomized trials resulted in a reduction in risk during an 11 month period in nursing homes to 0.44 [4] and 0.34 [44]. The two largest studies were based on intention to treat analysis, and when one consider treatment received, i.e., effect of protector when in the use, then the protective effect is high.

Home Dwellers

Trials with hip protectors among elderly subjects living at home are rare, although some compliance studies have been performed. In the Hvidovre study [46] the number of hip fractures avoided during an open intervention study among all elderly (> 75 years) orthopaedic patients was recorded in the intervention hospital (n = 1006) and compared with a control hospital (n = 678). The follow-up was 1–1½ years. Skewness in confounders between intervention group and controls was

Table 25.1. Randomized clinical studies in nursing homes with hip protectors: observed number of hip fractures occurring among nursing home residents in the intervention and control groups, and relative risk and estimated number of hip fractures saved

Study	Follow-up (months)	Intervention group	Control group	Relative risk	No. of hip fractures avoided
		(No. hip fractures/no. of subjects)			
Lauritzen et al. [4]	11	8/247	31/418	**0.44** 0.20–0.95 95% CI	10
Ekman et al. [44]	11	4/302	17/442	**0.34** 0.12–1.0 95% CI	8
Heikinheimo et al. [37]	12	1/36	5/36	**0.20**	4
Harada et al. [45]	19	0/30	4/24	**0.0**	5
All		13/615	57/920	**0.34**	27

Table 25.2. Nonrandomized observational studies with hip protectors: observed number of hip fractures associated with falls on a hip protector during prospective observational studies among nursing home residents [36,43].

	No. of hip fractures	No. of falls
Wortberg [36]		
10 months ($n = 28$)		
Falls with hip protector	0	16
Falls without hip protector	4	7
Parkkari et al. [43]		
6 months ($n = 12$)		
Falls on hip protector	0	6
Users ($n = 12$)	0	
Non-users ($n = 14$)	2	

accounted for in the analysis. All elderly orthopaedic patients who received and accepted the hip protectors and did not return them were defined as users.

During follow-up users reported 143 falls with impact on the hip protector, and no hip fractures occurred. Only two hip fractures occurred while the patients used their hip protectors, and in these cases no impact on the hip was reported [46]. Assuming each subject who had received a hip protector was a "user", the overall protective effect of the hip protectors was 12% and did not reach statistical significance.

The estimated numbers of hip fractures avoided in the elderly women and men with risk factors are given in Table 25.3. Only for patients with visual impairment did the prevention of hip fractures reach statistical significance. The confidence limits were rather wide due to the limited statistical power of the study.

Compliance

Based on a subgroup analysis in our early randomized nursing home study, hip protector wear compliance was 24% [4]. In this trial, the pads had to be retrieved and replaced in new sets of underwear for each change of underwear, and we believe this compromised compliance. The latest design of hip protectors are built into the

Table 25.3 Effect of hip protectors among elderly home dwellers included when admitted to an orthopaedic department [46]

	Relative risk	95% CI	No. of hip fractures avoided
All	0.88	0.5–1.5	3
Men	0.33	0.04–2.7	4
Demented	0.42	0.21–2.4	8
Admitted with fall	0.71	0.37–1.4	6
Admitted with hip fracture	0.67	0.19–2.4	2
Fall tendency	0.48	0.09–2.5	4
Dizziness	0.89	0.4–2.0	1
Help coming outdoor	0.82	0.28–2.3	1
Visual impairment, distance	0.25	0.08–0.85	9*
Reduced vision	0.25	0.06–1.11	6

*$p < 0.05$.

The numbers of hip fractures avoided in each risk group overlap each other.

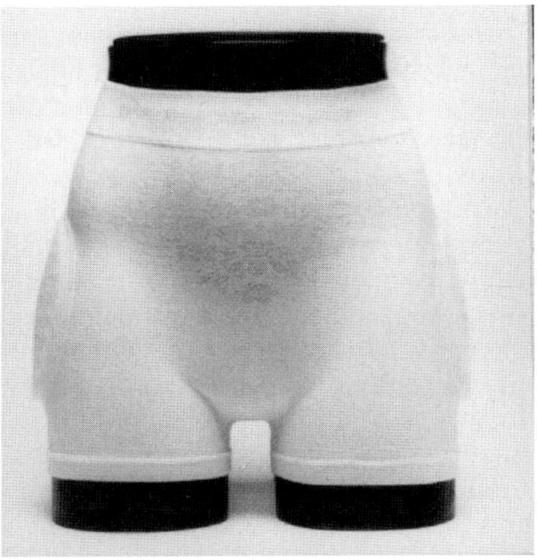

Fig. 25.1. The Safehip hip protector.

undergarment (Fig. 25.1) which can be washed and dried easily. The hip protectors can be worn at night. In the more recent community-based trials the initial rate of acceptance was 57% (572/1006). At 3 months the compliance was 75% [47]; at 2 years, the compliance was 40%. The compliance rate has been reported to be between 24% and 91% [4,36,37,43–45,47–49], reflecting a variety of compliance definitions ranging from primary compliance to compliance in recorded falls. Compliance rate must therefore be described properly when compliance rates are compared. In Table 25.4 the user rate is given for the two largest clinical studies.

Although the majority of elderly seems satisfied with the hip protectors, one-third of those who stop wearing them complain of discomfort or practical problems [47]. Fear of falling increases compliance, and this fear is reduced with the use of hip protectors. One-third feel more confident when walking, with an additional 15%

Table 25.4 Compliance rate with hip protectors in two large clinical studies

	Late compliance	Comments
Lauritzen et al. [4]	24%	Rate of users in registered falls, 11 months
Ekman et al. [44]	44%	Registered user rate, 11 months

of the elderly who use protectors spending more time outdoors [50]. Even though compliance may not reach 100%, the overall compliance of hip protectors has been high compared with other medical preventive modalities, and a 40% long-term compliance has been documented after 2 years (K. Hindsø, personal communication 1998). Primary acceptance and late compliance are important issues for the hip protection systems to work efficiently, and information and instructions including late follow-up may be necessary.

Cost-Effectiveness/Cost Savings

Hip protectors are cost-saving among frail elderly subjects in the community or in nursing homes [51]. The cost-saving ratio may be about 1 : 3 for nursing home residents. For elderly home dwellers with risk factors for hip fracture the cost-saving ratio may be 1 : 7. The ratio describes the relationship between costs spent for the intervention and money saved due to hip fractures avoided. Providing all Danish women older than 70 years of age and men over 80 years with hip protectors has been estimated to be cost-saving [51]. For clinical reasons, however, preventive efforts should focus on frail elderly subjects with a risk of falling and osteoporosis.

Besides the Municipality of Copenhagen, seven other municipalities in Denmark offer hip protectors to nursing home residents and frail elderly subjects with a propensity to fall. In Norway the health care system reimburses nursing home residents for the cost of hip protectors in one central municipality.

Discussion

Randomized clinical trials have shown a high efficacy of hip protectors among nursing home residents. The same has been shown for frail elderly home dwellers with visual impairment who were introduced to hip protectors when admitted to an orthopaedic department. Hip fracture has occurred even when wearing hip protectors, and the protectors have been said to induce hip fracture [52] due to the undergarment with hip protectors, which was placed at knee level and subsequently initiated the fall. Even though a hip fracture may occur in spite of the use of hip protectors, i.e., an indirect trauma or spontaneous fracture, it is a less frequent occurrence than would have been anticipated.

The benefit of hip protectors in relation to the prevention of periprosthetic hip fractures, luxation of hip arthroplasties and pelvic fractures, pressure sores and chronic bursitis is yet to be outlined and studied further.

Conclusion

Current evidence suggests that hip protectors are of benefit among nursing home residents and some frail elderly home dwellers. Thus, it seems realistic to expect a reduction in the occurrence of hip fractures by 15–25% when a systematic intervention among the frail elderly in nursing homes, hospitals and community is initiated.

References

1 Cummings SR, Nevitt MC. A hypothesis: the causes of hip fractures. J Gerontol 1989; 44:M107–M111.
2 Lauritzen JB, et al. Protection against hip fractures by energy absorption. Dan Med Bull 1998;39:91–93.
3 Hayes WC, et al. Relative risk of fall severity, body habitus and bone density in hip fracture among the elderly. Trans Orthop Res Soc 1991; 16: 70.
4 Lauritzen JB, Petersen MM, et al. Effect of external hip protectors on hip fractures. Lancet 1993;341:11–13.
5 Freeman MAR, et al. The role of fatigue in the pathogenesis of senile femoral neck fractures. J Bone Joint Surg Br 1974;56:698–702.
6 Sloan J, et al. Fractures neck of the femur: causes of the fall? Injury 1981;12:210–212.
7 Smith LD. Hip fractures: the role of muscular contraction or intrinsic forces in the causation of fractures of the femoral neck. J Bone Joint Surg Br 1953;35:367–383.
8 Hayes WC, et al. Impact near the hip dominates fracture risk in elderly nursing home residents who fall. Calcif Tissue Int 1993;52:192–198.
9 Campbell AJ, et al. Falls in old age: a study of frequency and related clinical factors. Age Ageing 1981;10:264–270.
10 Prudham D EJ. Factors associated with falls in the elderly: a community study. Age Aging 1981;10:141–146.
11 Blake AJ, et al. Falls by the elderly people at home: prevalence and associated factors. Age Ageing 1988;17:365–372.
12 Tinetti ME, et al. Risk factors for falls among elderly persons living in the community. N Engl J Med 1988;319:1701–1707.
13 Downton JH, et al. Prevalence, characteristics and factors associated with falls among the elderly living at home. Age Clin Exp Res 1991;3:219–228.
14 Berry G, et al. Detrimental incidents, including falls, in an elderly institutional population. J Am Geriatr Soc 1981;29:322–324.
15 Kiel DP. Falls. R I Med 1991;74:75–79.
16 Hindsø K, Lauritzen JB. Risk of subsequent hip fracture in elderly orthopaedic patients. Osteoporos Int 1998;8:18
17 Lotz JC, et al. The use of quantitative computed tomography to estimate risk of fracture from falls. J Bone Joint Surg AM 1990;72:689–700.
18 Robinovitch SN, et al. Prediction of femoral impact forces in falls on the hip. ASME Biomech Eng 1991;113:336–374.
19 Askegaard V, et al. Load on the hip in a stiff sideways fall. Eur J Exp Musculoskel Res 1995;4:111–116.
20 Adelsberg A, Pitman M, Alexander H. Lower extremity fractures: relationship to reaction time and coordination time. Arch Phys Med Rehabil 1989;79:737–739.
21 Stott S, et al. A prospective study of hip fracture patients. N Z Med J 1980;91:165–169.
22 Lauritzen JB, McNair P, et al. Risk factors for hip fractures. A review. Dan Med Bull 1993;40:479–485.

23 Lauritzen JB, et al. Estimate of hip fracture threshold adjusted for energy absorption in soft tissue. J Nucl Med 1994;21(Suppl):S48.

24 Elsasser U, et al. Deficit of trabecular and cortical bone in women with fracture of the femoral neck. Clin Sci 1980;59:393–395.

25 Lauritzen JB, et al. Body fat distribution and hip fractures. Acta Orthop Scand 1992; 63(Suppl):89.

26 Maitland LA, et al. Read my hips: measuring trochanteric soft tissue thickness. Calcif Tissue Int 1993;52:85–89.

27 DeVito CA, et al. Fall injuries among the elderly: community based surveillance. J Am Geriatr Soc 1988;36:1029–1035.

28 Maki BE, et al. Impact attenuation of floor coverings in simulated falling accidents. Appl Ergon 1990;21:107–114.

29 Pinella TP, et al. Impact direction from a fall influences the failure load of the proximal femur as much as age-related bone loss. Calcif Tissue Int 1996;58:231–235.

30 Courtney AC, et al. Age related reductions in the strength of the femur tested in fall loading configuration. J Bone Joint Surg AM 1995;77:387–395.

31 Cummings SR, et al. Risk factors for hip fracture in white women. N Engl J Med 1995; 332:767–773.

32 Greenspan SL, et al. Fall severity and bone mineral density as risk factors for hip fracture in ambulatory elderly. JAMA 1994;271:128–133.

33 Hayes WC, et al. Bone fracture prevention garment and method. Washington, DC: US Patent and Trademark Office 1992.

34 Lauritzen JB, et al. Impacts in patients with hip fractures and in vitro study of the padding effect: introduction of a hip protector. Acta Orthop Scand 1990;61(Suppl): 239.

35 Parkkari J, et al. Energy-shunting external hip protector attenuates the peak femoral impact force below the fracture threshold. An in vitro bimechanical study under typical falling conditions of the elderly. J Bone Miner Res 1995;10:1437–1442.

36 Wortberg WE. Hüft-Fraktur-Bandage zur Verhinderung von Oberschenkelhalsbrüchen bei älteren Menschen. Der Oberschenkelhalsbruch, ein biomechanisches Problem. Z Gerontol 1988;21:173.

37 Heikinheimo R, et al. To fall but not to break: safety pants. Proceeding of the 13th Triennial Congress of the International Ergonomics Association, Tampere, Finland, 1997: 576–578.

38 Sellberg MS, et al. The development of a passive protective device for the elderly to prevent hip fractures from accidental falls. Adv Bioe 1992;22:505–508.

39 Charpentier PJ. A hip protector based on airbag technology. Bone 1996;18(Suppl): 117S.

40 Hayes WC, et al. Energy shunting hip padding system reduces femoral impact force from a simulated fall to below fracture threshold. Proceedings of the third injury prevention through biomechanics CDC symposium, 1993.

41 Robinovitch SN, et al. Energy shunting hip padding system attenuates femoral impact force in a simulated fall. J Biomech Eng 1995;117:409–413.

42 Parkkari J, et al. Force attenuation properties of various trochanteric padding materials under typical falling conditions of the elderly. J Bone Miner Res 1994;9:1391–1396.

43 Parkkari J. Hip fractures in the elderly. Epidemiology, injury mechanisms, and prevention with an external hip protector. Acta Universitatis Tamperensis 1997;550: 1–85.

44 Ekman A, et al. External hip protectors to prevent osteoporotic hip fractures. Lancet 1997;350:563–564.

45 Harada A, et al. Hip fracture prevention trial using hip protector in Japanese elderly. Osteoporos Int 1998;8:121.

46 Hindsø K, et al. Intervention study with hip protectors. Osteoporos Int 1998;8:119.

47 Hindsø K, Lauritzen JB. Behavioral attitude towards hip protectors in elderly orthopedic patients. Osteoporos Int 1998;8:119.

48 Villar T, et al. Trochanteric hip protectors in the institutionalised elderly: a compliance study. Osteoporos Int 1996;6(Suppl):111.
49 Ross J-E, et al. Compliance by elderly in wearing hip joint protectors. In: Third international conference on injury prevention and control, Melbourne, 1996:no.298:73.
50 Hindsø K, Lauritzen JB. Effect of hip protectors on fear of falling. Osteoporos Int 1998; 8:119.
51 Lauritzen JB, Hindsø K, Singh G. Cost-effectiveness and external hip protectors. Osteoporos Int 1997;6:130.
52 Cameron I, et al. External hip protectors. [letter]. J Am Gerontol Soc 1997;45:1158.

26 Nutrition and Bone Health

J. Z. Ilich and J. E. Kerstetter

Introduction

Nutrition is important in the development and maintenance of bone mass and the prevention and treatment of osteoporosis. Approximately 80–90% of bone mineral content is composed of calcium (Ca) and phosphorus (P). Additional dietary components such as energy, protein, magnesium (Mg), zinc (Zn), copper (Cu), iron (Fe), fluoride (F), sodium (Na), and vitamins D, A, C and K, are required for normal calcium and bone metabolism, while other ingested compounds not usually categorized as nutrients (e.g., caffeine and phytoestrogens) may also affect bone health. This chapter reviews the role of these dietary components in bone health.

A new system of defining optimal nutrient intakes for healthy populations in the United States and Canada has been developed and is known as the Dietary Reference Intakes (DRIs) [1]. Unlike the previous Recommended Dietary Allowances (RDAs) [2] where only one level of a nutrient was defined, the DRIs delineate different levels of intakes including the Estimated Average Requirement (EAR), the Recommended Dietary Allowance (RDA), the Adequate Intake (AI), and the Tolerable Upper Intake Level (UL) (described in Table 26.1). The DRIs for the bone-related nutrients (Ca, P, Mg, F and vitamin D) were initially published in 1997 and will be updated as the scientific literature changes (Table 26.1) [1].

Calcium

The adult human body contains about 1000 g of calcium (Ca) of which 99% is found in bone in the form of hydroxyapatite. Therefore, the Ca requirement is determined mostly by skeletal needs. Dietary Ca exerts a threshold behavior, implying that skeletal Ca accumulation is a function of Ca intake only at intakes below the threshold. Ca intakes above the threshold have no effect on skeletal Ca accumulation. Matkovic and Heaney [3] determined the Ca threshold for different age groups based on a review of 34 balance studies. The threshold behavior of Ca in adolescents females was confirmed more recently in a study examining the relationship between Ca intake and urinary Ca excretion [4]. This study showed that at Ca intakes of about 1500 mg/day (threshold level for that age group), urinary Ca starts to rise more rapidly, indicating that skeletal saturation with Ca has been reached.

Table 26.1. Dietary Reference Intakes (DRI) for the bone-related nutrients

Life Stage Group	**Calcium** (mg)		**Phosphorus** (mg)		**Magnesium** (mg) (Male/Female)		**Vitamin D** (Fg) (Male/Female)		**Fluoride** (mg)	
	AI[a]	UL[b]	AI[a] or RDA[d]	UL	AI or RDA	UL	AI	UL	AI	UL
0–6 months	210	ND[c]	100[a]	ND	30/30 [a]	ND	5	25	0.01/0.01	0.7
7–12 months	270	ND	275[a]	ND	75/75[a]	ND	5	25	0.5/0.5	1.9
1–3 years	500	2500	460 [d]	3000	80/80[d]	65	5	50	0.7/0.7	1.3
4–8 years	800	2500	500 [d]	3000	130/130[d]	110	5	50	1.0/1.0	2.2
9–13 years	1300	2500	1250 [d]	4000	240/240[d]	350	5	50	2.0/2.0	10
14–18 years	1300	2500	1250 [d]	4000	410/360[d]	350	5	50	3.0/3.0	10
19–30 years	1000	2500	700 [d]	4000	400/310[d]	350	5	50	4.0/3.0	10
31–50 years	1000	2500	700 [d]	4000	420/320[d]	350	5	50	4.0/3.0	10
51–70 years	1200	2500	700 [d]	4000	420/320[d]	350	10	50	4.0/3.0	10
> 70 years	1200	2500	700 [d]	3000	420/320[d]	350	15	50	4.0/3.0	10
Pregnancy										
< 18 years	1300	2500	1250 [d]	3500	–/400[d]	350	5	50	–3.0	10
19–30 years	1000	2500	700 [d]	3500	–/350[d]	350	5	50	–3.0	10
31–50 years	1000	2500	700 [d]	3500	–/360[d]	350	5	50	–3.0	10
Lactation										
<18 years	1300	2500	1250 [d]	4000	–/360[d]	350	5	50	–3.0	10
19–30 years	1000	2500	700 [d]	4000	–/310[d]	350	5	50	–3.0	10
31–50 years	1000	2500	700 [d]	4000	–/320[d]	350	5	50	–3.0	10

DRI is a term that encompasses several levels of nutrient requirements including the Adequate Intake (AI), Recommended Dietary Allowance (RDA) and Upper Limit (UL).

[a] Adequate Intake (AI) is the goal intake for an individual or a group to sustain health and reduce disease risk.
[b] Tolerable Upper Intake Level (UL) is defined as the maximal level of daily nutrient intake that is unlikely to pose a risk of adverse health effects in almost all individuals within the life stage group. This term connotes the amount that, with high probability, can be safely tolerated.
[c] ND, not determined because of lack of data.
[d] Recommended Dietary Allowance (RDA) is the nutrient intake level that is sufficient to meet the requirements of 97–98% of the population.

Therefore, it is likely that below a certain level of Ca intake, young persons will not be able to reach their genetically predetermined peak bone mass, while adults will lose bone tissue at a faster rate than necessary.

Numerous studies in adults and children suggest that Ca is an important determinant of bone mass during skeletal formation and maintenance. Two epidemiological studies of an ecological nature examined bone mass in populations accustomed to different Ca intakes over a lifetime [5,6]. Both studies were cross-sectional: one conducted in a Croatian and another in a Chinese population. Differences in bone mass in both men and women living in regions of high and low Ca intake were present during young adulthood and continued into old age. These studies indicate that Ca is an important agent for skeletal formation affecting peak bone mass and subsequent rates of bone fracture. Retrospective studies in adults support the above conclusions. Dietary Ca from the distant past (childhood and adolescence) was a significant predictor of current adult bone mass [7–10].

A meta-analysis of the effect of Ca intake on bone mass in women and men (age 18–50 years) was performed by Welten et al. [11]. They analyzed 33 eligible, mostly cross-sectional and some interventional studies, and found a significant positive correlation between dietary Ca and bone mass. In a few interventional studies, supplementation of 1000 mg/day Ca in premenopausal women prevented bone loss of about 1% per year in all measured skeletal sites, except the ulna. (The overall bone loss for this population is about 0.5–1.5% per year.) A meta-analysis in postmenopausal women was performed by Cumming [12] and included 49 separate studies, again mostly cross-sectional. There was a positive correlation between bone mass and Ca intake. Calcium supplementation had a consistent preventive effect on the rate of bone loss. The effect was greatest when the baseline Ca intake was low, supporting the threshold hypothesis. More recently, Anderson and Rondano [13] summarized the effect of Ca on peak bone mass accumulation from both cross-sectional and longitudinal studies of postmenopausal women. The results again support the benefits of adequate Ca intake on the attainment of peak bone mass.

Most of the Ca studies performed in children and adolescents have shown a positive effect of Ca on bones. Those which did not, either were not specifically designed to determine the effect of Ca on bone or contained a small sample size in each age group [14,15]. Cross-sectional studies conducted in children of different races (Caucasians and Chinese) [16–18], adolescents [19,20], and young women [21] indicate that higher calcium intakes result in higher bone mass at almost all measured skeletal regions. African-American children and adolescents show higher Ca absorptive efficiency than Caucasians [22] which may contribute to their higher bone density [23].

The longitudinal clinical trials in children and adolescents showed that Ca intake close to the threshold level (as either food or supplement) was associated with higher bone mass [24–29]. However, the positive effect of Ca on bone mass diminishes when Ca supplementation is terminated. In other words, differences in bone mass between controlled and supplemented groups disappear when Ca supplementation ceases [30–32]. There are several explanations for this phenomenon. Heaney [33] proposed a bone remodelling transient hypothesis such that Ca supplement suppresses bone turnover, leading to an increase in measurable bone mass which then disappears after Ca is withdrawn. For the difference in bone mass to persist throughout puberty, high Ca intake should be maintained to suppress bone turnover within the expanding periosteal envelope. Another possible explanation for diminishing difference between placebo and Ca groups could be the threshold effect. With age, the threshold decreases (it is about 1000 mg Ca/day for adults, compared with 1500 mg Ca/day for adolescents), and once the adolescents reach maturity they do not need as much Ca to saturate their skeleton. Therefore, even with the lower Ca intake in the placebo groups, maximal saturation of the skeleton may still occur.

It is unclear which developmental phase (childhood, adolescence or young adulthood) is the most important when showing a nutritional affect on the accumulation of bone mass. The assumption is that dietary Ca at or above the threshold level is necessary throughout the entire bone modelling and consolidation phase (from childhood to young adulthood) if genetically predetermined peak bone mass is to be reached.

Likewise, during adulthood there is a continuous need for adequate Ca intake to compensate for obligatory Ca losses and to maintain bone mass. Gonadal hormones are primary determinants in regulating bone turnover, and the cessation of estrogen secretion in women or testosterone secretion in men contributes to increased bone loss. If untreated, a women can lose a substantial amount of bone during the early postmenopausal period due to estrogen withdrawal. If there is a concurrent deficiency in dietary Ca, the bone loss is exacerbated [34]. A substantial proportion of older women in the United States consume lower amounts of Ca than the former RDA (800 mg/day), and even more so in comparison with the new AIs for Ca (1200 mg/day for postmenopausal women). Many studies confirm the protective effect of Ca on bone turnover and bone mineral density [35–39] and the combination of estrogen and dietary Ca is more effective than either treatment alone [40].

It is likely that variations in Ca nutrition early in life can account for as much as a 5–10% difference in peak adult bone mass. Such a difference, although small, could potentially contribute to more than 50% of the difference in the hip fracture rates later in life [5,41] confirming the hypothesis that those with greater bone mass in early adulthood are resistant to osteoporotic bone fracture. However, national nutrition surveys indicate that Ca intakes in females of all age groups in the United States are consistently lower than current recommendations. In most young women, Ca intake is insufficient to optimize genetically programmed peak bone mass [42], and consequently, increases osteoporotic risk later in life. Increasing Ca intake was a primary objective in the Healthy People 2000 [43] which resulted in higher Ca standards [1,44]. Increasing Ca intake remains a primary objective in the newest version of Healthy People 2010 [43].

Vitamin D

The vitamin D endocrine system influences Ca and P metabolism by affecting the target organs: intestine, bone and kidney. The active metabolite, 1,25-dihydroxyvitamin D_3 (1,25$(OH)_2$-vitamin D_3; calcitriol) facilitates active Ca absorption in the intestine by stimulating the synthesis of Ca binding protein (calbindin). Vitamin D is also involved in bone turnover and a deficiency may cause rickets in children and osteomalacia in adults (both characterized by defective mineralization of bone). We recently demonstrated the important role of calcitriol in bone mass accretion in pubertal girls. Calcitriol concentration was the highest during peak growth (pubertal stages 3 and 4), probably due to the high skeletal demands for Ca. Baseline calcitriol levels also predicted annual change in total body and forearm bone mass [45].

Vitamin D status declines with age for many reasons: lower exposure to sunlight (particularly in the northern latitudes during winter months), decreased ability to activate precursors in the skin, decreased ability of the kidney and liver to hydroxylate vitamin D, use of anticonvulsant and steroid drugs, reduced dietary intake, and diminished absorption from food. Subsequently, vitamin D deficiency in the aged is not uncommon, particularly in the frail elderly living in northern industrialized cities. Approximately half the medical inpatients in the Boston area had low serum levels of 25-hydroxyvitamin D (25(OH)vitamin D) [46]. A similar trend was observed in the homebound elderly [47]. However, apparently healthy non-institutionalized adults in the US have a much lower incidence of hypovitaminosis D [48].

It is well established that the circulating 25(OH)vitamin D level (an indicator of vitamin D status) varies seasonally. As recently shown, the increase in 25(OH)vitamin D from winter to summer is much lower in black than in white women and inversely related to parathyroid hormone (PTH) [49]. Although black women have denser bones and lower 25(OH)vitamin D levels [50] there may be negative consequences later in life that contribute to higher rate of bone loss observed in the Study of Osteoporotic Fractures [51]. It was reported earlier that a substantial proportion of patients with hip fractures also have osteomalacia, caused by vitamin D deficiency [52]. Vitamin D deficiency may also be associated with reduced muscular function [53], which may increase the risk of falling and indirectly contribute to fractures.

There are a few foods which are natural sources of vitamin D, such as butter, margarine, liver, eggs. Therefore, milk in the United States is fortified with vitamin D to the level of 5 μg (200 IU) per serving. When compared with the previous RDAs, the 1997 Requirements [1] for vitamin D were decreased (by half) for adolescents and children; they were doubled or even tripled for the aged.

Vitamin K

Vitamin K is a coenzyme for γ-glutamate carboxylase, an enzyme that mediates the post-translational conversion of glutamate into gamma-carboxyglutamate (Gla). The specific Gla protein found in bone is osteocalcin, a small molecule that contains three gamma-carboxyglutamyl residues which transport Ca ions to the area of bone formation. Once the osteoblasts synthesize and secrete osteocalcin, most of the osteocalcin absorbs onto the hydroxyapatite matrix of bone. However, around 30% of the newly produced osteocalcin is released into the circulation and there it reflects bone formation.

Epidemiological studies show that low dietary or circulating vitamin K levels are associated with low bone mineral density (BMD) or increased fractures [54,55]. Warfarin, a vitamin K antagonist, should, in theory, lower BMD. There is scientific evidence to both support [56] and to refute this contention [57].

An increase in undercarboxylated osteocalcin is a sensitive marker for poor vitamin K status. In fact, high levels of undercarboxylated osteocalcin are associated with low BMD and increased hip fractures [58,59]. Vitamin K supplementation reduces undercarboxylated osteocalcin [60,61], reduces urinary Ca excretion [61] and improves bone turnover profile [62]. Vitamin K may also influence bone metabolism by inhibiting bone resorption agents such as prostaglandin E_2 [63] or interleukin 6 [64].

Vitamin K is supplied to the body from two sources: the diet and synthesis by intestinal bacteria. Dietary vitamin K is provided by plant foods, particularly broccoli, cabbage, spinach, brussels sprouts, turnip greens and lettuce, all of which contain more than 100 μg/100 g serving. The 1989 RDA for dietary vitamin K is 55–70 μg/day for the adult.

Antioxidant Vitamins

Vitamin C is required for collagen crosslinking and in the extreme case of vitamin C deficiency, scurvy, there is a weakening of the collagenous structure in bone [65]. Vitamin C along with other antioxidant vitamins may serve to protect the skeleton from the oxidative stress from smoking. Smoking is known to increase the relative risk of hip fracture between 1.5 and 2.0 times, possibly due to increased free radical generation and bone resorption. In a recent study of women, high intakes of vitamin E and C (but not beta-carotene or selenium) significantly decreased the odds ratio for hip fracture in current smokers [66], suggesting these antioxidant vitamins are protective against oxidant-mediated bone loss in smokers.

Vitamin A is important in the bone remodelling process. Osteoblasts and osteoclasts express nuclear receptors for retinoic acid [67,68]. Hypervitaminosis A in animals results in accelerated bone resorption, increased bone fragility and spontaneous fractures [69,70]. In a group of Swedish women, high dietary intake of retinol was negatively associated with BMD [71]. In vitamin A deficiency, osteoclasts are reduced in number, resulting in excessive deposition of periosteal bone from unchecked osteoblast activity [65]. As long as vitamin A is consumed within recommended levels, it is safe and beneficial to bone health [72].

Protein

We have known for around 50 years that increasing dietary protein increases urinary Ca loss such that for each 50 g increment of protein consumed, an extra 60 mg of urinary Ca is excreted [73]. It follows that the higher the protein intake, the more urinary Ca is lost, and the more negative Ca balance becomes. Since 99% of the body's Ca is in bone, one would hypothesize that protein-induced hypercalciuria would result ultimately in higher bone resorption and an increased prevalence of osteopenia or osteoporotis-related fractures.

The epidemiological and clinical data addressing this hypothesis are equivocal. On the one hand, many [74–76], but not all [77] epidemiological studies found a positive association between protein intake and BMD, thus generally not supporting the above hypothesis. On the other hand, many [78–80], but not all [81] studies report higher fractures in groups consuming a high protein diet, thus generally supporting the hypothesis. Clinical intervention trials generally support the hypothesis. Several [82–84], but not all [85] report an increase in bone resorption when animals or humans were fed a high protein diet. The effect on bone is likely to be small and difficult to detect experimentally given the complex nature of bone. A summary of the impact of dietary protein on Ca metabolism and bone health was presented by Massey and colleagues [86–88].

Attention has turned to the potential negative impact of low protein intake on bone health. We have reported that in healthy young women, acute intakes of low protein diets decreased urinary Ca excretion accompanied by secondary hyperparathyroidism (with 2- to 3-fold increases in serum PTH, 1,25$(OH)_2$-vitamin D and nephrogenous cyclic adenosine monophosphate excretion (a bio-index of PTH action)) [89]. The etiology of the secondary hyperparathyroidism is due, in part, to a significant reduction in intestinal Ca absorption during the low protein diet [90]. Another potential factor contributing to low bone mass during protein-restricted diets is alterations in insulin-like growth factor I (IGF-1), an important growth factor for bone. Protein restriction consistently reduces circulating IFG-I levels and this may lead to a series of catabolic events involving bone and Ca-P metabolism (reviewed in [91]).

Likewise, the addition of dietary protein in conditions of protein undernutrition improves bone health. Bonjour and colleagues studied the effects of 6 months of protein supplementation in a group of elderly subjects who had suffered osteoporotic hip fracture. The additional protein (+ 20 g) over a rather low baseline protein intake (approximately 40 g) in these subjects was associated with attenuation of proximal femur bone loss and almost a 50% reduction in proximal femur bone loss at 1 year [92].

Overall, it appears that both low and high protein diets may be detrimental to bone health. Low protein diets interfere with intestinal Ca absorption, and IGF-I levels and high protein diets induce excess urinary Ca loss. Diets containing moderate protein levels (approximately 1.0–1.5 g/kg) are probably optimal for bone health.

Phosphorus

As an inorganic element, phosphorus (P) is second to Ca in abundance in the human body, with 85% of the body's P being bound in the skeleton. P is widely distributed in foods including meat, poultry, fish, eggs, dairy products, nuts, legumes, cereals, grains and cola beverages. Phosphorus intakes have risen 10–15% over the past 20 years because of the increased use of phosphate salts in food additives [1]. Dietary P intakes in US adults range between 1000 and 1500 mg/day, a level generally well over recommendations (Table 26.1).

Although P is an essential nutrient, there is concern that excessive amounts may affect bone health. For example, a rise in dietary P increases serum P, which produces a transient fall in serum ionized Ca resulting in elevated PTH secretion. The typical diet that is moderately high in P and moderately low in Ca may potentially be detrimental to bone health. This hypothesis was tested in young adults consuming controlled diets containing 1660 mg P and 420 mg Ca per day. Within 24 h, this diet resulted in elevated indexes of PTH action [93], a change that persisted for 4 weeks [94] which could potentially decrease bone formation [95]. Animal data confirm that the combination of a high P, low Ca diet is deleterious to bone mass [96]. On the other hand, other data show that the transient decline in serum Ca induced by a P load is caused by an inhibition of PTH-mediated Ca release from bone, thus conferring beneficial effects on bone. Human studies using Ca kinetic methodology showed no effect on bone turnover from doubling P [97], a conclusion supported by a nonisotopic study done in young men [98].

Magnesium

There is approximately 25 g of magnesium (Mg) in the human body, two-thirds of which is present in the skeleton and the rest in soft tissue. The Mg in bone is not the integral part of the hydroxyapatite crystal structure (like Ca and P), but rather is adsorbed on the surface of the crystal. Only a small fraction of Mg in bone is freely exchangable with extracellular Mg [99]; however, it plays an important role in Ca and bone metabolism. Magnesium deficiency is frequently accompanied by hypocalcemia (due to the failure of bone to exchange Ca for Mg) and impaired secretory abilities of PTH [100]. With Mg deficiency, the osteoclastic receptor for PTH loses its responsiveness, resulting in a reduced bone resorption activity and restoration of serum Ca. As recently shown, there is a lower rate of bone loss immediately after cardiac transplantation in patients with low serum Mg [101]. Bone response to active vitamin D metabolites was impaired in Mg deficiency [102] along with decreased calcitriol activity. Several cases of rickets coincide with Mg-deficient states in children [103].

Magnesium concentration in bones is slightly higher in younger than older individuals [104] and osteoporotic patients have lower serum Mg than controls [105]. Recent studies showed a significant negative relationship between dietary Mg and BMD of different skeletal sites [106–108]. There is a higher incidence of osteoporosis in disease states where Mg deficiency is common, such as diabetes, alcoholism, malabsorption syndrome (see [109] for review) and gluten-sensitive enteropathy [110].

National surveys consistently show low intakes of Mg among females of all age groups, but particularly among teenagers [111]. This becomes even more pronounced with the new increased recommendations for Mg (Table 26.1). A recent report on Mg balance in teenage girls showed that those with low Mg intake (< 177 mg/day; RDA is 240 mg) were in negative Mg balance [112]. The same study did not show any adverse effect of Ca supplementation (total intake ~1700 mg Ca/day) on any components of Mg metabolism. Good sources of Mg in food are whole grains, vegetables (broccoli, squash), nuts and seeds. Dairy products and meats also contribute magnesium to a diet. "Hard" water contains high concentrations of Mg, and can be considered as a dietary source.

Sodium

Urinary sodium (Na) excretion parallels dietary Na intake. In animals and humans, dietary Na, in the form of NaCl, increases Ca loss in the urine [4,113,114]. On average, for every 100 mmol of Na excreted in the urine there is about 0.6–1 mmol loss of Ca in free-living healthy populations of various ages [4,115].

Although it is clear that Na is an important determinant of obligatory Ca loss in urine and causes bone loss in animals (especially at lower Ca intakes) [113,116], there are only a few studies examining its effect on bone mass in humans. Forearm BMD was significantly and negatively correlated with 24 h urinary Na excretion in a cross-sectional study of 440 healthy postmenopausal women [117]. Results from other cross-sectional studies, one in elderly men and women [118] and another in preadolescent females [4], show a strong correlation between urinary Na and Ca. However, there were no direct effects of urinary Na on BMD at the spine, hip, forearm or whole body [4,118]. In the only longitudinal study examining bone mass and urinary Na, Devine et al. [119] showed that changes in urinary Na were negatively correlated with changes in BMD of hip and ankle in postmenopausal women. Based on their data, halving dietary Na (from 3500 to 1750 mg) would have the same effect on the reduction of bone loss as increasing dietary Ca by 900 mg.

Other, indirect evidence of adverse effects of Na on bone originates from short-term interventional studies with Na loading or restriction and markers of bone turnover. Evans et al. [120] showed that postmenopausal, but not premenopausal, women, responded to a 1 week high Na intake of 300 mmol/day by an increase in deoxypyridinoline (bone resorption marker). Other studies investigating the effects of dietary Na on bone markers are inconclusive [121, 122].

The interaction between Ca and Na becomes even more important when considering the trends in intakes of each: Ca intake is lower than recommendations and Na intake remains consistently high. The estimated minimal requirements for adults are 500 mg Na/day [2] and the American Heart Association recommendations are at 2400 mg Na/day or less [123]. Yet dietary Na intake in the United States is generally much higher than recommendations [124].

Fluoride

Fluoride (F) is an ultratrace element, occurring in minute amounts in food and water supplies. It is completely and readily absorbed by passive diffusion. Once absorbed, F readily crosses cell membranes and becomes incorporated into the teeth and bones. It reacts instantaneously with Ca, and both are deposited in the hydration layer of hydroxyapatite and can replace other ions. There is a strong affinity for F in bones, particularly during the growing period. Because F is not easily released from bone, F toxicity may be a problem.

An early survey in North Dakota showed the incidence of osteoporosis was lower in an area where F was naturally high in the water [125]. F is a potent stimulator of bone formation, acting primarily on trabecular bone [126] and resulting generally in the 5–10% annual increase in spinal bone mass.

Although the precise mechanism of action of F on bones is not completely clear, it seems that it exerts its effect by sensitizing various skeletal growth factors through inhibition of osteoblastic acid phosphatase [127] or stimulation of osteoblastic replication [128] or both. Sodium fluoride (NaF) as a therapy for osteoporosis is used in many European countries; however, its approval in the United States by the Food and Drug Administration is still pending. Some of the earlier clinical trials with higher doses of NaF resulted in either unfavorable gastrointestinal side-effects, higher fracture rates despite increase in bone mass, or changes in bone structure [129]. This could have been due partially to inappropriate patient selection and the suboptimal designs of clinical trials.

Zinc

The human body contains 1–2 g of zinc (Zn), of which about 90% is found in muscle, bone, skin and hair, while blood contains less than 1%. Zinc plays an important role in connective tissue metabolism, acting as a cofactor for several enzymes, such as alkaline phosphatase (necessary for bone mineralization) and collagenase (essential for the development of the collagenous structure of bone) [130].

Zinc deficiency results in impaired DNA synthesis and protein metabolism which lead to negative effects on bone formation [130]. The role of Zn in bone formation is well documented in animal models [131] and low serum levels of Zn and excessive urinary excretion are related to osteoporosis in humans [132,133]. Zn concentration in bone is greatly reduced during Zn deficiency [134]. A beneficial effect of Zn supplementation was observed in vertebral and femoral bone mass in rats during strenuous treadmill exercise [135].

Zinc is abundant in animal protein foods (red meat, poultry, fish, oysters, eggs), legumes, whole grain breads and milk. The populations that may be susceptible to a mild or moderate Zn deficiency are infants and adolescents, due to increased requirements for growth and, in the case of the latter, poor eating habits [136, 137]. Several dietary constituents may decrease the bioavailability of Zn including phytic acid, dietary fiber, low dietary protein and Ca [138]. Although animal studies show that Ca interferes with the intestinal absorption of Zn [139], human studies have not been convincing [140–142]. Long-term Ca supplementation of 1000 mg Ca/day (from Ca citrate malate) did not affect any components of Zn metabolism (balance, urinary or fecal excretion) in adolescent girls already consuming low amounts of Zn [143].

Copper

The content of copper (Cu) in the body is about 75–100 mg, mostly accumulated during growth. Deficiency of Cu is rare as Cu is present in nearly all foods, particularly legumes, nuts, whole grains, beef liver and shellfish. The intake of Cu in the United States varies widely (from 0.7 to 7.5 mg/day) and the safe and adequate intake ranges from 2 to 3 mg/day [2]. Because Cu influences collagen maturation, it could influence bone composition and structure. The enzyme lysyl oxidase is a Cu-containing enzyme that catalyzes crosslinking of lysine and hydroxyproline in collagen, contributing to the mechanical strength of collagen fibrils [144]. Copper deficiency results in decreased bone strength in rats [145,146] and chicks [147].

Iron

Iron (Fe) may play an important role in bone formation, acting as a cofactor with enzymes involved in collagen synthesis [148]. It was reported recently that the bone breaking strength was lower in Fe deficient rats, suggesting that Fe deficiency may play a role in bone fragility [146].

Iron deficiency and Fe deficiency anemia is a prevalent nutrient deficiency, affecting about 11% of the US population. Iron deficiency is highest among toddlers, adolescent girls and women of child-bearing age [149]. Adolescent girls are particularly prone to developing Fe deficiency anemia due to increased demands for growth, loss of Fe with menstruation and poor dietary habits.

Iron absorption may be inhibited by the high intakes of other minerals and trace elements particularly Ca. Many studies suggest that Ca interferes with Fe absorption and that the effect is dose-dependent [150–154]. However, when Ca consumption occurs separately from the meal containing Fe, the effect is less clear [155,156]. It is also unclear to what extent, if any, higher Ca intake (even when it interferes with Fe absorption) might influence Fe stores and what the consequences would be of lower Fe stores on bone mass. There is no effect of Ca on serum ferritin (an indicator of Fe stores) in infants [157], adolescent girls (even after long-term supplementation with Ca) [158], adults [154] or lactating women [159].

We recently examined the relationship between bone mass and ferritin in a 4 year clinical trial of Ca supplementation in adolescent girls [158]. There was a trend for a positive association between BMD of the forearm and serum ferritin at baseline. A similar trend was noticed between the total-body BMD and BMC and serum ferritin in year 4 of the study, but only in the placebo group [158]. Further studies are necessary to clarify the above trend, particularly with regard to those subjects who suffer from the Fe deficiency anemia.

Energy Balance

There is a consistent positive association between body weight and BMD. Increased energy intake favors weight gain and higher BMD. The strong positive effect of excess weight on BMD may be due to weightbearing forces exerted on the skeleton [160,161]. Likewise, moderate weight loss of 10% typically results in 1–2% bone loss [162–164]. More severe weight loss, or conditions of malnutrition, are considered a risk factor for osteoporosis and there could be many contributing factors: low macronutrient intake (including protein), low micronutrient intake (including calcium, vitamin D, vitamin K), increased propensity to fall due to poor muscle strength, and less protective soft padding on the hip region (reviewed in [91]).

Phytochemicals

Phytochemicals are naturally occurring, plant-derived compounds that may have biological activity. One such group, the phytoestrogens, are a broad assortment of compounds, nonsteroidal in structure, that mimic estrogens. Because of their phenolic ring structure, phytoestrogens may act as estrogen agonists or antagonists [165]. Isoflavones, a type of phytoestrogen, of which soybeans are a rich source, are thought to have beneficial effects on bone. Soy protein or isoflavones added to the diets of ovariectomized rats prevented bone loss to varying degrees [166–168], perhaps by interfering with osteoclast acid transport [169] or by enhancing bone formation [168]. In a group of postmenopausal women, isoflavone supplementation increased BMC and BMD only in the lumbar spine [170].

The threshold intake in humans of dietary isoflavone to achieve biological activity is thought to be 30–50 mg/day, an amount that is attainable by the inclusion of several soy-containing foods per day [165]. Intakes in the 30–50 mg/day range may influence serum lipids, but higher doses may be required to influence bone. For example, moderate amounts of isoflavones (56 mg/day) did not affect BMD over a 6 month period; however, a 90 mg/day dose (taken as a supplement) was needed to show an effect on bone [170].

Caffeine

It was once thought that caffeine simply increased urinary loss of Ca and, as such, was considered a risk factor for bone loss. However, the long-term effect of caffeine on Ca and bone metabolism is more complex. In an analysis of 560 balance studies carried out in 190 adult women, caffeine surprisingly does little to affect either urinary Ca excretion or total Ca entry into the gut. Caffeine is, however, negatively correlated with intestinal Ca absorption, the net result being a more negative Ca balance. In adult women, for each 6 fl oz serving of caffeinated coffee (containing an estimated 103 mg of caffeine), Ca balance was more negative by 4.6 mg/day. Additionally, there was an inverse relationship between caffeine intake and Ca intake [171] such that as intake of caffeine-containing coffee increased, milk consumption decreased.

However, the epidemiological data addressing the association between coffee consumption and bone status are quite contradictory. Some studies show detrimental associations between caffeine consumption [172,173] and some do not [174–176]. It appears that the deleterious effect of caffeine becomes most pronounced when dietary Ca is inadequate and less harmful when dietary Ca is high [172,177,178].

Summary

With prolonged life expectancy and increasing number of elderly, it is predicted that osteoporotic fractures will reach epidemic proportions. Therefore, osteoporosis prevention and treatment as well as Ca nutrition remain a high priority in the latest health goals for the United States presented in Healthy People 2010 [43]. Osteoporosis is a multifactorial disorder and, despite the considerable influence of heredity on bone, environmental factors, such as nutrition, play an important role. A substantial effort has been made toward understanding the effect of nutrients, particularly Ca and vitamin D, on bone accretion during youth and bone loss during aging, and a wealth of new knowledge is now available. Yet in many populations within our society the intakes of Ca and vitamin D remain inadequate to meet skeletal demands. Health care professionals are encouraged to improve the dietary intakes of these two important nutrients, particularly among the young and the old. Meanwhile, our understanding of other nutrients or alternative food and nutrition components that affect bone health continues to grow.

References

1. Standing Committee on the Scientific Evaluation of Dietary Reference Intakes, FNB, Institute of Medicine. Dietary reference intakes for calcium, phosphorus, magnesium, vitamin D and fluoride. Washington, DC: National Academy Press, 1997.
2. National Research Council. Recommended dietary allowances, 10th ed. Washington, DC: National Academy Press, 1989.
3. Matkovic V, Heaney RP. Calcium balance during human growth: evidence for threshold behavior. Am J Clin Nutr 1992;55:992–996.
4. Matkovic V, Ilich JZ, Andon MB, Hsieh LC, Tzagournis MA, Lagger BJ, et al. Urinary calcium, sodium, and bone mass of young females. Am J Clin Nutr 1995;62:417–425.

5. Matkovic V, Kostial K, Simonovic I, Buzina R, Brodarec A, Nordin BE. Bone status and fracture rates in two regions of Yugoslavia. Am J Clin Nutr 1979;32:540–549.
6. Hu JF, Zhao XH, Jia JB, Parpia B, Campbell TC. Dietary calcium and bone density among middle-aged and elderly women in China. Am J Clin Nutr 1993;58:219–227.
7. Sandler RB, Slemenda CW, LaPorte RE, Cauley JA, Schramm MM, Barresi ML, et al. Postmenopausal bone density and milk consumption in childhood and adolescence. Am J Clin Nutr 1985;42:270–274.
8. Halioua L, Anderson JJ. Lifetime calcium intake and physical activity habits: independent and combined effects on the radial bone of healthy premenopausal Caucasian women. Am J Clin Nutr 1989;49:534–541.
9. Stracke H, Renner E, Knie G, Leidig G, Minne H, Federlin K. Osteoporosis and bone metabolic parameters in dependence upon calcium intake through milk and milk products. Eur J Clin Nutr 1993;47:617–622.
10. Murphy S, Khaw KT, May H, Compston JE. Milk consumption and bone mineral density in middle aged and elderly women. BMJ 1994;308:939–941.
11. Welten DC, Kemper HC, Post GB, van Staveren WA. A meta-analysis of the effect of calcium intake on bone mass in young and middle aged females and males. J Nutr 1995;125:2802–2813.
12. Cumming RG. Calcium intake and bone mass: a quantitative review of the evidence. Calcif Tissue Int 1990;47:194–201.
13. Anderson JJ, Rondano PA. Peak bone mass development of females: can young adult women improve their peak bone mass? J Am Coll Nutr 1996;15:570–574.
14. Glastre C, Braillon P, David L, Cochat P, Meunier PJ, Delmas PD. Measurement of bone mineral content of the lumbar spine by dual energy x-ray absorptiometry in normal children: correlations with growth parameters. J Clin Endocrinol Metab 1990;70:1330–1333.
15. Kroger H, Kotaniemi A, Kroger L, Alhava E. Development of bone mass and bone density of the spine and femoral neck- -a prospective study of 65 children and adolescents. Bone Miner 1993;23:171–182.
16. Chan GM. Dietary calcium and bone mineral status of children and adolescents. Am J Dis Child 1991;145:631–634.
17. Lee WT, Leung SS, Ng MY, Wang SF, Xu YC, Zeng WP, et al. Bone mineral content of two populations of Chinese children with different calcium intakes. Bone Miner 1993;23:195–206.
18. Lee WT, Leung SS, Lui SS, Lau J. Relationship between long-term calcium intake and bone mineral content of children aged from birth to 5 years. Br J Nutr 1993;70:235–248.
19. Ilich JZ, Skugor M, Hangartner T, Baoshe A, Matkovic V. Relation of nutrition, body composition and physical activity to skeletal development: a cross-sectional study in preadolescent females. J Am Coll Nutr 1998;17:136–147.
20. Ilich JZ, Hangartner TN, Skugor M, Roche AF, Goel PK, Matkovic V. Skeletal age as a determinant of bone mass in preadolescent females. Skeletal Radiol 1996;25:431–439.
21. Teegarden D, Lyle RM, McCabe GP, McCabe LD, Proulx WR, Michon K, et al. Dietary calcium, protein, and phosphorus are related to bone mineral density and content in young women. Am J Clin Nutr 1998;68:749–754.
22. Abrams SA, O'Brien K O, Liang LK, Stuff JE. Differences in calcium absorption and kinetics between black and white girls aged 5–16 years. J Bone Miner Res 1995;10:829–833.
23. Bell N, Shary J, Stevens J, Garza M, Gordon L, Edwards J. Demonstration that bone mass is greater in black than in white children. J Bone Miner Res 1991;6:719–723.
24. Johnston CC, Jr, Miller JZ, Slemenda CW, Reister TK, Hui S, Christian JC, et al. Calcium supplementation and increases in bone mineral density in children. N Engl J Med 1992;327:82–7.
25. Lloyd T, Andon MB, Rollings N, Martel JK, Landis JR, Demers LM, et al. Calcium supplementation and bone mineral density in adolescent girls. JAMA 1993;270:841–844.

26. Chan GM, Hoffman K, McMurry M. Effects of dairy products on bone and body composition in pubertal girls. J Pediatr 1995;126:551–556.
27. Bonjour JP, Carrie AL, Ferrari S, Clavien H, Slosman D, Theintz G, et al. Calcium-enriched foods and bone mass growth in prepubertal girls: a randomized, double-blind, placebo-controlled trial. J Clin Invest 1997;99:1287–1294.
28. Cadogan J, Blumsohn A, Barker ME, Eastell R. A longitudinal study of bone gain in pubertal girls: anthropometric and biochemical correlates. J Bone Miner Res 1998;13: 1602–1612.
29. Lee WT, Leung SS, Leung DM, Tsang HS, Lau J, Cheng JC. A randomized double-blind controlled calcium supplementation trial, and bone and height acquisition in children. Br J Nutr 1995;74:125–139.
30. Lee WT, Leung SS, Leung DM, Cheng JC. A follow-up study on the effects of calcium-supplement withdrawal and puberty on bone acquisition of children. Am J Clin Nutr 1996;64:71–77.
31. Lloyd T, Rollings N, Andon M, Eggli D, Mauger E, Chinchilli V. Enhanced bone gain in early adolescence due to calcium supplementation does not persist in late adolescence. J Bone Miner Res 1996;11:253–256.
32. Lee WT, Leung SS, Leung DM, Wang SH, Xu YC, Zeng WP, et al. Bone mineral acquisition in low calcium intake children following the withdrawal of calcium supplement. Acta Paediatr 1997;86:570–576.
33. Heaney RP. The bone-remodeling transient: implications for the interpretation of clinical studies of bone mass change. J Bone Miner Res 1994;9:1515–1523.
34. Heaney RP. Estrogen–calcium interactions in the postmenopause: a quantitative description. Bone Miner 1990;11:67–84.
35. Riggs BL, O'Fallon WM, Muhs J, O'Connor MK, Kumar R, Melton LJ, III. Long-term effects of calcium supplementation on serum parathyroid hormone level, bone turnover, and bone loss in elderly women. J Bone Miner Res 1998;13:168–174.
36. Michaelsson K, Bergstrom R, Holmberg L, Mallmin H, Wolk A, Ljunghall S. A high dietary calcium intake is needed for a positive effect on bone density in Swedish postmenopausal women. Osteoporos Int 1997;7:155–161.
37. Devine A, Dick IM, Heal SJ, Criddle RA, Prince RL. A 4-year follow-up study of the effects of calcium supplementation on bone density in elderly postmenopausal women. Osteoporos Int 1997;7:23–28.
38. Cepollaro C, Orlandi G, Gonnelli S, Ferrucci G, Arditti JC, Borracelli D, et al. Effect of calcium supplementation as a high-calcium mineral water on bone loss in early postmenopausal women. Calcif Tissue Int 1996;59:238–239.
39. Reid IR, Ames RW, Evans MC, Gamble GD, Sharpe SJ. Effect of calcium supplementation on bone loss in postmenopausal women [published erratum appears in N Engl J Med 1993;329:1281]. N Engl J Med 1993;328:460–464.
40. Prestwood KM, Thompson DL, Kenny AM, Seibel MJ, Pilbeam CC, Raisz LG. Low dose estrogen and calcium have an additive effect on bone resorption in older women. J Clin Endocrinol Metab 1999;84:179–183.
41. Matkovic V, Klisovic D, Ilich J. Epidemiology of fractures during growth and aging. In: Matkovic V, editor. Osteoporosis. Physical medicine and rehabilitation clinics of North America. Philadelphia: Saunders; 1995:415–439.
42. Matkovic V, Skugor M, Badenhop N, Landoll J, Ilich J. Skeletal development in young females: Endogenous vs exogenous factors. In: Burckardt P, Heaney R, Dawson-Hughes B, editors. Nutritional aspects of osteoporosis, 3rd ed. Berlin Heidelberg New York: Springer, 1998:26–41.
43. U.S. Department of Health and Human Services, Healthy People 2000 Homepage, http://odphp.osophs.dhhs.gov/pubs/hp2000/ accessed March 1999.
44. NIH consensus conference. Optimal calcium intake. NIH Consensus Development Panel on Optimal Calcium Intake. JAMA 1994;272:1942–1948.
45. Ilich JZ, Badenhop NE, Jelic T, Clairmont AC, Nagode LA, Matkovic V. Calcitriol and bone mass accumulation in females during puberty. Calcif Tissue Int 1997;61:104–109.

46. Thomas MK, Lloyd-Jones DM, Thadhani RI, Shaw AC, Deraska DJ, Kitch BT, et al. Hypovitaminosis D in medical inpatients. N Engl J Med 1998;338:777–783.
47. Gloth FM III, Gundberg CM, Hollis BW, Haddad JG, Jr, Tobin JD. Vitamin D deficiency in homebound elderly persons. JAMA 1995;274:1683–1686.
48. Looker AC, Gunter EW. Hypovitaminosis D in medical inpatients. N Engl J Med 1998;339:344–345.
49. Harris SS, Dawson-Hughes B. Seasonal changes in plasma 25-hydroxyvitamin D concentrations of young American black and white women. Am J Clin Nutr 1998;67: 1232–1236.
50. Kleerekoper M, Nelson DA, Peterson EL, Flynn MJ, Pawluszka AS, Jacobsen G, et al. Reference data for bone mass, calciotropic hormones, and biochemical markers of bone remodeling in older (55–75) postmenopausal white and black women. J Bone Miner Res 1994;9:1267–1276.
51. Cumming RG, Cummings SR, Nevitt MC, Scott J, Ensrud KE, Vogt TM, et al. Calcium intake and fracture risk: results from the study of osteoporotic fractures. Am J Epidemiol 1997;145:926–934.
52. Aaron JE, Gallagher JC, Anderson J, Stasiak L, Longton EB, Nordin BE, et al. Frequency of osteomalacia and osteoporosis in fractures of the proximal femur. Lancet 1974;I: 229–233.
53. Mowe M, Haug E, Bohmer T. Low serum calcidiol concentration in older adults with reduced muscular function. J Am Geriatr Soc 1999;47:220–226.
54. Kanai T, Takagi T, Masuhiro K, Nakamura M, Iwata M, Saji F. Serum vitamin K level and bone mineral density in post-menopausal women. Int J Gynaecol Obstet 1997; 56:25–30.
55. Feskanich D, Weber P, Willett WC, Rockett H, Booth SL, Colditz GA. Vitamin K intake and hip fractures in women: a prospective study. Am J Clin Nutr 1999;69:74–79.
56. Philip WJ, Martin JC, Richardson JM, Reid DM, Webster J, Douglas AS. Decreased axial and peripheral bone density in patients taking long-term warfarin. Q J Med 1995;88:635–640.
57. Jamal SA, Browner WS, Bauer DC, Cummings SR. Warfarin use and risk for osteoporosis in elderly women. Study of Osteoporotic Fractures Research Group. Ann Intern Med 1998;128:829–832.
58. Szulc P, Chapuy MC, Meunier PJ, Delmas PD. Serum undercarboxylated osteocalcin is a marker of the risk of hip fracture: a three year follow-up study. Bone 1996;18: 487–488.
59. Vergnaud P, Garnero P, Meunier PJ, Breart G, Kamihagi K, Delmas PD. Undercarboxylated osteocalcin measured with a specific immunoassay predicts hip fracture in elderly women: the EPIDOS Study. J Clin Endocrinol Metab 1997;82:719–724.
60. Douglas AS, Robins SP, Hutchison JD, Porter RW, Stewart A, Reid DM. Carboxylation of osteocalcin in post-menopausal osteoporotic women following vitamin K and D supplementation. Bone 1995;17:15–20.
61. Knapen MH, Jie KS, Hamulyak K, Vermeer C. Vitamin K-induced changes in markers for osteoblast activity and urinary calcium loss. Calcif Tissue Int 1993;53:81–85.
62. Craciun AM, Wolf J, Knapen MH, Brouns F, Vermeer C. Improved bone metabolism in female elite athletes after vitamin K supplementation. Int J Sports Med 1998;19: 479–484.
63. Hara K, Akiyama Y, Tajima T, Shiraki M. Menatetrenone inhibits bone resorption partly through inhibition of PGE2 synthesis in vitro. J Bone Miner Res 1993;8:535–542.
64. Reddi K, Henderson B, Meghji S, Wilson M, Poole S, Hopper C, et al. Interleukin 6 production by lipopolysaccharide-stimulated human fibroblasts is potently inhibited by naphthoquinone (vitamin K) compounds. Cytokine 1995;7:287–290.
65. Combs G. The vitamins, 2nd ed. San Diego: Academic Press; 1998.
66. Melhus H, Michalsson K, Holmberg L, Wolk A, Ljunghall S. Smoking, antioxidant vitamins, and the risk of hip fracture. J Bone Miner Res 1999;14:129–135.

67. Kindmark A, Torma H, Johansson A, Ljunghall S, Melhus H. Reverse transcription-polymerase chain reaction assay demonstrates that the 9-cis retinoic acid receptor alpha is expressed in human osteoblasts. Biochem Biophys Res Commun 1993;192: 1367–1372.
68. Saneshige S, Mano H, Tezuka K, Kakudo S, Mori Y, Honda Y, et al. Retinoic acid directly stimulates osteoclastic bone resorption and gene expression of cathepsin K/OC-2. Biochem J 1995;309:721–724.
69. Hathcock JN, Hattan DG, Jenkins MY, McDonald JT, Sundaresan PR, Wilkening VL. Evaluation of vitamin A toxicity. Am J Clin Nutr 1990;52:183–202.
70. Armstrong R, Ashenfelter K, Eckoff C, Levin A, Shapiro S. General and reproductive toxicology of retinoids. In: Sporn M, Roberts A, Goodman D, editors. The retinoids: biology, chemistry, and medicine, 2nd ed. New York: Raven Press, 1994:545–527.
71. Melhus H, Michaelsson K, Kindmark A, Bergstrom R, Holmberg L, Mallmin H, et al. Excessive dietary intake of vitamin A is associated with reduced bone mineral density and increased risk for hip fracture. Ann Intern Med 1998;129:770–778.
72. Arden N, Keen R, Arden E, Cooper C, Inskip H, Spector T. Dietary retinol intake and bone mineral density: a study of postmenopausal monozygous twins. J Bone Miner Res 1997;12:S485.
73. Kerstetter JE, Allen LH. Protein intake and calcium homeostasis. Adv Nutr Res 1994;9:167–181.
74. Cooper C, Atkinson EJ, Hensrud DD, Wahner HW, O'Fallon WM, Riggs BL, et al. Dietary protein intake and bone mass in women. Calcif Tissue Int 1996;58:320–325.
75. Michaelsson K, Holmberg L, Mallmin H, Wolk A, Bergstrom R, Ljunghall S. Diet, bone mass, and osteocalcin: a cross-sectional study. Calcif Tissue Int 1995;57:86–93.
76. Geinoz G, Rapin CH, Rizzoli R, Kraemer R, Buchs B, Slosman D, et al. Relationship between bone mineral density and dietary intakes in the elderly. Osteoporos Int 1993;3:242–248.
77. Metz JA, Anderson JJ, Gallagher PN Jr. Intakes of calcium, phosphorus, and protein, and physical-activity level are related to radial bone mass in young adult women. Am J Clin Nutr 1993;58:537–542.
78. Feskanich D, Willett WC, Stampfer MJ, Colditz GA. Protein consumption and bone fractures in women. Am J Epidemiol 1996;143:472–479.
79. Meyer HE, Pedersen JI, Loken EB, Tverdal A. Dietary factors and the incidence of hip fracture in middle-aged Norwegians. A prospective study. Am J Epidemiol 1997;145: 117–123.
80. Abelow B, Holford T, Insogna K. Cross-cultural association between dietary animal protein and hip fracture: a hypothesis. Calcif Tissue Int 1992;50:14–18.
81. Munger RG, Cerhan JR, Chiu BC. Prospective study of dietary protein intake and risk of hip fracture in postmenopausal women. Am J Clin Nutr 1999;69:147–152.
82. Schuette SA, Hegsted M, Zemel MB, Linkswiler HM. Renal acid, urinary cyclic AMP, and hydroxyproline excretion as affected by level of protein, sulfur amino acid, and phosphorus intake. J Nutr 1981;111:2106–2116.
83. Chan EL, Swaminathan R. The effect of high protein and high salt intake for 4 months on calcium and hydroxyproline excretion in normal and oophorectomized rats. J Lab Clin Med 1994;124:37–41.
84. Kerstetter J, Caseria D, Mitnick N, Ellison A, Liskov T, Carpenter T, et al. Bone turnover in response to dietary protein intake. J Clin Endocrinol Metab 1999;84:1052–1055.
85. Shapses SA, Robins SP, Schwartz EI, Chowdhury H. Short-term changes in calcium but not protein intake alter the rate of bone resorption in healthy subjects as assessed by urinary pyridinium cross-link excretion. J Nutr 1995;125:2814–2821.
86. Massey LK. Does excess dietary protein adversely affect bone? Symposium overview. J Nutr 1998;128:1048–1050.
87. Heaney RP. Excess dietary protein may not adversely affect bone. J Nutr 1998;128: 1054–1057.

88. Barzel US, Massey LK. Excess dietary protein can adversely affect bone. J Nutr 1998;128:1051–1053.
89. Kerstetter JE, Caseria DD, Mitnick ME, Ellison AF, et al. Increased circulating concentrations of parathyroid hormone in healthy, young women consuming a protein-restricted diet. Am J Clin Nutr 1997;66:1188–1196.
90. Kerstetter JE, O'Brien KO, Insogna KL. Dietary protein affects intestinal calcium absorption. Am J Clin Nutr 1998;68:859–865.
91. Bonjour JP, Schurch MA, Rizzoli R. Nutritional aspects of hip fractures. Bone 1996;18(Suppl 3):139S–144S.
92. Schurch MA, Rizzoli R, Slosman D, Vadas L, Vergnaud P, Bonjour JP. Protein supplements increase serum insulin-like growth factor-I levels and attenuate proximal femur bone loss in patients with recent hip fracture. A randomized, double-blind, placebo-controlled trial. Ann Intern Med 1998;128:801–809.
93. Calvo MS, Kumar R, Heath Hd. Elevated secretion and action of serum parathyroid hormone in young adults consuming high phosphorus, low calcium diets assembled from common foods. J Clin Endocrinol Metab 1988;66:823–829.
94. Calvo MS, Kumar R, Heath H. Persistently elevated parathyroid hormone secretion and action in young women after four weeks of ingesting high phosphorus, low calcium diets. J Clin Endocrinol Metab 1990;70:1334–1340.
95. Karkkainen M, Lamberg-Allardt C. An acute intake of phosphate increases parathyroid hormone secretion and inhibits bone formation in young women. J Bone Miner Res 1996;11:1905–1912.
96. Calvo MS. The effects of high phosphorus intake on calcium homeostasis. Adv Nutr Res 1994;9:183–207.
97. Heaney RP, Recker RR. Calcium supplements: anion effects. Bone Miner 1987;2: 433–439.
98. Bizik B, Ding W, Cerklewski F. Evidence that bone resorption of young men is not increased by high dietary phosphorus obtained from milk and cheese. Nutr Res 1996;16:1143–1146.
99. Broadus A. Mineral balance and homeostasis. In: Primer on the metabolic bone diseases and disorders of mineral metabolism, 3rd ed. Philadelphia: Lippincott-Raven, 1996:57–63.
100. Anast CS, Mohs JM, Kaplan SL, Burns TW. Evidence for parathyroid failure in magnesium deficiency. Science 1972;177:606–608.
101. Boncimino K, McMahon DJ, Addesso V, Bilezikian JP, Shane E. Magnesium deficiency and bone loss after cardiac transplantation. J Bone Miner Res 1999;14:295–303.
102. Carpenter TO. Disturbances of vitamin D metabolism and action during clinical and experimental magnesium deficiency. Magnes Res 1988;1:131–139.
103. Reddy V, Sivakumar B. Magnesium-dependent vitamin-D-resistant rickets. Lancet 1974;I:963–965.
104. Tsuboi S, Nakagaki H, Ishiguro K, Kondo K, Mukai M, Robinson C, et al. Magnesium distribution in human bone. Calcif Tissue Int 1994;54:34–37.
105. Reginster JY, Strause L, Deroisy R, Lecart MP, Saltman P, Franchimont P. Preliminary report of decreased serum magnesium in postmenopausal osteoporosis. Magnesium 1989;8:106–109.
106. Houtkooper LB, Ritenbaugh C, Aickin M, Lohman TG, Going SB, Weber JL, et al. Nutrients, body composition and exercise are related to change in bone mineral density in premenopausal women. J Nutr 1995;125:1229–1237.
107. New SA, Bolton-Smith C, Grubb DA, Reid DM. Nutritional influences on bone mineral density: a cross-sectional study in premenopausal women. Am J Clin Nutr 1997;65:1831–1839.
108. Dimai HP, Porta S, Wirnsberger G, Lindschinger M, Pamperl I, Dobnig H, et al. Daily oral magnesium supplementation suppresses bone turnover in young adult males. J Clin Endocrinol Metab 1998;83:2742–2748.
109. Rude R. Magnesium Metabolism. In: Bilezikian J, Raisz L, Rodau G, Markovac J, editors. Principles of bone biology. San Diego: Academic Press, 1996:277–293.

110. Rude RK, Olerich M. Magnesium deficiency: possible role in osteoporosis associated with gluten-sensitive enteropathy. Osteoporos Int 1996;6:453–461.
111. Federation of American Societies for Experimental Biology, Prepared for the Interagency Board for Nutrition Monitoring and Related Research. Vol. 1, Table A. T6–16 ed. Washington, DC: US Government Printing Office, Life Sciences Research Office, 1995.
112. Andon MB, Ilich JZ, Tzagournis MA, Matkovic V. Magnesium balance in adolescent females consuming a low- or high-calcium diet. Am J Clin Nutr 1996;63:950–953.
113. Goulding A, Campbell D. Dietary NaCl loads promote calciuria and bone loss in adult oophorectomized rats consuming a low calcium diet. J Nutr 1983;113:1409–1414.
114. Nordin BE, Need AG, Morris HA, Horowitz M. The nature and significance of the relationship between urinary sodium and urinary calcium in women. J Nutr 1993;123: 1615–1622.
115. Massey LK, Whiting SJ. Dietary salt, urinary calcium, and bone loss. J Bone Miner Res 1996;11:731–736.
116. Goulding A, Gold E. Effects of dietary sodium chloride loading on parathyroid function, 1,25-dihydroxyvitamin D, calcium balance, and bone metabolism in female rats during chronic prednisolone administration. Endocrinology 1986;119:2148–2154.
117. Nordin BE, Polley KJ. Metabolic consequences of the menopause. A cross-sectional, longitudinal, and intervention study on 557 normal postmenopausal women. Calcif Tissue Int 1987;41(Suppl 1):S1–S9.
118. Dawson-Hughes B, Fowler SE, Dalsky G, Gallagher C. Sodium excretion influences calcium homeostasis in elderly men and women. J Nutr 1996;126:2107–2112.
119. Devine A, Criddle RA, Dick IM, Kerr DA, Prince RL. A longitudinal study of the effect of sodium and calcium intakes on regional bone density in postmenopausal women. Am J Clin Nutr 1995;62:740–745.
120. Evans CE, Chughtai AY, Blumsohn A, Giles M, Eastell R. The effect of dietary sodium on calcium metabolism in premenopausal and postmenopausal women. Eur J Clin Nutr 1997;51:394–399.
121. Lietz G, Avenell A, Robins SP. Short-term effects of dietary sodium intake on bone metabolism in postmenopausal women measured using urinary deoxypyridinoline excretion. Br J Nutr 1997;78:73–82.
122. Ginty F, Flynn A, Cashman KD. The effect of dietary sodium intake on biochemical markers of bone metabolism in young women. Br J Nutr 1998;79:343–350.
123. Kolasa K. Summary of the sixth report of the joint national committee on prevention, detection, evaluation, and treatment of high blood pressure. J Nutr Edu 1998;30: 114B–115B.
124. Engstrom A, Tobelmann RC, Albertson AM. Sodium intake trends and food choices. Am J Clin Nutr 1997;65(Suppl 2):704S–707S.
125. Bernstein DS, Sadowsky N, Hegsted DM, Guri CD, Stare FJ. Prevalence of osteoporosis in high- and low-fluoride areas in North Dakota. JAMA 1966;198:499–504.
126. Resch H, Libanati C, Farley S, Bettica P, Schulz E, Baylink DJ. Evidence that fluoride therapy increases trabecular bone density in a peripheral skeletal site. J Clin Endocrinol Metab 1993;76:1622–1624.
127. Lau KH, et al. A proposed mechanism of the mitogenic action of fluoride on bone cells: inhibition of the activity of an osteoblastic acid phosphatase. Metabolism. 1989;38:858–868.
128. Caverzasio J, Imai T, Ammann P, Burgener D, Bonjour JP. Aluminum potentiates the effect of fluoride on tyrosine phosphorylation and osteoblast replication in vitro and bone mass in vivo. J Bone Miner Res 1996;11:46–55.
129. Kleerkoper M. The role of fluoride in the prevention of osteoporosis. Endocrinol Metab Clin North Am 1998;27:441–452.
130. Beattie J, Avenell A. Trace element nutrition and bone metabolism. Nutr Res Rev 1992;5:167–188.

131. Yamaguchi M, Yamaguchi R. Action of zinc on bone metabolism in rats. Increases in alkaline phosphatase activity and DNA content. Biochem Pharmacol 1986;35:773–777.
132. Herzberg M, Foldes J, Steinberg R, Menczel J. Zinc excretion in osteoporotic women. J Bone Miner Res 1990;5:251–257.
133. Atik OS. Zinc and senile osteoporosis. J Am Geriatr Soc 1983;31:790–791.
134. Calhoun NR, Smith JC Jr, Becker KL. The role of zinc in bone metabolism. Clin Orthop 1974;103:212–234.
135. Seco C, Revilla M, Hernandez ER, Gervas J, Gonzalez-Riola J, Villa LF, et al. Effects of zinc supplementation on vertebral and femoral bone mass in rats on strenuous treadmill training exercise. J Bone Miner Res 1998;13:508–512.
136. Skinner JD, Carruth BR, Houck KS, Coletta F, Cotter R, Ott D, et al. Longitudinal study of nutrient and food intakes of infants aged 2 to 24 months. J Am Diet Assoc 1997;97:496–504.
137. Donovan UM, et al. Iron and zinc status of young women aged 14 to 19 years consuming vegetarian and omnivorous diets. J Am Coll Nutr. 1995;14:463–472.
138. Cousins RJ. Absorption, transport, and hepatic metabolism of copper and zinc: special reference to metallothionein and ceruloplasmin. Physiol Rev 1985;65:238–309.
139. Dursun N, Aydogan S. Comparative effects of calcium deficiency and supplements on the intestinal absorption of zinc in rats. Jpn J Physiol 1994;44:157–166.
140. Wood RJ, Hanssen DA. Effect of milk and lactose on zinc absorption in lactose-intolerant postmenopausal women. J Nutr 1988;118:982–986.
141. Argiratos V, Samman S. The effect of calcium carbonate and calcium citrate on the absorption of zinc in healthy female subjects. Eur J Clin Nutr 1994;48:198–204.
142. Dawson-Hughes B, Seligson FH, Hughes VA. Effects of calcium carbonate and hydroxyapatite on zinc and iron retention in postmenopausal women. Am J Clin Nutr 1986;44:83–88.
143. McKenna AA, Ilich JZ, Andon MB, Wang C, Matkovic V. Zinc balance in adolescent females consuming a low- or high-calcium diet. Am J Clin Nutr 1997;65:1460–1464.
144. Tuderman L, et al. Mechanism of the prolyl hydroxylase reaction. I. Role of co-substrates. Eur J Biochem. 1977;80:341–348.
145. Jonas J, Burns J, Abel EW, Cresswell MJ, Strain JJ, Paterson CR. Impaired mechanical strength of bone in experimental copper deficiency. Ann Nutr Metab 1993;37:245–252.
146. Medeiros D, Ilich J, Ireton J, Matkovic V, Shiry L, Wildman R. Femurs from rats fed diets deficient in copper or iron have decreased mechanical strength and altered mineral composition. J Trace Elem Exp Med 1997;10:197–203.
147. Rucker RB, Riggins RS, Laughlin R, Chan MM, Chen M, Tom K. Effects of nutritional copper deficiency on the biomechanical properties of bone and arterial elastin metabolism in the chick. J Nutr 1975;105:1062–1070.
148. Prockop DJ. Role of iron in the synthesis of collagen in connective tissue. Fed Proc 1971;30:984–990.
149. Looker AC, Dallman PR, Carroll MD, Gunter EW, Johnson CL. Prevalence of iron deficiency in the United States. JAMA 1997;277:973–976.
150. Gleerup A, Rossander-Hulthen L, Gramatkovski E, Hallberg L. Iron absorption from the whole diet: comparison of the effect of two different distributions of daily calcium intake. Am J Clin Nutr 1995;61:97–104.
151. Deehr MS, Dallal GE, Smith KT, Taulbee JD, Dawson-Hughes B. Effects of different calcium sources on iron absorption in postmenopausal women. Am J Clin Nutr 1990;51:95–99.
152. Hallberg L, Brune M, Erlandsson M, Sandberg AS, Rossander-Hulten L. Calcium: effect of different amounts on nonheme- and heme-iron absorption in humans. Am J Clin Nutr 1991;53:112–119.
153. Cook JD, Dassenko SA, Whittaker P. Calcium supplementation: effect on iron absorption. Am J Clin Nutr 1991;53:106–111.
154. Minihane AM, Fairweather-Tait SJ. Effect of calcium supplementation on daily nonheme-iron absorption and long-term iron status. Am J Clin Nutr 1998;68:96–102.

155. Turnlund JR, Smith RG, Kretsch MJ, Keyes WR, Shah AG. Milk's effect on the bioavailability of iron from cereal-based diets in young women by use of in vitro and in vivo methods. Am J Clin Nutr 1990;52:373–378.
156. Reddy MB, Cook JD. Effect of calcium intake on nonheme-iron absorption from a complete diet. Am J Clin Nutr 1997;65:1820–1825.
157. Dalton MA, Sargent JD, O'Connor GT, Olmstead EM, Klein RZ. Calcium and phosphorus supplementation of iron-fortified infant formula: no effect on iron status of healthy full-term infants. Am J Clin Nutr 1997;65:921–926.
158. Ilich-Ernst JZ, McKenna AA, Badenhop NE, Clairmont AC, Andon MB, Nahhas RW, et al. Iron status, menarche, and calcium supplementation in adolescent girls. Am J Clin Nutr 1998;68:880–887.
159. Kalkwarf HJ, Harrast SD. Effects of calcium supplementation and lactation on iron status. Am J Clin Nutr 1998;67:1244–1249.
160. Felson DT, Zhang Y, Hannan MT, Anderson JJ. Effects of weight and body mass index on bone mineral density in men and women: the Framingham study. J Bone Miner Res 1993;8:567–573.
161. Harris SS, Dawson-Hughes B. Weight, body composition, and bone density in postmenopausal women. Calcif Tissue Int 1996;59:428–432.
162. Hyldstrup L, Andersen T, McNair P, Breum L, Transbol I. Bone metabolism in obesity: changes related to severe overweight and dietary weight reduction. Acta Endocrinol (Copenh) 1993;129:393–398.
163. Svendsen OL, Hassager C, Christiansen C. Effect of an energy-restrictive diet, with or without exercise, on lean tissue mass, resting metabolic rate, cardiovascular risk factors, and bone in overweight postmenopausal women. Am J Med 1993;95:131–140.
164. Compston JE, Laskey MA, Croucher PI, Coxon A, Kreitzman S. Effect of diet-induced weight loss on total body bone mass. Clin Sci (Colch) 1992;82:429–432.
165. Setchell KD. Phytoestrogens: the biochemistry, physiology, and implications for human health of soy isoflavones. Am J Clin Nutr 1998;68(Suppl 6):1333S–1346S.
166. Arjmandi BH, Birnbaum R, Goyal NV, Getlinger MJ, Juma S, Alekel L, et al. Bone-sparing effect of soy protein in ovarian hormone-deficient rats is related to its isoflavone content. Am J Clin Nutr 1998;68(Suppl 6):1364S–1368S.
167. Arjmandi BH, Getlinger MJ, Goyal NV, Alekel L, Hasler CM, Juma S, et al. Role of soy protein with normal or reduced isoflavone content in reversing bone loss induced by ovarian hormone deficiency in rats. Am J Clin Nutr 1998;68(Suppl 6):1358S–1363S.
168. Anderson JJ, Ambrose WW, Garner SC. Biphasic effects of genistein on bone tissue in the ovariectomized, lactating rat model. Proc Soc Exp Biol Med 1998;217:345–350.
169. Williams JP, Jordan SE, Barnes S, Blair HC. Tyrosine kinase inhibitor effects on avian osteoclastic acid transport. Am J Clin Nutr 1998;68(Suppl 6):1369S–1374S.
170. Potter SM, Baum JA, Teng H, Stillman RJ, Shay NF, Erdman JW Jr. Soy protein and isoflavones: their effects on blood lipids and bone density in postmenopausal women. Am J Clin Nutr 1998;68(Suppl 6):1375S–1379S.
171. Barger-Lux MJ, Heaney RP. Caffeine and the calcium economy revisited. Osteoporos Int 1995;5:97–102.
172. Barrett-Connor E, Chang JC, Edelstein SL. Coffee-associated osteoporosis offset by daily milk consumption. The Rancho Bernardo Study. JAMA 1994;271:280–283.
173. Cummings SR, Nevitt MC, Browner WS, Stone K, Fox KM, Ensrud KE, et al. Risk factors for hip fracture in white women. Study of Osteoporotic Fractures Research Group . N Engl J Med 1995;332:767–773.
174. Lloyd T, Rollings N, Eggli DF, Kieselhorst K, Chinchilli VM. Dietary caffeine intake and bone status of postmenopausal women. Am J Clin Nutr 1997;65:1826–1830.
175. Lloyd T, Rollings NJ, Kieselhorst K, Eggli DF, Mauger E. Dietary caffeine intake is not correlated with adolescent bone gain. J Am Coll Nutr 1998;17:454–457.
176. Packard PT, Recker RR. Caffeine does not affect the rate of gain in spine bone in young women. Osteoporos Int 1996;6:149–152.

177. Massey LK, Whiting SJ. Caffeine, urinary calcium, calcium metabolism and bone. J Nutr 1993;123:1611–1614.
178. Harris SS, Dawson-Hughes B. Caffeine and bone loss in healthy postmenopausal women. Am J Clin Nutr 1994;60:573–578.

27 Physical Activity

P. Kannus and H. Sievänen

Introduction: Possibilities of Physical Activity in Prevention of Osteoporotic Fractures

The number and incidence of various fall-induced injuries of the elderly have dramatically increased all over the world during recent decades and without any population-level intervention the increasing trend is likely to continue – largely due to an increasing number of older persons in the population – thus creating a true public health problem [1–3]. Approximately two-thirds of these injuries are osteoporotic bone fractures, hip fracture being the most common, devastating and expensive fracture modern health care systems has to deal with [2,4].

Regular exercise is currently the only well-known method which may prevent osteoporotic fractures, the true end-point of the entire osteoporosis problem, by preventing *both osteoporosis and falls.* Exercise or mechanical loading of the skeleton may prevent osteoporosis in three ways. First, exercise early in life can considerably increase the maximal amount of bone a person will have at young adulthood [5–7], the peak bone mass normally occurring around the age of 20 years [8,9]. Second, exercise can slow down premenopausal bone loss, or even slightly increase the bone mass and areal bone mineral density in 20- to 50-year-olds [10–15]. Third, regular exercise is able to prevent the age-related bone loss in peri- and postmenopausal women [16–23] and alleviate symptoms and complaints related to osteoporosis [15].

Regarding the second option of fracture prevention or prevention of falls in older adults, exercise can be effective by positively affecting many obvious risk factors of falling, i.e., by improving gait, balance, coordination, proprioception, reaction time and muscle strength – even in the very old and frail elderly [14,18,24,25].

Physical Activity in Childhood and Adolescence

Bone tissue is able to show reasonable adaptation to increased loading of the skeleton by increasing its mass and density and by improving its structure (geometry, architecture) and material properties (strength, stiffness and energy-absorbing capacity) [26]. Both human and animal studies have unequivocally shown that physical activity

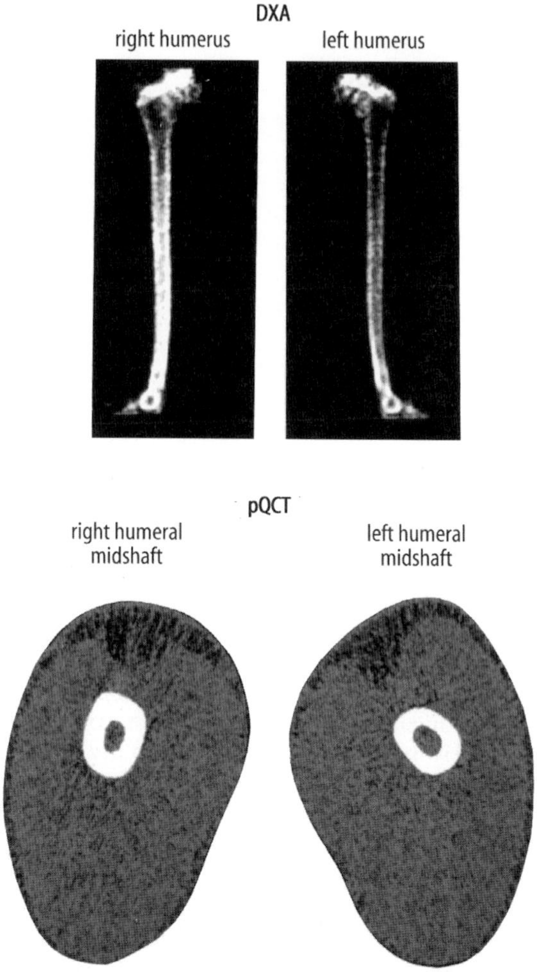

Figure 27.1. Dual energy X-ray absorptiometric (DXA) and peripheral quantitative computed tomographic (pQCT) images of the playing (*right*) and nonplaying (*left*) arm humeri of an adult male tennis player. The mineral content and cross-sectional area of the humerus are 32% and 40% higher on the playing than the nonplaying side.

or mechanical loading can considerably (up to 30–50%] increase bone mass, density and strength [5,27,28] (Fig. 27.1). The remodelling cycle of human bone tissue is, however, a slow process taking at least several months to complete.

To obtain maximal bone benefit, the starting age of activity is crucial. In female tennis players, the bone benefit is 2–4 times greater if the playing activity is started before or at puberty (12–45%) rather than after it (3–12%) [5,29] (Fig. 27.2). In addition, there seems to be a relative short age period – the period of rapid longitudinal growth at puberty or Tanner stages II–IV (corresponding approximately to ages 11–14 years in girls) – when the positive effects of exercise on bone are most pronounced [5, 7]. Before or after this period, the bone-loading activity

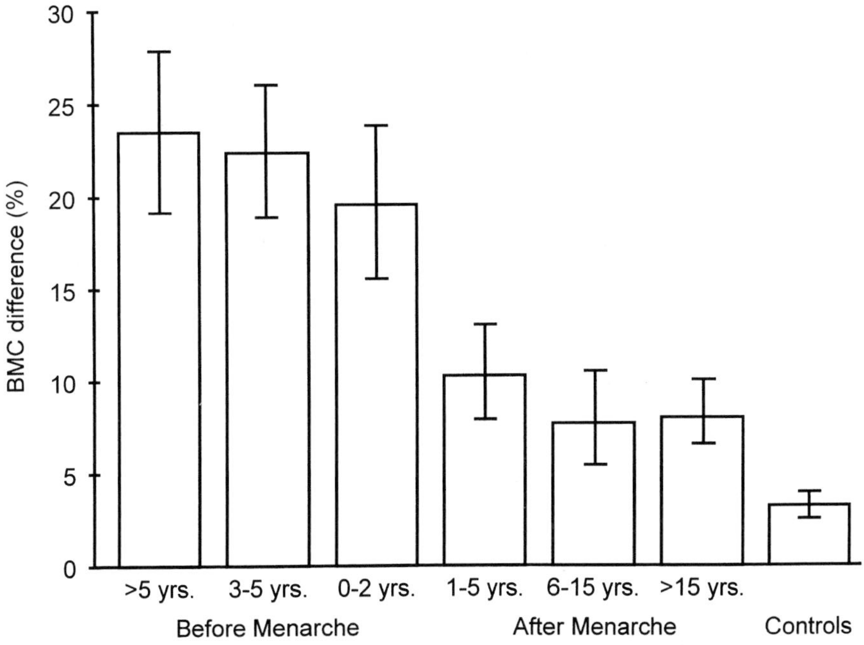

Figure 27.2. The mean (95% confidence interval) playing-to-nonplaying arm difference in the bone mineral content of the humeral shaft in 105 female tennis and squash players and their 50 controls according to the biological age at which training was started (i.e., starting age of playing relative to the age at menarche). Reprinted with permission from Kannus et al. [5].

most probably needs to be more frequent and intense to produce obvious effects on bone.

Compared with their mature counterparts, human growing bones seem to be more responsive to loading by changing not only their mass and density but also their geometry (increased bone size) due to loading [6,29]. This finding can be explained by the fact that the adolescent growth spurt is the only time in life when bone is added in substantial amounts to the inner and outer sides of the bone cortex by endosteal and periosteal apposition; quickly thereafter, endosteal apposition fades away [30]. It also seems logical that rising levels of estrogens during female puberty inhibit bone resorption and probably enhance bone formation in an additive manner with mechanical loading [28].

The public health importance of physical activity early in life originates from its above-noted considerable impact on peak bone mass. The higher the peak bone mass, the more bone an individual may lose in adulthood without risk of osteoporosis and subsequent fractures. In other words, a high peak bone mass in early adulthood is an important protective factor against osteoporotic fractures in later life – most probably at least as important as prevention of age-related bone loss [31–33]. Therefore, exercise during childhood and adolescence should be seen as a great opportunity for the prevention of osteoporosis and related fractures.

Physical Activity in Premenopausal Women

Bone tissue is also able to respond to exercise in adulthood. In general, however, training in adulthood preserves existing bone rather than adding new bone, the increase in bone mineral density normally being less than 5% [10–15]. Nevertheless, the bone-preserving action of adult-age exercise may be of great importance in maintaining bone strength and preventing age-related fractures, since only small percentage additions or avoided losses in bone mass and density are related to significant reductions in the risk of fracture [34,35].

The osteogenic effects of exercise are clearly site-specific, i.e., the training effect is normally seen in the loaded bone sites only [5,7,14,28]. Overactivity may, in turn, have a negative effect on bone mass (exercise-induced amenorrhea and bone loss) and the positive effect of exercise is likely to disappear if the subject returns to their previous level of activity [16,26,27]. The effects of deconditioning on bone will require more detailed studies, however. Our recent prospective 4-year follow-up of male tennis players provides preliminary evidence that if the exercise-induced bone gain is obtained in adolescence, the gain can be surprisingly resistant to deconditioning or reduced playing activity [36]. In this context it is also good to remember that in the case of immobility and limb immobilization, considerable bone loss occurs quickly and inevitably and good bony recovery can be expected with effective postimmobilization activity and undisturbed limb function only [37–39].

The type, frequency, intensity and duration of training that best produce the desired bone changes at each anatomical site are not well determined. Current knowledge suggests that impact-type loading (typically jumping or racket games) that creates high-magnitude strains and versatile strain distributions throughout the target bone structure can best improve bone strength [14,26,28]. Regular squash, tennis, aerobics, step exercises, volleyball, basketball, gymnastics, weight and power training or training for other similar sports may best fulfill these demands [26]. Of these, regular aerobic jumping exercise has also been proven to improve other risk factors for osteoporotic fractures, i.e., muscle strength, muscle power and dynamic body balance [14].

Physical Activity in Postmenopausal Women

In the postmenopausal period, too, physical activity has been shown to be beneficial for bone tissue by preventing age-related rapid bone loss [15–23]. Brisk walking, climbing up and down stairs, dancing, and gymnastics and calisthenics seem most suitable older-age activities, especially since they are easily available, safe, cheap and widely adopted [40,41]. In addition, postmenopausal women can safely and successfully take part in well-planned strength training regimens, as shown by Nelson et al. [18]. More detailed biomechanical analyses are, however, needed to clarify in each age group the loading patterns that are optimal for bone strength at clinically relevant sites, such as the lumbar spine and proximal femur [42].

Regarding the second option for fracture prevention or prevention of falls in older adults, exercise can improve many of the risk factors of falling, including gait, balance, coordination, proprioception, reaction time, and muscle strength and power [14,18,24,25]. Despite this, the ability of exercise to decrease the risk of falling in general, or the risk of injurious falling particularly, has remained questionable

[43], and in those exercise trials in which an effect has been seen, the effect has usually been relatively small, of the order of 10–15% [40,44,45].

In interpreting the above-noted results it has to be remembered, however, that the training methods used have shown considerable trial-to-trial variation and it is possible that an optimal training program has never been applied in these interventions. In other words, the type of activity may not have been optimal in improving the protective characteristics against falling and the frequency, intensity and duration of the training may have been insufficient in detecting any clear fall reduction in the intervention group of the elderly. Therefore, future exercise trials of older adults, prospective and randomized by nature, should be large, long-term and well designed in terms of the training methods used and their dosages. In addition, not only bone mineral parameters and falls but especially bone fractures should be considered as the primary end-point of the trial.

Lifelong Physical Activity and Risk of Osteoporotic Fractures

Although prevention of falls in the elderly by exercise has not yet been proven, epidemiological studies, case–control, nested case–control or prospective cohort follow-ups by nature, consistently suggest that both past and current physical activity is protective against hip fracture, the risk reduction being up to 50% [40,41,46–48]. Many of these studies have even found a dose–response relationship between the exercise exposure and the fracture risk. The best combination for prevention of hip fracture seems to be vigorous past activity and moderate recent activity (vigorous activity in old age may increase the predisposition to falling accidents) [41,49]. Of the various activity types, weightbearing activity seems the most protective and even daily walking and climbing stairs can be effective [40].

Only a few epidemiological studies have focused on physical activity and fractures other than hip fracture [40,48,50–53] and the findings have been partly contradictory, thus preventing any definitive conclusions concerning the relationship between activity and the risk of fracture. However, it seems that in these fractures, too, increased lifetime physical activity protects against fracture while vigorous current activity may increase the risk of fracture via an increased risk of falling [50,53]. Exercise programs for the elderly, therefore, must be undertaken with caution and proper training [41].

Conclusions

The available evidence suggests that regular physical activity, especially if started in childhood and adolescence, is the only cheap, safe, readily available and widely acceptable way to affect both bone strength and falling propensity. Therefore, physical activity should become an essential part of strategies that aim at controlling the alarming increase in osteoporotic fractures in our modern societies. It is also noteworthy that regular physical activity, unlike other methods of fracture prevention, provides many other health-related benefits: it decreases the risk of all-cause mortality, heart attack, hypertension, adult-onset diabetes, obesity, several types of cancer and functional and cognitive impairment [54,55]. For all these reasons, promotion of lifelong physical activity should be one of the most important goals in the public health programs of the new millennium.

References

1. Rubenstein LZ, Josephson KR, Robbins AS. Falls in the nursing home. Ann Intern Med 1994;121:442–451.
2. Kannus P, Niemi S, Palvanen M, Parkkari J. Fall-induced injuries among elderly people. Lancet 1997;350:1174.
3. Kannus P, Palvanen M, Niemi S, Parkkari J, Natri A, Vuori I, et al. Number and incidence of fall-induced severe head injuries among older adults. Am J Epidemiol, 1999;149:143–150.
4. Kannus P, Parkkari J, Niemi S. Age-adjusted incidence of hip fractures. Lancet 1995;346:50–51.
5. Kannus P, Haapasalo H, Sankelo M, Sievänen H, Pasanen M, Heinonen A, et al. Effect of starting age of physical activity on bone mass in the dominant arm of tennis and squash players. Ann Intern Med 1995;123:27–31.
6. Morris FL, Naughton GA, Gibbs JL, Carlson JS, Wark JD. Prospective ten-month exercise intervention in premenercheal girls: Positive effects on bone and lean mass. J Bone Miner Res 1997;12:1453–1462.
7. Haapasalo H, Kannus P, Sievänen H, Pasanen M, Uusi-Rasi K, Heinonen A, et al. Effect of long-term unilateral activity on bone mineral density of female junior tennis players. J Bone Miner Res 1998;13:310–319.
8. Matkovic V, Jelic T, Wardlaw GT, Ilich JZ, Goel PK, Wright JK, et al. Timing of peak bone mass in Caucasian females and its implications for the prevention of osteoporosis. J Clin Invest 1994;93:799–808.
9. Haapasalo H, Kannus P, Sievänen H, Pasanen M, Uusi-Rasi K, Heinonen A, et al. Development of mass, density and estimated mechanical characteristics of bones in Caucasian females. J Bone Miner Res 1996;11:1751–1760.
10. Snow-Harter C, Bouxsein ML, Lewis BT, Carter DR, Marcus R. Effect of resistance and endurance exercise on bone mineral status of young women: A randomized exercise intervention trial. J Bone Miner Res 1992;7:761–769.
11. Bassey EJ, Ramsdale SJ. Increase in femoral bone density in young women following high-impact exercise. Osteoporos Int 1994;4:72–75.
12. Friedlander AL, Genant HK, Sadowsky S, Byl NN, Gluer C-C. A two-year program of aerobics and weight training enhances bone mineral density of young women. J Bone Miner Res 1995;10:574–585.
13. Lohman T, Going S, Pamenter R, Hall M, Boyden T, Houtkooper L, et al. Effects of resistance training on regional and total bone mineral density in premenopausal women: a randomized prospective study. J Bone Miner Res 1995;10:1015–1024.
14. Heinonen A, Kannus P, Sievänen H, Oja P, Pasanen M, Rinne M, et al. Randomised controlled trial of effect of high-impact exercise on selected risk factors for osteoporotic fractures. Lancet 1996;348:1343–1347.
15. Ernst E. Exercise for female osteoporosis. A systematic review of randomised clinical trials. Sports Med 1998;25:359–368.
16. Dalsky GP, Stocke KS, Eshani AA, Slatopolsky E, Lee WC, Birge SJ. Weight-bearing exercise training and lumbar bone mineral content in post-menopausal women. Ann Intern Med 1988;108:824–828.
17. Grove KA, Londeree BR. Bone density in postmenopausal women: high impact vs low impact exercise. Med Sci Sports Exerc 1992;24:1190–1194.
18. Nelson ME, Fiatarone MA, Morganti CM, Trice I, Greenberg RA, Evans WJ. Effect of high-intensity strength training on multiple risk factors for osteoporotic fractures. A randomized controlled trial. JAMA 1994;272:1909–1914.

19. Prince R, Devine A, Dick I, Griddle A, Kerr D, Kent N, et al. The effects of calcium supplementation (milk powder or tablets) and exercise on bone density in postmenopausal women. J Bone Miner Res 1995;10:1068–1075.
20. Berard A, Bravo G, Gauthier P. Meta-analysis of the effectiveness of physical activity for the prevention of bone loss in postmenopausal women. Osteoporos Int 1997;7:331–337.
21. Kohrt WM, Ehsani AA, Birge SJ Jr. Effects of exercise involving predominantly either joint-reaction or ground-reaction forces on bone mineral density in older women. J Bone Miner Res 1997;12:1253–1261.
22. Kelley G. Aerobic exercise and lumbar spine bone mineral density in postmenopausal women: a meta-analysis. J Am Geriatr Soc 46: 1998;143–152.
23. Heinonen A, Oja P, Sievänen H, Pasanen M, Vuori I. Effects of two training regimens on bone mineral density of healthy perimenopausal women: a randomized controlled trial. J Bone Miner Res 1998;13:483–490.
24. Fiatarone MA, Marks EC, Ryan ND, Meredith CN, Lipsitz LA, Evans WJ. High- intensity strength training in nonagenarians: effects on skeletal muscle. JAMA 1990;263:3029–3034.
25. Fiatarone MA, O'Neill EF, Ryan ND, Clements KM, Solares GR, Nelson ME, et al. Exercise training and nurtitional supplementation for physical frailty in very elderly people. N Engl J Med 1994;330:1769–1775.
26. Kannus P, Sievänen H, Vuori I.. Physical loading, exercise, and bone [editorial]. Bone 1996;18:1S–3S.
27. Gutin B, Kasper MJ. Can vigorous exercise play a role in osteoporosis prevention. Osteoporos Int 1992;2:55–69.
28. Lanyon LE. Using functional loading to influence bone mass and architecture: objectives, mechanisms, and relationships with estrogen of the mechanically adaptive process in bone. Bone 1996;18:37S–43S.
29. Haapasalo H, Sievänen H, Kannus P, Heinonen A, Oja P, Vuori I. Dimensions and estimated mechanical characteristics of the humerus after long-term tennis loading. J Bone Miner Res 1996;11:864–872.
30. Parfitt AM. The two facets of growth: benefits and risks to bone integrity. Osteoporos Int 1994;4:382–398.
31. Seeman E, Tsalamandris C, Formica C, Hopper JL, McKay J. Reduced femoral neck bone density in the daughters of women with hip fractures: the role of low peak bone density in the pathogenesis of osteoporosis. J Bone Miner Res 1994;9:739–743.
32. Ribot C, Tremollières F, Pouilles JM. Late consequences of a low peak bone mass. Acta Paediatr Suppl 1995;411:31–35.
33. Riis BJ, Hansen MA, Jensen AM, Overgaard K, Christiansen C. Low peak bone mass and fast rate of bone loss at menopause. Equal risk factors for future fracture: a 15-year follow up study. Bone 1996;19:9–12.
34. Hui SL, Slemenda CW, Johnston CC. Age and bone mass as predictors of fracture in a prospective study. J Clin Invest 1988;81:1804–1809.
35. Cummings SR, Black DM, Nevitt MC, Browner W, Cauley J, Ensrud K, et al. Bone density at various sites for prediction of hip fractures. Lancet 1993;341:72–75.
36. Kontulainen S, Kannus P, Haapasalo H, Heinonen A, Sievänen H, Oja P, et al. Changes in bone mineral content with decreased training in competitive young adult tennis players and controls: a prospective 4-year follow-up. Med Sci Sports Exerc 1999;31: 646–652.
37. Kannus P, Järvinen M, Sievänen H, Oja P, Vuori I. Osteoporosis in men with a history of tibial fracture. J Bone Miner Res 1994;9:423–429.
38. Sievänen H, Heinonen A, Kannus P. Adaptation of bone to altered loading environment: biomechanical approach using x-ray absorptiometric data from the patella of a young woman. Bone 1996;19:55–59.
39. Järvinen M, Kannus P. Current concepts review. Injury of an extremity as a risk factor for the development of osteoporosis. J Bone Joint Surg Am 1997;79:263–276.

40. Joakimsen RM, Magnus JH, Fonnebo V. Physical activity and predisposition for hip fractures: a review. Osteoporos Int 1997;7:503–513.
41. Slemenda C. Prevention of hip fractures: risk factor modification. Am J Med 1997;103:65S–73S.
42. Snow CM. Exercise and bone mass in young and premenopausal women. Bone 1996;18:51S–55S.
43. Gillespie LD, Gillespie WJ, Cumming R, Lamb SE, Rowe BH. Interventions to reduce the incidence of falling in the elderly. The Cochrane Library 1997;4:1–33.
44. Province MA, Hadley EC, Hornbrook MC, Lipsitz LA, Miller JP, Mulrow CD, et al. The effects of exercise on falls in elderly patients. A preplanned meta-analysis of the FICSIT trials. JAMA 1995;273:1341–1347.
45. Oakley A, France-Dawson M, Fullerton D, Holland J, Arnold S, Cryer C, et al. Preventing falls and subsequent injury in older people. Effective Health Care 1996;2:1–16.
46. Cooper C, Barker DJ, Wickham C. Physical activity, muscle strength, and calcium intake in fracture of the proximal femur in Britain. BMJ 1988;297:1443–1446.
47. Law MR, Wald NJ, Meade TW. Strategies for prevention of osteoporosis and hip fracture. BMJ 1991;303:453–459.
48. Gregg EW, Cauley JA, Seeley DG, Ensrud KE, Bauer DC. Physical activity and osteoporotic fracture risk in older women. Ann Intern Med 1998;129:81–88.
49. Jaglal SB, Kreiger N, Darlington G. Past and recent physical activity and risk of hip fracture. Am J Epidemiol 1993;38:107–118.
50. Kelsey JL, Browner WS, Seeley DG, Nevitt MC, Cummings SR, for the Study of Osteoporotic Fractures Research Group. Risk factors for fractures of the distal forearm and proximal humerus. Am J Epidemiol 1992;135:477–489.
51. Mallmin H, Ljunghall S, Persson I, Bergström R. Risk factors for fractures of the distal forearm: A population based case control study. Osteoporos Int 1994;4:298–304.
52. Greendale GA, Barnett-Connor E, Edelstein S, Ingles S, Hailey S. Lifetime leisure exercise and osteoporosis: the Rancho Bernardo study. Am J Epidemiol 1995;141:951–959.
53. O'Neill TW, Marsden D, Adams JE, Silman AJ. Risk factors, falls, and fracture of the distal forearm in Manchester, UK. J Epidemiol Commun Health 1996;50:288–292.
54. Blair SN, Kohl HW, Gordon NF, Paffenbarger RSJ. How much physical activity is good for health? Annu Rev Public Health 1992;13:99–126.
55. US Department of Health and Human Services, Centers for Disease Control and Prevention, and National Center for Chronic Disease Prevention and Health Promotion. Physical activity and health: a report of the Surgeon General. US Department of Health and Human Services, Atlanta, GA, 1996.

Part V

Pharmacological Prevention of Osteoporotic Fractures

28 Calcium and Vitamin D

R. L. Prince

Introduction

The role of nutritional interventions for prevention of fracture relates to primary and secondary prevention, that is nutritional intervention before and after the first fracture. In the past, data on the efficacy of treatment with calcium and vitamin D have been controversial. In particular the epidemiological evidence that high dietary intakes of calcium can prevent fracture has been quite variable. With the advent of controlled clinical trials using bone density as an end-point it has become clear that calcium with or without vitamin D therapy can lead to reductions in the rate of bone loss. Furthermore calcium and vitamin D therapy in elderly women can lead to reductions in fracture rates in populations living in sunlight-deprived parts of the Northern Hemisphere. This chapter will review the physiological and cell biological basis of the effects of nutritional treatment with calcium and vitamin D and the effects on bone histology. The epidemiological data, bone density data and fracture end-point data will then be reviewed and clinical recommendations will be made.

Physiology and Cell Biology of Calcium Homeostasis

In the short term it is extracellular calcium balance that is much more important to the survival of the individual than total body calcium which includes the bone compartment where most calcium resides (1–2 kg). This is because of the vital role calcium pays in all cell signalling. In addition to the central role of calcium as a second messenger in the regulation of cell activity it also has a specific role in conduction of the action potential along nerves and in excitation–contraction coupling in striated and cardiac muscle. Often the requirements of maintenance of extracellular calcium balance are in conflict with maintenance of skeletal hydroxyapatite and thereby the skeletal structure. It is this tension between the requirements of separate body compartments that sets the scene for the importance of calcium nutrition in the prevention and treatment of age-related osteoporosis.

At an organ level the principal organs involved in extracellular calcium homeostasis are the bone, the gut and the kidney, as it is these structures that regulate the principal flow of calcium into or out of the extracellular space (Fig. 28.1). It is

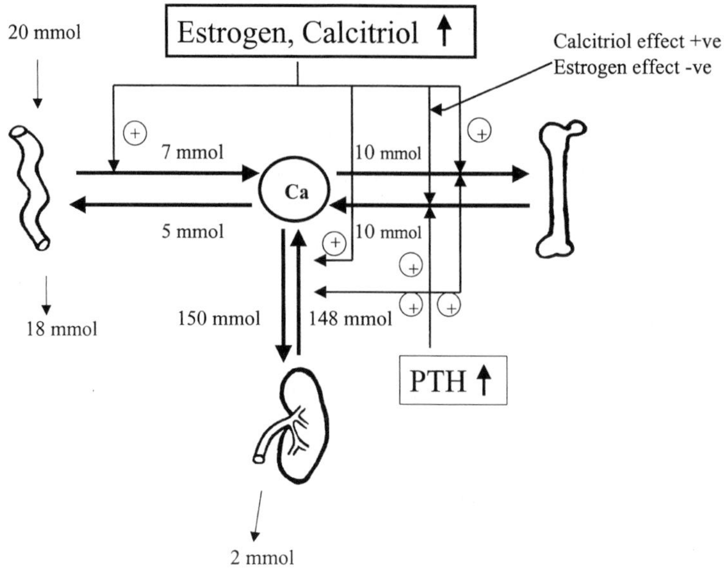

Figure 28.1. Regulation of organs involved in calcium transport.

critically important to realize that calcium is continually cycling in and out of the blood bathing these organs. In the kidney 98% of the dialyzed calcium filtered at the glomerulus is reabsorbed, i.e., approximately 150 mmol/day. In the bone it can be calculated that 5–10 mmol/day of calcium cycle into and out of the skeleton. In the bowel food adds about 20 mmol of calcium to intestinal calcium excretion of 5 mmol/day, approximately 7.0 mmol being reabsorbed. Thus calcium is continually fluxing in and out of these principal organs of extracellular calcium homeostasis. Similarly it is continually moving in and out of all the cells of the body. Thus the critical issue in the control of this system is to regulate the relative activity of the various organs and cells to optimize constancy of the internal environment.

Two hormones play a major role in regulating extracellular calcium concentrations (Fig. 28.2) these are parathyroid hormone (PTH) and the active form of vitamin D, i.e., calcitriol (1,25 dihydroxyvitamin D). Both are regulated by the concentration of calcium in the extracellular fluid, probably via a G-protein-linked calcium receptor in the membrane of PTH-secreting cells and proximal tubule cells of the kidney [1]. By feed back regulation between themselves they also influence the relative levels of the two hormones [2]. They also work in a coordinated way to influence the movement of calcium across membranes in the bowel, kidney or bone to maintain the calcium concentrations in the extracellular compartment. They have to respond to the many stresses that are placed on the requirement for calcium to maintain circulating concentrations of calcium. For example, if the dietary calcium intake goes down the coordinated action of PTH and calcitriol causes increased absorption of calcium from the bowel, urine and bone compartments to correct the extracellular deficit [3]. In this situation calcium cycles out of the bone compartment relative to the rate at which it enters the bone compartment. Estrogen is also important in determining the rate of flux of calcium into and out of the bone,

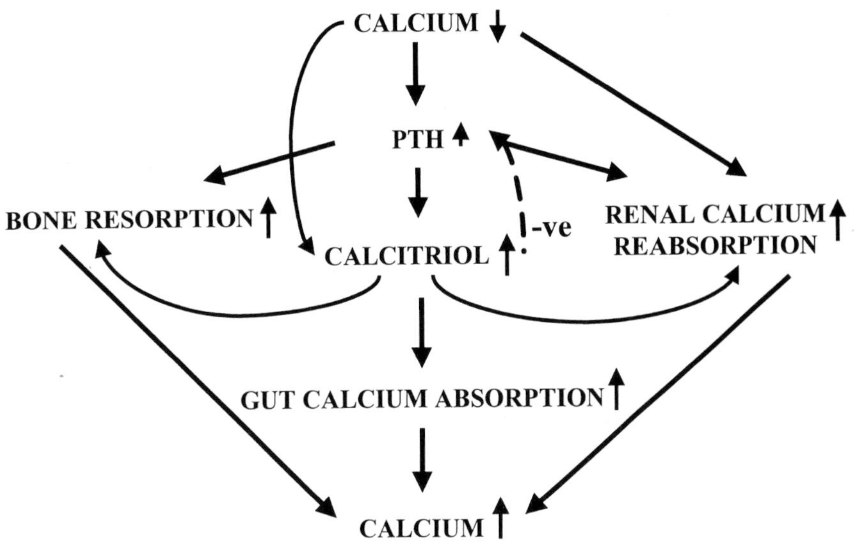

Figure 28.2. Parathyroid hormone (PTH) and calcitriol regulation of calcium homeostasis. Reprinted with permission from Marcus R. Atlas of Endocrinology. Philadelphia: Current Medicine (in press).

kidney tubule and bowel lumen and thus can indirectly determine circulating concentrations of PTH and calcitriol [4].

The Role of the Kidney in Extracellular Calcium Balance

The kidneys filter approximately 100–200 mmol of calcium per 24 h, of which about 98% is reabsorbed. Because of the high rate at which calcium is cycling across the renal tubular membrane it is possible for subtle variations in the rate of reabsorption to have profound effects on the extracellular calcium balance. The factors that increase calcium reabsorption are numerous and may include volume depletion, PTH, calcitriol and estrogen. The ways in which this may occur are outlined below.

Approximately 70% of calcium reabsorption occurs in the proximal tubule [5], reabsorption is largely passive and voltage dependent, and is associated with active reabsorption of sodium, glucose and other solutes. In the kidney, paracellular calcium transport is regulated by the extracellular ionized calcium concentration that acts on the calcium sensing receptor, this receptor has recently been cloned in human [6] and rat [7] kidney. In the distal tubule sodium and calcium reabsorption can be uncoupled, for instance with thiazide diuretics [8], and regulation by PTH and cAMP occurs [8].

The principal specific regulators of transcellular calcium transport are the plasma membrane calcium pump (PMCP), also known as calcium ATPase, and the sodium calcium exchanger (NCE). Fine regulation of calcium excretion by hormonal control of the NCE and the PMCP occurs in the distal tubule. In the kidney the NCE is located only in the distal tubule and has been shown to be the primary mechanism by which PTH modulates renal calcium reabsorption [9]. The PMCP is present in both proximal and distal tubules but with a higher affinity in the distal tubule, indicating that its role in the proximal tubule may be the maintenance of intracellular calcium levels rather than the translocation of large amounts of calcium [10]. Localization studies in the human kidney using monoclonal antibodies to the human red blood cell calcium pump could only detect the calcium pump in the distal tubule [11], indicating that lower-affinity plasma pump activity observed in proximal tubules is of a different type. We have recently shown that the PMCP of distal kidney tubule cells is directly regulated by estrogen and calcitriol.

It should be noted that sodium can compete with calcium for reabsorption in the proximal and distal tubule. This results in a strong association between sodium excretion and calcium excretion. In a 2 year prospective epidemiological study of the effects of sodium intake on bone mass in elderly postmenopausal women we were able to show a deleterious effect of sodium on the bone loss such that a high sodium intake was associated with a greater degree of bone loss [12]. In these same patients a high calcium intake prevented bone loss and the interaction of the two factors predicted the change in bone mass better than either alone.

The Role of the Intestine in Extracellular Calcium Balance

In the adult human, of the calcium consumed each day, 40–90% is excreted in feces, 10–60% is absorbed by the intestine and at normal calcium intakes "endogenous fecal calcium" is lost from pancreatic and bile secretions into the intestine. Under conditions of low calcium intake it is possible to excrete more calcium in the feces than is eaten in the diet. Under these circumstances the individual will be in negative calcium balance in the bowel compartment [13]. Net calcium absorption is the difference between the net amount of calcium absorbed and the amount excreted as fecal calcium excretion. Gut calcium absorption is determined firstly by the intraluminal concentration of calcium achieved at various points in the bowel and secondly by gut wall factors determining absorption efficiency, including the vitamin D status. The actual site of calcium absorption in the bowel varies dependent on the magnitude of the calcium load in the food and on its rate of transit through the bowel [14]. In general 95% of calcium absorption occurs in the small bowel [15]. Duodenal absorption, although having the highest rate of active absorption, is not the most important site for calcium absorption on a quantitative basis, except at very low calcium intakes. This is because the time that calcium resides within the duodenum is relatively short.

The absorption of calcium occurs by transcellular and paracellular mechanisms. In general the paracellular route is considered to be unregulated although there is some evidence that vitamin D can stimulate the nonsaturable phase of calcium transport [16]. The driving force behind the paracellular route is thought to be the concentration gradient and solvent drag driven. Paracellular movement of calcium takes place throughout the length of the intestine and may account for two-thirds of calcium flux in the rat intestine. In the human passive paracellular absorption appears to have an absorption efficiency of about 15%. Thus at high dietary intakes it would be possible to supply the calcium requirement to maintain extracellular homeostasis from this source. Paracellular movement favors absorption in the duodenum, with paracellular calcium secretion occurring in the jejunum and ileum, indicating that net calcium absorption is determined by transcellular mechanisms as well the net difference between paracellular absorption and secretion [17].

There are two mechanisms of transcellular transport: active transport and transcellular vesicular transport termed transcaltachia. Active transport involves both the NCE and the PMCP located on the basolateral membrane of the enterocyte. NCE activity has been shown in the intestine in both rats [18] and humans [19] and it appears to have approximately 20% of the calcium translocating activity of the PMCP in basolateral membrane preparations [18]. This suggests that the PMCP is the more important mechanism for translocation of calcium in the intestine. In support of this is the observation that the activity of the PMCP in the rat declines with age [20] and its activity and mRNA expression appear to be stimulated by calcitriol [20]. There is also evidence for an endocytotic, exocytotic vesicular transport mechanism (transcaltachia). Calcium transport into the cell may be increased by the opening of apical membrane calcium channels as the result of rapid, nongenomic stimulation by calcitriol [21]. In this mechanism, calcitriol stimulates calcium uptake into lysosomes at the apical membrane, with subsequent delivery to the basolateral membrane with a time course in the order of 30 min [22].

Determinants of Gut Calcium Absorption

Dietary Calcium Intake

The intraluminal factors affecting the magnitude of gut calcium absorption are related to the luminal concentration of calcium, which is determined by the frequency and magnitude of calcium intake, and the nature of the foods that it is consumed with. These factors are important when considering the clinical prescription of the calcium intake for the individual. Before considering methods of improving calcium balance by dietary means it would be desirable to know what the calcium intake of the individual patient actually is. Unfortunately it is difficult to assess dietary calcium intakes accurately, even in research studies in which weighed food records are used. This is because intakes vary from day to day and over the seasons quite considerably. Thus for research and clinical practice purposes it is difficult to define an individual's intake accurately, although mean calcium intakes in large groups of individuals can be measured reasonably accurately [23]. In terms of practical patient management it is reasonable to try to detect those with calcium intakes below 400 mg per day as they may respond best to calcium supplementation [24].

Effects of Lactose on Calcium Absorption

It is probably worth trying to determine whether milk products cause abdominal symptoms as this may be an indicator of lactose intolerance. Lactose intolerance has been associated with the development of osteoporosis [25] and more recently has been shown to be a predictor of fracture [26]. The connection between lactose intolerance and osteoporosis would appear to be due to a reduced calcium intake associated with avoidance of milk products [26]. In addition in subjects with lactose intolerance lactose will itself induce calcium malabsorption from about 25% to 20% [27]. Interestingly in normal subjects lactose may increase calcium absorption from 22 to 36%. Unfortunately lactose was not compared with other carbohydrates so it is uncertain as to whether this effect is specific to lactose as it is in animals.

Effects of Fibre on Calcium Absorption

High-fibre diets have been recommended for various benefits on the bowel and cardiovascular system. Studies that have examined the effects of these diets on calcium consumption have not found any significant deleterious effects, at least at moderate consumption of these foods [28]. However, at high fibre intakes calcium retention is reduced from 25% to 19% [29].

Role of Bone in Extracellular Calcium Balance

Bone structure can be divided into two types: trabecular and cortical bone. Each of these structures undergoes remodelling in which osteoclast-mediated bone resorption is followed by osteoblast-mediated bone formation. The combination of the osteoclast-induced Howship's lacuna and the consequent osteoblast-mediated bone formation to refill the pit is called the bone remodelling unit (BRU). The physiological rationale of this constant remodelling relates to removal of stress fractures in old bone and is also the physiological basis of maintenance of extracellular calcium homeostasis as regards the bone compartment. Evidence of the importance of osteoclast-mediated bone resorption in the maintenance of extracellular calcium levels is shown by the dramatic effects of bisphosphonates which directly inhibit osteoclast action. In Paget's disease of bone this results in low ionized calcium concentrations in plasma with consequent elevation of PTH and calcitriol [30]. There is also some evidence for regulated movement of calcium across a bone membrane made up of bone lining cells and osteoblasts. This may also play a role in the maintenance of extracellular calcium homeostasis.

It may well be that one of the functions of the BRU is to allow for the possibility of regeneration of bone calcium lost during the period of low calcium intake at the precise site of prior bone resorption. This occurs as a result of the linkage of bone formation to osteoclastic bone resorption within the bone remodelling unit. As indicated above calcium is cycling in and out of the skeleton on a continuous basis. If the individual is in calcium balance, over time the amount of bone removed during low calcium intakes must be matched by the amount of bone replaced during adequate calcium intake. During episodes of calcium deprivation there is a temporary imbalance in which bone resorption exceeds formation thus releasing calcium into the circulation [31]. During high calcium intakes the bone hydroxyapatite deficit is replaced by means of a relative increase in mineralized bone deposition [32]. This constitutes an elegant mechanism for smoothing out the intermittent demands on the skeleton for calcium during periods of dietary calcium deficiency without seriously impairing the mechanical function of the bone. This is because the bone is replaced exactly at the site it was removed from, ready to be available for the next episode of calcium deficiency.

The way in which the activity of the BRU is regulated to maintain extracellular calcium concentrations relates to the activity of PTH and calcitriol. Increased levels of both hormones induce osteoclast bone resorption by effects on osteoclast precursors and on mesenchymal stromal cells that produce cytokines such as interleukins 1 and 6 and tumor necrosis factor b that induce osteoclast differentiation. Other paracrine factors such as epidermal growth factor and insulin-like growth factor may also be important [33].

Causation of Bone Loss in Osteoporosis

There are a large number of causes of bone loss resulting in such a damaged skeletal structure that mechanical failure occurs. In general terms they all result in a negative whole-body calcium balance. However, if the primary cause of the bone loss is mechanisms originating in the skeleton itself then improvement in extracellular calcium balance only may result in hypercalcemia. Thus treatment with calcium is only of value where a reduction in calcium absorption in the intestine and reabsorption in the kidney is a cause of bone loss rather than a result of bone loss. There is now good evidence that the bone loss occurring in women after the age of 65 years is predominantly due to defects in intestinal calcium absorption and renal calcium reabsorption.

Age-Related Osteoporosis in Women: the Importance of Estrogen and Calcitriol Deficiency

An outline of the physiological interactions important in the development of a negative calcium balance in aging is shown in Fig. 28.3. In essence osteoporosis in these women could be regarded as a bi-hormonal deficiency disorder in which the importance of the estrogen deficiency is most marked close to the menopause and in which the calcitriol deficiency becomes more important as renal function declines with age. The principal causes of the decreased absorption of calcium with aging [34,35], are the effects of decreased concentrations of calcitriol and estrogen on the gut. In addition there may be an intrinsic age-related defect in the gut wall. The

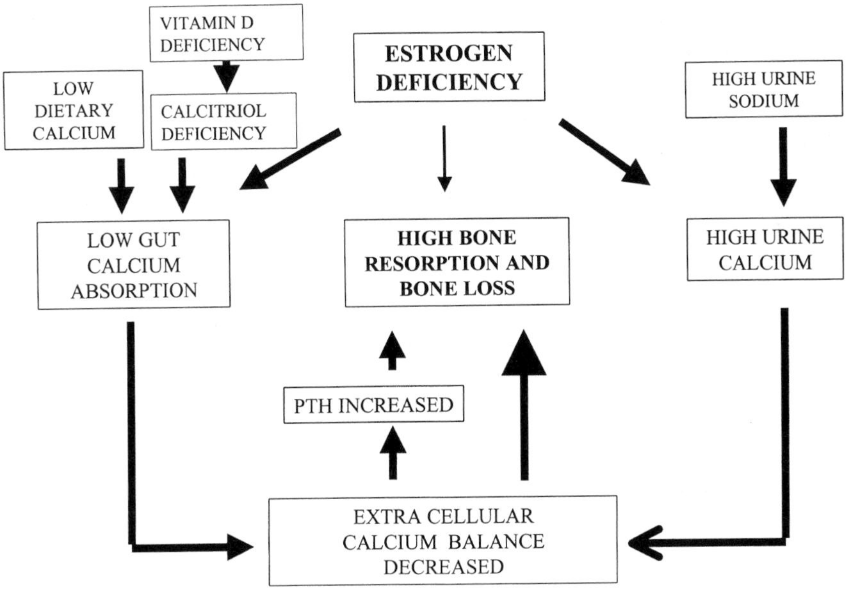

Figure 28.3. Role of estrogen in late postmenopausal bone loss. Reprinted with permission from Marcus R. Atlas of Endocrinology. Philadelphia: Current Medicine (in press).

principal cause of the decreased reabsorption of calcium in the kidney is estrogen deficiency [4, 36].

Dietary Factors

Under these circumstances dietary factors become important. In particular a low calcium intake exacerbates the intestinal calcium absorptive defect. A high salt intake exacerbates the renal calcium loss. Vitamin D deficiency due to lack of sunlight exposure and poor dietary intake will also exacerbate the calcitriol deficiency and impair gut calcium absorption. The combined problem of reduced intestinal calcium absorption and decreased renal calcium reabsorption results in a negative extracellular calcium balance that in turn results in increased bone resorption to maintain the calcium concentration in part by an increase in PTH [37–39]. The increased bone resorption results in trabecular plate perforation and endocortical bone resorption.

Osteoblast Defect

An important factor in age-related osteoporosis is the defect in osteoblastic bone formation that occurs with aging. In age-related osteoporosis, in addition to the potential for relative extracellular calcium deficiency causing increased bone resorption and consequent formation there is also evidence for a specific age-related defect in bone formation associated with osteoblast senescence [40,41]. Under these circumstances the temporary effects of calcium deprivation on the skeleton are converted into permanent bone loss. This may account for the greater sensitivity of the aging skeleton to calcium deprivation. The cause of the age-related osteoblast defect has not been elucidated. Possibilities include reduction of osteoblast activation as a result of decreases in activity and the stress/strain effects these induce at the bone surface. Certainly in animal experiments it is clear that mechanical effects stimulate periosteal bone formation [42]. It is possible that the strain-related increase in bone density in postmenopausal women [43] is due to stimulation of osteoblastic activity. Another potential mechanism for the osteoblast defect is the reduction in insulin-like growth factor I that occurs with aging [44]. Finally, as indicated above there may be an intrinsic cell senescence mechanism perhaps associated with impaired generation of osteoblast precursors. Thus the bone formation function of the BRU is deficient at a time when the increased remodelling due to the negative extracellular calcium balance is most marked. These interrelated defects result in a critically weakened bone structure which is more likely to fracture under normal daily stresses.

Vitamin D Intake and Osteoporosis

In subjects with low sunlight exposure there is a fall in vitamin D production in the skin with resulting fall in 25-hydroxyvitamin D, the substrate for the formation of calcitriol in the kidney [45]. This vitamin D deficiency may be compensated for by dietary vitamin D intake either in fish oils or in food fortification. It should be pointed out that although vitamin D as a compound was first described as a micronutrient, hence its name, the major physiological source is the skin. Because of difficulties with the assay of calcitriol it has not always been possible to show a fall in calcitriol in the presence of vitamin D deficiency. Vitamin D deficiency is, however, associated with a raised PTH and is thereby associated with bone loss [46, 47]. A comparison of treating vitamin-D-deficient elderly subjects with ultraviolet irradiation of the skin compared with oral therapy with vitamin D showed that calcitriol levels rose with skin irradiation but not with oral therapy [48]. This may be because the local concentration of vitamin D, the precursor of calcitriol, is high enough to modulate calcium absorption via a receptor-mediated mechanism [49].

Thus vitamin D deficiency and a negative calcium balance are intimately related at a mechanistic level. Arguments over the relative importance of vitamin D and calcium intake miss the main point, which is that adequate supplies of both are essential for maintenance of calcium balance and prevention of bone loss. Thus if an individual only has a deficient calcium intake, replacement of that nutrient will slow bone loss, whereas if that individual is short of both vitamin D and calcium then both will be required for an optimal effect on calcium balance.

Osteomalacia

Osteomalacia is a histopathological term referring to excessively thick osteoid seams on the surface of bone, due to a reduction in the rate of mineralization of the osteoid. This condition must be differentiated from high bone turnover in diseases such as Paget's disease of bone in which there is excess osteoid because of overactivity of osteoblasts.

Osteomalacia is often thought to be due only to vitamin D deficiency. However, in childhood and adolescence severe calcium deficiency is said to result in osteomalacia [50, 51] indicating that under these circumstances there is a mineralization defect. In the mature skeleton there is evidence that certain subjects with osteoporotic fracture have evidence of excess osteoid with high bone turnover [40, 52]. Although not clearly stated it is likely that a significant number of these subjects had calcium deficiency and secondary hyperparathyroidism. Certainly in primary hyperparathyroidism there is evidence of hyperosteoidosis and high bone turnover [53]. In addition to evidence of unmineralized osteoid it is clear that a specific mineralization defect can occur with vitamin D deficiency which can complicate the calcium deficiency. Thus the diagnosis of osteomalacia is not straightforward. Furthermore differentiating osteomalacia due to calcium deficiency from that due to vitamin D deficiency may not be easy. Histological evidence that osteomalacia is associated with fracture is quite variable, with evidence for very low levels in some studies and very high levels [54–57]in other studies of hip fracture.

Clinical Data on Dietary Vitamin D Supplementation

There are three sorts of data relevant to decision making on the role of vitamin D supplementation: epidemiological data, bone density data and fracture prevention data. The sum total of the data could be regarded as inadequate to make any definitive conclusions on the advantages of vitamin D supplementation.

Epidemiological data on the role of vitamin D intake in prevention of fracture independent of calcium intake has concentrated on the effects of circulating

25 hydroxyvitamin D (25OHD) levels on fracture rates [58]. 25OHD is of course an integral measure of vitamin D status, including as it does sunlight exposure as well as dietary intake. Indeed in the Lips et al. [58] study it was sunlight exposure that was lower in the fracture population not vitamin D intake. Thus these data do not assist in deciding whether to increase vitamin D supplementation by mouth.

Only a few clinical trials have been undertaken on the effects on bone density of vitamin D supplementation without calcium. In one study women over the age of 70 years received a vitamin D supplement of 400 IU per day or placebo. After 2 years the femoral neck bone density was 2% better in the vitamin-D-treated subjects. Bone density at other sites was no different [59].

Clinical data on the efficacy of vitamin D alone have been reported. One study reported a reduction in fractures with injections of vitamin D. Unfortunately this was not an intention-to-treat study and was not properly randomized or controlled [60]. A large randomized controlled trial of oral vitamin D supplementation with 400 IU of vitamin D per day for 2 years in elderly women has been reported. The supplemented group had no reduction in clinical fractures compared with the control group despite a rise in circulating vitamin D concentrations [61]. These data point to the fact that this group of subjects was not sufficiently vitamin D deficient for there to be a treatment effect of vitamin D alone. As indicated above, this supports the contention that a low vitamin D status alone is not usually a sufficient cause for an increased fracture rate. In addition there is also a negative calcium balance due to a defect in renal calcium reabsorption that is not corrected by vitamin D supplementation.

Calcium Intake and Osteoporosis

There are three sources of data relating to the potential for beneficial effects of increased calcium intake. There are a large number of epidemiological studies of calcium intake. These are of two sorts: case–control and cohort studies [62]. Most of the cohort studies show no beneficial effects of dietary calcium intake on fracture reduction (Table 28.1). Indeed some show an increase in fracture rate in subjects receiving calcium supplements [63] perhaps because the patients knew that they were at increased risk of fracture. Not surprisingly this has resulted in debate as to whether an increased dietary calcium intake will result in fewer fractures. The observational epidemiological approach has significant limitations in its sensitivity and specificity for the treatment effect under consideration. Thus it is accepted that measurement of dietary calcium intake using food frequency or weighed food records is an inaccurate estimate of calcium intake. Furthermore, as indicated above, dietary calcium intake is only one factor determining extracellular calcium balance and thus bone balance. Under these circumstances it is perhaps not surprising that calcium intake has proved to be only a weak predictor of fracture.

The data from randomized controlled trials of calcium supplementation have been much clearer, with all studies showing a reduction in bone loss with increased calcium intake at all skeletal sites at which the bone density was measured [70]. The current published data on long-term calcium trials are shown is Table 28.2. In three studies it is clear that over 3 or 4 years there is prevention of bone loss at all sites [71,72] except the whole-body site in the Reid study [73] which involved younger subjects. In addition there was a significant treatment benefit of a 1–3%

Table 28.1. Cohort and case control studies

Study	Baseline characteristics of subjects	Method of determination of calcium intake	Duration of study (years)	Fracture outcome	Comparative variable (mg Ca/day)	Relative risk of fracture high vs low calcium intake (risk = 1) (95% CI)
Cohort studies						
Holbrook et al., 1988 [63]	426 men, 531 women (age 50-79 years)	24 h recall/ caloric intake	14	33 hip fractures	Highest tertile of calcium intake > 765 vs lowest two < 765	0.4 ($p < 0.05$)
Wickham et al., 1989 [64]	542 men, 441 women (age > 64 years)	7 day record	15	44 hip fractures	Highest tertile of calcium intake > 802 vs lowest < 588	1.4 (0.26-10)
Kelsey et al., 1992 [65]	9704 women (age > 65 years)	Food frequency	2.2	250 wrist and humerus fractures	> 714 vs < 714	1.01 (0. 8-1.3)
Looker et al., 1993 [66]	2116 men, 2226 women (age 50-74 years)	24 hr recall and partial food frequency	16	Men 44 hip fractures Women 122 hip fractures	Highest quartile of calcium intake vs lowest: Men > 1004 vs < 405; Women > 707 vs < 292	Men 0.52 (0.2-1.2) Women 0.82 (0.5-1.4)
Cummings et al., 1995 [67]	9516 women (age > 65 years)	Food frequency	4.1	192 hip fractures	> 400 vs < 400	1.1 (0.5-2.3)
Meyer et al., 1997 [68]	1975 men and women (mean age 57 years)	Food frequency		150 hip fractures	Highest quartile of calcium intake vs lowest	0.7 (0.4-1.1)
Cumming et al., 1997 [69]	9704 women (aged > 65 years)	Food frequency	6.6	332 hip, 241 humerus, 210 ankle, 467 wrist, 389 vertebral fractures	Calcium supplements vs no calcium supplements	Hip 1.5 (1.1-2.0) Humerus 1.7 (1.3-2.4) Vertebrae 1.4 (1.1-1.9)

Table 28.2. Randomized controlled bone density studies over 2 years in duration

Study	Patient characteristics	Baseline calcium intake (mg/day)	Treatment calcium (mg/day)	Baseline mean BMD (mg/cm^2)	Overall % change in placebo group	Overall % change in calcium group	Overall mean % difference calcium-placebo (95% CI)	Later mean % difference calcium-placebo (95% CI)
Calcium								
Reid et al., 1995 [67]	Women (mean age 58 years, > 3 years postmenopause): 38 patients calcium, 40 patients placebo	750	Calcium lactate gluconate 1000	Total body 1060 Femoral neck 860 Spine 1060	Years 1-4 −3.4 −1.6 −1.47	Years 1–4 −2.16 +0.81 +0.79	Years 1-4 +1.4* +2.46* +2.27*	Years 2-4 +0.75* +0.30 NS +0.57 NS
Devine et al., 1997 [65]	63 women (mean age 66 years; mean years since menopause 18)	952	Calcium supplements > 1000	Ankle 680 Total hip 850 Spine 900	Years 1-4 −3.47 −1.13 +1.13	Years 1-4 −0.05 +1.58 +1.53	Years 1-4 +2.6(+0.4 to +4.7) +2.8(+0. 6 to +4.6) +0.2(−1.7 to +2.1)	Years 2-4 +0.4 (−1.7 to +2.7) +0.2(−1.4 to +1.9) −0.8 (−3.0 to +1.5)
Riggs et al., 1998 [66]	177 women (mean age 66 years; mean years since menopause 16)	710	Calcium citrate 1600	Total body 1020 Total hip 810 Spine 900	Years 1-4 +0.19 −1.23 +2.28	Years 1-4 +1.07 +0.37 +2.67	Years 1-4 +0.9* +1.3* +0.30 NS	
Calcium and vitamin D								
Dawson Hughes et al., 1997 [70]	213 women (mean age 72 years	700	Calcium citrate malate 500 Vitamin D 700 IU	Total body 1020 Femoral neck 800 Spine 1040	Years 1-3 −1.34 −0.09 +0.63	Years 1-3 +0.14 +0.71 +1.85	Years 1-3 +1.5(+1.1 to +1.9) −0.8(−2.0 to +0.3) +1.2(+0.2 to +2.2)	Years 2+3 +0.3(+0.1 to +0.5) +0.1(-07 to +0.8) −0.3(−0.8 to +0.3)

BMD, bone mineral density. *$p < 0.05$; NS, not significant.

Table 28.3. Effects on fracture rate of supplementation with calcium or calcium and vitamin D

Study	Baseline characteristics	Baseline calcium intake (mg/day)	Intervention	Fracture outcome in control group	Fracture outcome in treatment group	Relative risk	Absolute risk reduction (fractures per 100 patient years, 95 %CI)	No. needed to treat
Calcium supplementation								
Chevalley et al., 1994 [68]	11 males, 82 females (mean age 73 years) 44% prevalent vertebral fractures	650	$CaCO_3$ or osseino complex 800 mg/day for 1.5 years	New vertebral fractures 10.7%	New vertebral fractures 7.4%	0.69	3.3 (-7.8 to +14.3)	30
Reid et al., 1995 [67]	135 women baseline, 78 women completed (mean age 56 years); nonprevalent fractures	700	Calcium lactate gluconate 1000 mg/day for 4 years	New fractures 18%	New fractures 5%	0.3	3.1 (–0.4 to +6.5)	32
Recker et al., 1996 [69]	92 women (mean age 75 years); prevalent vertebral fractures	450	$CaCO_3$ 1200 mg/day for 4.3 years	New vertebral fractures 51%	New vertebral fractures 28%	0.55	5.3 (+0.7 to +9.8)	19
Recker et al., 1996 [69]	99 women (mean age 73 years); nonprevalent vertebral fractures	414	$CaCO_3$ 1200 mg/day for 4.3 years	New vertebral fractures 21%	New vertebral fractures 28%	1.33	–	
Calcium and vitamin D supplementation								
Chapuy et al., 1994 [72]	2303 women (mean age 84 years)	511	$Ca_3(PO_4)_2$ 1200 mg/day, vitamin D 800 IU for 3 years	Appendicular fractures 27.3%	Appendicular fractures 21.6%	0.72 (0.6-0.84)	1.9 (+0.7 to 3.1)	52
Chapuy et al., 1994 [72]	2303 women (mean age 84 years)	511	$Ca_3(PO_4)_2$ 1200 mg/day, vitamin D 800 IU for 3 years	Hip fractures 15.8%	Hip fractures 11.6%	0.73 (0.62-0.84)	1.4 (+0.4 to 2.3)	52
Dawson-Hughes et al., 1997 [70]	176 men; 213 women (mean age 72years)	700	Calcium citrate malate 500 mg/day, vitamin D 700IU/day for 3years	Appendicular fractures 12.8%	Appendicular fractures 5.9%	0.5 (0.2-0.9)	2.3 (+0.4 to 4.2)	43
Dawson Hughes et al., 1997 [70]	213 women (mean age 73 years)	700	Calcium citrate malate 500 mg/day, vitamin D 700IU/day for 3years	Appendicular fractures 19.6%	Appendicular fractures 11.6%	0.6 (0.2-0.8)	4.6 (+0.8 to 8.4)	22

increase in bone density over the placebo group which was most marked in the first 2 years but persisted after this time.

The data from a few small clinical trials of increased calcium intake on fracture rates in primary prevention trials [73,74] and one secondary prevention trial [75] have shown a beneficial effect for calcium (Table 28.3). However, the confidence interval on the size of the fracture reduction has often been wide. Nevertheless the size of the treatment effect gives rise to hope that calcium supplementation is an appropriate method of reducing fracture rates in the population who have not yet fractured and who have fractured.

Thus the clinical data on the biological and clinical effects of increased calcium supplementation suggest that many postmenopausal women would probably benefit from an increased calcium intake. However, the overall public health benefits of increased calcium intake all populations throughout the world still need more study before supplementation can be supported as a viable public health measure. Nevertheless a targeted approach to individual patients at high risk is probably warranted.

Calcium and Vitamin D Intake in Osteoporosis

The combined effects of calcium and vitamin D supplementation have also been studied in elderly populations in Northern latitudes where it is likely that vitamin D insufficiency and dietary calcium insufficiency are widespread. The epidemiological evidence that calcium with vitamin D is effective is rather weak presumably due the fact that dietary vitamin D intake in food is not a major determinant of circulating vitamin D levels. The bone density evidence is stronger and includes a 3 year bone density end-point study [76].

Clinical trial data using fracture as the primary outcome variable have been examined in two trials of primary prevention [76–78]. Both showed a reduction in clinical appendicular fractures in the population studied (Table 28.3). The size of the treatment effect was quite large in both studies amounting to a 30–50% reduction in fracture from rates of around 6–9% per year. Although not specifically studied there does not appear to have been an increase in unwanted side-effects in the populations studied. Thus in a population of women over the age of 70 years in northern latitudes primary prevention with calcium and vitamin D appears to be indicated as a cost-effective safe approach. The data can probably be extended to secondary prevention of fracture in these populations and should be introduced as part of practice guidelines for these individuals.

Conclusions

The basic mechanisms by which improvements in calcium balance prevent bone loss and fracture are beginning to be elucidated. The mechanisms are complex and still not fully understood. Nevertheless clinical trial data are now being collected which point to a significant beneficial action of calcium supplementation in the prevention of fracture of the appendicular and axial skeleton. As such it is appropriate to recommend calcium supplementation to individual patients at risk of further fracture. If there is a significant risk of vitamin D deficiency, vitamin D should also be administered.

References

1. Hebert SC, Brown EM, Harris HW. Role of the Ca^{2+} sensing receptor in divalent mineral ion homeostasis. J Exp Biol 1997;200:295–302.
2. Silver J, Russell J, Sherwood LM. Regulation by vitamin D metabolites of messenger ribonucleic acid for preproparathyroid hormone in isolated bovine parathyroid cells. Proc Natl Acad Sci USA 1985;82:4270–4273.
3. Prince RL, Dick I, Garcia-Webb P, Retallack RW. The effects of the menopause on calcitriol and parathyroid hormone: responses to a low dietary calcium stress test. J Clin Endocrinol Metab 1990;70:1119–1123.
4. Prince RL. Counterpoint: estrogen effects on calcitropic hormones and calcium homeostasis. Endocr Rev 1994;15:301–309.
5. Suki WN. Calcium transport in the nephron. Am J Physiol 1979;237:F1–F6.
6. Aida K, Koishi S, Tawata M, Onaya T. Molecular cloning of a putative Ca^{2+} sensing receptor cDNA from human kidney. Biochem Biophys Res Commun 1995;214:524–529.
7. Riccardi D, Park J, Lee WS, Gamba G, Brown EM, Hebert SC. Cloning and functional expression of a rat kidney extracellular calcium/polyvalent cation-sensing receptor. Proc Natl Acad Sci USA 1995;92:131–135.
8. Costanzo L, Windhager E. Calcium and sodium transport by the distal convoluted tubule in the rat. Am J Physiol 1978;235:F492–F506.
9. Bouhtiauy I, LaJeunesse D, Brunette MG. The mechanism of parathyroid hormone action on calcium reabsorption by the distal tube. Endocrinology 1991;128:251–258.
10. Tsukamoto Y, Saka S, Saitoh M. Parathyroid hormone stimulates ATP-dependent calcium pump activity by a different mode in proximal and distal tubules of the rat. Biochim Biophys Acta 1991;1103:163–171.
11. Borke JL, Minami J, Verma A, Penniston JT, Kumar R. Monoclonal antibodies to human erythrocyte membrane Ca^{2+}–Mg^{2+} adenosine triphosphate pump recognize an epitope in the basolateral membrane of human kidney distal tubule cells. J Clin Invest 1987;80:1225–1231.
12. Devine A, Criddle RA, Dick IM, Kerr DA, Prince RL. A longitudinal study of the effect of sodium and calcium intakes on regional bone density in postmenopausal women. Am J Clin Nutr 1995;62:740–745.
13. Hannan MT, Tucker K, Dawson-Hughes B, Felson DT, Kiel DP. Effect of dietary protein on bone loss in elderly men and women: the Framingham Osteoporosis Study. J Bone Miner Res 1997;12(Suppl 1):S194.
14. Wood RJ, Zheng JJ. High dietary calcium intakes reduce zinc absorption and balance in humans. Am J Clin Nutr 1997;65:1803–1809.
15. Reddy MB, Cook JD. Effect of calcium intake on nonheme-iron absorption from a complete diet. Am J Clin Nutr 1997;65:1820–1825.
16. Boyle IT, Omdahl JL, Gray RW, DeLuca HF. The response of intestinal calcium transport to 25-hydroxy- and 1,25-dihydroxyvitamin D in nephrectomized rats. Endocrinology 1972;90:605–608.
17. Karbach U. Paracellular calcium transport across the small intestine. J Nutr 1992;122: 641–643.
18. Hildmann B, Schmidt A, Murer H. Ca^{++} -transport across basal-lateral membranes from rat small intestinal epethelial cells. J Membrane Biol 1982;65:55–62.
19. Kikuchi K, Kikuchi T, Ghisan FK. Characterization of calcium transport by basolateral membrane vesicles of human small intestine. Am J Physiol 1988;255:G482–G489.
20. Armbrecht HJ, Boltz MA, Wongsurawat N. Expression of plasma membrane calcium pump mRNA in rat intestine: effect of age and 1,25-dihydroxyvitamin D. Biochim Biophys Acta 1994;1195:110–114.
21. Nemere I, Norman AW. Transcaltachia, vesicular calcium transport and microtubule-associated calbindin D28k: emerging views of 1,25-dihydroxyvitamin D_3-mediated intestinal calcium absorption. Miner Electrolyte Metab 1990;16:109–114.

22. Nemere I. Vesicular calcium transport in chick intestine. J Nutr 1992;122:657–661.
23. Heaney RP. Nutrient effects: discrepancy between data from controlled trials and observational studies. Bone 1997;21:469–471.
24. Dawson-Hughes B, Dallal GE, Krall EA, Sadowski L, Sahyoun N, Tannenbaum S. A controlled trial of the effect of calcium supplementation on bone density in postmenopausal women. N Engl J Med 1990;323:878–883.
25. Finkenstedt G, Skrabal F, Gasser RW, Braunsteiner H. Lactose absorption, milk consumption, and fasting blood glucose concentrations in women with idiopathic osteoporosis. BMJ 1986;292:161–162.
26. Honkanen R, Koger H, Alhava E, Tuppurainen M, Saarikoski S. Lactose intolerance associated with fractures of weight-bearing bones in Finnish women aged 38–57 years. Bone 1997;21:473–477.
27. Cochet B, Jung A, Griessen M, Bartholdi P, Schaller P, Donath A. Effects of lactose on intestinal calcium absorption in noormal and lactase-deficient subjects. Gastroenterology 1983;84:935–940.
28. Wisker E, Nagel R, Tanudjaja TK, Feldheim W. Calcium, magnesium, zinc, and iron balances in young women: effects of a low-phytate barley-fiber concentrate. Am J Clin Nutr 1991;54:553–559.
29. Knox TA, Kassarjian Z, Dawson-Hughes B, Golner BB, Dallal GE, Arora S, et al. Calcium absorption in elderly subjects on high- and low-fiber diets: effect of gastric acidity. Am J Clin Nutr 1991;53:1480–1486.
30. Devlin RD, Retallack RW, Fenton AJ, Grill V, Gutteridge DH, Kent GN, et al. Long-term elevation of 1,25-dihydroxyvitamin D after short-term intravenous administration of pamidronate (aminohydroxypropylidene bisphosphonate, APD) in Paget's disease of bone. J Bone Miner Res 1994;9:81–85.
31. Horowitz M, Need AG, Philcox JC, Nordin BEC. Effect of calcium supplementation on urinary hydroxyproline in osteoporotic postmenopausal women. Am J Clin Nutr 1984;3a:857–859.
32. Prince RL. The calcium controversy revisited: implications of new data. Med J Aust 1993;159:404–407.
33. Mundy GR. Cellular mechanism of bone resorption. In: Mundy GR editor.Bone remodelling and its disorders. London: Martin Dunitz, 1995:39–43.
34. Gallagher JC, Riggs BL, Eisman J, Hamstra A, Arnaud SB, DeLuca HF. Intestinal calcium absorption and serum vitamin D metabolites in normal subjects and osteoporotic patients. J Clin Invest 1979;64:729–736.
35. Devine A, Prince RL, Kerr DA, Dick IM, Kent GN, Price RI, et al. Determinants of intestinal calcium absorption in women ten years past the menopause. Calcif Tissue Int 1993;52:358–360.
36. McKane WR, Khosla S, Risteli J, Robins SP, Muhs JM, Riggs BL. Role of estrogen deficiency in pathogenesis of secondary hyperparathyroidism and increased bone resorption in elderly women. Proc Assoc Am Phys 1997;109:174–180.
37. Wiske PS, Epstein S, Bell NH, Queener SF, Edmondson J, Johnston CC. Increases in immunoreactive parathyroid hormone with age. N Engl J Med 1979;300:1419–1421.
38. Insogna KL, Lewis AM, Lipinski CB, Baran DT. Effect of age on serum immunoreactive parathyroid hormone and its biological effects. J Clin Endocrinol Metab 1981;53:1072–1075.
39. Prince RL, Dick I, Devine A, Price RI, Gutteridge DH, Kerr D, et al. The effects of menopause and age on calcitropic hormones: a cross sectional study of 655 healthy women aged 35 to 90. J Bone Miner Res 1995;10:835–842.
40. Eriksen EF, Hodgson SF, Eastell R, Cedel SL, O'Fallon WM, Riggs BL. Cancellous bone remodeling in type 1 (postmenopausal) osteoporosis: quantitative assessment of rates of formation, resorption, and bone loss at tissue and cellular levels. J Bone Miner Res 1990;5:311.
41. Parfitt AM, Villanueva AR, Foldes J, Sudhaker Rao D. Relationships between histological

indices of bone formation: implications for the pathogenesis of spinal osteoporosis. J Bone Miner Res 1995;10:446–473.
42. Rubin CT, Lanyon LE. Regulation of bone mass by mechanical strain magnitude. Calcif Tissue Int 1985;37:411–417.
43. Kerr D, Morton A, Dick I, Prince R. Exercise effects on bone mass in postmenopausal women are site-specific and load-dependent. J Bone Miner Res 1996;11:218–225.
44. Kelly PJ, Eisman JA, Stuart MC, Pocock NA, Sambrook PN, Gwinn TH. Somatomedin-C, physical fitness, and bone density. J Clin Endocrinol Metab 1990;70:718–723.
45. Krall EA, Sahyoun N, Tannenbaum S, Dallal GE, Dawson-Hughes B. Effect of vitamin D intake on seasonal variations in parathyroid hormone secretion in postmenopausal women. N Engl J Med 1989;321:1777–1783.
46. Dawson-Hughes B, Dallal GE, Krall EA, Harris S, Sokoll LJ, Falconer G. Effect of vitamin D supplementation on wintertime and overall bone loss in healthy postmenopausal women. Ann Intern Med 1991;115:505–512.
47. Khaw K-T, Sneyd M-J, Compston J. Bone density parathyroid hormone and 25-hydroxyvitamin D concentrations in middle aged women. BMJ 1992;305:273–276.
48. Chel VGM, Ooms ME, Popp-Snijders C, Pavel S, Schothorst AA, Meulemans CCE, et al. Ultraviolet irradiation corrects vitamin D deficiency and suppresses secondary hyperparathyroidism in the elderly. J Bone Miner Res 1998;13:1238–1242.
49. Heaney RP, Barger-Lux J, Dowell MS, Chen TC, Holick MF. Calcium absorptive effects of vitamin D and its major metabolites. J Clin Endocrinol Metab 1997;82:4111–4116.
50. Marie PJ, Pettifor JM, Ross FP, Glorieux FH. Histological osteomalacia due to dietary calcium deficiency in children. N Engl J Med 1982;307:584–588.
51. Okonofua F, Gill DS, Alabi ZO, Thomas M, Bell JL, Dandona P. Rickets in Nigerian children: a consequence of calcium malnutrition. Metabolism 1991;40:209–213.
52. Arlot ME, Delmas PD, Chappard D, Meunier PJ. Trabecular and endocortical bone remodeling in postmenopausal osteoporosis: Comparison with normal postmenopausal women. Osteoporos Int 1990;1:41–49.
53. Parisien M, Cosman F, Mellish RWE, Schnitzer M, Nieves J, Silverberg SJ, et al. Bone structure in postmenopausal hyperparathyroid, osteoporotic and normal women. J Bone Miner Res 1995;10:1393–1399.
54. Eventov I, Frisch B, Alk D, Eisenberg Z, Weisman Y. Bone biopsies and serum vitamin-D levels in patients with hip fracture. Acta Orthop Scand 1989;60:411–413.
55. Hoikka V, Alhava EM, Savolainen K, Parviainen M. Osteomalacia in fractures of the proximal femur. Acta Orthop Scand 1982;53:255–260.
56. Compston JE, Vedi S, Croucher PI. Low prevalence of osteomalacia in elderly patients with hip fracture. Age Ageing 1991;20:132–134.
57. Robinson CM, McQueen MM, Wheelwright EF, Gardner DL, Salter DM. Changing prevalence of osteomalacia in hip fractures in southeast Scotland over a 20 year period. Injury 1992;23:300–302.
58. Lips P, Ginkel FCV, Jongen MJM, Rubertus F, Vijgh WJFVD, Netelenbos JC. Determinants of vitamin D status in patients with hip fracture and in elderly control subjects. Am J Clin Nutr 1987;46:1005–1010.
59. Ooms ME, Roos JC, Bezemer PD, Vijgh WJFVD, Bouter LM, Lips P. Prevention of bone loss by vitamin D supplementation in elderly women: a randomized double-blind trial. J Clin Endocrinol Metab 1995;80:1052–1058.
60. Heikinheimo RJ, Inkovaara JA, Harju EJ, Haavisto MV, Kaarela RH, Kataja JM, et al. Annual injection of viamin D and fractures of aged bones. Calcif Tissue Int 1992;51:105–110.
61. Lips P, Graafmans WC, Ooms ME, Bezemer PD, Bouter LM. Vitamin D supplementation and fracture incidence in elderly persons. Ann Intern Med 1996;124:400–406.
62. Ott SM. Calcium and vitamin D in the pathogenesis and treatment of osteoporosis. In: Marcus R, editor. Osteoporosis.Oxford: Blackwell Scientific, 1994:227–292.
63. Holbrook TL, Barrett-Connor E, Wingard DL. Dietary calcium and risk of hip fracture: 14 year prospective population study. Lancet 1989;II:1046–1049.

64. Wickham CAC, Walsh K, Cooper C, Barker DJP, Margetts BM, Morris J et al. Dietary calcium, physical activity and risk of hip fracture: a prospective study. BMJ 1989;299: 889–892.
65. Kelsey JL, Browner WS, Seeley DG, Nevitt MC, Cummings SR. Risk factors for fractures of the distal forearm and proximal humerus. Am J Epidemiol 1992;135:477–489.
66. Looker AC, Harris TB, Madans JH, Sempos CT. Dietary calcium and hip fracture risk: the NHANES I epidemiologic follow-up study. Osteoporos Int 1993;3:177–184.
67. Cummings SR, Nevitt MC, Browner WS, Stone K, Fox KM, Ensrud KR, et al. Risk factors for hip fracture in white women. N Engl J Med 1995;332:767–773.
68. Meyer HE, Pedersen JL, Loken EB, Tverdal A. Dietary factors and the incidence of hip fractures in middle-aged Norwegians. Am J Epidemiol 1997;145:117–123.
69. Cumming RG, Cummings SR, Nevitt MC, Scott J, Ensrud KE, Vogt TM, et al. Calcium intake and fracture risk: results from the study of osteoporotic fractures. Am J Epidemiol 1997;145:926–934.
70. Cumming RG, Nevitt MC. Calcium for the prevention of osteoporotic fractures in postmenopausal women. J Bone Miner Res 1997;12:1321–1329.
71. Devine A, Dick IM, Heal SJ, Criddle RA, Prince RL. A 4-year follow up study of calcium supplementation on bone density in elderly postmenopausal women. Osteoporos Int 1997;7:23–28.
72. Riggs BL, O'Fallon WM, Muhs J, O'Connor MK, Kumar R, Melton LJ III. Long-term effects of calcium supplementation on serum parathyroid hormone level, bone turnover, and bone loss in elderly women. J Bone Miner Res 1998;13:168–174.
73. Reid IR, Ames RW, Evans MC, Gamble GD, Sharpe SJ. Long-term effects of calcium supplementation on bone loss and fractures in postmenopausal women: a randomized controlled trial. Am J Med 1995;98:331–335.
74. Chevalley T, Rizzoli R, Nydegger V, Slosman D, Rapin C-H, Michel J-P, et al. Effects of calcium supplements on femoral bone mineral density and vertebral fracture rate in vitamin-D-replete elderly patients. Osteoporos Int 1994;4:245–252.
75. Recker RR, Hinders S, Davies KM, Heaney RP, Stegman MR, Lappe JM, et al. Correcting calcium nutritional deficiency prevents spine fractures in elderly women. J Bone Miner Res 1996;11:1961–1966.
76. Dawson-Hughes B, Harris SS, Khall EA, Dallal GE. Effect of calcium and vitamin D supplementation on bone density in men and women 65 years of age or older. N Engl J Med 1997;337:670–676.
77. Chapuy MC, Arlot MF, Duboeuf F, Brun J, Crouzet B, Arnaud S, et al. Vitamin D_3 and calcium to prevent hip fractures in elderly women. N Engl J Med 1992;327:1637–1642.
78. Chapuy MC, Arlot ME, Delmas PD, Meunier PJ. Effect of calcium and cholecalciferol treatment for three years on hip fractures in elderly women. BMJ 1994;308:1081–1082.

29 Estrogen

A. Oladipo and J. C. Stevenson

Introduction

Osteoporosis is a condition which is caused primarily by estrogen deficiency in postmenopausal women. The underlying process is an excessive increase in bone resorption accompanied by an inadequate increase in bone formation. Estrogen is known to reduce bone resorption and turnover, and is widely used to prevent and treat osteoporosis. It is administered as hormone replacement therapy (HRT) as estrogen only or, when appropriate, as estrogen and progestogen.

Pharmacokinetics

Estrogen is a steroid hormone produced by the ovaries during a woman's reproductive life. It is produced in the body in various forms. Estradiol is the most important type of estrogen and is secreted by the granulosa cells of the ovarian follicle. The other important estrogens are estrone and estriol. Estradiol is 12 times more potent than estrone and 8 times more potent than estriol. Some estrogen is produced by the adrenal gland and some by aromatase activity in adipose tissues. At least 22 different other forms of estrogen are found in small quantities in the circulation [1].

The daily production of estradiol by the ovaries is between 0.07 and 0.8 mg/day, depending on the phase of the menstrual cycle [2]. Its level in serum varies from 150 to 200 pmol/l in the early follicular phase to a peak of 1200 to 2600 pmol/l in the mid-cycle and then drops to 700 pmol/l in the luteal phase. Estrogen is excreted following conjugation in the liver with glucuronate, and to a lesser extent with sulfate, and thereafter appears in the urine and intestine in inactive form. Seventy per cent of estrogen is excreted in urine and 30% in feces.

Estrogen is available for HRT mainly as conjugated equine estrogens (CEE) and 17β-estradiol. CEE are natural estrogens derived from the urine of pregnant mares. They comprise a combination of many different estrogens, the main ones being estrone sulfate and equilin sulfate. 17β-estradiol is the estrogen naturally produced by human ovaries.

Oral estradiol is well absorbed from the intestine and passes to the liver at a relatively high concentration. Up to 30–60% of the ingested dose is inactivated during this process. Extensive metabolism of this bolus of estrogen takes place in the liver leading to the activation of many enzyme systems which affect lipids and coagulation. Transdermal routes of administration avoid the first-pass effect. During one circuit of the body only 10–20% of blood passes through the liver. Thus with non-oral administration lower doses are required to achieve similar therapeutic effects, with less marked effects on lipids and coagulation.

Mechanism of Action

Estrogen exerts its effects via a specific estradiol receptor. Estrogen diffuses from the blood stream into the cell where it binds to the high-affinity estrogen receptor. Estrogen may have direct effects on bone cells. Estrogen binding and an estrogen-induced response have been reported in normal human osteoblast-like cell lines and in osteosarcoma cells [3,4]. The receptor is a ligand-activated transcription factor. Having undergone conformational change and dimerization, the hormone–receptor complex binds to specific sites on the nuclear DNA where it acts as a transcriptional factor. This initiates mRNA production, which translates over many hours into new protein synthesis and cell effects, including changes in cell function and metabolism [5,6].

Estrogen also acts indirectly on bone by regulating the production of local or systemic factors which directly affect bone remodelling. These include cytokines such as interleukins 1 and 6, tumor necrosis factors (TNF) α and β, and γ-interferon. These factors enhance the differentiation of osteoclasts [7] and hence influence bone resorption. Growth factors such as insulin-like growth factors (IGFs) and transforming growth factor β (TGF-β) are further factors through which estrogens act. In rats, prostaglandin E_2 is a potent stimulator of bone resorption [8] and estrogen inhibits its production.

Calcium homeostasis is affected by estrogen. Estrogen deficiency results in bone mobilization and thereby a reduction in parathyroid hormone and 1,25-dihydroxyvitamin D secretion.

Effect of Estrogen Deficiency on Bone

Albright [9] first noted the association between osteoporosis and the menopause in women in 1941. It is now clear that estrogen deficiency plays a very important role in the pathogenesis of bone loss. Until a century ago, only a small proportion of women lived long enough to experience the long-term consequences of estrogen deprivation on the skeleton. The average lifespan for women in industrialized nations is now 81 years. Women can thus expect to live over a third of their lives in the postmenopausal state. Immediately after the menopause, rates of bone loss in all areas of the skeleton are increased [10–12]. The most important risk factor for osteoporosis is estrogen deficiency which occurs at the menopause [12]. The greatest loss of bone may occur in the first 5 years after the menopause, when up to 50% of vertebral bone may be lost [13], but bone loss continues into old age. Bone resorption increases more suddenly after an artificial menopause than after a natural menopause due to the rapid decline of estrogen levels [14,15] Women who undergo an early menopause have a much lower bone density in the spine and

Table 29.1. Bone-conserving doses of estrogens

Conjugated equine estrogens	0.625 mg
17β estradiol (oral)	1 mg
17β estradiol (transdermal)	0.05 mg
17β estradiol (implant)	50 mg
Estrone	1.5 mg
Tibolone	2.5 mg
Raloxifene	60 mg

femur than in age-matched controls [16]. In addition, acute estrogen deficiency, following administration of gonadotropin-releasing hormone agonists for the treatment of endometriosis, leads to rapid trabecular bone loss of about 10% when measured by quantitative computed tomography (QCT) and about 5% when measured by dual-energy X-ray absorptiometry (DXA) [17,18] over a period of a few months. Compared with women, men lose bone at a much slower rate. The incidence of vertebral fractures in women rises steadily from the age of 50 years onwards and, by the age of 70 years almost a third of Caucasian women will have at least one vertebral fracture. After the age of 65 years, there is a more marked rise in femoral neck fractures in women compared with men.

The loss of bone following estrogen deficiency results from increased bone turnover. Whilst there is also a compensatory increase in bone formation, this fails to match the excessive bone resorption and the net result is loss of bone. These changes are reflected by increases in the biochemical markers of bone formation such as osteocalcin, and increases in markers of bone resorption such as urinary collagen cross-linked peptide excretion [19]. Not only do these increases in bone turnover result in generalized bone loss, but also the increased number of remodelling sites increases the likelihood of trabecular perforation. This disruption of the underlying bone microarchitecture itself increases the risk of mechanical failure, namely fracture. Thus, loss of estrogen production at the menopause results in loss of bone mass and increased risk of fracture.

Effect of Estrogen on Bone Density

Estrogen therapy is well known to prevent bone loss in the wrist, spine and hip after the menopause. Long-term prospective studies with mestranol versus placebo showed a maintenance of bone mass in estrogen users compared with a 16% loss in placebo [20]. Similar results were obtained in the spine and femur using natural estrogens [21–23]. Transdermal or percutaneous estrogen with patches or gels appears to be as effective as oral estrogen [23–25]. The addition of sequential or continuous progestogen may have a synergistic effect on bone [26,27]. The bone-conserving doses of different estrogens given by a variety of routes of administration (Table 29.1) have now been established [28]. However, up to 12% of women treated with bone-conserving doses of HRT still lose bone from the hip [23]. Furthermore, these doses were mainly determined in women during the early postmenopause, and it is thought that older women may conserve bone with lower doses.

Effect of Estrogen on Fractures

The most important fractures clinically are those of the femoral neck, distal radius and vertebral bodies. Fractures of the femoral neck are the most important in terms of morbidity, loss of independence, cost and mortality. The incidence of radial and vertebral fractures is higher between the ages of 50 and 75 years while those of the femoral neck are higher at a later age.

Estrogen is the best established prophylactic treatment which reduces the frequency of osteoporotic fractures [29]. Kanis et al. [30] compared a number of drugs affecting bone metabolism and observed the greatest effect on hip fracture risk amongst those who had taken estrogen. Estrogens are effective in preventing bone loss in the elderly [31] and in those who have already sustained an osteoporotic fracture [32–34]. Several studies have demonstrated a reduction in fracture incidence with estrogen use [30,35–37]. Compared with controls, HRT users have shown reduction in the risk of fractures of 20–60%. Naesson et al. [38] carried out a prospective population-based cohort study in 23 000 women. The reduction in hip fractures was significant with estrogen/progestogen combinations. The study of Kiel et al. [39] based on the Framingham population also showed a significant reduction in the incidence of hip fractures in HRT users. Estrogen also reduces the incidence of radial and vertebral fractures [35,36,40–42].

With 5 or more years of use, estrogen appears to lower the rate of fracture of the forearm or hip by 60% [37]. The reduction in risk of fractures is identical in users of CEE at a dose of either 0.625 mg/day or 1.25 mg/day after controlling for duration for exposure. Framingham data also demonstrated a protective effect of estrogen with respect to subsequent hip fracture in elderly postmenopausal women [39]. Estrogen, both alone and in combination with progestogen, reduces the risk of both cervical and trochanteric hip fracture within the first decade of the menopause [38].

Identifying Whom to Treat

The single most useful means of identifying whom to treat is measurement of bone density. Such measurements can predict fracture and the site-specific measurements are best for predicting site-specific fractures. Thus whilst bone density measurements at a variety of skeletal sites will identify those at risk of future hip fracture, the best discriminator is hip bone density measurement. The World Health Organization defines osteoporosis as a bone mineral density of more than 2.5 standard deviations (SD) below the mean of a young normal range [43]. This means that more than 70% of women 80 years and above have osteoporosis, 60% of whom will have suffered one or more fractures of the proximal femur, vertebrae, distal forearm, proximal humerus and pelvis [44]. In addition, 40% of 70- to 79-year-olds, 22% of 60- to 69-year-olds and 10% of 50- to 59-year-olds have osteoporosis and are at risk of developing an osteoporotic fracture. The relative risk for fracture doubles with each 1 SD decrease in bone mineral density. However, fracture incidence, though proportional to severity of osteoporosis, is also affected by other factors. The subsets of women with osteoporosis who also have one or more fragility fractures are said to have severe or established osteoporosis. Bone mass and loss is best assessed by measurements of bone mineral density, and a variety of techniques are now available [45].

Table 29.2. Identifiable risk factors for osteoporosis

Bone densitometry
Bone density measurement
Menstrual history
Premature menopause
Secondary amenorrhoea (excluding pregnancy)
Endometriosis treatment with gonadotropin-releasing hormone agonists
Irregular periods
Nulliparity
Medical History
Prolonged immobilization
Anorexia nervosa
Malignant diseases
Hyperparathyroidism
Hyperthyroidism
Type 1 diabetes mellitus
Genetic
Family history
Ethnic origin
Drugs
Glucocorticoids
Anti-epileptic therapy
Heparin

Measurements of biochemical markers may be of value for identifying patients with increased bone turnover, since high bone turnover is a determinant of osteoporosis. Markers of bone formation include serum osteocalcin and bone-specific alkaline phosphatase isoenzyme; markers of bone resorption include urinary pyridinoline and deoxypyridinoline crosslinks, and the N- and C-terminal collagen crosslinked peptides [19]. There is some evidence that such biochemical measurements will identify patients at increased fracture risk, and it may be that the combination of measurements of bone density and bone turnover will be a better predictor of future fracture [46]. Further studies are required to establish the precise role of these measurements in the clinical management of osteoporosis.

The problem arises in deciding which women require treatment. Population screening by bone densitometry is not cost-effective, but targeted screening of those deemed at increased risk is very desirable. It is commonly believed that women at risk can be identified from clinical history and observation [47]. A detailed personal, family and medical history will identify risk factors (Table 29.2). Probably the most important risk factor is a previous fragility fracture. A physical examination of gait, posture, spinal tenderness, spinal deformity and range of movement should be performed on all people identified as being at risk [48]. However, risk factor profiles alone, without bone density measurements, are not able to identify individuals with osteoporosis.

Estrogen Therapy

The types of estrogen first discovered to conserve bone were the synthetic estrogens mestranol, ethinylestradiol and stilboestrol. Their adverse effects on coronary heart disease and venous thromboembolism obtained from data on the contraceptive pill resulted in a search for more natural and less potent types of estrogen. The natural types of estrogen, such as CEE, 17β-estradiol and estrone, are now used for estrogen replacement in older women. When unopposed estrogen is used to treat menopausal symptoms or conserve bone in women with an intact uterus, the risk of endometrial hyperplasia and carcinoma rises with increasing dose and duration of use [49–51]. This risk can be nullified by the addition of progestogen sequentially for 10–14 days of a cycle or continuously combined with estrogen [52,53]. The use of unopposed estrogen is contra-indicated in postmenopausal women with a uterus [54]. Women who have had a hysterectomy with cervical conservation may have a remnant of endometrial tissue left and should be given progestogen.

Estrogen for HRT is available in Europe as tablets, patches, gels or subcutaneous implants. In young premenopausal women, estrogen for osteoporosis, for example secondary to anorexia nervosa or glucocorticoid use, may be offered in the form of the combined oral contraceptive pill.

Different treatment strategies for osteoporosis prevention may be considered [55]. Estrogen therapy, with the addition of progestogen when appropriate, may be commenced at, or soon after, the menopause in women at increased risk for osteoporosis. The advantage to this strategy is that the maximum amount of bone mass will be conserved as postmenopausal bone loss will be avoided. The disadvantage to this strategy is that treatment will need to be continued in the long term, perhaps for 20–30 years. Thus there are major cost implications as well as any risks involved with long-term HRT use. Furthermore, the chance of a woman aged 50 years sustaining a fracture over the next 10–15 years is relatively low even in those at increased risk. An alternative strategy, therefore, is to wait until the woman is much older, in her late sixties or seventies, when her risk of osteoporotic fracture is much higher. An early effect of estrogen on reducing fracture risk will then be seen as bone turnover is reduced, and treatment even in the short term will be cost-effective. The disadvantage to this strategy is that delaying the start of treatment might result in women sustaining a fracture before HRT is actually commenced. Furthermore, the acceptability of HRT, as well as other osteoporosis treatments, is much lower in older women. The use of HRT which avoids cyclical bleeding may be particularly useful in these women.

Tolerance and Compliance

Many intellectual and emotional issues are involved in the decision as to whether or not HRT should be commenced. Questions such as benefits and risks, and duration of use need to be discussed fully. Some women, especially the elderly who are many years past the menopause, do not want to take hormones. Estimates of current use of HRT vary by geographical regions throughout Europe. Substantial numbers of women who start HRT stop within a year [56–58]. Long-term use of HRT remains too low. If women are to commence and continue using HRT, this requires them receiving accurate information about HRT. Interestingly, women's sources of information about HRT differ by country. In the UK, 28% of women obtain information from their physicians, 20% from women's magazines, 11% from television and 18% from friends. Over 60% of women in France, Germany and Spain obtain information from their doctor [59]. The reasons why so many women choose not to start or stop HRT are varied. The common reasons are:

- Cancer phobia
- Return of monthly bleeds
- Concerns about weight gain
- Thought to be too old to start HRT
- Unwillingness to interfere with a "natural" event such as the menopause
- A desire not to take hormones
- Physician not willing to prescribe HRT.

Currently, very few women beyond the age of 65 years are treated with HRT [60]. Some physicians believe that HRT is less effective in older women, they fear it may be less tolerable because of side-effects, and therefore do not prescribe it. A survey in 1995 [61] showed that physicians are not fully aware of the therapeutic role of estrogen in preventing osteoporosis and coronary heart disease. Of the physicians who responded to the survey, 75% were aware of a possible role for estrogen in osteoporosis whilst only 7% were aware of a role in preventing coronary heart disease. In addition, less than 50% of physicians informed patients that osteoporosis and coronary heart disease were related to the menopause.

Compliance with HRT can largely be improved by disseminating accurate information to women. Many studies have reported that women who are concerned about osteoporosis are likely to start using HRT [60]. Educating both women and physicians about HRT will improve use and compliance rates. Scientists and the pharmaceutical industry are faced with the task of addressing the concerns and needs of women to improve patient satisfaction and produce estrogen therapy which is more acceptable. The development of tibolone, continuous combined HRT and selective estradiol receptor modulators (SERMs) offer alternatives to women who find a return of monthly bleeds unacceptable. Careful follow-up is necessary in the small minority of women who have persistent breakthrough bleeding in order to exclude endometrial hyperplasia.

Adverse Events of HRT

Estrogen is known to be currently the most effective therapy for the prevention and treatment of osteoporosis. However, as mentioned earlier, adverse events result in poor compliance. Up to 46% of women may discontinue HRT primarily for "minor" complaints such as physical uneasiness/bloating (22%), weight gain (15%) and mastodynia (9%). Other important side-effects are breakthrough bleeding (17%), return of monthly periods (12%), headaches (7%), fear of breast cancer (8%), doctor's negative attitude towards HRT (8%), and cost (2%) [62]. The adverse events associated with HRT are listed in Table 29.3.

Symptoms such as breast enlargement and tenderness, headaches and bloating may be reduced by starting with the lowest dose of HRT and gradually increasing it to the minimum effective dose for bone conservation. Such strategies include giving oral estradiol 1 mg on alternate days increasing after a few weeks to once daily or using 25 μg estradiol patches eventually increasing to 50 μg.

The unwanted return of cyclical bleeding may be prevented by the use of continuous combined HRT, tibolone or SERMs. If persistent bleeding occurs, investigation of the endometrium and pelvic organs with a transvaginal ultrasound and endometrial biopsy or hysteroscopy is recommended [63–65].

Table 29.3. Adverse events associated with HRT

Estrogen-related adverse effects
Breast enlargement and tenderness
Headache (especially with high doses)
Muscle cramps in legs
Cancer of the uterus
Venous thromboembolism
?Cancer of the breast
Progestin-related adverse events
Headaches
Breast tenderness
Bloating
Weight gain
Abdominal cramps
Irritability, depression and anxiety
Breakthrough bleeding

References

1. Chamberlain G, editor. Gynaecology by 10 teachers. Oxford: Oxford University Press, 1995:25.
2. Carr BR. The ovary. In: Blackwall RE, Carr BR, editors. Textbook of reproductive medicine. Norfolk, VA: Appleton and Lange, 1993:199–200.
3. Eriksen EF, Colvard DS, Berg NJ, et al. Evidence of estrogen receptors in normal human osteoblast-like cells. Science 1988;241:84–86.
4. Komm BS, Tarpening CM, Benz DJ, et al. Estrogen binding, receptor, mRNA and biologic response in osteoblast-like osteosarcoma cells. Science 1988;241:81–84.
5. Speroff L Glass RH, Kase NG. Hormone biosynthesis, metabolism and mechanism of action. In: Clinical gynaecological endocrinology and fertility. Baltimore: Williams and Wilkins, 1978:19.
6. Lordoso DW, Kearney M, Kim EA, Jekanowski J, Isner JM. Variable expression of estrogen receptor in normal and atherosclerotic coronary arteries of premenopausal women. Circulation 1994;89:1501–1510.
7. Bertolini DR, Nedwin GE, Bringman TS, Smith DD, Mundy GR. Stimulatin of bone resorption an inhibition of bone formation in vitro by human tumour necrosis factors. Nature 1986;319:516–521.
8. Raisz LG. Local and systemic factors in the pathogenesis of osteoporosis. N Engl J Med 1988;318:818–828.
9. Albright F, Smith PH, Richardson AM. Postmenopausal osteoporosis. JAMA 1941; 116:2465–2474.
10. Hui SL, Slemenda CW, Johnston CC, Appledorn CR. Effects of age and menopause on vertebral bone density. Bone Miner 1987;2:141–146.
11. Hedlund CR, Gallagher JC. The effect of age and menopause on bone mineral density of the proximal femur. J Bone Miner Res 1988;4:639–641.
12. Stevenson JC, Lees B, Davenport M, Cust MP, Ganger KF. Determinants of bone density in normal women: risk factors for future osteoporosis? BMJ 1989;298:924–928.
13. Ribot C, Tremollieres F, Pouilles JM, Louvet JP, Guiraud R. Influence of the menopause and ageing on spinal density in French women. Bone Miner 1988;5:89–97.
14. Ohta H, Masuzala T, Ineda T, Swa Y, Maruta K, Nozarra S. Which is more osteoporosis producing: menopause or oopherectomy? Bone Miner 1992;22:273–285.
15. Pansini F, Bagri B, Bonaccossi G, et al. Oophorectomy and spine bone density. Evidence

of a higher rate of bone loss in surgical compared with spontaneous menopause. Menopause 1995;2:109–115.
16. Richelson LS, Wahner HL, Melton LJ, Riggs BL. Relative contributions of ageing and estrogen deficiency to postmenopausal bone loss. N Engl J Med 1984;311:1273–1275.
17. Gallagher JC. Effect of gonadotrophin-releasing hormone agonist on bone metabolism. Semin Reprod Endocrinol 1993;11:201–208.
18. Howell R, Edmonds DK, Dowsett, M, Crook D, Lees B, Stevenson JC. Gonadotropin-releasing hormone analogue (goserilin) plus hormone replacement therapy for the treatment of endometriosis: a randomized controlled trial. Fertil Steril 1995;64:474–481.
19. Delmas PD, Garnero. Biochemical markers of bone turnover in osteoprosis. In: Stevenson JC, Lindsay R, editors. Osteoporosis. London: Chapman & Hall Medical, 1998:117–136.
20. Lindsay R, Hart DM, Forrest C, Baird C. Prevention of spinal osteoporosis in oophorectomised women. Lancet 1980;II:1151–1154.
21. Nachtigall LE, Nachtigall RH, Nachtigall RD, Beckman EM. Estrogen replacement therapy. A 10 year prospective study in relationship to osteoporosis. Obstet Gynecol 1979;53:277–281.
22. Christiansen C, Christiansen MS, McNair P, Hagen C, Stocklund KE, Transbol I. Prevention of early postmenopausal bone loss: controlled 2 year study in 315 normal females. Eur J Clin Invest 1980;10:273–279.
23. Hillard TC, Whitcroft SJ, Marsh MS, et al. Long-term effects of transdermal and oral hormone replacement therapy on postmenopausal bone loss. Osteoporos Int 1994;4:341–348.
24. Riis BJ, Thomsen K, Strøm V, Christiansen C. The effects of percutaneous estradiol and natural progesterone on postmenopausal bone loss. Am J Obstet Gynecol 1987;156:61–65.
25. Lufkin EG, Wahner HW, O'Fallon WM, et al. Treatment of postmenopausal osteoporosis with transdermal estrogen. Ann Intern Med 1992;117:1–9.
26. Christiansen C, Riis BJ. Five years with continuous combined estrogen/progestogen therapy. Effects on calcium metabolism, lipoproteins and bleeding pattern. Br J Obstet Gynaecol 1990;97:1087–1092.
27. Nielson SP, Barenholdt O, Hermansen F, Munk-Jensen N. Magnitude and pattern of skeletal response to long-term continuous and cyclical sequential estrogen/progestogen treatment. Br J Obstet Gynecol 1994;101:319–324.
28. Stevenson JC. Gonadal hormones. Osteoporos Int 1997;7(Suppl 1):58–60.
29. Consensus Development Conference. Prophylaxis and treatment of osteoporosis. BMJ 1987;295:914–915.
30. Kanis JA, Johnell O, Gulberg B, et al. Evidence for efficacy of drugs affecting bone metabolism in preventing hip fractures. BMJ 1992;305:1124–1128.
31. Quigley MET, Martin PL, Burnier AM, Brooks P. Estrogen therapy arrests bone loss in elderly women. Am J Obstet Gynecol 1987;156:1516–1523.
32. Nordin BEC, Horseman A, Crilly RG, Marshall DH, Simpson M. Treatment of spinal osteoporosis in postmenopausal women. BMJ 1980;1:451–454.
33. Civitelli R, Agnusdei D, Nardi P, Zacchei F, Avioli LV, Gennari C. Effects of one year treatment with estrogens on bone mass and intestinal calcium absorption and 25-hydroxyvitamin D 1-alpha hydroxylase reserve in postmenopausal osteoporosis. Calcif Tissue Int 1987;42:77–86.
34. Lindsay R, Tohme J. Estrogen treatment of women with established osteoporosis. Obstet Gynecol 1990;76:1–6.
35. Gordan GS, Picchi J, Roof BS. Antifracture efficacy of long-term estrogens for osteoporosis. Trans Assoc Am Physicians 1973;86:326–332.
36. Hutchinson TA, Polansky SM, Feinstein AR. Postmenopusal estrogens prevent against fractures of the wrist and distal radius. Lancet 1979;II:706–710.
37. Weiss NS, Ure CL, Ballard JH, et al. Decreased risk of fracture of the hip and lower forearm with postmenopausal estrogen use. N Engl J Med 1980;303:1195–1198.

38. Naesson T, Persson I, Adami HO, Bergstrom R, Bergkvist L. Hormone replacement therapy and the risk of first hip fracture: a prospective population-based cohort study. Ann Intern Med 1990;113:95–103.
39. Kiel DP, Felson DT, Andersson JJ, Wilson PWF, Moskowitz MA. Hip fracture and the use of estrogens in postmenopausal women. N Engl J Med 1987;317:1169–1174.
40. Paganini-Hill A, Ross RK, Gerkins VR, Henderson BE, Arthur M, Mack TM. Menopausal estrogen therapy and hip fractures. Ann Intern Med 1981;95:28–31.
41. Ettinger B, Genant HK, Cann CE. Long-term estrogen replacement therapy prevents bone loss and fractures. Am Int Med 1985;102:319–24.
42. Cauley JA, Seeley DG, Ensrud K, Ettinger B, Black D, Cummings SR. Study of osteoporotic fractures group. Estrogen replacement therapy and fractures in older women Ann Intern Med 1994;12:9–16.
43. WHO. Assessment of fracture risk and its application to the screening of postmenopausal osteoporosis. WHO technical report series. Geneva: WHO, 1994.
44. Melton LJ III. How many women have osteoporosis now? J Bone Miner Res 1995; 10:175–177.
45. Lees B, Banks LM, Stevenson JC. Bone mass measurements. In: Stevenson JC, Lindsay R, editors. Osteoporosis. London: Chapman & Hall Medical, 1998:137–160.
46. Garnero P, Hausherr E, Chapuy MC, et al. Markers of bone resorption predict hip fracture in elderly women. J Bone Miner Res 1996;11:1531–1138.
47. Turner LW, Taylor BE, Hunt S. Predictors for osteoporosis diagnosis among postmenopausal women: results from a national survey. J Women Aging 1998;10:79–96.
48. Gardsell P, Johnell O, Nilsson BE. Predicting fractures in women using forearm bone densitometry. Calcif Tissue Int 1989;44:355–361.
49. Noyes RW, Hertig AT, Rock J. Dating the endometrial biopsy. Fertil Steril 1950;1:3–25.
50. Ziel HK, Finkle WD. Increased risk to endometrial carcinoma among users of conjugated estrogens. N Engl J Med 1975;293:1167–1170.
51. Smith DC, Prentice R, Thompson DJ, Hermann WL. Association of exogenous estrogen and endometrial cancer. N Engl J Med 1975;293:1164–1167.
52. Grady D, Grebestsadik T, Kerlikowise K. Hormone replacement therapy and endometrial cancer risk; a meta-analysis. Obstet Gynecol 1991;85:304–313.
53. Voigt LF, Weiss NS, Chu J. Progestogen supplementation of exogenous estrogen and risk of endometrial cancer. Lancet 1991;338:274–277.
54. Leather AT, Studd JWW. Can the withdrawal bleeding following estrogen replacement therapy be avoided? Br J Obstet Gynaecol 1990;97:1071–1079.
55. Stevenson JC. Is there a case for targeting hormone replacement therapy for osteoporosis at the menopause? Osteoporos Int 1998;8(Suppl 1):47–50.
56. Kaufert PL. The menopausal transition: the use of estrogen. Can J Public Health 1986;77(Suppl 1):86–91.
57. McKinlay JB, McKinlay SM, Brambilla DJ. Health status and utilisation behaviour associated with menopause. Am J Epidemiol 1987;125:110–121.
58. Hemminki E, Brambilla DJ, McKinlay SM, Posner JP. Use of estrogen amongst middle-aged Massachusetts women. Drug Intell Clin Pharm 1991;25:418–423.
59. Schneider HPG. How to improve compliance with HRT. In: Birkhauser M, Rozenbaum H, editors. Proceedings of IV European Congress on menopause, 1998:105–110.
60. Rozenberg S, Vandromme J, Knoll M. Compliance of hormone replacement therapy. Int J Fertil Men Studies 1995;40:123–132.
61. Griffith F. Women's health concern: is the promotion of hormone replacement therapy for prevention important to women? Fam Pract Man 1995;1:54–59.
62. Grazziotin A. HRT: from motivation to compliance. In: Paoletti R, Crosignani PG, Kenemans P, Samisioe G, Soma G, Jackson AS, editors. Women's health and menopause: risk reduction strategies. Dordrecht: Kluwer Academic, 1997:263–273.
63. Karlsson B, Granberg S, Ridell B, Wikland M. Endometrial thickness as measured by transvaginal sonography. Ultrasound Obstet Gynecol 1994;4:320–325.

64. Granberg S, Ylostalo P, Wikland M, Karlsson B. Endometrial sonographic and histological findings in women with and without hormone replacement therapy suffering from postmenopausal bleeding. Maturitas 1997;27:35–40.
65. Hanggi W, Bersinger N, Altermatt HJ, Birkhauser MH. Comparison of transvaginal ultrasonography and endometrial biopsy in endometrial surveillance in postmenopausal HRT users. Maturitas 1997;27:133–143.

30 Bisphosphonates

H. Fleisch

Introduction

The bisphosphonates, in the past erroneously called diphosphonates, have been known to the chemists since the middle of the nineteenth century, the first synthesis dating back to 1865 in Germany. Their use was industrial, mainly in the textile, fertilizer and oil industries, and, because of their property of inhibiting calcium carbonate precipitation, as preventors of scaling. Our knowledge of the biological characteristics of bisphosphonates dates back 30 years, the first report on them being produced by the author's group in 1968.

Chemistry

Bisphosphonates are compounds characterized by two C–P bonds. If the two bonds are located on the same carbon atom, the compounds are called geminal bisphosphonates and are analogs of pyrophosphate which contain an oxygen instead of a carbon atom. They are in general simply called bisphosphonates. The P–C–P structure allows a great number of possible variations, mostly by changing the two lateral chains on the carbon. Many bisphosphonates have been investigated in humans with respect to their effects on bone, and seven of them are commercially available today for treatment of bone disease (Fig. 30.1).

Each bisphosphonate has its own chemical, physicochemical and biological characteristics, which implies that it is not possible to extrapolate from the results of one compound to others with respect to their actions.

Biological Effects

The bisphosphonates have two fundamental biological effects: inhibition of bone resorption and, when given at high doses, inhibition of calcification.

Inhibition of Bone Resorption

Bisphosphonates can be very powerful inhibitors of bone resorption [1], their potency varying according to their structure. This was shown in vitro in cell and organ culture, as well as in vivo in both animals and humans. In animals the effect is present in normal animals, as well as in conditions where resorption is experimentally increased.

Effects In Vivo

Intact Animals. In growing intact rats, the bisphosphonates block the degradation of both bone and cartilage, thus arresting the remodelling of the metaphysis, which becomes club-shaped and radiologically denser than normal [2]. This effect is often used as a model to study the potency of new compounds. The inhibition of endogenous bone resorption has also been documented by ^{45}Ca kinetic studies [3], by markers of bone resorption [3] and by morphology. It leads secondarily to a decrease in bone formation, thus resulting in diminished bone turnover. The decrease in resorption is accompanied by an increase in calcium balance [3] and in the mineral content of bone. This is possible because of an increase in intestinal absorption of calcium [3], consequent on an elevation of 1,25-dihydroxyvitamin D. This increased balance is the reason for administering these compounds to humans suffering from osteoporosis.

The inhibition of bone resorption reaches a certain steady level even when the compounds are given continuously [4]. This level depends on the administered dose. This fact, which has also been described in humans [5], shows that there is no accumulation of effect with time and suggests that, at the therapeutic dosage, there is no danger of a continuous decrease in bone turnover which might result in osteopetrosis and brittle bone.

Animals with Experimentally Increased Resorption. Bisphosphonates can also prevent experimentally induced increases in bone resorption. They impair, for example, resorption induced by agents such as parathyroid hormone [1,6], 1,25dihydroxyvitamin D, and retinoids, as well as in various models mimicking human diseases, including osteoporosis and tumor bone disease [7].

Many osteoporosis models have been investigated. They include sciatic nerve section, which was the first model to be studied [8], spinal cord section, hypokinesis, ovariectomy, orchidectomy, heparin, lactation, low calcium diet and corticosteroids. All bisphosphonates investigated have been effective, examples being alendronate, clodronate, etidronate, ibandronate, incadronate, olpadronate, pamidronate, risedronate, tiludronate and YH 529. The inhibition of bone loss leads to reduced trabecular thinning, a decreased number of trabecular perforations, a decreased reduction in connectivity and a smaller erosion of the cortex [9,10], thus slowing down the decrease in bone strength. Indeed, if not given in excess, bisphosphonates improve biomechanical properties both in normal animals and in experimental models of osteoporosis [9,11].

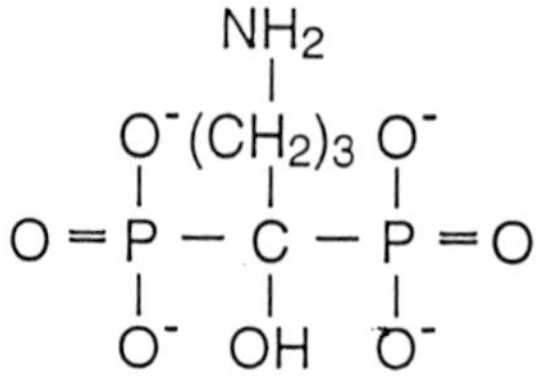

(4-Amino-1-hydroxybutylidene)bis-phosphonate
alendronate*
Gentili; Merck Sharp & Dohme

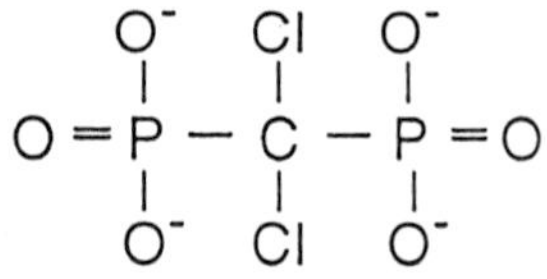

(Dichloromethylene)-bis-phosphonate
clodronate*
Astra; Gentili; F. Hoffmann-La Roche; Leiras; Rhône-Poulenc Rorer

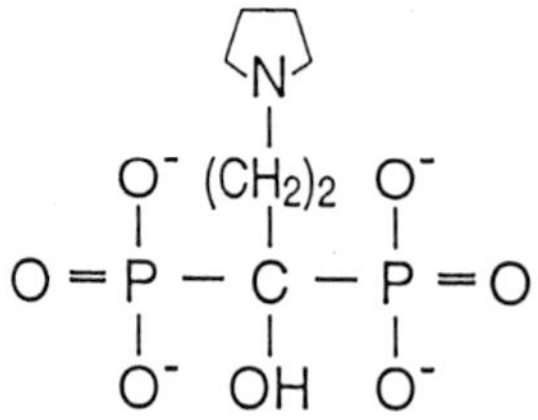

[1-Hydroxy-3-(1-pyrrolidinyl)-propylidene]bis-phosphonate
EB-1053
Leo

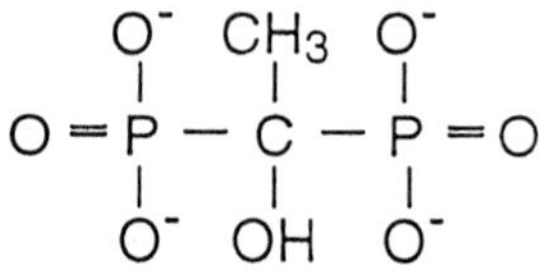

(1-Hydroxyethylidene)-bis-phosphonate
etidronate*
Gentili; Procter & Gamble

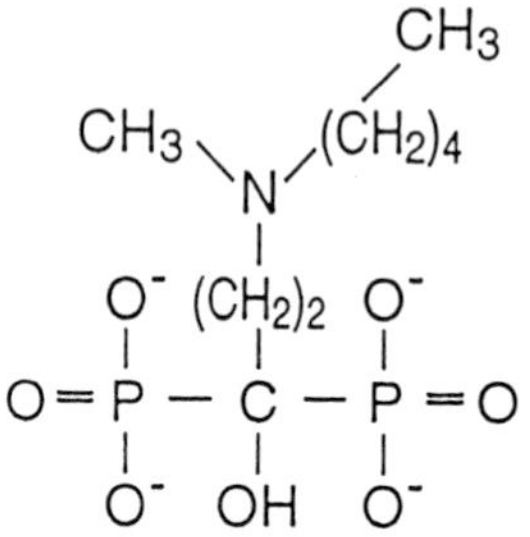

[1-Hydroxy-3-(methylpentylamino)propylidene]bis-phosphonate
ibandronate*
F. Hoffmann-La Roche

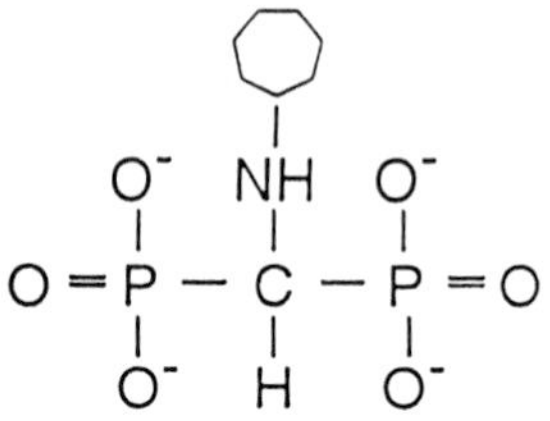

[(Cycloheptylamino)-methylene]bis-phosphonate
incadronate
Yamanouchi

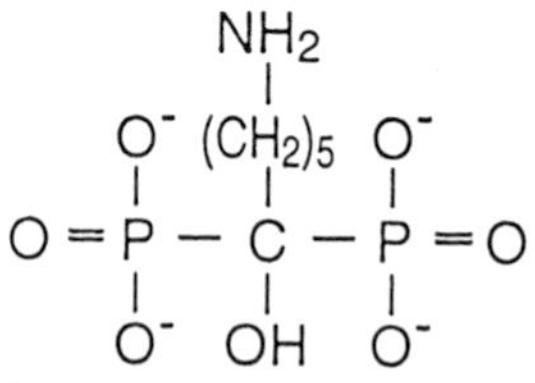

(6-Amino-1-hydroxyhexylidene)bis-phosphonate
neridronate
Abiogen

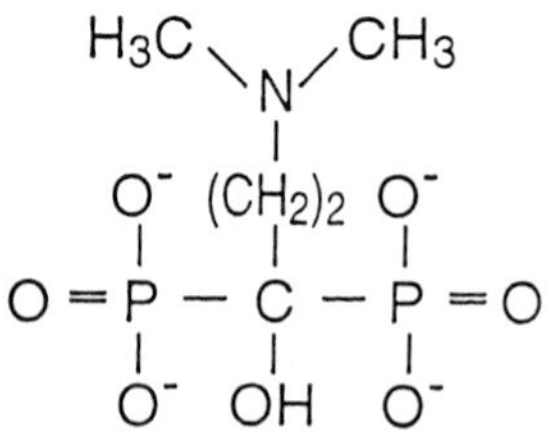

[3-(Dimethylamino)-1-hydroxypropylidene]bis-phosphonate
olpadronate
Gador

Figure 30.1. Chemical structure of bisphosphonates investigated in humans.

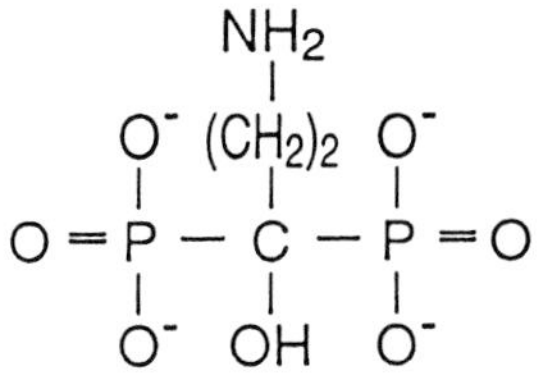

(3-Amino-1-hydroxypropylidene)bis-phosphonate
pamidronate*
Gador, Novartis

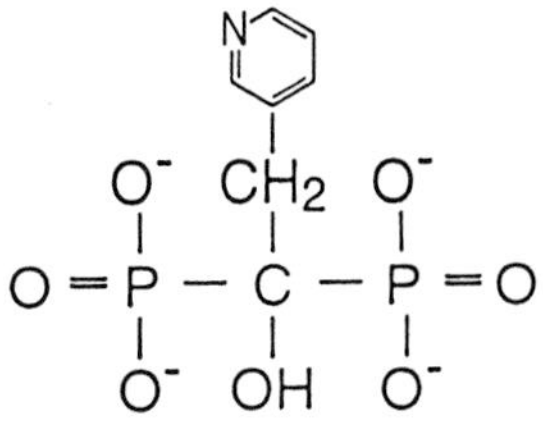

[1-Hydroxy-2-(3-pyridinyl)-ethylidene]bis-phosphonate
risedronate *
Procter & Gamble

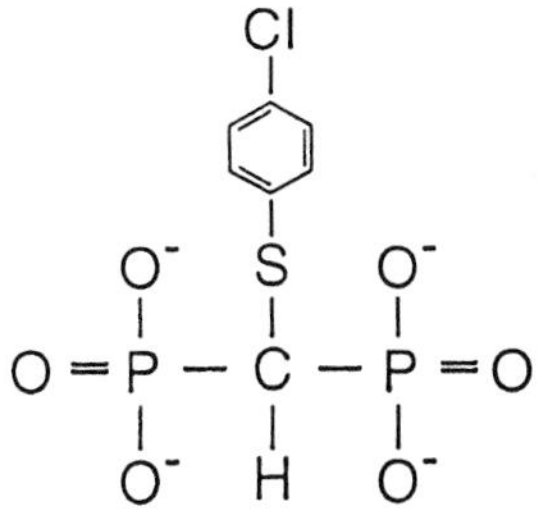

[[(4-Chlorophenyl)thio]-methylene]bis-phosphonate
tiludronate*
Sanofi

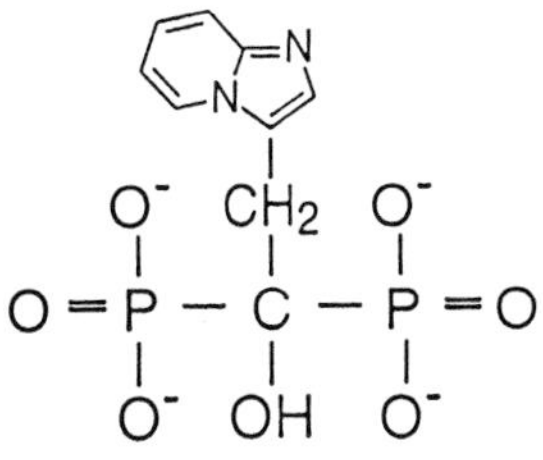

[1-Hydroxy-2-imidazo-(1,2-a) pyridin-3-ylethylidene]bis-phosphonate
minodronate
Yamanouchi–Hoechst

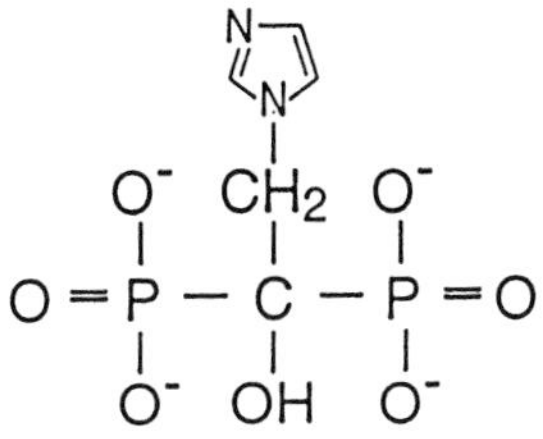

[1-Hydroxy-2-(1H-imidazole-1-yl)ethylidene]bis-phosphonate
zoledronate
Novartis

Figure 30.1. (*continued*)

Effects on Organ and Cell Culture

Bisphosphonates block bone resorption induced by various means in organ culture [12]. Inhibition can also be found when the effect of isolated osteoclasts is investigated on various mineralized matrices in vitro [13]. Under bisphosphonate treatment the osteoclasts form fewer erosion cavities and these are of smaller size.

Structure–Activity Relationship

The activity of bisphosphonates on bone resorption varies greatly from compound to compound. Bisphosphonates 5000–10 000 times more powerful in inhibiting bone resorption than etidronate, the first bisphosphonate investigated, have now been developed. The gradation of potency evaluated in rats corresponds quite well with that found in humans.

However, no clearcut relationship between structure and activity has yet been demonstrated. The length of the aliphatic carbon is important since up to a certain length the activity first increases and then decreases. Adding a hydroxyl group to the carbon atom at position 1 increases its potency [14]. Derivatives with an amino group at the end of the side chain are very active. A primary amine is not necessary for this activity since adding certain groups to the amino nitrogen increases its efficacy. Cyclic geminal bisphosphonates are also very potent, as long as they contain a nitrogen atom in the ring. It is now clear that a three-dimensional structural requirement is involved.

Mechanisms of Action

The inhibition of bone resorption is explained largely, if not entirely, by cellular mechanisms. The mechanism initially proposed of inhibition through crystal dissolution, which is observed in vitro [1,6], probably has a negligible effect, if any. The terminal effect is on the osteoclasts which show morphological changes both in vitro and in vivo [2,15], including alterations of the cytoskeleton, especially actin and vinculin, and of the ruffled border. The effect may be a direct one, which is supported by the fact that, under certain conditions, bisphosphonates can enter cells [16], particularly osteoclasts [17]. Furthermore the concentration of bisphosphonate can also attain very high values under osteoclasts, where they deposit preferentially [15,17]. They would be released from the mineral due to the acid pH level prevailing at this location.

Four mechanisms appear to be involved in the inhibition of resorption: (1) inhibition of osteoclast recruitment [18]; (2) possibly inhibition of osteoclastic adhesion [19], since bisphosphonates in vitro can inhibit the adhesion of other cells, such as tumor cells [20]; (3) shortening of the lifespan of osteoclasts by inducing osteoclast programmed cell death (apoptosis), both in vitro and in vivo [21]; and (4) inhibition of osteoclast activity. Indeed, the cells are sometimes more numerous but look inactive [2]. All four effects could be due either to a direct action on the osteoclast or its precursors, or indirectly through action on cells which modulate the osteoclast, most likely osteoblastic lineage cells. Thus bisphosphonates, when added even in low concentrations to osteoblasts, stimulate these cells to produce an inhibitor of osteoclast formation and hence of bone resorption in vitro [22,23].

The molecular and biochemical events leading to these effects have not been fully elucidated. It has been known for a long time that bisphosphonates decrease acid production of various cells [24] as well as of calvaria. Recently, bisphosphonates were shown to decrease the release of acid through a sodium-independent mechanism by osteoclasts [25]. Possibly part of this effect is due to the decrease in proton transport by the vacuolar-type proton ATPase. Certain bisphosphonates, such as clodronate and etidronate, also inhibit prostaglandin synthesis by bone cells or calvariae, both in vitro and in vivo [26]. Since prostaglandins are involved in bone resorption, this inhibition may play a role in the resorption process.

Various enzymes are modulated by bisphosphonates. Bisphosphonates inhibit lysosomal enzymes in vitro, in cultured calvariae, or when given in vivo. In view of the homology between pyrophosphate and bisphosphonates, enzymes involving pyrophosphate or ATP have been examined. Thus, some protein-tyrosine phosphatases are inhibited in vitro by micromolar concentrations [27,28] of biphosphonate. These effects might be relevant since protein-tyrosine phosphorylation is important in the signal transduction pathways which control cell growth, differentiation and activity.

Recent evidence indicates that not all bisphosphonates act by the same mechanism. Thus, the compounds containing a nitrogen atom can inhibit the mevalonate pathway which leads to an inhibition of the isoprenylation of GTP-binding proteins. This can cause apoptosis and possibly decrease function of the osteoclasts [29]. On the other hand, etidronate, clodronate and tiludronate are incorporated into adenine nucleotides to make nonhydrolyzable ATP analogs and may then act via a different pathway [30].

Unfortunately, no individual mechanism shows a good correlation with the potency in vivo when different bisphosphonates of various potencies are investigated. This confirms the above-mentioned hypothesis that the mechanisms might be dissimilar for different bisphosphonates and suggests that, if any of the above mechanisms is relevant for bone resorption, it is not the only one.

Inhibition of Calcification

Ectopic and Normal Mineralization and Ossification

Bisphosphonates can very efficiently inhibit ectopic calcification in vivo. Thus, they prevent experimentally induced calcification of many soft tissues when given either parenterally or orally [31].

Unfortunately, when administered in doses approximating those which inhibit soft tissue calcification, bisphosphonates can impair the mineralization of normal calcified tissues such as bone and cartilage [2] and, when given in higher amounts, also that of dentine, enamel and cementum. Inhibition of the mineralization of bone and cartilage is also seen in humans when biphosphonates are given in larger amounts, which has hampered the therapeutic use of these compounds in ectopic calcification.

The mechanism of the inhibition of both normal and ectopic mineralization is most likely to be due, at least in part if not entirely, to a physicochemical mechanism. Indeed, bisphosphonates are powerful inhibitors of the formation and aggregation of calcium phosphate crystals, even at very low concentrations [31]. This effect is related to the marked affinity of these compounds for the surface of solid phase calcium phosphate where they bind onto the calcium [32].

Pharmacokinetics

Bisphosphonates have a very low bioavailability, from a few percent to below 1% for the newer more potent ones, which are given in lower quantities. This is partly explained by their low lipophilicity which hampers transcellular transport, and their high negative charge which hampers paracellular transport. Furthermore, they may be partly in an insoluble form in the gut, due to chelation to calcium.

Once in the blood, bisphosphonates disappear very rapidly, mostly into bone. This might be explained by their strong binding to hydroxyapatite crystals [32]. Consequently, soft tissues are exposed to these compounds for only short periods, explaining their bone-specific effects and their low toxicity. It was generally thought that the bisphosphonates deposit in those locations within the bone where new bone is formed. Recently, however, they have been found to deposit also under osteoclasts [15,17].

Once the bisphosphonates are buried in the skeleton, they will be released to a significant extent only when the bone is destroyed in the course of its turnover. The skeletal half-life of various bisphosphonates is therefore long, between 3 months and 1 year for mice and rats, and much longer, sometimes over 10 years, for humans.

Lastly, the bisphosphonates are not metabolized in vivo, and up to now all the bisphosphonates investigated have been found to be excreted unaltered. More detailed preclinical information can be obtained from a recent review [33].

Clinical Effects

Bisphosphonates are used clinically as: (1) skeletal markers in the form of ^{99m}Tc derivatives; (2) antiosteolytic agents in patients with increased bone destruction, especially Paget's disease, tumor bone disease and osteoporosis; (3) inhibitors of calcification in patients with ectopic calcification and ossification; and (4) antitartar agents when added to toothpaste. Only their use in osteoporosis will be discussed here.

Use in Osteoporosis

Many studies show clearly that various bisphosphonates not only stop the decrease in bone mineral density (BMD) in various types of osteoporosis, but actually induce an increase of a few percent in this parameter. A substantial amount of data is now available for [in alphabetical order]: alendronate, clodronate, etidronate, ibandronate, pamidronate, risedronate and tiludronate. Since only alendronate and etidronate are commercially available today for osteoporosis, emphasis will mainly be placed on these, the others being only superficially reviewed. In most of the trials two main parameters have been assessed, namely bone turnover and BMD. BMD can, but does not necessarily, faithfully represent bone mass. Indeed part of the increase can be due to an increase in mineralization of the bone because the osteons become older and more mineralized due to the decrease in turnover. This has recently been shown to be the case in baboons treated with alendronate [34]. "Bone mass" is the term commonly used in the literature, which is not entirely correct. We shall use the term BMD, which is the measured parameter.

Alendronate

A large number of studies have demonstrated the effectiveness of alendronate in inhibiting the decrease in BMD after the menopause and in other conditions. The first multicenteric, randomized and placebo-controlled studies investigated the dose-effect of this bisphosphonate, administered orally at doses between 5 mg and 40 mg daily to postmenopausal osteoporotic patients. The drug not only prevented the decrease in BMD, but led to an increase at both lumbar spine and hip, as opposed to the drop or no change in BMD seen in the controls [35]. Since 10 mg were more active than 5 mg, but not less active than 20 mg, 10 mg appears to be the most favorable dose. These results were later confirmed by two much larger studies on 994 osteoporotic patients [36] and 2027 patients [37], respectively. Later, many other studies reported similar data [e.g., 38,39]. Alendronate is also active in the elderly [40] and in nonosteoporotic women [41], 5 mg daily being more effective than 2.5 mg in these two studies. Of interest is the recent finding that the effect on BMD is partially additive to that of hormone replacement therapy (HRT).

Not only postmenopausal osteoporosis is prevented: alendronate given at 5 and 10 mg daily also led to an increase instead of a small decrease in BMD in patients given corticosteroids [42].

The patients showed a dramatic decrease in both bone resorption and bone formation as assessed by biochemical markers. It is interesting that, analogous to what has been seen in rats, the inhibitory effect on bone turnover reaches a plateau even if administration of the drug is pursued, and that this plateau depends on the dose administered. With a dosage of 10 mg daily, premenopausal levels were reached [5]. Turnover increases again when the drug is discontinued although in one investigation prestudy levels were not quite reached after 1 year [43]. The difference in BMD between the treated and untreated patients was maintained for at least 1 year with doses of 5 and 10 mg daily and for at least 2 years with 20 and 40 mg daily [43]. Similar results are seen with other bisphosphonates, although initial turnover is usually attained after only one year, and BMD starts to decrease in the first year after discontinuation. It seems likely that this evolution depends on the dosage given.

It must be noted that the effective dose appears to be lower in Asians. Thus, as shown in a recent study on Japanese postmenopausal osteoporotic patients, 2.5 mg given daily by mouth was as effective on BMD as 10 mg, although the effect on bone turnover was smaller [44].

The studies with alendronate also showed for the first time with certainty that fracture incidence is decreased by bisphosphonates. Thus, the administration of alendronate led to a decrease of 48% in vertebral fractures [36] in osteoporotic patients with or without fractures. This was accompanied by a decreased loss of stature of the patients. In addition, also non-vertebral fractures diminished significantly. These results were later confirmed in another study on 2027 osteoporotic patients, all of them with fractures [37]. The oral administration of 5 mg alendronate daily for 2 years, followed by 10 mg for 1 year, reduced the risk of vertebral fractures by about 50% and the risk of sustaining multiple fractures by 89%. Furthermore, both hip and wrist fractures were also decreased by about 50%.

Morphologically, alendronate given at doses between 5 and 20 mg orally per day for 24 or 36 months produced a dramatic decrease in bone turnover of about 90% as analyzed in transiliac bone biopsies. Mineralization was normal. Interestingly there was an increase in the thickness of the packets, suggesting that local bone formation might have been increased [45].

Thus, alendronate given at oral doses of 10 mg daily or, in certain cases, 5 or 2.5 mg daily, not only prevents a further decrease in BMD but increases BMD by a few percent. Furthermore, it decreases the risk of fractures.

Etidronate

Up to now, the only dosage of etidronate which has been adequately studied and which is recommended by the manufacturer is the discontinuous administration of 400 mg orally. Two controlled double-masted studies on postmenopausal women [46,47] investigated the effect of discontinuous oral administration of this dose for 2 weeks, followed in both the etidronate and the placebo groups by either 10 or 13 weeks of 500 mg daily of calcium. The cycle was repeated over a period of 3 years or more. Both studies showed a significant increase in vertebral and hip BMD. Some of the patients were further investigated for up to 5 years [48] or 7 years [49,50] in the first and second study, respectively. It was clear that the treatment was well tolerated throughout this time. Furthermore, the BMD was maintained or even somewhat increased. These results were confirmed by many other studies. Etidronate is also active in the early postmenopausal period [51]. In addition the effect is partially additive with that seen with HRT [52]. Etidronate also induces an increase in BMD of the spine and hip rather than a decrease, and it decreases fracture incidence in patients receiving corticosteroids [53,54].

Some decrease in vertebral fractures was found in both etidronate studies [46,47] but, although the data looked promising, the significance of this result was not clearly established. As the study progressed, the vertebral fracture incidence seemed to decrease further [48,50].

Therefore, etidronate is also active in preventing the loss of BMD and, at least in certain conditions, in decreasing fracture risk. However, the latter is not as well documented as in alendronate.

Other Bisphosphonates

Clodronate

Various regimens of clodronate given either orally [55] or intravenously [56] have been found to be effective in influencing BMD. Furthermore, clodronate is also active in corticosteroid-treated patients [57]

Pamidronate

This bisphosphonate also prevents the loss of BMD and can induce an actual increase in this parameter, both when the compound is given orally [58] [59] [60], most often at a dose of 150 mg, or intravenously, most often as an infusion of 30 mg every 3 months [61]. Pamidronate is also effective in corticosteroid-induced bone loss [62].

Tiludronate

In a first study 100 mg of tiludronate given orally every day for 6 months also induced an increase in BMD as opposed to a decrease after 2 years [63]. Despite discontinuation of the drug, the effect appeared to be maintained over the entire study period of 2 years. This bisphosphonate was also active in the bone loss induced by immobilization [64]. However, in a recent large study where tiludronate was given at 50 mg or 200 mg daily for the first 7 days of each month for up to 36 months to a large number of patients with or without fractures, no clinically relevant effect on either BMD or fractures was seen [65].

Ibandronate

Ibandronate given either orally at doses up to 5 mg daily [66] or by intravenous bolus injections at doses up to 2 mg every 3 months [67] also increased BMD. The optimal dose seemed to be 2.5 mg orally, and possibly 2 mg intravenously.

Risedronate

Risedronate prevents the decrease in BMD when given by mouth daily at 30 mg for 2 weeks on and 10 weeks off for a period of 2 years to women with artificial menopause induced by chemotherapy for breast cancer [68]. It was also effective in postmenopausal women with normal BMD when given for 2 years either as 5 mg daily, or as 5 mg daily for 2 weeks of each month. Continuous administration was more effective than on-and-off therapy [69]. Risedronate has just been shown to decrease both vertebral and non-vertebral fractures when given at 5 mg per day orally [70].

In practically all the studies with various bisphosphonates bone turnover was assessed with various biochemical markers. At the doses which were effective on BMD, both bone resorption and bone formation were always decreased.

Use in Localized Bone Loss

It has been suggested that bisphosphonates might also be used to advantage in diseases characterized by localized bone loss, such as periprosthetic osteolysis, Sudeck's disease and perionditis. Clinical trials in this direction are under way.

Adverse Events

Bisphosphonates have relatively few adverse events. Care must be taken when administering bisphosphonates intravenously, which is now done mostly in cases of tumor bone disease and Paget's disease. Indeed when infused in the large amounts that are necessary, especially with the less potent compounds, bisphosphonates can form a solid phase in the blood which may induce renal failure. It is generally suggested that etidronate, clodronate and pamidronate are diluted in at least 250 ml and infused no faster than over a period of 2 h. Smaller amounts will be needed for the more powerful bisphosphonates. Recently injections of up to 3 mg [67] have been used for ibandronate.

The most common adverse events of the bisphosphonates, especially the derivatives with a nitrogen atom, are gastrointestinal disturbances such as discomfort, pain and diarrhea, and sometimes even ulcerations. There are fewer problems with etidronate and clodronate. In order to avoid these side-effects, the bisphosphonates should always be taken with a large glass of water in an erect position, and the patient should not recline until food has been taken.

Some of the bisphosphonates, such as etidronate, when given in large amounts, can inhibit normal skeletal mineralization, leading to osteomalacia. For etidronate this effect is present at oral dosages above 800 mg given over prolonged periods. The dosage and regimen suggested by the manufacturer, namely 400 mg orally every day for 2 weeks, to be repeated every 3 months, does not have this inhibitory effect. Inhibition of mineralization has also been observed with pamidronate in a few patients when large amounts were infused. However, no such effect has been described so far for the more powerful bisphosphonates, since the window between the amount inhibiting bone resorption and mineralization is much larger in these compounds.

The derivatives with a nitrogen atom, when given intravenously at higher doses, but not when given orally, lead to a transient pyrexia which is, however, usually observed only once. It is accompanied by changes in blood lymphocytes and other serum alterations, suggesting an acute-phase reaction. These events appear to have no clinical relevance, except for minor discomfort lasting for a few days [71].

A concern has been whether bisphosphonates would inhibit bone healing of fractures or after implants. This does not seem to be the case at the doses administered in osteoporosis [72].

In general it can be stated that the various bisphosphonates have very few adverse events at the dosage used for osteoporosis. For a review see Adami and Zamberlan [73].

Conclusion

The bisphosphonates are compounds characterized by a very potent capacity to inhibit bone resorption. They have therefore been developed as drugs to treat various diseases characterized by high bone turnover, among them osteoporosis. For a review of both preclinical and clinical aspects see Fleisch [74].

References

1. Fleisch H, Russell RGG, Francis MD. Diphosphonates inhibit hydroxyapatite dissolution in vitro and bone resorption in tissue culture and in vivo. Science 1969;165: 1262–1264.
2. Schenk R, Merz WA, Mühlbauer R, Russell RGG, Fleisch H. Effect of ethane-1-hydroxy-1,1-diphosphonate (EHDP) and dichloromethylene diphosphonate (Cl2MDP) on the calcification and resorption of cartilage and bone in the tibial epiphysis and metaphysis of rats. Calcif Tissue Res 1973;11:196–214.
3. Gasser AB, Morgan DB, Fleisch HA, Richelle LJ. The influence of two diphosphonates on calcium metabolism in the rat. Clin Sci 1972;43:31–45.
4. Reitsma PH, Bijvoet OLM, Verlinden-Ooms H, van der Wee-Pals LJA. Kinetic studies of bone and mineral metabolism during treatment with (3-amino-1-hydroxypropylidene)-1,1-bisphosphonate (APD) in rats. Calcif Tissue Int 1980;32:145–157.
5. Garnero P, Shih WJ, Gineyts E, Karpf DB, Delmas PD. Comparison of new biochemical markers of bone turnover in late postmenopausal osteoporotic women in response to alendronate treatment. J Clin Endocrinol Metab 1994;79:1693–1700.

6. Russell RGG, Mühlbauer RC, Bisaz S, Williams DA, Fleisch H. The influence of pyrophosphate, condensed phosphates, phosphonates and other phosphate compounds on the dissolution of hydroxyapatite in vitro and on bone resorption induced by parathyroid hormone in tissue culture and in thyroparathyroidectomised rats. Calcif Tissue Res 1970;6:183–196.
7. Martodam RR, Thornton KS, Sica DA, D'Souza SM, Flora L, Mundy GR. The effects of dichloromethylene diphosphonate on hypercalcaemia and other parameters of the humoral hypercalcemia of malignancy in the rat Leydig cell tumor. Calcif Tissue Int 1983;35:512–519.
8. Mühlbauer RC, Russell RGG, Williams DA, Fleisch H. The effects of diphosphonates, polyphosphates and calcitonin on "immobilisation osteoporosis" in rats. Eur J Clin Invest 1971;1:336–344.
9. Balena R, Toolan BC, Shea M, Markatos A, Myers ER, Lee SC et al. The effects of 2-year treatment with the aminobisphosphonate alendronate on bone metabolism, bone histomorphometry, and bone strength in ovariectomized non human primates. J Clin Invest 1993;92:2577–2586.
10. Boyce RW, Paddock CL, Gleason JR, Sletsema WK, Eriksen EF. The effects of risedronate on canine cancellous bone remodelling: Three-dimensional kinetic reconstruction of the remodelling site. J Bone Miner Res 1995;10:211–221.
11. Ferretti JL. Effects of bisphosphonates on bone biomechanics. In: Bijvoet OLM, Fleisch HA, Canfield RE, Russell RGG, editors. Bisphosphonate on bones, Amsterdam: Elsevier, 1995:211–229.
12. Reynolds JJ, Minkin C, Morgan DB, Spycher D, Fleisch H. The effect of two diphosphonates on the resorption of mouse calvaria in vitro. Calcif Tissue Res 1972;10: 302–313.
13. Flanagan AM, Chambers TJ. Dichloromethylenebisphosphonate (Cl_2MBP) inhibits bone resorption through injury to osteoclasts that resorb Cl_2MBP-coated bone. Bone Miner 1989;6:33–43.
14. Shinoda H, Adamek G, Felix R, Fleisch H, Schenk R, Hagan P. Structure–activity relationships of various bisphosphonates. Calcif Tissue Int 1983;35:87–99.
15. Sato M, Grasser W, Endo N, Akins R, Simmons H, Thompson DD, et al. Bisphosphonate action. Alendronate localization in rat bone and effects on osteoclast ultrastructure. J Clin Invest 1991;88:2095–2106.
16. Felix R, Guenther HL, Fleisch H. The subcellular distribution of (^{14}C)dichloromethylenebisphosphonate and (^{14}C)1-hydroxyethylidene-1,1-bisphosphonate in cultured calvaria cells. Calcif Tissue Int 1984;36:108–113.
17. Masarachia P, Weinreb M, Balena R, Rodan GA. Comparison of the distribution of ^3H-alendronate and ^3H-etidronate in rat and mouse bones. Bone 1996;19:281–290.
18. Hughes DE, MacDonald BR, Russell RGG, Gowen M. Inhibition of osteoclast-like cell formation by bisphosphonates in long-term cultures of human bone marrow. J Clin Invest 1989;83:1930–1935.
19. Colucci S, Minielli V, Zambonin G, Grano M. Etidronate inhibits osteoclast adhesion to bone surfaces but does not interfere with their specific recognition of single bone proteins. It J Miner Electrolyte Metab 1995;9:159–164.
20. Van der Pluijm G, Vloedgraven H, van Beek E, van der Wee-Pals L, Löwik C, Papapoulos S. Bisphosphonates inhibit the adhesion of breast cancer cells to bone matrices in vitro. J Clin Invest 1996;98:698–705.
21. Hughes DE, Wright KR, Uy HL, Sasaki A, Yoneda T, Roodman GD, et al. Bisphosphonates promote apoptosis in murine osteoclasts in vitro and in vivo. J Bone Miner Res 1995;10:1478–1487.
22. Sahni M, Guenther HL, Fleisch H, Collin P, Martin TJ. Bisphosphonates act on rat bone resorption through the mediation of osteoblasts. J Clin Invest 1993;91:2004–2011.
23. Vitté C, Fleisch H, Guenther HL. Bisphosphonates induce osteoblasts to secrete an inhibitor of osteoclast-mediated resorption. Endocrinology 1996;137:2324–2333.

24. Fast DK, Felix R, Dowse C, Neuman WF, Fleisch H. The effects of diphosphonates on the growth and glycolysis of connective-tissue cells in culture. Biochem J 1978; 172:97–107.
25. Zimolo Z, Wesolowski G, Rodan GA. Acid extrusion is induced by osteoclast attachment to bone: inhibition by alendronate and calcitonin. J Clin Invest 1995;96:2277–2283.
26. Ohya K, Yamada S, Felix R, Fleisch H. Effect of bisphosphonates on prostaglandin synthesis by rat bone cells and mouse calvaria in culture. Clin Sci 1985;69:403–411.
27. Endo N, Rutledge SJ, Opas EE, Vogel R, Rodan GA, Schmidt A. Human protein tyrosine phosphatase-σ: alternative splicing and inhibition by bisphosphonates. J Bone Miner Res 1996;11:535–543.
28. Schmidt A, Rutledge SJ, Endo N, Opas EE, Tanaka H, Wesolowski G et al. Protein-tyrosine phosphatase activity regulates osteoclast formation and function: inhibition by alendronate. Proc Natl Acad Sci USA 1996;93:3068–3073.
29. Luckman SP, Hughes DE, Coxon FP, Russell RGG, Rogers MJ. Nitrogen-containing bisphosphonates inhibit the mevalonate pathway and prevent post-translational prenylation of GTP-binding proteins, including Ras. J Bone Miner Res 1998;13:581–589.
30. Rogers MJ, Brown RJ, Hodkin W, Blackburn GM, Russell RGG, Watts DJ. Bisphosphonates are incorporated into adenine nucleotides by human aminoacyl-tRNA synthetase enzymes. J Bone Miner Res 1996;11:1482–1491.
31. Fleisch H, Russell RGG, Bisaz S, Mühlbauer RC, Williams DA. The inhibitory effect of phosphonates on the formation of calcium phosphate crystals in vitro and on aortic and kidney calcification in vivo. Eur J Clin Invest 1970;1:12–18.
32. Jung A, Bisaz S, Fleisch H. The binding of pyrophosphate and two diphosphonates by hydroxyapatite crystals. Calcif Tissue Res 1973;11:269–280.
33. Fleisch H. Bisphosphonates: mechanisms of action. Endocrinol Rev 1997;19:80–100.
34. Meunier PJ, Boivin G. Bone mineral density reflects bone mass but also the degree of mineralization of bone: therapeutic implications. Bone 1997;21:373–377.
35. Chesnut CH III, McClung MR, Ensrud KE et al. Alendronate treatment of the postmenopausal osteoporotic woman: effect of multiple dosages on bone mass and bone remodelling. Am J Med 1995;99:144–152.
36. Liberman UA, Weiss SR, Bröll J et al. Effect of oral alendronate on bone mineral density and the incidence of fractures in postmenopausal osteoporosis. N Engl J Med 1995;333:1437–1443.
37. Black DM, Cummings SR, Karpf DB, Cauley JA, Thompson DE, Nevitt M, et al. Randomised trial of effect of alendronate on risk of fracture in women with existing vertebral fractures. Lancet 1996;348:1535–1541.
38. Devogelaer JP, Broll H, Correa-Rotter R, Cumming DC, Nagant de Deuxchaisnes C, Geusens P, et al. Oral alendronate induces progressive increase in bone mass of the spine, hip, and total body over 3 years in postmenopausal women with osteoporosis. Bone 1996;18:141–150.
39. Tucci JR, Tonino RP, Emkey RD, Peverly CA, Kher U, Santora II AC. Effect of three years of oral alendronate treatment in postmenopausal women with osteoporosis. Am J Med 1996;101:488–501.
40. Bone HG, Downs RW, Tucci JR, Harris ST, Weinstein RS, Licata AA, et al. Dose-response relationships for alendronate treatment in osteoporotic elderly women. J Clin Endocrinol Metab 1997;82:265–274.
41. Hosking D, Chilvers CED, Christiansen C, Ravn P, Wasnich R, Ross P, et al. Prevention of bone loss with alendronate in postmenopausal women under 60 years of age. N Engl J Med 1998;338:485–492.
42. Saag KG, Emkey R, Schnitzer TJ, Brown JP, Hawkins F, Goemaere F, et al. Alendronate for the prevention and treatment of glucocorticoid-induced osteoporosis. N Engl J Med 1998;339:292–299.
43. Stock JL, Bell NH, Chesnut CH, Ensrud KE, Genant HK, Harris ST, McClung MR, et al. Increments in bone mineral density of the lumbar spine and hip and suppression

of bone turnover are maintained after discontinuation of alendronate in postmenopausal women. Am J Med 1997103:291–297.
44. Shiraki M, Kushida K, Fukunaga M, Kishimoto H, Kaneda K, Minaguchi H, et al. A placebo-controlled, single-blind study to determine the appropriate alendronate dosage in postmenopausal Japanese patients with osteoporosis. Endocrinol J 1998;45:191–201.
45. Chavassieux PM, Arlot ME, Reda C, Wei L, Yates J, Meunier PM. Histomorphometric assessment of the long-term effects of alendronate on bone quality and remodelling in patients with osteoporosis. J Clin Invest 1997;100:1475–1480.
46. Storm T, Thamsborg G, Steiniche T, Genant HK, Sorensen OH. Effect of intermittent cyclical etidronate therapy on bone mass and fracture rate in women with postmenopausal osteoporosis. N Engl J Med 1990;322:1265–1271.
47. Watts NB, Harris ST, Genant HK, et al. Intermittent cyclical etidronate treatment of postmenopausal osteoporosis. N Engl J Med 1990;323:73–79.
48. Storm T, Kollerup G, Thamsborg G, Genant HK, Sorensen OH. Five years of clinical experience with intermittent cyclical etidronate for postmenopausal osteoporosis. J Rheumatol 1996;23:1560–1564.
49. Harris ST, Watts NB, Jackson, et al. Four-year study of intermittent cyclic etidronate treatment of postmenopausal osteoporosis: Three years of blinded therapy followed by one year of open therapy. Am J Med 1993;95:557–567.
50. Miller PD, Watts NB, Licata AA, Harris ST, Genant HK, Wasnich RD, et al. Cyclical etidronate in the treatment of postmenopausal osteoporosis: efficacy and safety after seven years of treatment. Am J Med 1997;103:468–476.
51. Meunier PJ, Confavreux E, Tupinon I, Hardouin C, Delmas PD, Balena R. Prevention of early postmenopausal bone loss with cyclical etidronate therapy (a double-blind, placebo-controlled study and 1-year follow-up). J Clin Endocrinol Metab 1997;82: 2784–2791.
52. Wimalawansa SJ. A four-year randomized controlled trial of hormone replacement and bisphosphonate, alone or in combination, in women with postmenopausal osteoporosis. Am J Med 1998;104:219–226.
53. Struys A, Snelder AA, Mulder H, Mulder H. Cyclical etidronate reverses bone loss of the spine and proximal femur in patients with established corticosteroid-induced osteoporosis. Am J Med 1995;99:235–242.
54. Adachi JD, Bensen WG, Brown J, Hanley D, Hodsman A, Josse R, et al. Intermittent etidronate therapy to prevent corticosteroid induced osteoporosis. N Engl J Med 1997;337:382–387.
55. Giannini S, D'Angelo A, Malvasi L, et al. Effects of one-year cyclical treatment with clodronate on postmenopausal bone loss. Bone 1993;14:137–141.
56. Filipponi P, Cristallini S, Rizzello E, et al. Cyclical intravenous clodronate in postmenopausal osteoporosis: results of a long-term clinical trial. Bone 1996;18:179–184.
57. Herrala J, Puolijoki H, Lippo K, Raitio M, Impivaara O, Tala E, et al. Clodronate is effective in preventing corticosteroid-induced bone loss among asthmatic patients. Bone 1998;22:577–582.
58. Reid IR, Wattie DJ, Evans MC, Gamble GD, Stapleton JP, Cornish J. Continuous therapy with pamidronate, a potent bisphosphonate, in postmenopausal osteoporosis. J Clin Endocrinol Metab 1994;79:1595–1599.
59. Landman JO, Hamdy NAT, Pauwels EKJ, Papapoulos SE. Skeletal metabolism in patients with osteoporosis after discontinuation of long-term treatment wit oral pamidronate. J Clin Endocrinol Metab 1995;80:3465–3468.
60. Lees B, Garland SW, Walton, C, Ross D, Whitehead MI, Stevenson JC. Role of oral pamidronate in preventing bone loss in postmenopausal women. Osteoporos Int 1996;6:480–485.
61. Thiébaud D, Burckhardt P, Melchior J, et al. Two years' effectiveness of intravenous pamidronate (APD) versus oral fluoride for osteoporosis occurring in the postmenopause. Osteoporos Int 1994;4:76–83.

62. Reid IR, King AR, Alexander CJ, Ibbertson HK. Prevention of steroid-induced osteoporosis with (3-amino-1-hydroxypropylidene)-1,1-bisphosphonate (APD). Lancet 1988;I:143–146.
63. Reginster JY, Lecart MP, Deroisy R, Sarlet N, Denis D, Ethgen D, et al. Prevention of postmenopausal bone loss by tiludronate. Lancet 1989;II:1469–1471.
64. Chappard D, Minaire P, Privat C, Bérard E, Mendoza-Sarmiento J, Tournebise H, et al. Effects of tiludronate on bone loss in paraplegic patients. J Bone Miner Res 1995;10:112–118.
65. Genant HK, Chesnut CH III, Eisman JH, Harris ST, McClung MR, Prince RL, et al. Chronic intermittent cyclic administration of tiludronate in postmenopausal osteoporosis: report of two multicenter studies in 2317 patients. Bone 1998;23(Suppl 5):S175.
66. Ravn P, Clemmesen B, Riis BJ, Christiansen C. The effect on bone mass and bone markers of different doses of ibandronate: a new bisphosphonate for prevention and treatment of postmenopausal osteoporosis. A 1-year randomized, double-blind, placebo-controlled dose-finding study. Bone 1996;19:527–533.
67. Thiébaud D, Burckhardt P, Kriegbaum H, Huss H, Mulder H, Juttmann JR, et al. Three monthly intravenous injections of ibandronate in the treatment of postmenopausal osteoporosis. Am J Med 1997;103:298–307.
68. Delmas PD, Balena R, Confravreux E, Hardouin C, Hardy P, Bremond, A. Bisphosphonate risedronate prevents bone loss in women with artificial menopause due to chemotherapy of breast cancer: a double-blind placebo-controlled study. J Clin Oncol 1997;15:955–962.
69. Mortensen L, Charles P, Bekker PJ, Digennaro J, Johnston CC. Risedronate increases bone mass in an early postmenopausal population: two years of treatment plus one year of follow-up. J Clin Endocrinol Metab 1998;83:396–402.
70. Harris ST, Watts NB, Genant HK, McKeever CD, Hangartner D, Keller M, et al. Effects of risedronate treatment on vertebral and nonvertebral fractures in women with post-menopausal osteoporosis. JAMA 1999;14:1344–1352.
71. Adami S, Bhalla AK, Dorizzi R, Montesanti F, Rosini S, Salvagno G, Lo Cascio V. The acute-phase response after bisphosphonate administration. Calcif Tissue Int 1987;41: 326–331.
72. Peter CP, Cook WO, Nunamaker DM, Provost MT, Seedor JG, Rodan GA. Effect of alendronate on fracture healing and bone remodelling in dogs. J Orthop Res 1996;14:74–79.
73. Adami S, Zamberlan N. Adverse effects of bisphosphonates. Drug Safety 1996;14: 158–170.
74. Fleisch H. Bisphosphonates in bone disease. From the laboratory to the patient, 4th edition. San Diego: Academic Press, 2000.

31 Calcitonin

V. Halkin and J.-Y. Reginster

Introduction

Fractures are common complications of osteoporosis and frequently constitute the inaugural event leading to the discovery of severe osteoporosis. Pain is a prominent symptom of these fractures. Calcitonin possesses multiple therapeutic properties including a specific inhibition of bone resorption and an important analgesic effect. Because of these properties, calcitonin is a first-line treatment in the early management of osteoporotic fractures.

Pharmacological Properties

Calcitonin is a natural hormone found throughout the body. In humans, calcitonin is mainly produced by the C cells of the thyroid [1] and is a polypeptide containing 32 amino acid residues. The differences in the amino acid composition of the calcitonin from different species explain their different potencies [2]. Salmon calcitonin was developed for clinical use because, at an equivalent dose, it has a greater hypocalcemic activity than the human type.

Effects on Bone

All calcitonins have an anti-osteoclastic property. Osteoclasts possess specific receptors that bind calcitonin. Administration of calcitonin causes brush borders of the osteoclast to disappear and the osteoclast to move away from the bone resorption site. Calcitonin radically alters the internal structure of isolated osteoclasts, inhibiting cytoplasmic mobility, which is essential for bone resorption. Finally, calcitonin reduces both the lifespan and number of osteoclasts, probably by decreasing their rate of formation by blocking the fusion of mononuclear marrow cells, the committed progenitors of the osteoclasts that are known to possess calcitonin receptors.

Nonskeletal Effects

Although calcitonin is usually thought of in terms of its skeletal effects, it has many actions elsewhere in the body. The most noteworthy extraskeletal effect of calcitonin is the hormone's analgesic activity, which is particularly important in osteoporosis because of bone pain associated with fractures.

At pharmacological doses, calcitonin has been reported to inhibit many endocrine and exocrine secretions of the digestive tract. Calcitonin also affects the cardiovascular system, decreasing blood pressure and causing vasodilation.

Clinical Aspects

Skeletal Effects

Currently, salmon calcitonin is being tested in the prevention and treatment of postmenopausal osteoporosis and in acute postovariectomy osteoporosis. Prospective studies suggest that salmon calcitonin is effective in the treatment of established osteoporosis with a specific action on both cortical and trabecular bone. Calcitonin was also shown to be effective in senile, immobilization-induced and corticosteroid-induced forms of osteoporosis [3]. The two current methods used for calcitonin delivery (injectable and intranasal spray) have been extensively tested.

The efficacy of the injectable forms of calcitonin has been confirmed in the treatment of postmenopausal osteoporosis in short-term and controlled studies [4,5], as well as in long-term studies [6]. In an open prospective study, Rico et al. [7] suggested that injectable calcitonin is effective in the treatment of osteoporosis with a specific action on both cortical and trabecular bone.

The large PROOF study [8] evaluated the outcome of salmon calcitonin nasal spray therapy in a well-designed 5 year double-masked randomized placebo-controlled study of 1255 postmenopausal women with established osteoporosis randomized to either placebo or 100, 200 or 400 IU/day nasal salmon calcitonin. In this analysis the 5 year data demonstrate a statistically significant reduction in the relative risk of new vertebral fractures (39%) in women treated with 200 IU/day nasal salmon calcitonin compared with placebo. The 100 IU and 400 IU groups showed improvements with respect to the fracture indices but the data did not reach a level of stastistical significance.

Some authors have tested, more specifically, the effect of calcitonin on bone following a fracture. One of these studies is evaluating the effect of short-term calcitonin administration on biochemical bone markers in patients with acute immobilization following hip fractures [9]. Forty elderly patients with recent hip fracture who underwent surgery were randomly divided in two equal groups: one received no treatment and one received 100 IU/day salmon calcitonin intramuscularly for 2 weeks starting at admission. The study concludes that immobilization resulting from a hip fracture and, possibly, surgery itself causes significant changes in biochemical markers of bone resorption. Calcitonin successfully reverses these changes and may also be effective in preventing subsequent bone loss, particularly in patients who cannot be remobilized immediately.

Crespo et al. [10] compared in a randomized longitudinal study two types of complementary medical treatment (calcitonin with calcium and calcium alone) versus placebo in 45 women with Colles' fracture. Biochemical and radiogrammetic studies were made at baseline and after 1 year of treatment. Calcium alone at the dosage used here (1200 mg of elemental calcium for 10 days each month) inhibited bone loss after Colles'fracture. The addition of salmon calcitonin (100 IU/day intramuscularly for 10 successive days each month) not only slowed bone loss but significantly increased cortical bone mass.

Two studies employing animal models investigated the effect of calcitonin on bone quality in vivo. In adult ewes, intermittent calcitonin treatment from the time of ovariectomy was associated with a significant preservation of both cancellous bone strength and strain in trabecular bone of the femoral neck without affecting the crystalline properties of bone [11]. Similarly, it was demonstrated that the administration of salmon calcitonin in rabbits improves the biochemical properties of normal bone and bone after osteotomy [12].

Analgesic Effect

Calcitonin has been observed to have an analgesic effect for painful bone conditions. There is increasing clinical evidence supporting this phenomenon, though few rigorously controlled studies exist. Calcitonin may have an advantage over other analgesics in the treatment of bone pain resulting from an osteoporotic fracture, since, in addition to the observed analgesic effect, it is useful in treating the underlying disorder. However, there is presently no consensus among researchers concerning the mechanism of action involved in the analgesic effect which has been shown with human, salmon and eel calcitonins [13–16].

A double-masked controlled clinical trial compared the effect of 100 IU injectable calcitonin given daily, and placebo injections given daily, for a period of 14 days among patients who had recently suffered an osteoporotic vertebral fracture. The results showed a significant difference in pain intensity between the calcitonin group and the placebo group. This beneficial effect was generally apparent from the second day of treatment onward. It allowed the patients to sit, stand and gradually walk again. It can therefore be concluded that calcitonin exerts a beneficial effect on back pain following a vertebral crush fracture [17].

Nasal salmon calcitonin 200 IU/day in established osteoporosis cases possesses a potent analgesic effect, reduces the duration of bed confinement, and decreases the number of concomitant analgesic medications [18,19].

Nasal salmon calcitonin has also been tested in the treatment of osteoporotic vertebral crush fractures, in a double-masked, placebo-controlled, clinical study of patients with acute pain due to recent, nontraumatic osteoporotic vertebral crush fractures [20]. Patients received 200 IU of nasal salmon calcitonin daily or, alternatively, a placebo nasal spray. Patients receiving the calcitonin treatment for a period of 20 days had a dramatic decrease in spinal pain. This analgesic effect was accompanied by early mobilization and restoration of locomotive function. Nasal salmon calcitonin and early mobilization also reduced hydroxyproline excretion, preventing bone loss during the period of bed rest [20]. Finally, the consumption of high doses of paracetamol did not reduce the bed confinement of placebo patients during the 4 weeks of hospitalization.

Therefore, the analgesic property of calcitonin allows earlier mobilization of patients suffering from crush fractures and limits bone resorption linked to reduced mobility.

Tolerability and Safety

The current delivery mechanisms of calcitonin are subcutaneous or intramuscular injections and intranasal spray. Unfortunately, there remain several drawbacks to injections. In some cases, calcitonin injections produce unpleasant reactions.

The most frequently reported adverse effect is nausea, which occurs shortly after injection in up to 30% of patients. Evening administration with concomitant antiemetics can bring relief to some extent. Other symptoms include local pain at the injection site, flushing, diarrhea and vomiting, and collectively are the cause for stopping long-term treatment in approximately 45% of patients.

In contrast, administration by nasal spray is well tolerated and none of the adverse effects experienced during parenteral administration of the hormone are observed, even in patients who had discontinued the drug when it was previously administered by injection [21]. Nasal spray administration does not cause pathological abnormalities at the site of administration [22]. This hormone has an excellent safety profile, and, to date, there is no evidence of systemic toxicity.

Dosage and Administration

The dosage frequency and amount of calcitonin used in the treatment of osteoporosis and bone pain therapy (i.e., analgesic properties exhibited to date) remains an open debate among clinicians. It appears evident that, in the case of established osteoporosis, there is indeed a dose-dependent effect on the trabecular [23,24] and cortical bone mass [24]. The PROOF study suggests that the combination of 200 IU of calcitonin, 1000 mg of calcium and 400 IU of vitamin D daily is able significantly to reduce the relative risk of new fractures compared with placebo [8].

Concerning the analgesic property of calcitonin, no large-scale trials have been performed. Evidence suggests, though, that 100 IU of injectable calcitonin daily [17] or 200 IU intranasal salmon calcitonin daily can have a very important analgesic effect. The nasal bioavailability of calcitonin is only 10–25 % in comparison with subcutaneous or intramuscular injections, while the biological effects of the nasal spray of calcitonin represent 40% of those observed with the injectable form [18,19,25,26]. The ability of salmon calcitonin to cross the nasal mucosa was demonstrated immunologically by the generation of specific salmon calcitonin antibodies in the plasma. In healthy volunteers these alternative routes of administration do not decrease the anti-osteoclastic activity of calcitonin, as demonstrated by a significant decrease in biochemical parameters that reflect bone turnover [27].

Conclusion

The specific therapeutic effects of calcitonin combining both analgesic and anti-osteoclastic properties, allow this molecule to treat fracture-related pain as well as underlying osteoporosis. Being a very potent analgesic, calcitonin is a first-line treatment for acute pain following a fracture. With respect to the treatment of underlying osteoporosis, the chronic nature of this disease and the subsequent necessity for long-term pharmacological intervention requires an acceptable route of delivery which minimizes side-effects. Nasal salmon calcitonin fulfills the requirements discussed above, allowing successful long-term treatment.

References

1. Wolffe HJ. Calcitonin: perspective in current concepts. J Endocrinol Invest 1982; 5:523–530.
2. MacIntyre I, Craig R. Molecular evolution of the calcitonins. In: Fink G, Whalley J, editors. Neuropeptides: basic and clinical aspects. Edinburgh: Churchill Livingstone, 1982:255–258.
3. Reginster JY. Ostéoporose postménopausique: traitement prophylactique. Paris: Masson, 1993:127–137.
4. Cannigia A, Gennari C, Bencini M, et al. Calcium metabolism and 47-calcium kinetics before and after long-term thyrocalcitonin treatment in senile osteoporosis. Clin Sci 1970;38:397–407.
5. Milhaud G, Talbot JN, Coutris G. Calcitonin treatment of postmenopausal osteoporosis, evaluation of efficacy by principal component analysis. Biomedicine 1975;23:223–232.
6. Reginster JY. Calcitonin for prevention and treatment of osteoporosis. Am J Med 1993;95:44–47.
7. Rico H, Revilla M, Hernandez ER, et al. Total and regional bone mineral content and fracture rate in postmenopausal osteoporosis treated with salmon calcitonin: a prospective study. Calcif Tissue Int 1995;56:181–185.
8. Silverman SL, Chesnut C, Andriano K, Genant H, Gimona A, Maricic M, et al. Salmon calcitonin nasal spray (NS-CT) reduces risk of vertebral fracture(s) (VF) in established osteoporosis and has continuous efficacy with prolonged treatment. Accrued 5 year worldwide data of the PROOF study. Bone 1998;23:174.
9. Tsakalakos N, Magiasis B, Tsekoura M, Lyritis G. The effect of short-term calcitonin administration on biochemical bone markers in patients with acute immobilization following hip fracture. Osteoporos Int 1993;3:337–340.
10. Crespo R, Revilla M, Crespo E, Villa LF, Rico H. Complementary medical treatment for Colles' fracture: a comparative, randomized, longitudinal study. Calcif Tissue Int 1997;60:567–570.
11. Geusens P, Boonen S, Nijs J. Effect of salmon calcitonin on femoral bone quality in adult ovariectomized ewes. Calcif Tissue Int 1996;59:315–320.
12. Karachalios T, Lyritis GP, Giannarakos DG. Calcitonin effects on rabbit bone. Acta Orthop Scand 1992;63:615–618.
13. Guidobono F, Netti C, Villani P, et al. Antinociceptive activity of eel calcitonin, injected into the inflamed paw in rats. Neuropharmacology 1991;30:1275–1278.
14. Ljunghall S, Gardsell P, Johnell O, et al. Synthetic human calcitonin in postmenopausal osteoporosis: a placebo-controlled, double-blind study. Calcif Tissue Int 1991;49:17–19.
15. Lyritis GP, Tsakalakos N, Magiasis B, et al. Analgesic effect of salmon calcitonin in osteoporotic vertebral fractures: a double-blind placebo-controlled clinical study. Calcif Tissue Int 1991;49:369–372.
16. Pun KK, Shan LW. Analgesic effect of salmon calcitonin in the treatment of osteoporotic vertebral fractures. Clin Ther 1989;11:205–209.
17. Lyritis GP, Tsakalakos N, Magiasis B, Karachalios T, Yiatzides A, Tsekoura M. Analgesic effect of salmon calcitonin in osteoporotic vertebral fractures: a double-blind placebo-controlled clinical study. Calcif Tissue Int 1991;49:369–372.
18. Nagant de Deuxchaisnes C, Devogelaer JP, Huaux JP, et al. New modes of administration of salmon calcitonin in Paget's disease. Clin Orthop 1987;217:56–71.
19. Reginster JY, Denis D, Albert A, et al. Assessment of the biological effectiveness of nasal synthetic salmon calcitonin (SSCT) by comparison with intramuscular (im) or placebo injection in normal subjects. Bone Miner 1987;2:133–140.
20. Lyritis GP, Paspati I, Karachalios T, Ioakimidis D, Skarantavos G, Lyritis PG. Pain relief from nasal calcitonin in osteoporotic vertebral crush fractures. A double-blind, placebo-controlled clinical study. Acta Orthop Scand 1997;275:112–114.

21. Reginster JY, Franchimont P. Side-effects of synthetic salmon calcitonin given by intranasal spray compared with intramuscular injection. Clin Exp Rheumatol 1985;3:155–157.
22. Foti R, Martorana U, Broggini M. Long-term tolerability of nasal spray formulation of salmon calcitonin. Curr Ther Res 1995;56:429–435.
23. Overgaard K, Hansen MA, Jensen SB, et al. Effect of salcatonin given intranasally on bone mass and fracture rates in established osteoporosis: a dose–response study. BMJ 1992;305:556–561.
24. Thamsborg G, Storm TL, Sykulski R, et al. Effect of different doses of nasal salmon calcitonin on bone mass. Calcif Tissue Int 1991;41:302–307.
25. Overgaard K, Agnusdei D, Hansen Ma, et al. Dose–response bioactivity of salmon calcitonin in premenopausal and postmenopausal women. J Clin Endocrinol Metab 1991;72:344–349.
26. Mazzuoli GF, Passeri M, Gennari C, et al. Effects of salmon calcitonin in postmenopausal osteoporosis; a controlled double-blind study. Calcif Tissue Int 1986;38:3–8.
27. Reginster JY, Gaspard S, Deroisy R. Prevention of osteoporosis with nasal salmon calcitonin: effect of anti-salmon calcitonin antibody formation. Osteoporos Int 1993;3:261–264.

32 Fluoride Therapy of Established Osteoporosis

K.-H. W. Lau

Introduction

A well-known characteristic associated with aging is the age-dependent decrease in bone density. Significant reductions in bone density may cause deterioration of microarchitectural integrity of bone tissues, leading to decreased biomechanical properties and strength. Accordingly, when the bone density is reduced to a level that is below the putative "fracture threshold" [1], the risk for fragility (nontraumatic) fractures is increased, and osteoporosis develops. If a patient has a bone density that is near the "fracture threshold" and has only a modest decrease in bone density, what this patient needs is an antiresorptive therapy, such as bisphosphonate, estrogen or calcitonin, essentially to maintain bone mass by preventing further bone loss. These antiresorptive therapies are very effective in this regard. On the other hand, if a patient has a bone density that is very much below the "fracture threshold" (i.e., established osteoporosis), this patient would still be at high fracture risk even if she takes an antiresorptive drug. Such a patient would need an osteogenic agent to increase bone formation and bone mass to the level that is above the "fracture threshold". To date, among the potential osteogenic agents, fluoride is the only orally active and bone-specific agent that produces a substantial increase in spinal bone density in humans [2–4].

While fluoride is an investigational drug in North America, it has been approved for treating osteoporosis for many years in several European countries. Hence, there is a large amount of information regarding the use of fluoride therapy in humans. This chapter will review some of the key findings of the fluoride therapy of established osteoporosis. The discussion will focus on the clinical aspects of the therapy, such as fluoride's pharmacokinetics, side-effects and clinical efficacy. And because it appears, for most part, that fluoride therapy has an unfavorable benefit-to-risk profile, a proposed strategy to improve the benefit-to-risk ratio is also included. Although an understanding of its molecular mechanism of action is essential for the appropriate use of fluoride, this issue has been discussed in detail in our recent review [5] and, therefore, will not be addressed here.

Fluoride Pharmacokinetics

There is strong circumstantial evidence that fluoride pharmacokinetics and bioavailability are important determining factors of skeletal responses to fluoride therapy in humans. For instance, patients who responded well to fluoride therapy exhibited a decrease in renal fluoride clearance and an increase in skeletal fluoride deposition [6]. A strong correlation between urinary fluoride level and lumbar bone mineral content is noted in patients who responded well to fluoride therapy [7]. Moreover, the fluoride-mediated increase in bone mineral content was associated with the age-related reduction in renal function [8]. In addition to the dosage and body size of the patient, the bioavailability of fluoride is influenced by (a) fluoride salts and forms, (b) gastrointestinal fluoride absorption, (c) fluoride tissue deposition and (d) fluoride renal clearance.

Fluoride Salts and Forms

Currently, two types of fluoride salts, i.e., sodium fluoride (NaF) and sodium monofluorophosphate (MFP), are used for osteoporosis in humans. Both fluoride salts are available in enteric-coated and/or sustained-release preparations. Enteric-coated forms of fluoride salts minimize gastrointestinal irritation, whereas the sustained-release preparations enable a gradual release of fluoride ion, allowing the maintenance of serum fluoride at the therapeutic level without sharp post-absorption peaks [9,10]. This is desirable since the post-absorption peak is not essential for in vivo efficacy [11–13] but would increase the amount of fluoride deposited in bone, which may have detrimental effects on bone quality.

Fluoride Absorption

The fluoride ion is rapidly and extensively (i.e., almost 100% of ingested fluoride salts) absorbed, primarily through passive mechanisms, from the gastrointestinal tract into the circulation [14]. Although the majority of the fluoride ion is absorbed in the duodenum and jejunum [15], a significant amount can also be absorbed in the stomach [16]. The rate of gastric fluoride absorption is inversely proportional to the pH of the gastric contents [14,15]. The efficacy of intestinal fluoride absorption is influenced by three factors: (1) the type and galenic formulation of fluoride salt [17–19]; (2) the presence of other ions (i.e., Ca^{2+}, Mg^{2+}, Al^{3+}, other di- or trivalent cations, and Cl^{-}) that would influence fluoride absorption [20]; and (3) the physiological and pathological state (e.g., age, body acid–base equilibrium, gastric and urine pH, renal function) of the individual [21].

Tissue Distribution of Fluoride

The absorbed fluoride ion is distributed into three major tissue compartments: (1) extracellular fluids, (2) soft tissues and (3) hard tissues (i.e., bone, calcified cartilages and teeth). The biological half-life of fluoride in extracellular fluids and soft tissues is relatively short, i.e., a few hours, whereas the fluoride ion in hard tissues has a much longer half-life of up to several years. The predominant deposition site for fluoride ion is the skeleton, where the fluoride ion is exchanged for hydroxyl groups in hydroxyapatite to form fluoroapatite. However, fluoride ions are not homogeneously distributed in bone, but are deposited primarily in areas that are actively mineralizing (i.e., bone formation sites) during fluoride treatment [22]. Accordingly, in addition to the serum fluoride concentration (influenced by the dosage) and the exposure time (related to the treatment duration), the amount of fluoride deposition in bone is also determined by the bone formation rate. The removal of bone fluoride ion is primarily mediated by osteoclastic resorption during remodelling. A significant proportion of the released bone fluoride is recycled into newly formed bone minerals, while the rest is excreted in the urine. Consequently, upon discontinuation of fluoride therapy the bone fluoride content would only drop slowly but progressively [23]. This slow release may account for the relatively long half-life of fluoride in the skeleton.

Renal Clearance of Fluoride

Fluoride ion is filtered freely in the kidney and excreted in the urine. The amount of renal fluoride clearance is primarily determined by the filtered load (the glomerular filtration rate × blood fluoride concentration) and free water clearance (the greater the free water clearance, the greater the fluoride excretion) [24]. Approximately 75% of the excreted fluoride ion in humans is found in the urine, 12–20% in feces, and 5–13% in sweat [25]. Because the kidney is the major excretory route for fluoride, even a moderate impairment of renal function could predispose to excessive fluoride retention during fluoride therapy [26]. Since increased fluoride retention increases the risk of skeletal fluorosis, fluoride therapy should only be used with great caution, or not at all, in patients with renal insufficiency.

Therapeutic Fluoride Dosage and Regimen

There are several pieces of strong circumstantial evidence that the serum level of fluoride ion is the key determinant of the skeletal response. First, in vitro studies indicate that fluoride ion acts directly on osteoblast-line cells [27,28]; thus, the circulating fluoride ion, rather than bone matrix bound fluoride, is likely to be the biologically active species. Second, the optimal in vitro osteogenic doses of fluoride were similar to the effective serum fluoride concentrations in fluoride-treated patients [27,28]. Third, good fluoride responders had a higher serum fluoride level than poor responders [6]. In addition, the osteogenic response (increases in spinal bone density) correlated positively with the daily dose (Fig. 32.1) [29]. Because the serum fluoride level is related to the oral dose, it is concluded that the serum fluoride level is probably the most important index for monitoring the therapeutic dose.

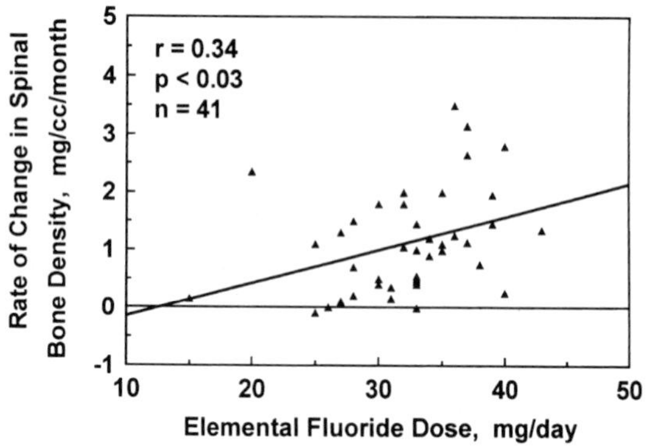

Figure 32.1. The daily dose of fluoride was related to the rate of change in spinal bone density in 41 osteoporotic patients receiving fluoride (range 15–43 mg/day) and calcium carbonate (1500 mg/day). Adapted from figure 1 of [29] with permission of Springer-Verlag New York.

Therapeutic Serum Fluoride Level

Taves [30] proposed a "therapeutic window" for fluoride therapy in that fasting serum fluoride levels should be maintained between 5 and 10 μM. There is circumstantial evidence arguing for these proposed limits. Accordingly, anecdotal data indicate that serum fluoride levels below 5 μM rarely produce an increase in bone mass in humans. Thus, it is reasonable to set this level as the minimal level. In vitro studies show that the dose-dependent stimulation of human osteoblast proliferation persists at fluoride concentrations of 10–30 μM but is linear only up to 10 μM [28]. Although higher serum fluoride levels would produce greater osteogenic responses in humans (Fig. 32.1), it is conceivable that the greater increases in bone formation caused by higher fluoride doses would be offset by a greater incidence of harmful side-effects. Thus, the optimal upper limit of fluoride dose should be one that yields the highest benefit-to-risk ratio, which, unfortunately, is lacking. It is reasonable to suspect that an appropriate fluoride dose should be one that yields a blood fluoride level that stays within the linear portion of the mitogenic dose–response curve, i.e., ≤ 10 μM. A serum fluoride level of 5–10 μM would be a reasonable therapeutic range for adults with established osteoporosis, since consistent stimulation of bone formation was seen in patients when fasting serum fluoride levels were maintained at 5–10 μM [31], and since no serious side-effects were observed at these serum fluoride levels.

Because the putative "therapeutic window" is relatively narrow, regular monitoring of fasting serum fluoride levels in fluoride-treated patients is highly recommended to detect abnormally high or subtherapeutic fluoride levels. The timing of serum fluoride measurements is an important issue since oral intake of fluoride often produces acute post-absorption peaks, which can be as much as 3 times the morning pre-dose level. Measurements during the post-absorption peak period could yield misleading information. On the other hand, the morning pre-dose level would most likely represent the steady-state serum fluoride level and as such would be an acceptable estimate of the mean serum level throughout the 24-h dosing period.

Dosage and Regimen of Fluoride Therapy

A typical daily fluoride dose for established osteoporosis is 20–30 mg of elemental fluoride. This dosage range usually produces a morning pre-dose serum fluoride level between 5 and 10 μM (i.e., the putative "therapeutic window"). However, the required oral fluoride dose that would achieve optimum serum fluoride concentrations within the putative "therapeutic window" is influenced by the patient's age, intestinal and renal function, and other clinical factors [8]. Thus, it is likely to vary from one individual to another. Consequently, it may require some adjustments in the oral fluoride dosage in order to keep serum fluoride levels within the "therapeutic window".

There is evidence that higher doses do not necessarily yield better clinical efficacy. In the randomized placebo controlled study of Riggs et al. [32], postmenopausal women who were treated with 75 mg/day plain NaF (or 34 mg/day elemental fluoride) for 4 years showed no significant reduction in spinal fracture rate (compared with the placebo-treated subjects), despite a highly significant increase in spinal bone density. However, an extended analysis of the study found that a subgroup of 50 patients, who had received lower fluoride doses (< 75 mg/day), showed significant decreases in spinal fracture rate [33]. This indicates that an appropriate dosage is essential for clinical efficacy and suggests that higher doses of fluoride, while showing rapid increases in bone density and larger increments in serum fluoride levels, do not necessarily reduce spinal fracture rate. Conversely, lower doses of fluoride, which yield lesser increments in serum fluoride levels and bone density, could be effective in fracture rate reduction.

There are two potential explanations why higher doses of fluoride do not produce a beneficial effect on fracture risks. First, if higher fluoride doses produce larger increases in bone formation, it follows that the higher the increment in bone formation (due to higher doses), the greater the demand for calcium. A large calcium demand may lead to osteomalacia. Patients with smaller increases in bone formation (with lower doses) would have a lesser tendency toward osteomalacia. Accordingly, it is possible that the lack of a significant reduction in spinal fracture rate with higher fluoride doses may be attributed to the osteomalacia. Consistent with this speculation, histomorphometric evaluation of iliac biopsy samples from the study of Riggs et al. [32] has shown clear evidence for osteomalacia, even though these patients had received daily supplementation of 1500 mg calcium carbonate during the study [34]. The second potential explanation relates to the fact that higher fluoride doses result in increased fluoride incorporation into bone minerals, which can have deleterious effects on bone quality and strength. Thus, it may be possible that high fluoride deposition into bone (due to higher doses) contributes to the lack of fracture rate reduction in spite of an increase in bone density.

The recent randomized prospective, placebo-controlled study of Pak et al. [11,12] raises the possibility that dosage regimen and scheduling is also an important factor. In this regard, postmenopausal osteoporotic women who were treated for 4 years with an intermittent slow-release NaF (50 mg NaF/day (23 mg/day of elemental fluoride) and 800 mg/day calcium citrate) in a dosage regimen consisting of 14-month cycles (12 months receiving fluoride and 2 months off therapy) showed a marked decrease in spinal fracture rate accompanying a moderate increase in bone density. There was no evidence for osteomalacia and secondary hyperparathyroidism in patients treated with the intermittent regimen [11,12]. Thus, it has been speculated that the 2 month "off fluoride" period together with the use of the more soluble calcium citrate facilitated the resolution of any potential osteomalacia that might have occurred during the therapy. The "off fluoride" period is believed to reduce the amount of fluoride deposited in bone. Thus, the lack of osteomalacia, along with the reduction in fluoride incorporation in bone, may lead to a significant reduction in fracture rate as was seen in the study of Pak et al. [11,12]. Regimens containing moderate and cyclic doses of fluoride may therefore have advantages over continuous fluoride regimens for therapy of established osteoporosis.

Side-Effects of Fluoride Therapy

Gastrointestinal Irritation

When plain NaF was used in fluoride therapy in the past, gastrointestinal irritation was a common side-effect (i.e., in > 25% of fluoride-treated patients) [24]. This gastrointestinal irritation is caused by hydrofluoric acid (an irritant) formed from free fluoride and the gastric acid, and by gastric absorption of free fluoride ion. The common symptoms include epigastric pain, nausea and vomiting, which can be effectively treated with antiacids or H2 blockers. Since the severity of this side-effect is dose-related, it can also be treated by decreasing the fluoride dose. In rare cases, patients who are treated with large doses of plain NaF may develop duodenal ulceration and bleeding which requires temporary discontinuation of the therapy. With the recent use of new galenic sustained-release or enteric-coated formulations of fluoride, the gastrointestinal irritation side-effect is virtually eliminated.

Peripheral Bone Pain

In 10–40% of patients receiving fluoride therapy, severe pain may develop at peripheral joints such as knees, ankles or feet [35]. The pain usually subsides within a few days when the therapy is discontinued. This side-effect is dose-related, and is much less frequent in patients receiving relatively low daily doses (< 20 mg of elemental fluoride), especially when the drug is given in a cyclic regimen [36].

Calcium Deficiency

Although early clinical studies included daily supplementation of a large dose of calcium carbonate, some fluoride-treated elderly osteoporotic patients still developed calcium deficiency and osteomalacia [37–39]. This is presumably because elderly subjects have reduced calcium absorption efficiency such that calcium supplementation alone is insufficient to overcome the calcium deficiency resulting from exuberant bone formation caused by the fluoride therapy. Calcium deficiency is a serious side-effect because it would lead to secondary hyperparathyroidism, increased bone resorption and, perhaps, also peripheral bone loss and osteomalacia [37,39]. There is evidence that calcium deficiency may also promote deposition of fluoride in bone since it has been reported that, in rats fed a low calcium diet, there was a greater increase in fluoride deposited in bone compared with rats fed a normal calcium diet [40]. Osteomalacia can impair the healing of microdamage in the bone and, thereby, may lead to an accumulation of microdamage in the skeleton. High incorporation of fluoride in bone matrix has a negative effect on bone quality. Hence, calcium deficiency and osteomalacia can have a significant adverse impact on bone strength and, as such, may increase fracture risk. To avoid the potential complications of calcium deficiency it is necessary to routinely monitor patients for signs of calcium deficiency, such as low urinary calcium, a high serum parathyroid hormone level, and a large increase in bone formation [39]. Calcium deficiency (and osteomalacia) can easily be corrected by treatment with effective doses of calcitriol or 1α-hydroxyvitamin D_3 and calcium.

Stress Fractures

Fluoride therapy may increase the prevalence of stress fractures in the weightbearing appendicular skeleton [32]. Peripheral stress fractures are found almost exclusively in patients with severe osteoporosis [41]. However, this complication may be considered relatively benign since these stress fractures are incomplete fractures and, in all cases, they healed after a transitory drug discontinuation [41,42].

Hip Fractures

The most serious of all potential side-effects of fluoride therapy is the possibility that the treatment may increase the incidence of hip fractures [43,44]. Theoretically, fluoride may increase the risk of hip fracture through three mechanisms: (1) fluoride-induced calcium deficiency can cause significant peripheral cortical bone loss as a consequence of increased bone resorption due to the secondary hyperparathyroidism; (2) osteomalacia impairs healing of microdamage, and accumulation of significant amounts of unrepaired microdamage can lead to stress and hip fractures; (3) high bone fluoride deposition can cause deterioration in bone quality and strength which, in turn, could increase the risk for stress and hip fractures.

The contention that fluoride therapy can cause hip fractures, however, has not been confirmed and is not universally accepted. Accordingly, a retrospective analysis of more than 1000 patient-years of fluoride therapy by five international medical centers indicated that hip fracture risk in osteoporotic patients was because of the bone deficit and that the risk was unaffected by fluoride therapy [45]. Moreover, a study of more than 250 patients followed for over 5 years showed that fluoride did not increase the frequency of hip fractures [46]. Similarly, treatment with intermittent slow-release fluoride also did not show evidence of an increase in the incidence of hip or stress fractures [11,12]. To add to the controversy, a recent report indicates that fluoridation of drinking water not only did not increase, but also appears to significantly reduce, hip fracture incidence [47]. Accordingly, much additional work is needed to resolve the issue whether fluoride therapy indeed causes hip fractures.

Clinical Efficacy of Fluoride Therapy

The ultimate clinical objectives of fluoride therapy of established osteoporosis are: (1) to reduce clinical symptoms; (2) to increase bone mass (bone density); (3) to improve bone strength and quality; and (4) to reduce fracture risks. Thus, clinical efficacy of fluoride therapy is assessed according to its ability to achieve these goals.

Symptoms

A significant clinical symptom of osteoporosis is back pain. There is now abundance of evidence that fluoride therapy significantly reduces back pain [3,48–50]. This is an important benefit since it gives the patient the feeling of increased strength and reduced morbidity. It also allows the patient to become more physically active and participate in physical therapy and exercise programs. Accordingly, this significantly improves the quality of life of patients.

Bone Density

There is unequivocal evidence that fluoride therapy produces a marked increase in spinal bone density in good responders. Lateral lumbar spine radiographs (Fig. 32.2) show that treatment of an osteoporotic patient with fluoride causes an increase in spinal bone density that is accompanied by a coarsening of vertebral trabeculae and an increased prominence of the vertebral end plates. Measurements of bone density by dual-energy X-ray absorptiometry (DXA) and quantitative computed tomography (QCT) confirm marked increases in the spinal bone density in fluoride-treated patients.

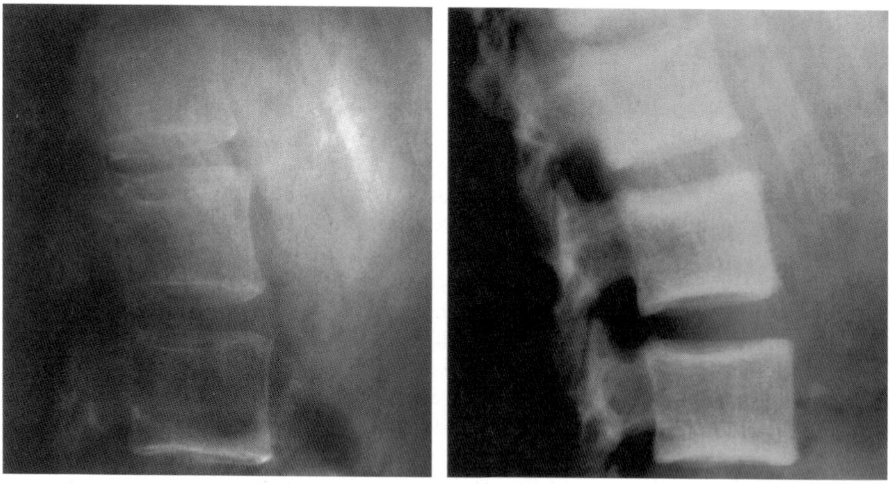

Figure 32.2. Lateral lumbar spinal radiograph of a 60-year-old postmenopausal woman before (*left panel*) and after (*right panel*) 3.5 years therapy with fluoride (30 mg elemental fluoride per day) and calcium carbonate (1500 mg per day). Reproduced from figure 7 of [77] with permission of Academic Press.

The increase in spinal bone density in postmenopausal osteoporotic women is proportional to the duration on fluoride therapy for at least 5 years [4,32,42]. Although the dose–response has not been rigorously evaluated with prospective controlled studies, there seems to be a dose–response in spinal bone density between 5 and 40 mg/day of elemental fluoride (Fig. 32.1). The response in spinal bone density to fluoride therapy is not related to the severity of osteoporosis, the patient's age, or the cause of the disease [8]. The gain in spinal bone density during fluoride therapy is, however, not maintained after discontinuation of the therapy [51]. In addition, not all patients respond to fluoride therapy, in that 20–25% of treated patients do not manifest an increase in spinal bone density [3,52,53]. A better understanding of the molecular mechanism whereby fluoride exerts its osteogenic actions could shed light on the cause of the nonresponsiveness and/or individual variability in response to fluoride therapy.

There is bone scintigraphic [54], radiological [55] and bone density [32,54,56] evidence that, in addition to increasing bone formation in the axial skeleton, fluoride therapy also increases bone formation in the appendicular skeleton. The magnitude of the increases at appendicular sites is much smaller than that seen in the axial skeleton [29]. The relative differences in bone density gains in response to fluoride between the appendicular and axial skeleton may be due, in part, to the lower inherent turnover of cortical bone compared with that of trabecular bone. On the other hand, Riggs et al. [32] showed a significant (7.7% per year) decrease in the forearm bone density in the fluoride-treated patients in spite of a marked increase in spinal bone density. This was interpreted to mean that the increase in spinal trabecular bone density might occur at the expense of the cortical bone of the peripheral skeleton. However, there was unambiguous evidence for severe osteomalacia in these fluoride-treated patients [37], suggesting that these patients might have developed calcium deficiency. It is conceivable that the calcium deficiency and secondary hyperparathyroidism could, to some extent, be responsible for this observed peripheral cortical bone loss [34]. Consistent with this speculation, Pak et al. [21,22] showed that patients, who were treated with low doses of intermittent fluoride and who showed no evidence for osteomalacia or calcium deficiency, did not lose bone mass at peripheral bone sites.

Bone Quality and Strength

Fluoride therapy increases the incorporation of fluoride into bone minerals. A survey of past human studies for which bone fluoride content data are available reveals that the amount of fluoride in bone ash is proportional to the total amount of fluoride ingested by the patients (Fig. 32.3), indicating that the dosage and duration of the therapy determine the amount of fluoride that is deposited in bone. There is evidence that deposition of a large amount of fluoride in bone significantly reduces bone quality and strength in rats [57] and humans [58]. Studies in rodents suggested that deleterious effects of fluoride on cortical bone quality and strength could be seen only when the bone fluoride level exceeds 0.5% [59]. These findings led to the suggestion that the bone fluoride level should be kept below 0.45% (putative "maximum safe level") to avoid harmful effects on bone strength.

There is circumstantial evidence supporting a putative "safe bone fluoride level" (Fig. 32.3). Sögaard et al. [58] showed that there was a 45% reduction in trabecular bone strength and a 58% decrease in trabecular bone quality in 12 osteoporotic

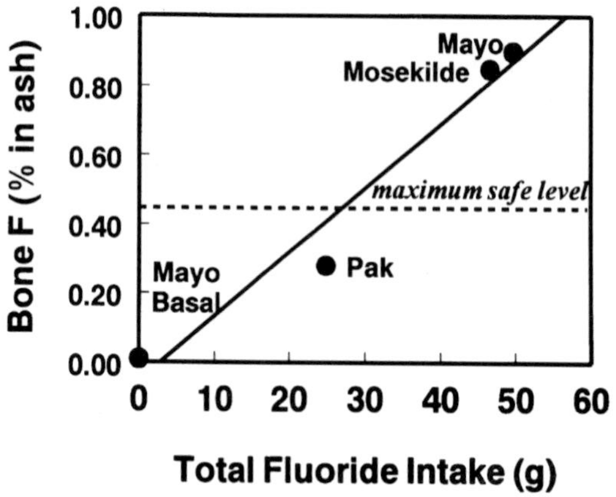

Figure 32.3. Relationship between total elemental fluoride taken orally in clinical trials and the corresponding subsequent bone fluoride concentrations. The total oral fluoride intake and bone fluoride concentrations are calculated from data obtained from references [12], [34] and [58], respectively. The putative "maximum safe level" of bone fluoride (0.45% in bone ash) was suggested by Turner et al. [59]. Reproduced from figure 13 of [78] with permission of Academic Press.

patients after 5 years of NaF therapy (with an accumulated oral dose of approximately 45 g of elemental fluoride), which led to an accumulation of bone fluoride of approximately 0.85%. Patients in the Mayo Clinic study [32,33], who received an accumulated fluoride dose of approximately 50 g and deposited a bone fluoride level of approximately 0.95%, showed increased peripheral fracture rates and had no significant reduction in spinal fracture rates. On the other hand, the fluoride-treated patients in Pak's slow-release intermittent dosage study [11,12], where the bone fluoride level of the treated patients was less than 0.3%, exhibited an impressive reduction in spinal fracture rates without an increase in peripheral fracture rates.

A high level of bone fluoride may act through three mechanisms to reduce bone strength and quality. First, fluoride deposition may alter the physicochemical properties of bone mineral crystals [60,61]. Incorporation of a high level of fluoride in bone minerals in vivo significantly increased bone material density (i.e., calcium content/unit dry bone weight) and microhardness in cortical bones [62,63], which, in turn, increases compressive strength but reduces bending strength of the bone. Second, fluoride incorporation can produce histologically abnormal bone, as it results in distinct hypermineralized areas as well as undermineralized areas in cortical bones [61,62]. The increased variability of bone mineral content with areas of high and low mineral density could weaken the integrity of the bone [64]. Third, large doses of fluoride may cause calcium deficiency and osteomalacia. Calcium deficiency and the accompanying secondary hyperparathyroidism would increase bone resorption and promote trabecular perforation which, in turn, leads to deterioration of trabecular microarchitecture and bone quality, resulting in a reduction in bone strength. Osteomalacia would impair the repair of microdamage, the accumulation of which will further corrupt the trabecular integrity, causing a significant reduction in bone strength and bone quality.

Spinal Fracture Rate

Several uncontrolled studies have suggested that a significant reduction in vertebral fracture rate is associated with an increase in spinal bone density in fluoride therapy [2,3,36,65–68], and that there appears to be a strong inverse relationship between spinal bone density and vertebral fracture rate [1,68]. However, recent randomized, prospective, placebo-controlled clinical trials have produced conflicting results with respect to spinal fracture rate reduction. In this regard, the two studies which employed an intermittent "cyclic" regimen with a low fluoride dose showed a significant reduction in spinal fracture rate [11,12,50]. Conversely, three other studies, including the recently completed FAVOS study, which utilized a continuous regimen, demonstrated no significant reduction in spinal fracture rate [32,69,70]. Consequently, the issue concerning the efficacy of fluoride therapy in reducing spinal fracture rate is highly controversial [71,72]. On the other hand, these prospective, controlled, clinical studies have clearly indicated that a significant reduction in spinal fracture rate can be achieved with fluoride therapy under appropriate conditions. However, the question is what would be considered the optimum conditions for fluoride therapy, such that a reduction in spinal fracture reduction can be consistently achieved.

To better define the optimal conditions it would be essential to understand the cause of the contrasting effects of these prospective controlled studies on spinal fracture rates. Theoretical assessments of skeletal responses of the fluoride therapy suggest three potential causes. First, loss of trabecular connectivity and number is a characteristic of established osteoporosis. Although it is clear that fluoride treatment increases the thickness and volume of remaining trabeculae, there is no convincing evidence that fluoride therapy can restore the trabecular number and connectivity. It is possible that, while the thickened but less connected trabeculae in the fluoride-treated skeleton may increase the biomechanical strength compared with the osteoporotic trabeculae, the strength per unit of bone mass would still be less than that of normal skeleton. Consequently, the number and connectivity of the remaining trabeculae in patients before fluoride therapy could be a significant variable in determining the efficacy of the therapy on fracture risk. In other words, the more severe the disease, the less likely fluoride would be to completely correct the fracture risk. The fact that patients enrolled in the intermittent slow-release fluoride trial [11,12] appeared to have less severe osteoporosis (i.e., higher basal spinal bone density) than those who participated in studies with continuous fluoride therapy [32,69,70], may, in part, be responsible for the observed reduction in spinal fracture rate in the intermittent studies. Second, fluoride-induced calcium deficiency and osteomalacia may contribute to increases in vertebral fragility and fractures. Accordingly, there was clear evidence for osteomalacia and calcium deficiency in patients in studies with the continuous fluoride regimen [34], but no evidence of osteomalacia and calcium deficiency in the intermittent slow-release fluoride study [11,12]. Thus, the observed differences with respect to spinal fracture risks may also, in part, be attributed to whether or not patients developed calcium deficiency and osteomalacia. Third, the total oral fluoride dose in the continuous fluoride therapy was higher than the accumulated dose in the intermittent-dose slow-release study. As discussed earlier, a high level of deposition of fluoride in bone mineral crystals can adversely affect bone quality and strength. Therefore, the difference in bone fluoride level may, to some extent, account for the different efficacy with respect to spinal fracture risk in these clinical trials.

Strategies to Improve Fluoride Therapy

Two serious disadvantages of fluoride therapy, namely calcium deficiency and reduced bone quality and strength, give fluoride therapy an unfavorable benefit-to-risk profile and, thereby, diminish its therapeutic value. We propose a strategy to improve the benefit-to-risk profile of fluoride therapy. We reason that, by avoiding calcium deficiency and high fluoride deposition in bone during therapy, the benefit-to-risk profile of fluoride therapy will be improved. Because further loss of trabecular connectivity and number could have an adverse effect on bone quality and strength, we further propose that combination therapy of fluoride with an antiresorption therapy may be necessary, especially when the patient has an elevated bone resorption rate.

Strategy to Avoid Calcium Deficiency

Calcium deficiency is the cause of two significant side-effects of fluoride therapy, i.e., osteomalacia and stress fracture. To avoid potential complications of calcium deficiency, it is recommended that the fluoride-treated patient should be monitored regularly for signs of calcium deficiency, such as a low urinary calcium, a high serum parathyroid hormone level, and a marked increase in bone formation [39]. Regular monitoring of signs of calcium deficiency could alert physicians to undertake the necessary interventions. To treat calcium deficiency it would be necessary to give calcitriol (in a dosage of 0.25–0.5 μg/day) or alfacalcidol (in a dosage of 0.5–1.0 μg/day) to enhance intestinal calcium absorption. These steps, when taken together, should minimize the occurrence of calcium deficiency and the associated side-effects, such as secondary hyperparathyroidism, osteomalacia, stress fractures and peripheral bone loss.

Strategy to Reduce Fluoride Deposition in Bone

As discussed earlier, poor bone quality and reduced bone strength may result, in part, from high fluoride deposition in bone matrix. Accordingly, it is very important to minimize the amount of bone fluoride deposition. There are four ways to reduce fluoride deposition in bone: reduce the fluoride dosage, use a slow-release fluoride formulation, use cyclic or intermittent fluoride therapy and avoid calcium deficiency.

Reduce the Fluoride Dosage

One of the key determinants of fluoride deposition in bone is fluoride intake (Fig. 32.3). Thus, the fluoride dosage becomes an important issue. Although it is necessary to give the patient a sufficient fluoride dose to effectively increase bone density, the dose should not be so high that it will cause an excessive accumulation of fluoride in bone. Because the in vitro mitogenic dose–response curve of fluoride indicates that there is no additional increase in mitogenic activity at doses above 10 μM [28], we speculate that, when the blood fluoride level increases above a certain level (e.g., 10 μM) there would also not be any proportionally greater increase in bone cell mitogenic activity. On the other hand, higher fluoride doses would significantly increase the amount of bone fluoride deposition, since there is a proportionality between the serum fluoride level and the amount of fluoride deposited in bone [57,59]. As discuss earlier, we believe the optimal bone fluoride level would be between 5–10 μM. Thus, we recommend that patients be given an appropriate fluoride dose to yield a morning pre-dose, fasting serum level that is maintained between 5 and 10 μM.

Use a Slow-Release Fluoride Formulation

The amount of fluoride deposition in bone is directly proportional to the circulating fluoride concentration. Accordingly, the greater the area under the serum fluoride curve, the more fluoride will be deposited in bone. In this regard, the formulation of fluoride salt can be important. Fig. 32.4 illustrates the differences in pharmacokinetics of giving patients a plain MFP formulation and a 12-h slow-release MFP formulation (MFP-SR). There was a large post-absorption peak in serum fluoride level in patients treated with the plain MFP. In contrast, there was only one point along the time course curve that was significantly above the 5–10 μM fluoride level when the MFP-SR formulation was given to the patients. Because of this post-absorption peak, the area under the curve of plain MFP was much greater than the area under the curve of the slow-release formulation. The post-absorption peak of fluoride is undesirable since it is not essential for in vivo efficacy [11–13], and serves only to increase the amount of bone fluoride deposition. Thus, it seems advisable to use slow-release or sustained-release formulations to avoid post-absorption peaks in order to limit the amount of fluoride deposited in bone. Consequently, we recommend that a slow-release or sustained-release formulation of fluoride salt be used in fluoride therapy.

Use a Cyclic or Intermittent Fluoride Therapy

Previous studies in the rat have shown that the bone formation effect of fluoride on the osteoblast persists for weeks even after fluoride withdrawal [73]. In humans

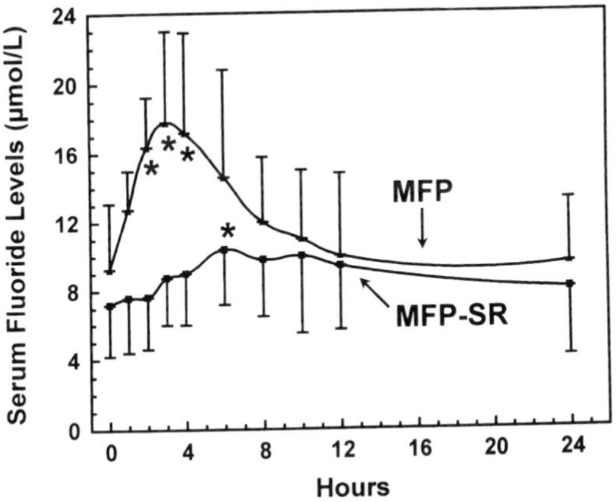

Figure 32.4. Serum fluoride levels (mean and SD) over 24 h in six osteoporotic patients following a single 76 mg dose of either plain monofluorophosphate (MFP) or 12-h slow release MFP (MFP-SR). $*p < 0.05$. Reproduced from figure 2 of [9] with permission of Springer-Verlag New York.

(following discontinuation of fluoride therapy), the half-life for the disappearance of the increase in bone formation, as measured by bone formation markers, was much slower than that for the disappearance of serum fluoride [9]. Therefore, it is likely that cyclic (intermittent) fluoride therapy would considerably decrease the exposure to fluoride and, thereby, reduce the amount of fluoride incorporation into bone without impairing the osteogenic effect. This principle has been confirmed by the study of intermittent fluoride administration by Pak et al. [11,12] and also recently by that of Ringe et al. [50]. For instance, the patients in the study of Pak et al. [11,12] received a daily dose of 23 mg elemental fluoride only for 12 months in each 14 month cycle. These patients showed the same increase in bone density as if the drug had been given continuously throughout the study. They had a 15% less exposure to fluoride and, as shown in Fig. 32.3, also had significantly less bone fluoride deposition compared with patients on a continuous fluoride regimen. More importantly, the benefit of intermittent, slow-release fluoride therapy of established osteoporosis on spinal fracture rates has been convincingly demonstrated by these studies [11,12,50]. In addition, a recent study also indicates that intermittent slow-release NaF therapy produced bone with normal histomorphometric parameters [74], in contrast to continuous fluoride therapy, where calcium deficiency and osteomalacia were evident [34]. Therefore, we consider that the use of cyclic (intermittent) therapy instead of continuous fluoride therapy would be a logical approach to reduce high accumulation of fluoride in bone.

Although the intermittent regimen used by Pak et al. (12 months on, 2 months off fluoride) and that by Ringe et al. (3 months on, 1 month off fluoride) appeared to be successful, there is no compelling evidence that either of these regimens is the most appropriate intermittent schedule. Ideally, the optimum cyclic regimen would be one that contains the shortest possible fluoride treatment period with the longest possible "off fluoride" period without a sacrifice in therapeutic efficacy. To this end, the optimum cyclic regimen would probably depend on the half-lives of serum fluoride level and the fluoride-induced bone formation. Accordingly, a better understanding of appropriate rate constants between the persistence of osteogenic effects of fluoride and the duration of fluoride treatment would help to design more optimized cyclic regimens.

Avoid Calcium Deficiency

As discussed earlier, there is evidence that calcium deficiency can enhance fluoride deposition in bone. Therefore, it is essential to avoid calcium deficiency during fluoride therapy in order to reduce the possibility of increased bone fluoride incorporation.

Combination Therapy with an Antiresorptive Therapy

If the patient is treated with fluoride to increase bone formation when she is also experiencing an increase in bone resorption, which increases perforations of the trabeculae, this would not be an optimum therapy for osteoporosis. Accordingly, it would seem reasonable to include an antiresorptive agent with fluoride therapy if the bone resorption rate of the patient is elevated above the premenopausal level. The goal of the combination therapy is to decrease bone resorption, and thereby, further loss of trabeculae, with an antiresorptive agent such as estrogen, bisphosphonate or calcitonin, at the same time to increase the thickness of the remaining trabeculae with fluoride therapy. On the other hand, because fluoride acts only at remodeling sites to increase wall thickness and does not stimulate bone formation on a neutral surface, there is a concern that the decrease in remodelling sites by an antiresorptive agent may impair the effect of fluoride to incease bone density. However, this concern is probably not valid since there is evidence that significant increases in spinal bone density were observed with the combination of estrogen (or etidronate) and fluoride [75,76]. Therefore, the combination therapy of fluoride and an antiresorptive agent has a good rationale as a therapy of osteoporosis, and may improve the benefit-to-risk ratio of fluoride therapy.

Concluding Remarks

It has been well recognized for decades that fluoride has both beneficial and detrimental effects on the skeleton. On the one hand, it is well documented that fluoride is an orally active, bone-cell-specific anabolic agent that effectively stimulates bone formation at appropriate skeletal sites, i.e., trabecular and cortical-endosteal bone sites, and increases spinal bone density, without an increase in bone resorption. On the other hand, fluoride therapy may have detrimental effects on bone quality and bone strength. Accordingly, fluoride therapy of established osteoporosis has been highly controversial. Because there is a great need for an effective bone-specific anabolic agent for treatment of established osteoporosis, and because no better osteogenic therapy is currently available, I believe a reasonable option is to take advantage of the benefits (i.e., bone-specific anabolic actions) of fluoride and to improve the therapy to minimize its adverse side-effects. I have described in this chapter a set of strategies to improve the benefit-to-risk profile of fluoride therapy. I believe that these strategies, if appropriately applied, should increase the therapeutic efficacy of fluoride therapy, i.e., increase bone density without impairment of bone quality and reduce fracture risks. In this regard, some of the concepts in these strategies have been incorporated in studies of Drs Pak [11,12] and Ringe [50], which have shown beneficial results with respect to fracture risk reduction.

Acknowledgements. This work was supported in part by a research grant from the National Institute of Dental Research (DE08681).

References

1. Odvina CV, Wergedal JE, Libanati CR, Schulz EE, Baylink DJ. Relationship between trabecular body density and fractures: a quantitative definition of spinal osteoporosis. Metabolism 1988;37:221–228.
2. Rigg BL, Hodgson JF, Hoffman DL, Kelly PJ, Johnson KA, Taves D. Treatment of primary osteoporosis with fluoride and calcium: clinical tolerance and fracture occurrence. JAMA 1980;243:446–449.
3. Briancon D, Meunier PJ. Treatment of osteoporosis with fluoride, calcium, and vitamin D. Orthop Clin North Am 1981;12:629–648.
4. Farley SMG, Libanati CR, Mariano-Menez MR, Tudtud-Hans LA, Schulz EE, Baylink DJ. Fluoride therapy for osteoporosis promotes a progressive increase in spinal bone density. J Bone Miner Res 1990;5(Suppl 1):S37–S42.

5. Lau KHW, Baylink DJ (1998) Molecular mechanism of action of fluoride on bone cells. J Bone Miner Res 13:1660–1667.
6. Kraenzlin ME, Kraenzlin C, Farley SMG, Fitzsimmons RJ, Baylink DJ. Fluoride pharmacokinetics in good and poor responders to fluoride therapy. J Bone Miner Res 1990;5(Suppl 1):S49–S52.
7. Duursma SA, Raymakers JA, de Raadt ME, Karsdorp NJGH, van Dijk A, Glerum J. Urinary fluoride excretion in responders and nonresponders after fluoride therapy in osteoporosis. J Bone Miner Res 1990;5(Suppl 1):S43–S47.
8. Murray TM, Harrison JE, Bayley TA, Josse RG, Sturtridge WC, Chow R, et al.. Fluoride treatment of postmenopausal osteoporosis: age, renal function, and other clinical factors in osteogenic response. J Bone Miner Res 1990;5(Suppl 1):S27–S35.
9. Resch H, Libanati C, Talbot J, Tabuenca M, Farley S, Bettica P, et al. Pharmacokinetic profile of a new fluoride preparation: sustained-release monofluorophosphate. Calcif Tissue Int 1994;54:7–11.
10. Erlacher L, Templ H, Magometschnigg D. A comparative bioavailability study on two new sustained-release formulations of disodiummonofluorophosphate verse a nonsustained-release formulation in healthy volunteers. Calcif Tissue Int 1995;56: 196–200.
11. Pak CY, Sakhaee K, Piziak V, Peterson RD, Breslau NA, Boyd P, et al. Slow-release sodium fluoride in the management of postmenopausal osteoporosis. A randomized controlled trial. Ann Intern Med 1994;120:625–632.
12. Pak CY, Sakhaee A, Adams-Huet B, Piziak V, Peterson RD, Poindexter JR. Treatment of postmenopausal osteoporosis with slow-release sodium fluoride. Final report of a randomized controlled trial. Ann Intern Med 1995;123:401–408.
13. Battman A, Resch H, Libanati CR, Ludy D, Fischer M, Farley S, et al. Serum fluoride and serum osteocalcin levels in response to a novel sustained release monofluorophosphate preparation, comparison with plain monofluorophosphate. Osteoporos Int 1997;7:48–51.
14. Cremer HD, Butner W. Absorption of fluorides. In: Fluorides and human health, WHO monograph series. Geneva: WHO, 1970:75–80.
15. Whitford GM. Intake and metabolism of fluoride. Adv Dent Res 1994;8:5–14.
16. Whitford GM. Effects of plasma fluoride and dietary calcium concentrations on GI absorption and secretion of fluoride in the rat. Calcif Tissue Int 1994;54:421–425.
17. Jowsey J, Riggs BL. Effect of concurrent calcium ingestion on intestinal absorption of fluoride. Metabolism 1978;27:971–974.
18. Ekstrand J, Ehrnebo M. Influences of milk products on fluoride bioavailability in man. Eur J Clin Pharmacol 1979;16:211–215.
19. Duursma SA, Raymakers JA, Fakkeldij TMV, van Asten P. Pharmacokinetics of monofluorophosphate. Res Clin Forums 1993;15:21–31.
20. Richards A, Kragstrup J, Nielsen-Kudsk F. Pharmacokinetics of chronic fluoride ingestion in growing pigs. J Dent Res 1985;64:425–430.
21. Rao GS. Dietary intake and bioavailability of fluoride. Annu Rev Nutr 1984;4:115–136.
22. Boivin G, Chavassieux P, Chapuy MC, Meunier PJ. Skeletal fluorosis: histomorphometric analysis of bone changes and bone fluoride content in 29 patients. Bone 1989;10:89–99.
23. Boivin G, Chapuy MC, Baud CA, Meunier PJ. Fluoride content in the human iliac bone, results in controls, patients with fluorosis, and osteoporotic patients treated with fluoride. J Bone Miner Res 1988;3:497–502.
24. Pak CYC. Fluoride and osteoporosis. Proc Soc Exp Biol Med 1989;191:278–286.
25. Gabovich RD, Ovrutsky GD. Fluorine in stomatology and hygiene. NIH Publication 78-785. Bethesda, MD: National Institutes of Health, 1977.
26. Ekstrand J, Spak C-J. Fluoride pharmacokinetics: its implications in the fluoride treatment of osteoporosis. J Bone Miner Res 1990;5(Suppl 1):S53–S61.
27. Farley JR, Wergedal JR, Baylink DJ. Fluoride directly stimulates proliferation and alkaline phosphatase activity of bone forming cells. Science 1983;222:330–332.

28. Wergedal JE, Lau K-HW, Baylink DJ. Fluoride and bovine bone extract influence cell proliferation and phosphatase activities in human bone cell cultures. Clin Orthop 1988;233:274–282.
29. Dure-Smith BA, Kraenzlin ME, Farley SM, Libanati CR, Schulz EE, Baylink DJ. Fluoride therapy for osteoporosis: a review of dose response, duration of treatment, and skeletal sites of action. Calcif Tissue Int 1991;49(Suppl):S64–S72.
30. Taves DR. New approach to the treatment of bone disease with fluoride. Fed Proc 1970;29:1185–1187.
31. van Kesteren RG, Duursma SA, Visser WJ, van der Sluys V, Backer Dirks O. Fluoride in serum and bone during treatment of osteoporosis with sodium fluoride, calcium, and vitamin D. Metab Bone Dis Rel Res 1982;4:31–37.
32. Riggs BL, Hodgson SF, O'Fallon WM, Chao EY, Wahner HW, Muhs JM, et al. Effect of fluoride treatment on the fracture rate in postmenopausal women with osteoporosis. N Engl J Med 1990;322:802–809.
33. Riggs BL, O'Fallon WM, Lane A, Hodgson SF, Wahner HW, Muhs J, et al. Clinical trial of fluoride therapy in postmenopausal osteoporotic women: extended observations and additional analysis. J Bone Miner Res 1994;9:265–275.
34. Lundy MW, Stauffer M, Wergedal JE, Baylink DJ, Featherstone JD, Hodgson SF, et al. Histomorphometric analysis of iliac crest bone biopsies in placebo-treated versus fluoride-treated subjects. Osteoporos Int 1995;5:115–129.
35. Riggs B. Treatment of osteoporosis with sodium fluoride: an appraisal. In: Peck WA, editor. Bone and Mineral Research, Amsterdam: Elsevier, 1983:366–393.
36. Pak CYC, Sakhaee K, Zerwekh JE, Parcel C, Peterson R, Johnson K. Safe and effective treatment of osteoporosis with intermittent slow-release sodium fluoride argumentation of vertebral bone mass and inhibition of fractures. J Clin Endocrinol Metabol 1989;68:150–159.
37. Duursma SA, Glerum JH, van Dijk A, Bosch R, Kerkhoff H, van Putten J, Raymakers JA. Responders and nonresponders after fluoride therapy in osteoporosis. Bone 1987; 8:131–136.
38. Compston JE, Chadha S, Merrett AL. Osteomalacia developing during treatment of osteoporosis with sodium fluoride and vitamin D. BMJ 1980;281:910–911.
39. Dure-Smith BA, Farley SM, Linkhart SG, Farley JR, Baylink DJ. Calcium deficiency in fluoride treated osteoporotic patients despite calcium supplementation. J Clin Endocrinol Metabol 1996;81:269–275.
40. Beary D. The effects of fluoride and low Ca on the physical properties of the rat femur. Anat Rec 1969;164:305–316.
41. Devogelaer JP, Nagant de Deuxchaisnes C. Fluoride therapy of type I osteoporosis. Clin Rheumatol 1995;14(Suppl 3);26–31.
42. Kleerekoper M. Fluorides and the skeleton. Crit Rev Clin Lab Sci 1996;33:139–161.
43. Hedlund LR, Gallagher JC. Increased incidence of hip fracture in osteoporotic women treated with sodium fluoride. J Bone Miner Res 1989;4:223–225.
44. Gutteridge DH, Price RI, Kent GN, Prince RL, Mitchell PA. Spontaneous hip fractures in fluoride-treated patients: potential causative factors. J Bone Miner Res 1990;5 (Suppl 1):205–212.
45. Riggs BL, Baylink DJ, Kleerekoper M, Lane JM, Melton LJ, Meunier PJ. Incidence of hip fractures in osteoporotic women treated with sodium fluoride. J Bone Miner Res 1987;2:123–126.
46. Farrerons J, Rodriguez de la Serna A, Guanabens N, Armadans L, Lopez-Navidad A, Yoldi B, et al. Sodium fluoride treatment is a major protector against vertebral and nonvertebral fractures when compared with other common treatments of osteoporosis: a longitudinal, observational study. Calcif Tissue Int 1997;60:250–254.
47. Lehmann R, Wapniarz M, Hofmann B, Pieper B, Haubitz I, Allolio B. Drinking water fluoridation: bone mineral density and hip fracture incidence. Bone 1998;22:273–278.
48. Farley SMG, Wergedal JE, Smith LC, Lundy MW, Farley JR, Baylink DJ. Fluoride therapy

for osteoporosis: characterization of the skeletal response by serial measurements of serum alkaline phosphatase activity. Metabolism 1987;36:211–218.
49. Bernstein DS, Cohen P. use of sodium fluoride in the treatment of osteoporosis. J Clin Endocrinol 1967;27:197–210.
50. Ringe JD, Dorst A, Kipshoven C, Rovati LC, Setnikar I. Avoidance of vertebral fractures in men with idiopathic osteoporosis by a three year therapy with calcium and low-dose intermittent monofluorophosphate. Osteoporos Int 1998;8:47–52.
51. Talbot JR, Fischer MM, Farley SM, Libanati C, Farley J, Tabuenca A, et al. The increase in spinal bone density that occurs in response to fluoride therapy for osteoporosis is not maintained after the therapy is discontinued. Osteoporos Int 1996;6:442–447.
52. Harrison JE, Bayley TA, Josse RG, Murray TM, Sturtridge W, Williams C, et al. The relationship between fluoride effects on bone histology and on bone mass in patients with postmenopausal osteoporosis. Bone Miner 1986;1:321–333.
53. Budden FH, Bayley TA, Harrison JE, Josse RG, Murray TM, Sturtridge WC, et al. The effect of fluoride on bone histology depends on adequate fluoride absorption and retention. J Bone Miner Res 1988;3:127–132.
54. Resch H, Libanati C, Farley S, Bettica P, Schulz E, Baylink DJ. Evidence that fluoride therapy increases trabecular bone density in a peripheral skeletal site. J Clin Endocrinol Metabol 1993;76:1622–1624.
55. Schulz EE, Engstrom H, Sauser DD, Baylink DJ. Osteoporosis: radiographic detection of fluoride-induced extra-axial bone formation. Radiology 1986;159:457–462.
56. Dambacher MA, Ittner J, Ruegsegger P. Long-term fluoride therapy of postmenopausal osteoporosis. Bone 1986;7:199–205.
57. Turner CH, Akhter MP, Heaney RP. The effects of fluoridated water on bone strength. J Orthop Res 1992;10:581–587.
58. Sögaard CH, Mosekilde L, Richards A, Mosekilde L. Marked decrease in trabecular bone quality after five years of sodium fluoride therapy – assessed by biomechanical testing of iliac crest bone biopsies in osteoporotic patients. Bone 1994;15:393–399.
59. Turner CH, Hasegawa K, Zhang W, Wilson M, Li Y, Dunipace AJ. Fluoride reduces bone strength in older rats. J Dent Res 1995;78:1475–1481.
60. Eanes ED, Reddi AH. The effect of fluoride on bone mineral apatite. Metab Bone Dis 1979;2:3–11.
61. Singer L, Armstrong WD, Zipkin I, Frazier PD. Chemical composition and structure of fluorotic bone. Clin Orthop Rel Res 1974;99:303–312.
62. Franke J, Runge H, Grau P, Fengler F, Wanka C, Rempel H. Physical properties of fluorosis bone. Acta Orthop Scand 1976;47:20–27.
63. Yamamoto K, Wergedal JE, Baylink DJ. Increased bone microhardness in fluoride treated rats. Calcif Tissue Res 1974;15:45–54.
64. Carter DR, Beaupre GS. Effects of fluoride treatment on bone strength. J Bone Miner Res 1990;5(Suppl 1):S177–S184.
65. Riggs BL, Seeman E, Hodgson SF, Taves DR, O'Fallon WM. Effect of fluoride/calcium regimen on vertebral fracture occurrence in postmenopausal osteoporosis: comparison with conventional therapy. N Engl J Med 1982;306:446–450.
66. Lane JM, Healey JH, Schwartz E, Vigorita VJ, Schneider R, Einhorn TA, et al. Treatment of osteoporosis with sodium fluoride and calcium: effects on vertebral fracture incidence and bone histomorphometry. Orthop Clin North Am 1984;15:728–745.
67. Mamelle N, Meunier PJ, Dusan R, Guillaume M, Martin JL, Gaucher A, et al. Fluoride therapy for the vertebral crush fracture syndrome (a status report). Ann Intern Med 1988;111:678–680.
68. Farley SM, Wergedal JE, Farley JR, Javier GN, Schulz EE, Talbot JR, et al. Spinal fractures during fluoride therapy for osteoporosis: relationship to spinal bone density. Osteoporos Int 1992;2:213–218.
69. Kleerekoper M, Peterson EL, Nelson DA, Phillips E, Schork MA, Tilley BC, et al. A randomized trial of sodium fluoride as a treatment for postmenopausal osteoporosis. Osteoporos Int 1991;1:155–161.

70. Meunier PJ, Sebert J-L, Reginster J-Y, Briancon D, Appelboom T, Netter P, et al. for the FAVOStudy Group. Fluoride salts are no better at preventing new vertebral fractures than calcium-vitamin D in postmenopausal osteoporosis: the FAVOStudy. Osteoporos Int 1998;8:4–12.
71. Pak CYC, Zerwekh JE, Antich PP, Bell NH, Singer FR. Slow-release sodium fluoride in osteoporosis. J Bone Miner Res 1996;11:561–564.
72. Kleerekoper M. Fluoride: the verdict is in, but the controversy lingers. J Bone Miner Res 1996;11:565–567.
73. Chavassieux P, Boivin G, Serre CM, Meunier PJ. Fluoride increases rat osteoblast function and population after in vivo administration but not after in vitro exposure. Bone 1993;14:721–725.
74. Schnitzler CM, Wing JR, Raal FJ, van der Merwe MT, Mesquita JM, Gear KA, et al. Fewer bone histomorphometric abnormalities with intermittent than with continuous slow-release sodium fluoride therapy. Osteoporos Int 1997;7:376–389.
75. Libanati CR, Baylink DJ. Fluoride and estrogen combination therapy for osteoporosis. J Bone Miner Res 1993;8(Suppl 1):S335.
76. Lems WF, Jacobs JW, Bijlsma JW, van Veen GJ, Houben HH, Haanen HC, et al. Is addition of sodium fluoride to cyclical etidronate beneficial in the treatment of corticosteriod induced osteoporosis? Ann Rheum Dis 1997;56:357–363.
77. Libanati C, Lau K-HW, Baylink DJ. Fluoride therapy for osteoporosis. In: Marcus R, Feldman D, Kelsey J, editors. Osteoporosis. San Diego: Academic Press, 1996:1259–1277.
78. Lau K-HW, Baylink DJ. Fluoride therapy of established osteoporosis. In: Rosen C, Glowacki J, Bilezikian JP (eds) The aging skeleton. San Diego: Academic Press, 1999: 587–612.

33 Androgens and Anabolic Steroids

P. Geusens, D. Vanderschueren and S. Boonen

Androgen Replacement Therapy

Skeletal Effects of Androgens

A number of in vitro studies have provided evidence for the involvement of androgens in bone metabolism. These studies provide a consistent basis for the potential role of androgens in skeletal homeostasis in vivo. In particular, androgens have been shown to have stimulatory effects on osteoblast proliferation and differentiation [1,2], and androgen receptors have been demonstrated in primary human osteoblasts [3,4]. Receptor concentrations are lower than those found in typical androgen target tissues such as the prostate but the affinity of the receptor is similar. In both men and women, human cortical bone seems to express more androgen receptors than trabecular bone. In osteoclasts, on the other hand, androgen receptors have not been identified. In addition to androgen receptors, human osteoblasts from both sexes also express estrogen receptors [5], suggesting that androgens may partially affect skeletal homeostasis following aromatization into estrogens. In line with the concept that testosterone functions as a prohormone for estrogens in skeletal tissue, aromatase activity has recently been demonstrated in both female and male bone tissue and in human osteoblast-like cells [6,7]. A further possible mode of action is the conversion of testosterone into the nonaromatizable androgen dihydrotestosterone which binds to the androgen receptor with higher affinity. A number of cell lines have recently been shown to express both aromatase and reductase activity, suggesting that, in addition to direct binding of testosterone to the androgen receptor, aromatization and reduction of androgens may affect bone metabolism as well. Recent in vivo studies using various orchidectomized rat models provide further evidence that androgens may affect bone metabolism in different ways and, more importantly, strongly support the concept that androgen exposure may be critically involved in skeletal maintenance [8-11]. Although it is beyond the scope of this chapter to discuss these studies, it should be emphasized that these different pathways for androgen involvement in skeletal homeostasis are not mutually exclusive.

Androgen Replacement Therapy in Men

Potential Candidates for Androgen Replacement Therapy

The aging process in normal men has been shown to be associated with declining levels of circulating androgens in a number of studies [12-14], an observation commonly referred to as the *partial androgen deficiency of the aging male* (PADAM). The mechanisms inducing androgen deficiency include decreased responsiveness of Leydig cells to luteinizing hormone (LH) as well as a blunted compensatory elevation of LH to the prevailing hypoandrogenic state [15]. Although the precise mechanisms for the blunted LH response to diminished steroid feedback inhibition in elderly men are yet to be defined, several observations suggest the involvement of alterations at the hypothalamic level. However, the variability in these hormonal alterations is substantial, such that even in very old age some men have values which fall well within the range for young adults, while others have levels corresponding to a frankly hypogonadal state. When compared with the young adult reference range, only about 20% of men older than 60 years and 30% of men older than 80 years will experience (partial) androgen deficiency. Most of these hypogonadal men will have concentrations of testosterone between 250 and 300 ng/dl although levels below 200 ng/dl have been reported in some. In most aging men, androgen concentrations remain within the normal range [16]. It is clear, however, that the limits of normality are rather arbitrary and that the sensitivity threshold for androgens might vary from tissue to tissue and, possibly, also according to age [17].

In view of the expanding evidence for the involvement of androgens in bone remodelling, it is tempting to speculate that bone loss in aging men might be the result, at least in part, of androgen deficiency. Androgens may indeed be essential for the maintenance of skeletal integrity in adult men, as the development of hypogonadism in mature men is associated with osteopenia [11]. In addition, there have been several reports of (modest) increases in bone mineral density with androgen replacement in adult men with hyperprolactinemic or idiopathic hypogonadotropic hypogonadism [18,19]. However, the extent to which the partial androgen deficiency associated with normal aging affects skeletal maintenance remains to be established.

Various cross-sectional studies have shown a weak positive association between androgen levels and bone mass at different skeletal sites, even after adjusting for the effects of age and body mass index (for references see [20]). However, as both androgen levels and bone density are known to decline with age, it is not possible to establish a causal relationship with certainty from these studies. In a recent cross-sectional study involving 534 community-dwelling men with a mean age of 69 years, the relation between osteoporosis and both total and bioavailable sex steroids was explored after adjustment for various other major determinants of bone mineral density [21]. In this large population-based sample of older men, directly measured free testosterone was positively associated with bone density at the ultradistal radius, spine and hip whereas no relationship was observed between dihydrotestosterone and bone density. Interestingly, bioavailable estrogen was even more strongly associated with density than bioavailable testosterone, supporting the concept that at least part of the complex effects of androgen status on skeletal maintenance in aging men may depend on their aromatization. However, the effect of endogenous sex steroid levels on bone loss in older men has not been investigated in prospective studies. Therefore, it remains unclear what proportion of the variance in bone density in elderly males is accounted for by androgen status.

More importantly, it remains to be determined whether androgen status has an impact on osteoporotic fracture risk. In a number of case–control studies, reduced serum levels of free testosterone were observed in male hip fracture patients compared with age- and sex-matched controls [22-25]. In a population of severely osteoporotic fracture patients, we were able to demonstrate (cross-sectionally) an inverse association between free testosterone and biochemical markers of bone resorption [26], suggesting that androgen deficiency may predispose to bone resorption in elderly men and in turn to remodelling imbalance and fracture risk. However, these patients had a substantial degree of androgen deficiency (serum concentrations of testosterone invariably below 200 ng/dl) and may not be representative of the majority of older men with less severe degrees of partial androgen deficiency. Nevertheless, these results suggest that the partial androgen deficiency of the aging male might contribute to the age-related osteoporotic syndrome in men.

Skeletal Impact of Androgen Administration in Aging Men

As indicated, there have been several reports of increases in bone mineral density with androgen replacement in clinically differentiated groups of hypogonadal males. However, the effects of androgen substitution on bone loss were mostly documented in uncontrolled studies and often based on small numbers [18,19,27–32]. Moreover, the methods used to assess bone density were quite variable (Table 33.1) and, more importantly, the response of bone mineral density to androgen replacement was modest and could not be consistently documented. Nevertheless, it is generally accepted that the management of adult-onset hypogonadism should include androgen replacement therapy, regardless of the underlying cause.

Few studies have addressed the effects of androgen replacement in partially androgen-deficient elderly men. In an earlier attempt to test the hypothesis that relative androgen deficiency has a skeletal impact in older men, Tenover [32] reported in a preliminary study that parenteral testosterone supplementation in 13 elderly men aged 57–76 years reduced urinary hydroxyproline excretion. Bone mineral density was not assessed. Although consistent with a suppressive effect of testosterone on bone resorption, it could not be excluded that the urinary hydroxyproline changes were caused by the effects of testosterone on the skin. More recently, Tenover presented data from a much larger 3 year randomized controlled substitution trial in partially androgen-deficient elderly men, showing increases in bone density at all measured sites (L. Tenover, 1998, personal communication) and supporting the view that reversing the partial androgen deficiency associated with normal aging may prevent bone loss. However, the extent to which these effects on bone density will be paralleled by similar effects on fracture incidence remains unknown. Only long-term randomized controlled fracture endpoint trials can provide an answer to that important question.

Modalities of Androgen Substitution

In view of the lack of data both on the consequences of the relative hypoandrogenism of the elderly and on the effects of androgen replacement therapy, it would certainly not be justified to propose a strategy of systematic androgen supplementation in elderly men presenting with only moderately decreased serum testosterone levels. Meanwhile, treatment should probably not be withheld from selected

Table 33.1. Androgen replacement studies in hypogonadal men

Author	Year	Study group	Duration	Type of replacement	Method of measurement	Effect
Finkelstein et al. [33]	1989	Idiopathic hypo-gonadotrophic hypogonadism ($n = 21$)	12–31 months	Testosterone enanthate 200 mg IM/2 weeks	QCT spine	+ ($n = 6$, 19–26 years) No effect ($n = 15$, 24–52 years)
Greenspan et al. [34]	1989	Hyperprolactinemia ($n = 8$)	6–48 months	Correction of hyperprolactinemia and hypogonadism by bromocryptine	SPA radius SPA radius	+ +
Diamond [26]	1991	Hemochromatosis ($n = 6$)	24 months	Sustanon 250 mg IM/3 weeks	DPA spine	+
De Vogelaer [27]	1992	Mixed ($n = 16$)	55 (9 months	Sustanon 250 mg IM/3 weeks	SPA radius	+ (only at trabecular site when closed epiphysis)
Isaia [29]	1992	Mixed (n= 6)	3 months	Sustanon 250 mg IM/3 weeks	DPA spine	+
Wang [29]	1996	Mixed ($n = 34$)	6 months	Testosterone cyclodextrine 5 mg 3×/d	DXA spine, hip, total body	No effect
Katznelson [30]	1996	Mixed ($n = 36$)	24 months	Testosterone enanthate 200 mg IM/2 weeks	DXA spine SPA radius	+ No effect
Behre et al. [35]	1997	Mixed ($n = 77$)	1–16 years (retrospective androgen therapy)	Testosterone enanthate 200 mg IM/2 weeks or transdermal or scrotal testosterone patch	QCT spine	+

IM, intramuscularly; +, increase; QCT, quantitative computed tomography; SPA, single photon absorptiometry; DPA, dual photon absorptiometry; DXA, dual-energy X-ray absorptiometry.

Reproduced with permission from the International Society for the Study of the Aging Male and Parthenon Publishing [43]

osteoporotic patients presenting with clinically and biochemically manifest hypogonadism, after careful screening for contraindications.

The testosterone esters enanthate and cyprionate, preparations for intramuscular injection, have been used in most studies but result in widely fluctuating levels of testosterone. New delivery systems are already commercially available and several others are under development. In particular, patches for transdermal testosterone administration have been developed, aimed at achieving more physiological profiles of circulating testosterone concentrations [17]. Daily renewed patches applied to the shaved scrotal skin can produce plasma testosterone levels around mid-normal values 4–8 h following application to hypogonadal men. The more recently introduced permeation-enhanced non-scrotal patch produces mid-normal range testosterone levels 8–12 h following nightly application. Unfortunately, because of the lack of relevant controlled clinical trials of sufficient duration, it is not possible to propose an optimal therapeutc regimen for androgen substitution in elderly osteoporotic men.

As to the potential risks of androgen replacement in elderly men, again data from controlled trials are scarce. Androgen replacement therapy in aging men may be associated with weight gain due to the anabolic effects on lean mass and sodium retention, and patients with congestive cardiac failure may have worsening edema. Aromatization of testosterone to estradiol may result in (painful or painless) gynecomastia. In addition, some men may develop polycythemia [32]. Effects of androgen treatment on lipoprotein profiles in elderly men, on the other hand, have been rather modest. A subject of more concern in terms of safety is the possibility of exacerbation of pre-existent malign or benign prostatic disease, known to be androgen sensitive. To date, most studies in elderly men have failed to observe clinically important changes at the level of the prostate [32], but these studies included only small numbers of carefully prescreened subjects treated for relatively short periods of time. Prostatic cancer and prostatic hypertrophy should be regarded as contraindications, along with sleep apnea syndrome and severe pre-existent cardiovascular pathology. Monitoring of elderly men under androgen substitution should mainly be based on careful clinical evaluations but may include measurements of hematocrit or prostate-specific antigen in selected patients. Physicians considering androgen therapy for an osteoporotic man should be aware that the potential risks of androgen replacement therapy, particularly in the elderly, are still uncertain in relation to the possible skeletal benefits to be gained.

Conclusion

Androgen therapy is indicated in hypogonadal men, irrespective of their degree of osteoporosis, and the concern of bone loss and fractures should represent one of the indications for androgen therapy of gonadal failure. However, the use of testosterone therapy in osteoporotic men without frank hypogonadism – for instance, the older man with low normal testosterone levels – remains highly speculative. Whether this relative hypoandrogenism of elderly men contributes to the development of age-related osteopenia and osteoporosis is an intriguing, but not fully explored, possibility. The association between bone loss and androgen status in older men has only been studied cross-sectionally and no attempts have been made to examine the antifracture efficacy of androgen substitution. Future studies are needed to assess the impact of different degrees of androgen deficiency on skeletal maintenance in aging men and to define the clinical potential of testosterone substitution in attenuating bone loss and reducing fracture risk. Available data on the effects of androgen treatment on bone mass and bone turnover in elderly men are at present too limited to allow for any valid conclusion. The safety profile of androgen replacement therapy should be an additional focus of future large-scale controlled trials of long duration.

Androgen Replacement Therapy in Postmenopausal Women

Androgens and Bone Loss in Aging Women

The primary change in endocrine function that occurs across the menopause is loss of secretion of estrogens and progesterone from the ovary. However, these are not the only alterations in ovarian endocrine function in postmenopausal women. Androgens, in particular testosterone, also decrease across menopause, by about 30–50% [36]. Circulating testosterone may continue to be secreted by the postmenopausal ovary in some individuals, but the major source in the menopause is conversion from dihydroepiandrostenedione in peripheral tissues. Although the main alteration, failure of the ovary to secrete estradiol, is considered to be the dominant effect on the skeleton in postmenopausal women, recent evidence suggests that the lack of production of other steroids, especially androgens, may contribute to bone loss in older women.

The association between endogenous testosterone and bone density in postmenopausal women has mostly been studied in cross-sectional studies. In a small study of peri- and postmenopausal women, Johnston and colleagues [37]reported a weak and statistically unadjusted correlation between circulating testosterone and vertebral density. In a similar attempt involving 16 postmenopausal women, on the other hand, no association was observed between lumbar bone density and endogenous testosterone [38]. More recently, the associations between endogenous sex steroids and bone mineral density were studied in a large sample of 456 community-dwelling women aged 50–89 years [21]. In this study, total testosterone was again unrelated to bone mineral density in postmenopausal women. An association between bioavailable testosterone and bone density was evident at all sites but, after accounting for age, body mass index and other covariates, statistical significance remained only at the ultradistal radius. These results apparently contrast with those observed by Slemenda and co-workers [39], who reported positive correlations between total and bioavailable testosterone and *longitudinal* change in bone density in postmenopausal women. However, in multivariate models, unbound testosterone was related only to change in femoral neck density and not to bone loss at other sites. Further studies are clearly needed to establish the impact of circulating androgens on skeletal maintenance in postmenopausal women.

Women to be Considered for Androgen Replacement Therapy

To date, no controlled, prospective studies have been performed to establish the effects of androgen replacement on postmenopausal bone loss. Although androgen substitution might have a positive impact on bone loss, changes in sexuality and other aspects of menopause, it is clear that this therapeutic strategy suffers because of a lack of long-term data that state physiological replacement doses, modalities of administration, risks and benefits, and indications for therapy. In view of the risk of unwanted lipoprotein changes, the potential prevention of desirable estrogen effects on cardiovascular health, the uncertain risks of endometrial or breast neoplasms, and the potential virilizing effects [40], androgen replacement therapy cannot yet be recommended as a strategy to restore bone mass in osteoporotic postmenopausal women.

Conclusion

Few studies have examined the relationship between endogenous androgens and bone density in older women, and a coherent conclusion has not emerged. While androgen therapy may favorably affect several aspects of health in postmenopausal women, many issues remain unanswered. Long-term well-designed androgen replacement studies should be performed to obtain the knowledge needed to guide this type of therapy in selected postmenopausal women.

Anabolic Steroid Therapy

Skeletal Effects of Anabolic Steroids

Anabolic steroids are synthetic derivatives of testosterone that have been developed in attempt to dissociate the anabolic effects of testosterone from its virilizing effects. These derivatives can be administered either orally (stanozole) or intramuscularly (nandrolone) and have been shown to have a positive impact on bone density in osteoporotic women in a number of studies. Although these positive effects may be related in part to a stimulatory effect on bone formation [1], anabolic steroid agents are likely to exert an inhibitory effect on bone turnover and bone resorption as well. Furthermore, nandrolone positively influences calcium balance by increasing gastrointestinal calcium absorption and renal tubular reabsorption [41].

In postmenopausal osteoporotic women, studies using stanozole [42] and nandrolone [43] have provided evidence for a preserving effect on bone mass at different sites. These effects are generally consistent with a preferential effect on cortical bone, although various studies indicate effects on cancellous bone as well. These effects, however, should be interpreted with caution because of the effects of anabolic steroids on other components of body composition [44]. Indeed, nandrolone increases lean body mass and decreases fat mass [44]. This decrease of the ratio of fat to lean body mass introduces errors into the measurement of spinal bone density using absorptiometry. In a 4 year study of osteoporotic women, we observed a sustained effect on forearm bone density for 2 years after discontinuing treatment with nandrolone [45], suggesting that the effects on skeletal mass may persist in time after withdrawal of anabolic steroid treatment (Fig. 33.1). Nandrolone also increases cortical width at the radius, which could result in a major increase in biomechanical competence [45]. In addition, the impact of these agents on body composition suggests a beneficial effect on muscle mass and, by implication, muscle function. In line with these effects, many patients on anabolic steroids report an improved mobility and may be less at risk for falls. Finally, a retrospective survey in six European countries has provided evidence to suggest an effect of anabolic steroid therapy on the risk of hip fracture after adjusting for potential confounding factors (relative risk: 0.66, 95% confidence interval: 0.29–1.22) [46]. Seventy percent

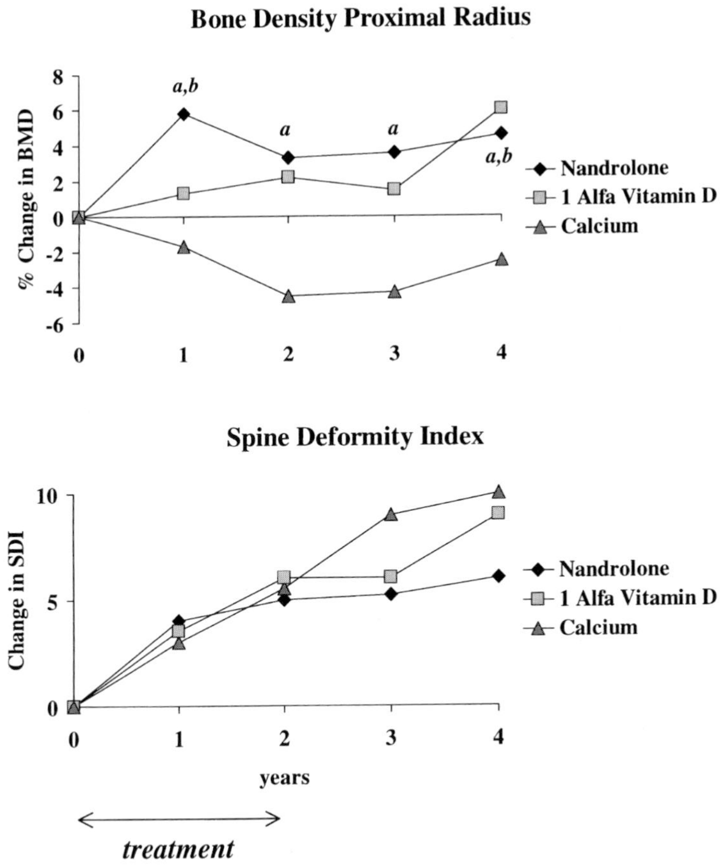

Figure 33.1. Effect of nandrolone decanoate 50 mg intramuscularly every 3 weeks compared with 1α-vitamin D 1 μg per day and intermittent calcium infusions (mean percentage changes from baseline). [a]$p < 0.05$ versus baseline; [b]$p < 0.05$ versus calcium.

of the use of all anabolic steroids in that study was in Italy. In that country, the use of anabolic steroids was related to a significant decrease in the relative risk of hip fracture (0.55, 95% confidence interval: 0.31–0.85, $p < 0.01$) [46]. There are, however, no prospective controlled studies demonstrating an effect of anabolic steroids on vertebral or hip fracture.

Modalities of Anabolic Steroid Therapy

A number of systemic side-effects have been reported during anabolic steroid therapy, although it should be emphasized that, in the majority of osteoporotic patients, both stanozole and nandrolone are well tolerated. The mean incidence of voice changes is up to 38%, mostly reversible [41]. In addition to liver function test abnormalities (when using orally administered agents), sodium retention may occur in some patients. An additional side-effect is the (potentially atherogenic)

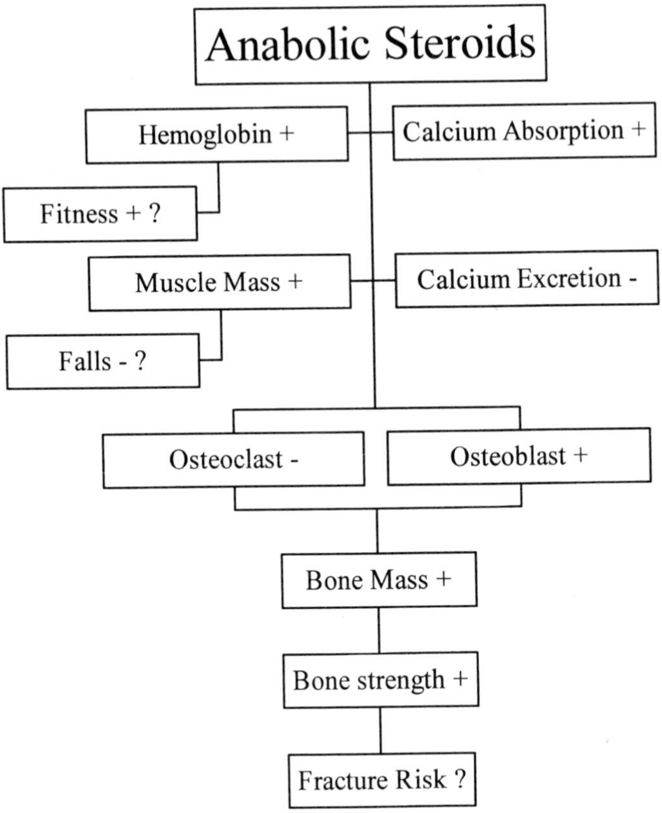

Figure 33.2. Overview of possible mechanisms of action of nandrolone decanoate.

reduction in high-density lipoproteins and elevation in low-density lipoproteins during stanozole therapy. Nandrolone, on the other hand, has a lower propensity for introducing an atherogenic lipid profile. Significant virilizing effects have been noted in some women receiving (oral or parenteral) anabolic steroids. Because of these side effects, patients on anabolic steroids should be closely monitored. Anabolic steroids are contraindicated early after menopause, in patients with liver disease or abnormal lipids, and in men with breast or prostate carcinoma.

Clinical Use of Anabolic Steroids in the Management Of Patients with Osteoporosis

The side-effects of anabolic steroids limit their use. Because of their concomitant effects on bone and muscle tissue, these agents are particularly suitable in the frail and elderly, based on possible mechanisms of action (Fig. 33.2). They should preferably be used on a short- or medium-term basis (6–12 months) in the treatment of patients with severe osteoporosis. Prolonged treatment is only indicated if the treatment is well tolerated and no contraindications are present.

Conclusions

Among other factors, variation in endogenous sex steroid levels has recently been implicated as a major factor underlying individual differences in age-related bone loss in women and men. The concept that androgens may indeed be essential for the maintenance of bone mass in adult men is supported by observations of osteopenia in mature men with adult-onset hypogonadism. In view of the expanding evidence for the involvement of androgens in bone remodelling, it is tempting to speculate that age-associated changes in androgen status might contribute to the determination of the rate of bone loss, and fractures, in older individuals. In a subset of normal men, aging is indeed associated with partial androgen deficiency but the skeletal impact of this deficiency remains to be clarified. Similarly, a reduction in blood androgen levels is noted in women who enter menopause. However, the extent to which age-related bone loss in both sexes is accounted for by androgen status has been studied only cross-sectionally and no attempts have been made as yet to examine the antifracture efficacy of androgen substitution. It therefore remains for future studies to assess the impact of different degrees of androgen deficiency on skeletal maintenance and to identify those elderly individuals who would benefit most from androgen administration. In addition, there is an urgent need for clinical trials to define the optimal timing, dosage schedule and mode of administration of testosterone substitution and to address its long-term safety and antifracture efficacy. The role of anabolic steroids in the treatment of osteoporosis, on the other hand, continues to be a matter of debate, although a number of studies have demonstrated positive results. Because of the side-effects of these agents and the lack of definitive data on their ability to reduce fracture frequency, anabolic steroids should probably be targeted to frail and elderly patients with severe osteoporosis.

References

1. Kasperk C, Wergedal J, Farley J, Linkhart T, Turner R, Baylink D. Androgens directly stimulate proliferation of bone cells in vitro. Endocrinology 1989;124:1576–1579.
2. Gray C, Colston K, MacKay A, Taylor L, Arnett T. Interaction of androgen and 1,25-dihydroxyvitamin D_3: effects on normal rat bone cells. J Bone Miner Res 1989;7: 41–46.
3. Colvard D, Eriksen E, Keeting P, Wilson E, Lubahn D, French F, Riggs B, Spelsberg T. Identification of androgen receptors in normal human osteoblast-like cells. Proc Natl Acad Sci USA 1989;86:854–857.
4. Orwoll E, Stribrska L, Ramsey E, Keenan E. Androgen receptors in osteoblast-like cells. Calcif Tissue Int 1991;49:183–187.
5. Eriksen E, Colvard D, Berg N, Graham M, Mann K, Spelsberg T, Riggs B. Evidence of estrogen receptors in normal human osteoblast-like cells. Science 1988;241: 84–86.
6. Tanaka S, Haji M, Nishi Y, Yanase T, Takayanagi R, Nawata H. Aromatase activity in human osteoblast-like osteosarcoma cell. Calcif Tissue Int 1993;52:107–109.
7. Purohit A, Flanagan A, Reed M Estrogen synthesis by osteoblast cell lines. J Clin Endocrinol Metab 1992;61:152–157.
8. Vanderschueren D, Van Herck E, Suiker A, Visser W, Schot L, Bouillon R. Bone and mineral metabolism in aged male rats: short- and long-term effects of androgen deficiency. Endocrinology 1992;130:2906–2916.

9. Vanderschueren D, Van Herck E, Schot L, Rush E, Einhorn T, Geusens P, et al. The aged male rat as a model for human osteoporosis: evaluation by nondestructive measuremens and biomechanical testing. Calcif Tissue Int 1993;53:342–347.
10. Hodgkinson A. Effects of calcium deprivation and orchidectomy on bone composition in the rat. Horm Metab Res 1979;11:516–519.
11. Vanderschueren D, Van Herck E, Nijs J, Ederveen A, De Coster R, Bouillon R. Aromatase inhibition impairs skeletal modeling and decreases bone mineral density in growing male rats. Endocrinology 1997;138:2301–2307.
12. Kalu D, Hardin R, Cockerman R. Evaluation of the pathogenesis of skeletal changes in ovariectomized rats. Endocrinology 1984;115:507–512.
13. Orwoll E, Klein R. Osteoporosis in men. Endocr Rev 1995;16:87–116.
14. Gray A, Feldman H, McKinlay J, Longcope C. Age, disease, and changing sex hormone levels in middle-aged men: results of the Massachusetts male aging study. J Clin Endocrinol Metab 1991;73:1016–1025.
15. Veldhuis R, Urban R, Lizarralde G, Johnson M, Iranmanesh A. Attenuation of luteinizing hormone secretory burst amplitude as a proximate basis for the hypoandrogenism of healthy aging in men. J Clin Endocrinol Metab 1992;75:707–713.
16. Abassi A, Drinka P, Mattson D, Rudman D. Low circulating levels of insulin-like growth factors and testosterone in chronically institutionalized elderly men. J Am Geriatr Soc 1993;41:975–982.
17. Kaufman JM, Vermeulen A. Declining gonadal function in elderly men. Baillieres Clin Endocrinol Metab 1997;11:289–309.
18. Vermeulen A. Androgens in the aging male. J Clin Endocrinol Metab 1991;73:221–224.
19. Kaufman JM, Vermeulen A. Androgens in male senescence. In: Nieschlag E, Behre HM, editors. Testosterone: action, deficiency, substitution, 2nd edition. Berlin Heidelberg New York: Springer, 1998:437–471.
20. Boonen S, Vanderschueren D, Geusens P, Bouillon R. Age-associated endocrine deficiencies as potential determinants of femoral neck (type II) osteoporotic fracture occurrence in elderly men. Int J Androl 1997;20:134–134.
21. Greendale G, Edelstein S, Barrett-Connor E. Endogenous sex steroids and bone mineral density in older women and men: the Rancho Bernardo Study. J Bone Miner Res 1997;12:1833–1843.
22. Cooper C, Campion G, Melton L. Hip fractures in the elderly: A world-wide projection. Osteoporos Int 1992;2:285–289.
23. Poor G, Atkinson E, O'Fallon W, Melton L. Prediction of hip fractures in elderly men. J Bone Miner Res 1995;10:1900–1907.
24. Stanley HL, Schmitt BP, Poses RM, Deiss WP. Does hypogonadism contribute to the occurrence of a minimal trauma hip fracture in elderly men? J Am Geriatr Soc 1991;39:766–771.
25. Jackson J, Riggs M, Spiekerman A. Testosterone deficiency as a risk factor for hip fractures in men: a case-control study. Am J Med Sci 1992;304:4–8.
26. Boonen S, Vanderschueren D, Cheng X, Verbeke G, Dequeker J, Geusens P, Broos P, Bouillon R. Age-related (type II) femoral neck osteoporosis in men: biochemical evidence for both hypovitaminosis D- and androgen deficiency-induced bone resorption. J Bone Miner Res 1997;12:2119–2126.
27. Diamond T, D Stiel, S Posen. Effects of testosterone and venesection on spinal and peripheral bone mineral in six hypogonadal men with hemochromatosis. J Bone Miner Res 1991;6:39–43.
28. Devogelaer JP, Decooman S, Dedeuxchaines C. Low bone mass in hypogonadal males. Maturitas 1992;15:17–21.
29. Isaia G, Mussetta M, Pecchio F, Sciolla A, Distefano M, Molinatti G. Effect of testosterone on bone in hypogonadal males. Maturitas 1992;15:47–51.
30. Wang C, Eyre DR, Clark R, Kleinberg D, Newman C, Iranmanesh A, et al. Sublingual testosterone replacement improves muscle mass and strength, decreases bone resorption, and increases bone formation markers in hypogonadal men-a clinical research

center study. J Clin Endocrinol Metab 1996;81:3654–3662.
31. Katznelson L, Finkelstein JS, Schoenfeld DA, Rosenthal DI, Anderson EJ, Klibanski A. Increase in bone density and lean body mass during testosterone administration in men with acquired hypogonadism. J Clin Endocrinol Metab 1996;81:4358–4365.
32. Tenover JS. Effect of androgen supplementation in the aging male. In Oddens B, Vermeulen A, editors. Androgens and the aging male. New York: Parthenon, 1996: 191–221.
33. Finkelstein J, Klibanski A, Neer R, Greenspan S, Rosenthal D, Crowley W.Osteoporosis in men with idiopathic hypogonadotropic hypogonadism. Ann Intern Med 1987;106: 354–361.
34. Greenspan S, Oppenheim S, Klibanski A. Importance of gonadal steroids to bone mass in men with hyperprolactinemic hypogonadism. Ann Intern Med 1989;110:526–531.
35. Behre HM; Kliesch S, Leifke E, Link TM, Nieschlag E. J Clin Endocrinol Metab 1997;82:2386–2390.
36. Longcope C, Hunter R, Franz C. Steroid secretion by the postmenopausal ovary. Am J Obstet Gynecol 1980;138:654–568.
37. Johnston CC, Hui S, Witt R, Apledorn R, Baker R, Longcope C. Early menopausal changes in bone mass and sex steroids. J Clin Endocrinol Metab 1985;61:905–911.
38. Deutsch S, Benjamin F, Seltzer V, Tafreshi M, Kocheril G, Frank A. The correlation of serum estrogens and androgens with bone density in the late menopause. Int J Gynecol Obstet 1987;25:217–222.
39. Slemenda C, Longcope C, Peacock M, Hui S, Johnston CC. Sex steroids, bone mass, and bone loss. J Clin Invest 1996;97:14–21.
40. Devaprabu A, Carpenter P. Issues concerning androgen replacement therapy in postmenopausal women. Mayo Clin Proc 1997;72:1051–1055.
41. Geusens P. Nandrolone decanoate: pharmacological properties and therapeutic use in osteoporosis. Clin Rheumatol 1995;14(Suppl 3):32–39.
42. Chesnut C, Ivey J, Gruber H, Matthews M, Nelp W, Sisom K, et al. Stanozole in postmenopausal osteoporosis. Metabolism 1983;32:571–580.
43. Need A, Horowitz M, Bridges A, Morris H, Nordin B. The effects of nandrolone decanoate and antiresorptive therapy on vertebral density in osteoporotic menopausal women. Arch Intern Med 1989;149:57–60.
44. Hassager C, Podenphant J, Riis B. Changes in soft tissue body composition and plasma lipid metabolism during nandrolone decanoate therapy in postmenopausal osteoporotic women. Metab Clin Exp 1989;38:238–242.
45. Geusens P, Dequeker J, Verstraeten A, Nijs J, Van Holsbeeck M. Bone mineral content, cortical thickness and fracture rate in osteoporotic women after withdrawal of treatment with nandrolone decanoate, 1-alpha hydroxyvitamin D or intermittent calcium infusions. Maturitas 1986;8:281–289.
46. Kanis J, Johnell O, Gulberg B, Allander E, Dilsen G, Gennari C, et al. Evidence for efficacy of drugs affecting bone metabolism in preventing hip fracture. BMJ 1992;305: 1124–1128.

34 Selective Estrogen Receptor Modulators (SERMs)

J. E. Compston

Introduction

Selective estrogen receptor modulators are compounds which bind to the estrogen receptor and exhibit tissue-specific effects [1–3]. The ability of some compounds to exert both anti-estrogenic and estrogenic actions has been recognized for some years; in particular, the example of tamoxifen, which acts as an anti-estrogen in the breast but has bone-preserving properties, has stimulated the search for agents which possess an optimal combination of agonistic and antagonistic effects. The wide range of physiological actions of estrogen throughout the body provides considerable potential for such agents to prevent many of the major illnesses resulting from estrogen deficiency in the postmenopause, namely coronary heart disease, osteoporosis, breast cancer and declining cognitive function.

Raloxifene is currently the only SERM licenced for prevention and treatment of osteoporosis. Tamoxifen, which is widely used in the treatment of breast cancer, has been shown to have partial estrogenic effects in the skeleton, at least in postmenopausal women [4,5]. However, it is not licenced for prevention or treatment of osteoporosis and in view of its adverse effects on the endometrium should not be used for this indication.

Mechanism of Action

The estrogen receptor belongs to a family of nuclear receptors which include cortisol, testosterone, progesterone, thyroid hormone and retinoic acid. Following binding of estrogen to the estrogen receptor in the cell nucleus, dimerization and conformational change in the ligand-binding domain of the receptor occurs; the resulting receptor/ligand complex then initiates or enhances the transcription of genes containing specific response elements (Fig. 34.1).

The complexity of estrogen signalling pathways is increasingly being recognized [6,7]. Two receptor subtypes have been identified – estrogen receptor α and β – and, at least in vitro, these have the ability to form either the α/α or β/β homodimers or the a/β heterodimer [8,9]. The tissue distribution of the two subtypes is overlapping but not identical; current information is based mainly on localisation of mRNA and further studies are required. In addition to the classical estrogen

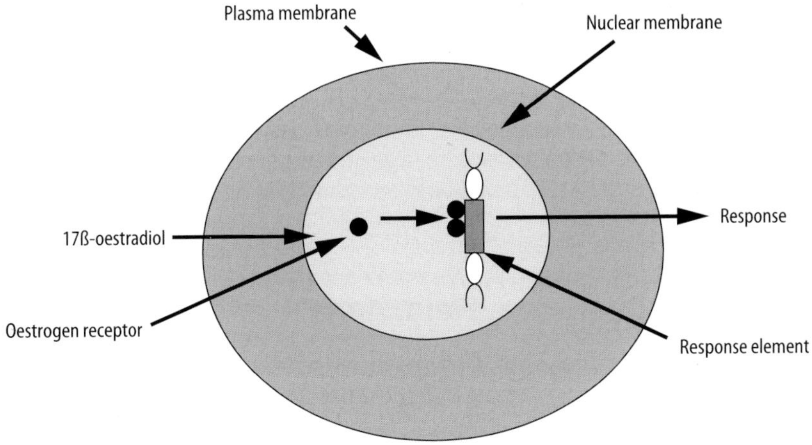

Figure 34.1. Schematic representation of estrogen receptor/ligand interaction. 17ß-estradiol is transported across the nuclear membrane and binds to the estrogen receptor. The receptor/ligand complex then undergoes dimerization and conformational change before binding to a response element within the promotor area of an estrogen-responsive gene, hence activating its transcription.

response element, other estrogen-dependent genes may contain alternative promotor regions, including the AP-1 response element which requires the protein transcription factors c-*jun* and c-*fos* for activity. The transcriptional response may also be modulated by the presence of cell-specific coactivators and corepressors. Finally, the recent resolution of the crystal structure of the ligand-binding domain of the estrogen receptor [10] has provided new insights into the molecular mechanisms by which estrogenic and anti-estrogenic effects may be achieved. In the case of raloxifene, the presence of a side-chain prevents the conformational change required to initiate signal transduction at the activation function-2 (AF2) site.

Skeletal Effects of Raloxifene

Raloxifene is a synthetic benzothiophene derivative (Fig. 34.2) which has recently been licenced for the prevention and treatment of spinal osteoporosis in postmenopausal women. It is administered as a 60 mg tablet, taken orally once daily. It can be taken at any time of day without special regard to meals and dose adjustment is not required in the elderly. Calcium supplements are recommended in women with a low dietary calcium intake; although there is no accepted threshold for this, an intake of less than 500 mg/day would be regarded as low and between 500 and 750 mg/day may be considered as borderline.

Estrogenic effects of raloxifene in the skeleton have been demonstrated in animal models [11] and, more recently, in postmenopausal women. Clinical studies have included postmenopausal women with and without vertebral osteoporosis and have used biochemical markers of bone turnover, bone mineral density measurements and vertebral fracture as end-points. In a short-term, randomized double-masked placebo-controlled study in healthy early postmenopausal women two oral doses of raloxifene, 200 or 600 mg/day, were compared with placebo and with premarin

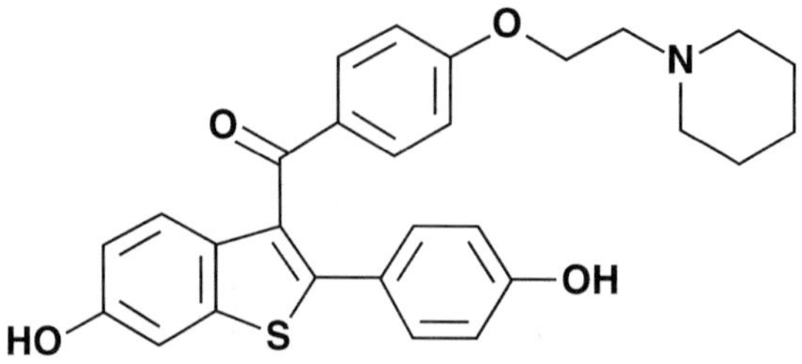

Figure 34.2. Chemical structure of raloxifene.

0.625 mg daily [12]. Biochemical markers of bone resorption and formation showed a significant and quantitatively similar decrease in the estrogen- and raloxifene-treated groups, providing support for the contention that raloxifene induces similar skeletal benefits to those of estrogen. It should be noted, however, that the doses of raloxifene used in this study were considerably in excess of that subsequently recommended for prevention of osteoporosis, namely 60 mg daily.

The effects of raloxifene on bone mineral density were reported by Delmas et al. [13] in a multicenter randomized controlled study in 601 postmenopausal women within 2–8 years of their menopause. The study included women with both normal and low bone mineral density (lumbar spine *T*-score between +2 and −2.5). Three doses of raloxifene were tested – 30, 60 and 150 mg daily – and all groups (including the placebo group) received 400–600 mg daily of a calcium supplement. After 2 years of treatment, bone mineral density had increased significantly at the lumbar spine, total hip, femoral neck and total body with all doses of raloxifene, whereas bone loss occurred in the placebo group (Fig. 34.3).

In general, a dose effect was seen for the changes in bone mineral density, the greatest increase (except in the total hip) occurring in women receiving 150 mg daily. Biochemical markers of bone resorption and formation decreased significantly in all three treatment groups and by 12 months of treatment were within the normal premenopausal range.

The effects of raloxifene have also been assessed in women with osteoporosis, defined as a spine or hip bone mineral density *T*-score below −2.5, with or without prevalent vertebral fracture. In a multinational placebo-controlled, double-masked study, 7705 postmenopausal women were randomly assigned to placebo, 60 mg or 120 mg of raloxifene daily; all subjects also received vitamin D and calcium supplementation (400–600 IU and 500 mg daily respectively).

After three years treatment, the percentage of women who had sustained at least one new vertebral fracture was 10.1% in the placebo group compared with 6.6% and 5.4% of women treated with 60 and 120 mg daily of raloxifene [20]. The relative risk of vertebral fracture in women receiving 60mg daily was 0.7 (95% confidence intervals 0.5–0.8) and, in those receiving 120 mg daily, 0.5 (0.4–0.7). This beneficial effect was seen both in women with and without prevalent vertebral fracture(s) at baseline. Significant treatment benefits were seen at three years on bone mineral density, the mean difference from placebo being 2.1% and 2.4% in the femoral neck for the 60mg and 120 mg doses and 2.6% and 2.7% respectively in the spine.

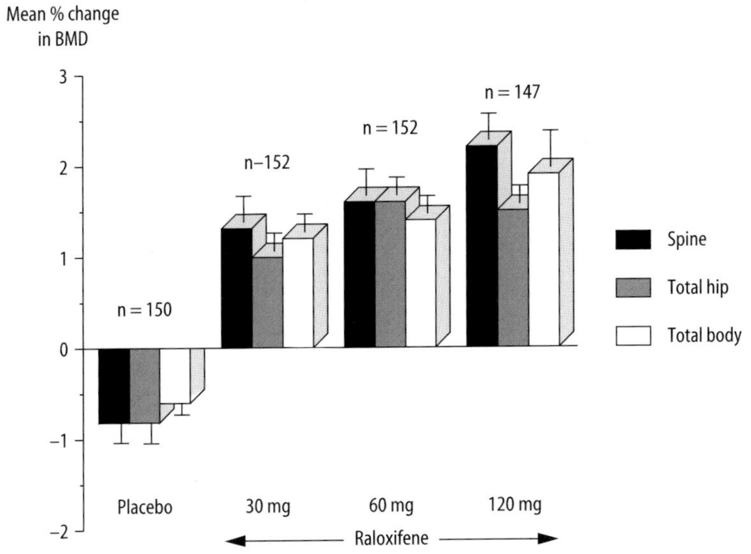

Figure 34.3. Effect of three doses of raloxifene on bone mineral density in the spine, total hip and total body in early postmenopausal women. Values are shown as the mean ± SD. Data from Delmas et al. [13].

Suppression of biochemical markers of bone turnover to normal premenopausal values was also demonstrated.

In this study no significant reduction in the risk of hip or other non-vertebral fracture was demonstrated; the relative risk of all non-vertebral fractures after three years treatment was 0.9 in women receiving 60 or 120 mg daily raloxifene (95% confidence intervals 0.8–1.1) and, for hip fracture, 1.1 (0.6–1.9). However, the study was not powered to demonstrate a reduction in non-vertebral fractures and the use of vitamin D supplementation in all patients at doses of up to 600 IU/day would be expected to reduce the rate of these fractures, thus decreasing the likelihood of showing any significant benefit of raloxifene. Moreover, the mean age of women in this study was 67 years, considerably lower than that at which the incidence of hip fracture is greatest. In addition, ethically driven protocol requirements resulted in the withdrawal from the study of patients who either sustained a fracture or who exhibited high rates of bone loss; as expected, the majority of such patients were receiving placebo, thus further reducing the chance of demonstrating significant protection against non-vertebral fracture. Nevertheless, the maintained treatment benefit on bone mineral density in the femoral neck, suppression of bone biomarkers and absence of adverse neuromuscular effects which might increase risk of falling would all be consistent with benefits on fracture risk at non-vertebral sites.

In a smaller randomized double-masked study in 143 postmenopausal women with at least one prevalent vertebral fracture and low bone mineral density at the spine and/or hip, the effects of 60 mg and 120 mg daily of raloxifene were evaluated over the course of 1 year [15]. All women were also given vitamin D and calcium supplements (400 IU and 750 mg/day respectively). At the end of the treatment period significant increases in bone mineral density at the total hip (for the group receiving 60 mg/day) and ultradistal radius (for both raloxifene doses) were seen with nonsignificant increases at the lumbar spine and total body (and total hip for the 120 mg/day raloxifene group). These changes were accompanied by suppression of biochemical markers of bone resorption and formation.

Currently available data thus indicate that raloxifene has estrogen-like effects on bone turnover and preserves bone mass at the hip, spine and total body. The observed treatment effect of raloxifene on bone mineral density is slightly less than that demonstrated in most studies of conventional estrogen replacement therapy, raising the possibility that the skeletal actions of raloxifene may be weaker than those of estrogen. Nevertheless, the reduction in vertebral fracture risk demonstrated after 3 years treatment with raloxifene is similar to that observed with another antiresorptive agent, alendronate, in a randomized controlled trial and to that reported for hip fracture in observational studies of hormone replacement therapy.

Extraskeletal Effects of Raloxifene

Effects on the Breast

Raloxifene acts as an anti-estrogen in breast tissue. Unlike conventional hormone replacement with estrogen, with or without a progestin, its use is not associated with breast discomfort, swelling or tenderness.

In the MORE (Multiple Outcomes of Raloxifene Evaluation) study referred to earlier [20], the effect of raloxifene on breast cancer risk was assessed in 7705 postmenopausal women after a median follow-up period of 40 months [21]. Raloxifene use was associated with a 76% decrease in the risk of breast cancer overall (95% confidence intervals 0.13–0.44). For estrogen receptor positive tumours, the reduction in risk was 90% (0.04–0.24) whereas risk of estrogen negative tumours was unaffected (relative risk 0.8 (0.2–2.7). These data confirm a highly significant protective effect of raloxifene against breast cancer in postmenopausal women, at least for the first 3–4 years of therapy.

Effects on the Endometrium

Raloxifene does not stimulate the endometrium and its use in clinical trials has not been associated with vaginal bleeding or endometrial hyperplasia. Transvaginal ultrasound measurements have not demonstrated any increase in endometrial thickness attributable to raloxifene [13] and, in those women in whom endometrial biopsies were performed, no evidence of endometrial proliferation was observed. Finally, no increase in the risk of endometrial cancer has been documented in women treated with raloxifene. Vaginal bleeding during raloxifene therapy is therefore not expected and, if it occurs, should be thoroughly investigated.

Effects on Serum Lipids, Coagulation Factors and Risk of Cardiovascular Disease

The effects of raloxifene on cardiovascular disease have not yet been established and information is only available on some surrogate markers, mainly serum lipids.

In general, these show similar changes to those observed in women on conventional hormone replacement therapy and may thus indicate cardioprotection. However, it should be noted that although substantial protection against heart disease has been demonstrated in observational studies of hormone replacement a recent prospective study of the effects of hormone replacement therapy in the secondary prevention of coronary heart disease did not reveal any such benefit despite favorable effects on lipid profile [17]. These findings emphasize the need for prospective studies and the potential limitations of commonly used surrogate markers of cardiovascular risk.

Several studies have demonstrated a significant reduction in serum total cholesterol levels in women treated with raloxifene and in low density lipoprotein (LDL) cholesterol, similar to that observed with conventional hormone replacement therapy [12,13,18]. There is also a decrease in lipoprotein (a) which, however, is less than that seen with hormone replacement therapy. In contrast to hormone replacement therapy, raloxifene does not significantly affect serum high density lipoprotein (HDL) cholesterol (although a relatively small increase is seen in HDL2-cholesterol) and does not increase serum triglycerides. Raloxifene therapy is also associated with a small increase in apolipoprotein A-1, significantly less than the increase seen with hormone replacement therapy. With respect to coagulation factors, raloxifene significantly lowers serum fibrinogen levels but does not affect plasminogen activator inhibitor-1.

Overall, these effects of raloxifene on serum lipid and coagulation factor profile are favorable and may indicate decreased risk of cardiovascular disease, although, as noted above, caution is required in the use of these indices as surrogate markers of disease. Although similar in many respects to estrogen in terms of its effects on serum lipids and coagulation factors, raloxifene exhibits both qualitative and quantitative differences, possibly reflecting only partial agonistic effects. Interestingly, the raloxifene-induced effects are more similar to those of tamoxifen, which has been reported to show a cardioprotective effect in women undergoing treatment for breast cancer [19]. However, prospective studies are required to establish the effects of raloxifene on coronary heart disease; a large multicenter trial is currently being initiated and results are expected in approximately 5 years.

Vasomotor and Urogenital Effects

Raloxifene does not alleviate vasomotor symptoms associated with the menopause and its use is associated with a small but significant increase in the frequency of hot flushes. Its effects on urogenital menopausal manifestations and sexual function are not well defined but significant adverse effects have not emerged in clinical trials. Although co-administration of raloxifene and systemic estrogens is not recommended, topical vaginal preparations can be used in raloxifene-treated women who complain of vaginal dryness.

Effects on Cognitive Function

In view of the potential benefits on cognitive function and reduction in risk of Alzheimer's disease documented in observational studies of hormone replacement therapy, the effects of raloxifene are of considerable interest. However, at present no information is available other than the lack of any significant adverse effects of raloxifene on cognitive function in clinical trials.

Adverse Effects

Raloxifene appears to be well tolerated and no serious adverse effects have been reported in clinical trials. Increased frequency of hot flushes has been reported in healthy postmenopausal women receiving 600 mg raloxifene daily [12] and in a subsequent study of the impact of raloxifene on quality of life in women treated with lower doses, but this finding has not been universal. In general, when hot flushes occur in women treated with raloxifene they are not severe and do not significantly impair quality of life, at least in the long term. Leg cramps have been reported to occur with increased frequency in women taking raloxifene. There is also an increase in the risk of venous thromboembolism, similar in magnitude to that observed with hormone replacement therapy. This most commonly occurs soon after treatment is commenced and is particularly likely to affect women with a predisposition to or past history of venous thromboembolism. An increase in peripheral edema has also been reported in women receiving raloxifene.

Contraindications to Raloxifene

Raloxifene should not be given to women of child-bearing potential and there are no indications for its use in men. In view of the increased risk of thromboembolic disorders associated with raloxifene therapy, it should be avoided in women with a past history of or risk factors for this condition – for example immobilization, thrombophlebitis, obesity, or disorders of coagulation which predispose to thrombosis. Raloxifene is mainly metabolized in the liver and plasma concentrations are increased in patients with liver dysfunction when compared with normal subjects; it should therefore be avoided in patients with hepatic dysfunction and is also contraindicated in patients with severe renal impairment. Although, as discussed below, raloxifene acts as an anti-estrogen in the endometrium and breast, there is no experience of its use in patients with current endometrial or breast cancer and it should therefore not be advised in such patients, or in those with unexplained uterine bleeding. Finally, there are no data on the effects of co-administration of systemic estrogens and raloxifene and such use is thus not recommended.

Drug Interactions

There are relatively few drug interactions with raloxifene. Modest increases in the prothrombin time have been reported with co-administration of raloxifene and warfarin and careful monitoring of the prothrombin time is advised in patients receiving raloxifene and warfarin or other coumarin derivatives. Cholestyramine significantly reduces the intestinal absorption and enterohepatic cycling of raloxifene and for this reason concurrent administration of these two drugs is not recommended.

The Role of Raloxifene in the Management of Osteoporosis

A number of agents are currently licenced for the prevention and treatment of osteoporosis and positioning of raloxifene with respect to other interventions is thus required. Other options include hormone replacement therapy, bisphosphonates, calcitonin, calcitriol, and calcium and vitamin D. Robust evidence from randomized controlled trials for fracture reduction at both vertebral and non-vertebral sites is only available for two bisphosphonates, namely alendronate and risedronate. In the case of hormone replacement therapy, evidence for reduction in fracture risk has been obtained almost exclusively from observational studies, which are likely to be biased. As discussed earlier in this chapter, although raloxifene has only been shown to have anti-fracture efficacy at the spine, the available data would also be consistent with beneficial effects at non-vertebral sites and this agent is licensed for use in all types of postmenopausal osteoporosis.

Raloxifene therapy may be particularly appropriate for certain patient groups. These include women who are intolerant of bisphosphonates and are unwilling to take hormone replacement therapy because of vaginal bleeding, breast tenderness or fear of breast cancer. Raloxifene should also be considered in women who wish to stop hormone replacement therapy after long-term use for osteoporosis, but still require treatment to prevent bone loss. The good safety profile of raloxifene with respect to breast cancer is likely to be a positive advantage for women with high levels of concern about this disease, particularly in view of the intended long-term use of raloxifene.

Raloxifene does not alleviate vasomotor menopausal symptoms such as hot flushes and is not suitable for women with menopausal symptoms, in whom hormone replacement therapy remains the treatment of choice. At present there are no data on the effects of raloxifene on glucocorticoid-induced bone loss and it is therefore not indicated for prevention or treatment of glucocorticoid-induced osteoporosis.

The Future of SERMs

SERMs provide an exciting approach not only to the treatment of osteoporosis but also to the management of many of the major illnesses of the postmenopause. The example of raloxifene has demonstrated the potential of these compounds to have beneficial skeletal effects without adverse actions on the breast and uterus; effects on cardiovascular disease and cognitive function require further research before the risk benefit ratio of raloxifene can be accurately evaluated. Recent advances in our knowledge of estrogen signalling and, in particular, the structure and diversity of estrogen receptors, should facilitate the design of new SERMs which possess the "ideal" pharmacological profile and maintain health in the postmenopausal era, which now occupies one-third of the lifespan of women.

References

1. Compston JE. Designer estrogens: fact or fantasy? Lancet 1997;350:676–677.
2. Baynes KCR, Compston JE. Selective estrogen receptor modulators: a new paradigm for HRT. Curr Opin Obstet Gynecol 1998;10: 189–192.

3. Compston JE. Selective estrogen receptor modulators: potential therapeutic applications. Clin Endocrinol 1998;48:389–391.
4. Love RR, Mazess RB, Barden HS, Epstein S, Newcomb PA, Jordan VC, et al. Effects of tamoxifen on bone mineral density in postmenopausal women with breast cancer. N Engl J Med 1992;326:852–856.
5. Wright CDP, Garrahan NJ, Stanton M, Gazet J-C, Mansell RE, Compston JE. Effect of long-term tamoxifen therapy on cancellous bone remodelling and structure in women with breast cancer. J Bone Miner Res 1994;9:153–159.
6. MacGregor JI, Jordan VC. Basic guide to the mechanisms of antiestrogen action. Pharmacol Rev 1998;50:151–196.
7. Jordan VC. Antiestrogenic action of raloxifene and tamoxifen: today and tomorrow. J Natl Cancer Inst 1998;90:967–971.
8. Kuiper GGJM, Enmark E, Pelto-Huikko M, Nilsson S, Gustafsson J-A. Cloning of a novel estrogen receptor expressed in rat prostate and ovary. Proc Natl Acad Sci USA 1996;93:5925–5930.
9. Kuiper GGJM, Gustafsson J-A. The novel estrogen receptor-β subtype: potential role in the cell- and promotor-specific actions of estrogens and anti-estrogens. FEBS Lett 1997;410:87–90.
10. Brzozowski AM, Pike ACW, Dauter Z, Hubbard RE, Bonn T, Engstrom O, et al. Molecular basis of agonism and antagonism in the estrogen receptor. Nature 1997; 389:753–758.
11. Bryant HU, Glasebrook AL, Yang NN, Sato M. A pharmacological review of raloxifene. J Bone Miner Metab 1996;14:1–9.
12. Draper MW, Flowers DE, Huster WJ, Neild JA, Harper KD, Arnaud C. A controlled trial of raloxifene (LY139481) HCL: impact on bone turnover and serum lipid profile in healthy postmenopausal women. J Bone Miner Res 1996;11:835–842.
13. Delmas PD, Bjarnason NH, Mitlak BH, Ravoux AC, Shah AS, Huster WJ, et al. Effects of raloxifene on bone mineral density, serum cholesterol concentrations and uterine endometrium in postmenopausal women. N Engl J Med 1997;337:1641–1647.
14. Ettinger B, Black D, Cummings S, Genant H, Glüer C, Lips P, et al. Raloxifene reduces the risk of incident vertebral fractures: 24-month interim analysis (abstract). Osteoporos Int 1998;8(Suppl 3):11).
15. Lufkin EG, Whitaker MD, Nickelson T, Argueta R, Caplan RH, Knickerbocker RK, et al. Treatment of established postmenopausal osteoporosis with raloxifene: a randomized trial. J Bone Miner Res 1998;13:1747–1754.
16. Jordan VC, Glusman JE, Eckert S, Lippman M, Powles T, Costa A, et al. Incident primary breast cancers are reduced by raloxifene: integrated data from multicenter, double-blind, randomized trials in 12 000 postmenopausal women (abstract). Proc Am Soc Clin Oncol 1998;17:122a.
17. Hulley S, Grady D, Bush T, Furberg C, Herrington D, Riggs B, Vittinghoff E. Randomized trial of estrogen plus progestin for secondary prevention of coronary heart disease in postmenopausal women. JAMA 1998;280:605–613.
18. Walsh BW, Kuller LH, Wild RA, Paul S, Farmer M, Lawrence JB, et al. Effects of raloxifene on serum lipids and coagulation factors in healthy postmenopausal women. JAMA 1998;279:1445–1451.
19. McDonald CC, Stewart HJ, for the Scottish Breast Cancer Committee. Fatal myocardial infarction in the Scottish adjuvant tamoxifen trial. BMJ 1991;303:435–437.
20. Ettinger B, Black DM, Mitlak BH, Knickerbocker RK, Nickelsen T, Genant HK et al Reduction of vertebral fracture risk in postmenopausal women with osteoporosis treated with raloxifene. JAMA 1999; 282: 637–645.
21. Cummings SR, Eckert S, Krueger KA, Grady D, Powles TJ, Cauley JA et al. The effect of raloxifene on risk of breast cancer in postmenopausal women. JAMA 1999; 281: 2189–2197.

35 Evolving Therapies: PTH, IGF, GH, Ipriflavone

C. Wüster

Introduction

The management of osteoporotic fractures is multifactorial and pharmacological strategies consist of acute management of pain and complications resulting from the fractures rather than building up new, strong bone. This challenge to increase bone density can be achieved at a later stage after fracture healing has already occurred as this usually takes more than 5 years to be efficient. However osteoporotic patients with acute vertebral fractures have an increased risk for further new vertebral fractures at a given bone density level compared with those without prevalent fractures. Thus the management of patients with multiple acute vertebral fractures and very low bone density is the most difficult problem in osteoporosis.

Osteoporosis is a complex, multifactorial, chronic disease which can progress without any symptoms for decades, until the loss of bone in an individual finally reaches a point at which fractures occur [1]. Due to the great number of fractures and to the clinical symptoms, osteoporosis is an enormous public health problem and impairs the patients' quality of life.

Since fracture rates increase with advancing age, this problem will be further aggravated in the future. This is due not only to the aging population but also to the rising incidence of fractures caused by increasing risk factors. To date, many studies have been carried out which show that the risk of fractures increases with lower bone density. Often, other bone-loss-inducing risk factors are added [2]. However, independently of risk factors, bone density as measured by quantitative ultrasonography, quantitative computed tomography or dual x-ray absorptiometry are independent, equivalent predictive variables for future fractures [3].

Role of PTH, GH AND IGF-I in the Regulation of Bone Metabolism

The physiology of bone turnover is a very complex cycle occurring at all skeletal sites [4–6]. Old bone is regularly replaced by new bone in well-defined quantities: the basic multicellular unit (BMU). Osteoclasts originating from hematopoietic stem cells are activated by an as yet unknown resorption stimulus. One might speculate that, for example, growth hormone (GH) or parathyroid hormone (PTH) may be required as systemic hormonal stimuli. Osteoclasts need about 5–7 days to produce a resorption lacuna. Osteoblasts which are derived from mesenchymal cells move onto this freshly resorbed bone surface and produce new bone matrix which subsequently mineralizes within 100 days. Some osteoblasts are incorporated into bone and become differentiated into osteocytes. They probably possess the location of the mechanoreceptors responsible for perception of physical and mechanical stress on bone. Skeletal growth factors (GFs) are stored within bone and released during the resorption process. They are needed to stimulate differentiation of preosteoblasts into mature osteoblasts. During osteoblastic matrix deposition GFs are again incorporated within bone. The amount of GFs deposited is dependent on the level of bone turnover, which is under hormonal control (e.g., of GH and sex steroid). Activity of GFs is regulated by the presence of specific binding proteins and binding protein proteases which are important for control of the local concentrations of GFs within a BMU. The amount of transforming growth factor-ß (TGF-ß) released from bone originating from adult patients with GH deficiency of juvenile onset after 1,25-vitamin D administration in vitro is diminished; however, this phenomenon is not reversible after GH treatment of the patients before taking the bone biopsy. The release of cytokines such as interleukins 1 and 6 known to stimulate bone resorption is increased after acute estrogen deprivation in human bone marrow cells in vitro. GFs might reflect a memory of previous hormonal disturbances within the skeleton. Together with possible variations at the local hormone receptor level these changes might explain changes in bone turnover and density seen with aging or in hormone deficiency states (menopause, somatopause).

PTH exerts its actions via its receptor it shares with PTH-related peptide (PTHrP). These receptors are not found on osteoclasts, increased bone resorption driven by PTH is thought be mediated via the coupling factor between blasts and clasts, a factor which is probably a secondary messenger or GF but still unknown. However, PTH can inhibit bone formation (long-term treatment) and stimulate it (transient treatment) [8] possibly via insulin-like growth factor I (IGF-I) (Fig. 35.1). Other mechanisms include prostaglandins and effects on generation of preosteoblasts and inhibition of apoptosis of osteoblasts [9].

GH is responsible for longitudinal bone growth via its direct stimulatory effect on chondrocytes and osteoblasts. GH acts directly on osteoblasts via its own receptor and via IGF-I which acts in an auto- and paracrine fashion (Fig. 35.1). This mechanism of action has been described as the dual effector theory. The GH receptor belongs to a receptor superfamily which includes the prolactin receptor and several cytokine receptors and has a soluble form such as the GH binding protein (GHBP) which might also regulate GH action. Osteoclasts are stimulated by GH and/or IGF-I. Nishiyama et al. [10] showed that bovine GH (bGH; 1–100 ng/ml) significantly stimulated bone resorption by pre-existent osteoclasts in stromal-cell-containing mouse bone cell cultures, whereas it did not affect the bone-resorbing activity of isolated rabbit osteoclasts. GH also enhanced 1,25-dihydroxyvitamin D_3-induced osteoclast-like cell formation. Moreover, osteoclast-like cells newly formed from unfractionated bone cells in the presence of bGH possessed the ability to form pits on dentine slices. GH concentration dependently stimulated osteoclast-like cell formation from these hematopoietic blast cells in the absence of stromal cells, and these osteoclast-like cells formed pits on dentine slices in the presence of MC3T3-G2/PA-6 stromal cells. This study indicated for the first time that GH stimulates osteoclastic bone resorption through both its direct and indirect actions on

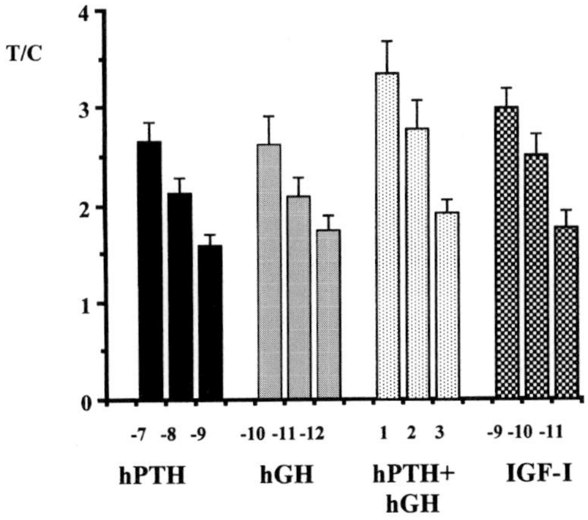

Figure 35.1. Stimulation of human osteoblasts in vitro using human growth hormone (hGH), human parathyroid hormone (hPTH), insulin-like growth factor-I (IGF-I) and a combination. See [11] for details.

osteoclast differentiation and through its indirect activation of mature osteoclasts, possibly via stromal cells, including osteoblasts [10]. The osteoclastic stimulation by GH/IGF-I is supported by in vivo data in mice, dogs and humans (see below). Osteoblasts have own GH- and IGF-I and -II receptors. They are stimulated to produce IGFs when GH is given in vitro [7,11], although these cells make greater amounts of IGF-II than IGF-I.

In contrast to liver, where GH is the principal regulator of IGF-I production, osteoblastic IGF-I gene transcription is influenced by both paracrine and endocrine factors. IGF concentrations in the rest of the skeleton are produced by bone marrow stromal cells, which are rich sources of cytokines for hematopoietic progenitors and actively synthesize IGF-I and various IGF-binding proteins (IGFBPs) Other IGFBPs regulate IGF action, such as IGFBP-4 which inhibits the stimulatory effect of IGF-I on mouse osteoblasts as described above. GH, IGF-I and IGF-II have a potent stimulatory effect of cell growth in a dose-dependent manner. GH-induced cell growth can be blocked by the the simultaneous addition of a specific monoclonal antibody to IGF-I. IGF-II is also a potent mitogen; IGF-II stimulates mitogenesis even when high doses of IGF-I are also administered. This suggests that IGF-II regulates osteoblastic proliferation via the IGF type 2 receptor. The role of IGF-I and IGF-II in the coupling of bone resorption and formation is extensively reviewed by Mohan and Baylink [12]. IGF-II stimulates type I collagen synthesis in human osteoblast-like cells. IGF-I and IGF-II stimulate alkaline phosphatase activity. Both IGFs act synergistically with 1,25-vitamin D to increase the osteocalcin production.

The intraosseous concentrations of IGF-I, IGF-II, IGFBP-3 and IGFBP-5 in cortical bone decrease with age. Another role of IGF-I becomes apparent in the regulation of bone remodelling by in response to physical stress. IGF-I mRNA expression is increased in osteocytes after application of mechanical stress before initiation of bone formation.

GH has several other target organs apart from bone. These effects might indirectly influence bone metabolism. Its predominant action is the anabolic effect stimulating muscle mass, strength and exercise capacity. The same applies to the effects of GH on improving quality of life and cardiac function, which increases mobility and thus stimulates bone turnover. Interactions of GH with sex steroids are multiple. GH influences their secretion in testes and ovaries and potentiates their effects on bone. Furthermore GH has enteral and renal effects which influence calcium metabolism. Whether GH has a daily regulatory effect on bone turnover is a new speculative thought. There is evidence that bone resorption is increased during night and this increase in nightly bone resorption is preceded by the midnight GH peak [13]. Whether this is a direct link between bone resorption and GH secretion or coincidence has to be investigated further. GH also has effects on mechanical properties and biochemical composition of rat bones [14]. It increases external diameters of long bones whereas the internal diameters were unaffected or increased as well [15]. It thus improved the mechanical properties of the cortical femur and tibia although bone density, bone collagen content and bone ash weight remained unchanged.

Pathophysiology of Osteoporosis: Role of Endogenous PTH, GH AND IGFs. Changes in Serum PTH, GH AND IGF-I in Patients with Osteoporosis

GH secretion in patients with osteoporosis was found to be reduced after stimulation with L-arginine in comparison with patients with osteoarthritis. Wüster et al. [16] have shown low serum IGF-I, IGF-II and IGFBP-3 as measured by radioimmunoassays in 98 women with postmenopausal osteoporosis compared with 59 normals and 91 patients with osteoarthrosis or degenerative bone disease. Results are shown in Fig. 35.2. Similar results were measured in males with osteoporosis and serum IGF-I as well as IGFBP-3 concentrations were positively correlated with lumbar bone mineral density (BMD) in osteoporotic patients. Comparable results

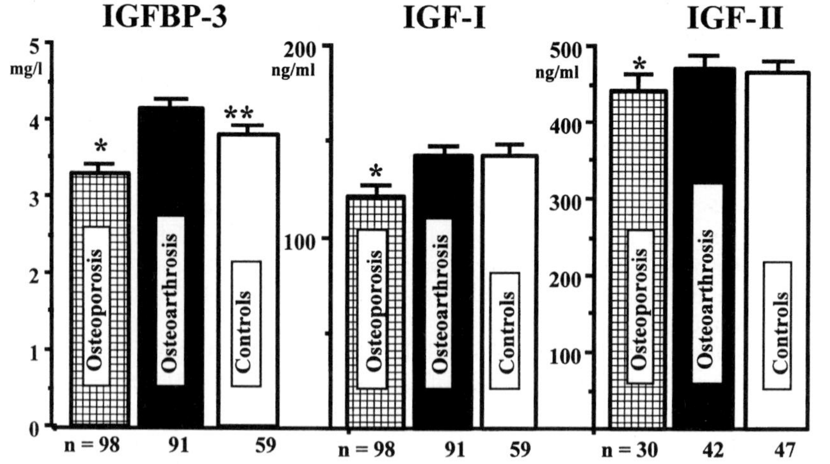

Figure 35.2. Serum concentrations of IGF-I, IGF-II and IGFBP–3 in males and females with primary osteoporosis, with degenerative spine disease (osteoarthrosis) and in controls in relation to age. Adapted from [16].

have been found by others for IGF-I. Patients with osteoarthrosis seemed to have higher values. This is consistent with results from studies on IGF-II concentrations in bones from patients with osteoarthrosis. Human marrow stromal osteoblast-like cells from 9 patients with osteoporosis did not show reduced responsiveness to in vitro stimulation with GH. An age-related decline in the content of growth factors and their binding proteins such as IGFBP-5, IGF-I and TGF-ß has been shown. It remains to be determined whether there is a difference between patients with and without osteoporosis from the same age. Low IGF-I levels correlate significantly with osteoblastic surface in 18 males and 12 females with idiopathic osteoporosis. Own data do not support the hypothesis that low serum IGF-I is due to diminished secretion of endogenous GH [17]. So at present one might explain the low serum IGF-I levels by decreased osseous production of IGF-I in osteoporosis patients with low-turn over and diminished osteoblastic activity or simply a reflection of low BMD looking at the high correlation between serum IGF-I and BMD. This hypothesis is supported by data showing diminished intraosseous GF concentrations in patients with osteoporosis and increased GF concentrations in osteoarthritis. Endogenous serum PTH concentrations are often increased due to diminished calcium intake or resorption in vitamin D deficiency or enteral calcium depletion. However, in low turnover osteoporosis low PTH pulsatility was shown by several investigators [17].

PTH Treatment

Various fragments of PTH and recombinant hPTH(1–84) alone and in combination with antiresorptive agents continuously and cyclically (according to the ADFR concepts) are under investigation at various stages of clinical and preclinical research. First studies in aged, ovariectomized rats showed impressive effects on trabecular connectivity, increases in trabecular thickness and also cortical thickness [18] (Fig 35.3). New data suggest that the increase in cortical thickness might be threatened by cortical tunnelling due to increased bone resorption. Data from other animal studies suggest that bone-selective analogs of hPTH(1–34) such as [His3]hPTH(1–34) or [Leu(3)]hPTH(1–34) maintain the ability to induce bone formation but are less potent than hPTH(1–34) [19].

PTH needs to be administered parenterally; however, all researchers so far have reported good cooperation and compliance with daily injection regimens. Side-effects include pain in the tibiae, development of autoantibodies, reddening around the injection site and hypercalcemia.

PTH therapy increases bone turnover, renal calcium excretion, increased bone perfusion as measure with the ^{18}F technique and, especially, axial (spinal and hip) bone volume and bone mass. Early studies showed that this anabolic effect was derived from the peripheral skeleton and that there was no increase in enteral calcium absorption.

Other studies have determined that intermittent PTH therapy increases bone mass and improves biomechanical strength in osteopenic animal models. hPTH(1–34) at medium and high doses significantly increased trabecular bone volume and trabecular thickness compared with ovariectomized animals treated with vehicle ($p < 0.05$). The trabecular bone volume was equal to or greater than that in the sham-operated animals in both hPTH(1–34) 40 and 400 microg/kg of BW treatment groups. Trabecular bone connectivity decreased by nearly 50%

a 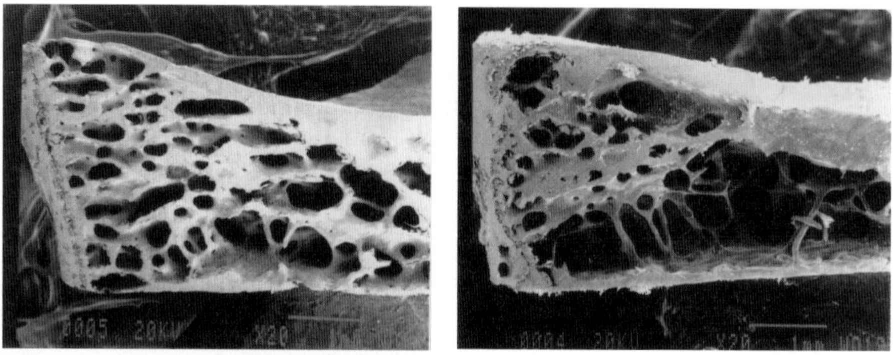 b

c 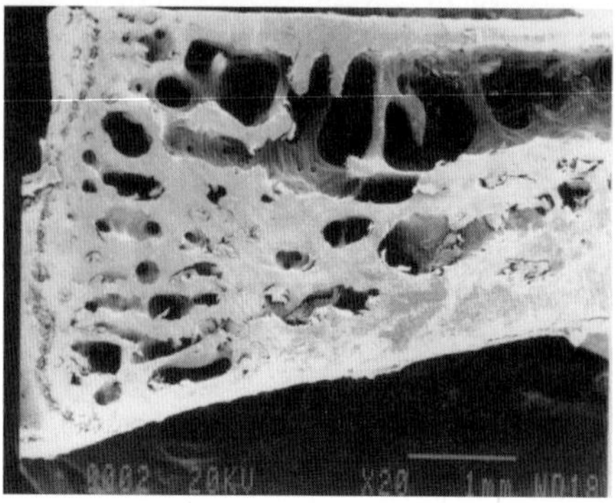

Figure 35.3. PTH maintains trabecular connectivity, increases trabecular thickness and also cortical thickness in aged ovariectomized rats. From [18] with permission from Lis Mosekilde. **a** Sham animal. **b** OVX animal. **c** OVX animal treated with PTH (1–38).

compared with the Sham-operated group at day 84 post-OVX and did not increase with any of the hPTH(1–34) treatments. Intermittent hPTH(1–34) treatment in osteopenic ovariectomized rats increased trabecular bone volume to control levels or higher by thickening existing trabeculae. Human PTH(1–34) did not re-establish connectivity when therapy was started after 50% of the trabecular connectivity was lost. We hypothesize that to re-establish trabecular connectivity, a therapeutic intervention would have to be given before a significant distance between trabeculae has developed. Further studies will need to be done to refute or confirm our hypothesis [20]. Other investigators have shown that PTH is a powerful agent in an animal model of immobilization osteoporosis and can accelerate the recovery and add extra bone to osteopenic cancellous bone in rats [21]. Former studies with PTH(1–34) 500 IU/day by Reeve et al. [22] showed increases in bone density at the lumbar spine as measured by quantitative computed tomography (QCT); however, no data were given on hip and total-body BMD. New unpublished studies by Lindsay et al. (presented at the ASBMR 1998) using rhPTH(1–84) showed 7% per year increases in spine BMD and 2% per year increase in spinal bone area, no change in femoral neck BMD and 2% per year decrease in total-body BMD, suggesting a decrease in BMD at arms and legs.

GH Treatment

Andreassen et al. [23] conducted a study treating aged rats with 2.7 mg/kg per day rhGH (1mg = 3 IU) for 80 days. A significant increase in the cortical bone volume,

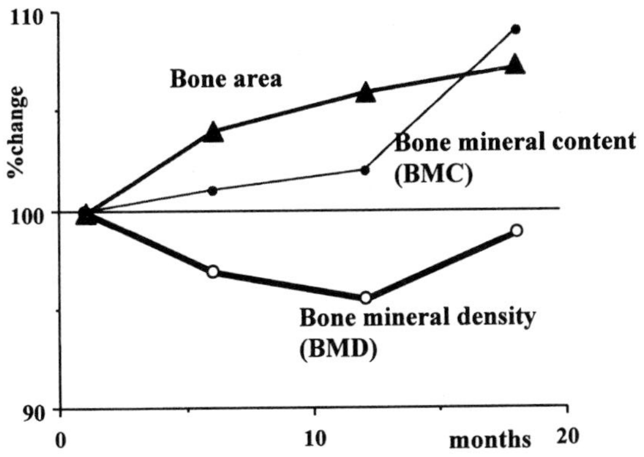

Figure 35.4. Increased bone area and BMC and decreased BMD in the first months of treatment with rhGH. Adapted from [59].

mineralizing surface/total surface, mineral apposition rate, and mineralized bone formation rate was found. Furthermore the transversal and midsagittal diameters were increased by GH. The compressive mechanical strength of the vertebral body specimens was increased, and this increase most likely could be explained by formation and deposition of cortical bone [23]. This is shown in vivo in patients with pituitary insufficiency under GH substitution (Fig. 35.4). However, treatment with 5 mg/kg per day of rhGH in glucocorticoid-treated rats (5 mg/kg per day prednisolone) was not able to inhibit loss of body weight, decrease in bone length, and diameters, or decreased bone strength induced by glucocorticoid administration [24]. Elevated levels of GH in metallothionein promotor-GH-transgenic mice increased the amounts of vertebral bone and tibia bone in young mice. Intact ovaries are a prerequisite for the stimulatory effect of elevated levels of GH. The fact that ovariectomy decreased the stimulatory effect of elevated GH levels suggested that this GH effect is dependent on the presence of endogenous sex steroid secretion [25]. Denis et al. [26] treated growing pigs with 40 μg porcine GH/kg body weight or its vehicle twice daily for 2 months. GH accelerated growth, with greater tibial and metacarpal weights, greater tibial length and diameters and greater tibial ash weight in GH-treated pigs than in controls. The similar values of apparent bone density in the two groups suggest adequate coupling between bone growth and mineralization in GH-treated pigs. Histomorphometric data for the distal metacarpal metaphysis indicated greater trabecular bone volume, osteoblastic surface and mineral apposition rate in GH-treated pigs. The osteoclast surface, lacuna depth and osteoid-related parameters in GH-treated and control pigs were similar. The plasma PTH levels of the two groups of pigs were similar throughout the experiment. These data and the elevated plasma alkaline phosphatase activity in GH-treated pigs suggest that GH specifically affects bone formation. GH had no effect on the plasma 25-hydroxyvitamin D_3 but 1,25-hydroxyvitamin D_3 (calcitriol) was higher in treated pigs throughout the experiment. This suggests that calcitriol may help adapt bone mineralization to accelerated bone formation during growth hormone treatment. Effects of rhGH on bone formation are blunted in unloaded hypophysectomized rats indicating that the physiological stimulus of bone turnover has always the most predominant effect on bone formation.

GH has been given to young males [27] and to healthy elderly people [28] for short periods. The effects seen were similar to those seen in GH deficiency. Rudman et al. [29] treated old men with low IGF-I levels with 0.03 mg/kg of rhGH three times per week for 1 year. They also reported on the known effects of GH on muscle and fat mass. Furthermore they showed a significant increase in lumbar BMD which was not seen at any other sites (hip and radius) and might be due to a statistical problem as no multivariate analysis was shown in their report. It is doubtful whether this effect can be reproduced and whether it would last for a longer period. Holloway et al. [30] reported a longer study of GH treatment in 27 healthy postmenopausal elderly women, 8 of whom took a stable dose of estrogen throughout the study. Thirteen women completed 6 months of treatment and 14 women completed 6 months in the placebo group. Side-effects prompted a 50% reduction in the original dose of rhGH (from 0.043 mg/kg body weight or approximately 0.3 mg rhGH/kg per week to 0.02 mg/kg per day) and led to several drop-outs in the treatment group. Although fat mass and percentage body fat declined in the treatment group there was no significant effect on BMD at spine or hip after 6 months or 1 year of treatment [30]. Although bone mass did not change, there were some changes in biochemical markers, particularly markers of bone resorption, the urinary pyridinolines. The effects on markers of bone formation were more variable: osteocalcin increased, type I procollagen peptide levels did not change. For women taking estrogen replacement therapy, indices of bone turnover were blunted.

Treatment of osteoporotic patients with GH has not been successful in the past. As early as 1975, two patients with osteogenesis imperfecta and one patient with involutional osteoporosis were treated with GH [30] and an increase of serum and histology markers of bone turnover was achieved. Subsequent studies employed GH with and without antiresorptive agents [32–34]. Aloia et al. [33] administered between 2 and 6 U/day of GH for 12 months to 8 patients with postmenopausal osteoporosis (the first 6 months of treatment featured low-dose GH; the last 6 months consisted of high-dose GH, (6 U/day). Radial bone mineral content dropped slightly and histomorphometric parameters did not change during treatment. However, severity of back pain decreased considerably in several patients [32]. Daily GH injections (4 U/day) combined with alternating doses of calcitonin produced an increase in total-body calcium but a decline in radial bone mass after 16 months [33]. In a separate trial, 14 postmenopausal women were given 2 months of GH then 3 months of calcitonin in a modified form of coherence therapy [34]. Total-body calcium increased 2.3% per year and there were few side-effects, but there were no changes in BMD or histomorphometric indices. Dambacher et al. [35] administered 16 U of rhGH every other day along with daily sodium fluoride to 6 women with postmenopausal osteoporosis. On histomorphometric analysis there was a significant increase in the number of osteoblasts and osteoclasts but bone mass was unchanged. Johannsen et al. [36] conducted a placebo-controlled, double-masked crossover trial of rhGH and IGF-I in 14 men with idiopathic osteoporosis. In this 7 day trial with rhGH (2 IU/m^2), procollagen peptide and osteocalcin levels increased after treatment as did urinary markers of bone resorption. The changes in osteocalcin were relatively small, however, and were not sustained after discontinuation of GH treatment. Erdtsieck et al. [37] treated 21 postmenopausal women with osteoporosis with the aminobisphosphonate pamidronate for 12 months. During the initial 6 months rhGH (0.0675 IU/kg, 3 times/week) was administered in a placebo-controlled fashion [37]. Bone mineral content (BMC) of the lumbar spine and femoral neck using dual-energy X-ray absorptiometry (DXA) and BMC of the radius using singlr photon absorptiometry (SPA) showed no change in the rhGH group; however, a consistent increase of about 5% at the lumbar spine and somewhat less in the distal forearm was reached from 6 months onward in women treated with pamidronate. Compared with baseline, the biochemical measurements of bone turnover showed a decrease of about 50% in the pamidronate group, but this was blunted in the group additionally treated with rhGH. The body composition measurements showed clear effects of rhGH administration: a decrease in fat mass of about 5% and an increase in lean body mass of about 3%. However, these effects disappeared after the treatment with rhGH was stopped and both fat mass and lean body mass returned to initial values. Thus, rhGH blunted both the pamidronate-induced accumulation of bone mineral mass and the reduction of biochemical markers of bone turnover.

New studies combined PTH and GH treatment in males with osteoporosis [38], but these have been solely published as abstracts. Finally, Gonelli et al. [39] compared three sequential treatment regimens in a single-masked, randomized study involving 30 women with postmenopausal osteoporosis. Treatments were (a) GH for 7 days, calcitonin for 21 days and a drug-free period of 61 days, (b) GH for 7 days, placebo for 21 days and a drug-free period of 61 days and (c) placebo for 7 days, calcitonin for 21 days and a drug-free period of 61 days. These cycles were repeated eight times over 24 months. GH was given at 12 IU/day (4 mg/day) and salmon calcitonin at 50 IU/day. A significant increase in BMD of the lumbar spine (2.5% per year) was seen in group (a), but this was accompanied by a significant decrease in the BMD of the femoral shaft.

IGF Treatment

Treatment with rhIGF-I has been conducted for other indications apart from osteoporosis, including diabetes mellitus, cachexia (after severe operations or burns) and amyotrophic lateral sclerosis. Compared with GH there are potential benefits from IGF-I: (1) more direct stimulation of bone formation, (2) bypass of skeletal resistance and (3) reduction in GH-induced side-effects such as diabetes mellitus and symptoms arising from GHs antinatriuretic effects such as edema and muscle pain.

Most post-oophorectomy studies in rats reported partial restoration of trabecular bone volume, increased mid-shaft tibial BMD, enhanced periosteal bone apposition, an increase in lumbar and trochanteric BMD, but no change in bone strength and stiffness during treatment with rhIGF-I. Other studies investigated the effects of rhIGF-I on osteopenia in diabetic rats, although the pathophysiology of diabetic osteopathy remains unknown. These studies failed to show that IGF-I administration could correct any inherent defect in bone formation. Development of immobilization osteopenia was thought to due to decreased IGF-I activity; however, IGF-I infusion during hindlimb elevation did not reverse the cessation in linear growth induced by immobilization, suggesting resistance to IGF-I bioactivity. However, these studies were contradicted by other investigators showing effects on bone formation by IGF-I. A complex of IGF-I/IGFBP-3 was used to treat osteopenic rats, and showed positive effects on bone formation and density having the advantage of only 10% hypoglycemia in these trials compared with 50% with rhIGF-I alone.

In normal postmenopausal women administration of rhIGF-I caused a dose-dependent increase in serum type I procollagen carboxyl-terminal propeptide

(PICP), osteocalcin and urinary deoxypyridinolines [40]. Johansson et al. [41] administered subcutaneous rhIGF-I to a man with idiopathic osteoporosis and low serum IGF-I level. Both markers of bone formation and resorption increased. Subsequently they treated several osteoporotic men with rhIGF-I; however, bone resorption increased as well as formation. There are no data on bone density or fracture rates so far, as production of stable rhIGF-I seems to be difficult and therapy results in severe side-effects such as hypoglycemia which need to be dealt with.

Ipriflavone Treatment

In contrast to the other three agents described in this chapter the flavonoid ipriflavone (7-isopropoxyisoflavone) is an antiresorptive drug. It inhibits osteoclastic resorption by potentiating estrogenic bioeffects and estrogen binding to receptor.

The mechanism of its action was investigated using highly purified chicken osteoclast precursors, which spontaneously differentiate into multinucleated osteoclasts in 3–6 days. [^{3}H]Ipriflavone binding studies indicated the presence of specific ipriflavone binding sites (two classes), both in precursor cells and in mature osteoclasts. Specific ipriflavone binding was not displaced by various modulators of avian osteoclast function, such as estradiol (10^{-8} M) or retinoic acid (10^{-6} M), indicating that ipriflavone receptors differed from the receptors for these calcium-regulating hormones. The fusion of osteoclast precursor cells was significantly inhibited by ipriflavone, which led to dose-dependent inhibition of bone resorption and tartrate-resistant acid phosphatase activity. Novel specific ipriflavone receptors that were coupled to Ca^{2+} influx were demonstrated in osteoclasts and their precursor cells. These ipriflavone receptors might provide a mechanism for regulating osteoclast differentiation and function [42]. Studies using fetal rat long bones in stationary cultures indicated that metabolites of ipriflavone, in particular M3 and M2, inhibited bPTH(1–34)-induced bone resorption. Accordingly, they might play an important role in the pharmacological effects of the drug [43]. In 10-week-old, intact and ovariectomized (OVX) rats, prelabelled from birth with [^{3}H]tetracycline, ipriflavone can decrease bone resorption in both intact and OVX animals given a purified diet as a single daily meal. In the OVX model, ipriflavone mimics the osteoprotective effect of estrogen. However, the lack of a uterotropic effect suggests that the compound can discriminate between bone and reproductive tissues [44]. Ghezzo et al. [45] found that short-term treatment with high doses of ipriflavone increased bone density and improved the biomechanical properties of adult male rat bones, without altering their mineral composition. A 12 week treatment with ipriflavone at high doses does not induce significant modifications of bone "crystallinity".

The positive effect of ipriflavone on BMD appears to be associated with an increased apatite crystal formation rather than an increase in crystal size [45]. Recently, 149 elderly, osteoporotic women (65–79 years) with prevalent vertebral fractures were enrolled in two Italian, multicenter, double-masked, 2 year studies. Women were randomly allocated to receive either oral ipriflavone (200 mg t.i.d. at meals) or matching placebo, plus 1 g oral calcium daily. A significant increase in forearm BMD was obtained after treatment. A reduction in incident vertebral fractures was observed in ipriflavone-treated women compared with control subjects. A significant improvement in bone pain and mobility has also been pointed out in one of the studies. To date, 2769 patients have been treated with ipriflavone, for a total of 3132 patient-years, in 60 clinical studies performed in Italy, Japan and

Hungary and reviewed for long-term safety assessment. The incidence of adverse reactions in ipriflavone-treated patients (14.5%) was similar to that observed in subjects receiving the placebo (16.1%). Side-effects were mainly gastrointestinal. Few patients presented reversible modifications of laboratory parameters. The data from the above studies show that long-term treatment with ipriflavone may be considered safe, and may increase bone density and possibly prevent fractures in elderly patients with established osteoporosis [46]. In another 12 month study ipriflavone increased BMD by 3-5% in the lumbar spine and in the femur neck. Significant decrease of pain was observed in 55% of the patients. The number of side-effects was low [47]. In another multicenter study a bone-sparing effect of 1.6% at the lumbar spine and of 3.5% at the radius after 2 years in 453 postmenopausal women with low bone mass was seen. Biochemical markers of bone turnover decreased in patients treated with ipriflavone [48]. Ipriflavone plus low-dose hormone replacement therapy (HRT) in the prevention of postmenopausal bone loss was unable to increase the antiresorptive effect of ipriflavone and did not exert any further action in the prevention of postmenopausal osteopenia [49]. A large multicenter European study was designed to determine the risk of vertebral fracture in postmenopausal, osteoporotic women [50].

Summary and Conclusions

GH is a potent anabolic hormone for almost all systems including bone and calcium metabolism. This has been previously discussed in numerous excellent reviews [51–58]. Patients with hypopituitarism have signs and symptoms of osteoporosis and increased fracture rate [59]. Most of the signs and symptoms in the syndrome of GH deficiency can be restored by substitution of the necessary hormones including GH. Initial effects have been published in numerous reviews [6,57]. Effects on bone density and size are shown in Fig. 35.4 [60]. Similar effects are seen with PTH. It is important to note that calculated effects on bone densitometry measurements might be influenced by changes in bone size induced by PTH or GH. Whereas increased effects on BMC induced by GH are not due to losses in peripheral bones but newly formed bone, PTH induces a reduction in peripheral BMD. The combination of GH or PTH with antiresorptive agents has been tried in several studies. The effects with PTH were promising, whereas GH was not able to promote its anabolic effects in the presence of antiresorptive agents. Recent studies have shown the effect of exercise or loading in combination with GH treatment. As for any anti-osteoporotic drug, rhGH is not able to stimulate bone formation in an unloaded state. Thus vigorous exercise in combination with muscle training and rhGH treatment might be an option to treat osteoporosis still to be studied. However, it is interesting to wait for the results of long-term studies on the effects on BMD and fracture rates in studies with PTH or GH. As GH and IGF-I seems to reverse some signs of old age such as muscle weakness and reduced exercise capacity, one might speculate that GH could prevent the occurrence of hip fractures in elderly people.

Ipriflavone is another antiresorptive drug and an alternative to estrogens and SERMs (selective estrogen receptor modulators); however, studies on fracture rates have not been published.

Acknowledgements. I wish to thank my wife and my children for their patience with me while I was writing and being in a different world.

References

1. Wüster C, Heilmann P, Pereira-Lima J, Schlegel J, Anstätt K, Soballa T. Quantitative ultrasonometry (qus) for the evaluation of osteoporosis risk: reference data for various measurement sites, limitations and application possiblities. Exp Clin Endocrinol Diabetes 1998;106:277–288.
2. Kanis JA. Assessment of fracture risk and its application to screening for postmenopausal osteoporosis : synopsis of a WHO report. Osteoporos Int 1994;4:368–381.
3. Cummings SR, Nevitt MC, Browner WS, et al. Risk factors for hip fractures in white women. N Engl J Med 1995;332:767–773.
4. Wüster C.. Growth hormone and ageing. In: Scherbaum W, Rossmanith WG, editors. Endocrinology of aging, W. Berlin: De Gruyter, 1995:95–112.
5. Wüster C. Growth hormone, insulin-like growth factors and bone metabolism. Endocrinol Metab 1995;2:3–12.
6. Rosen C, Wüster C. Growth hormone, insulin-like growth factors: potential applications and limitations in the management of osteoporosis. In: Marcus R, Feldman D, editors. Osteoporosis. San Diego: Academic Press, 1996:1313–1333.
7. Carlsson B, Eden S, Nilsson A, Ohlsson C, Törnell J, Vikman K, et al. Expression and physiological significance of grwoth hormone receptors and growth hormone binding protein in rat and man. Acta Pediatr Scand 1991;379(Suppl):70–76.
8. Canalis E, Centrella M, Burch W, McCarthy T. Insulin-like growth factor I mediates selective anabolic effects of parathyroid hormone in bone cultures. J Clin Invest 1989;83:60–65.
9. Harrington EA, Fanidi A, Evan GI. Oncogenes and cell death. Genet Dev 1994;4:120–129.
10. Nishiyama K; Sugimoto T; Kaji H; Kanatani M; Kobayashi T; Chihara K Stimulatory effect of growth hormone on bone resorption and osteoclast differentiation. Endocrinology 1996;137:35–41.
11. Wüster C. Osteoporose durch Mangel an Calcitonin und Wachstumshormon: Untersuchungen mittels Knochenzellkultur, Tiermodell und Osteodensitometrie. Thesis of habilitation at the Faculty of Clinical Medicine I, Ruprecht-Karls-Universität Heidelberg, 1993:79–82.
12. Mohan S, Baylink DJ. The role Of IGF-II in the coupling of bone formation to resorption. In: Spencer EM, editor. Modern concepts of insulin-like growth factors. New York: Elsevier, 1991:169–184.
13. Müller C, Wüster C, Seibel M, Knauf K, Ziegler R. Cosecretion of human growth hormone and bone markers. Thesis, University of Heidelberg, 1998.
14. Jørgensen PH, Bak B, Andreassen TT. Mechanical properties and biochemical composition of rat cortical femur and tibia after long-term treatment with biosynthetic human growth hormone. Bone 1991;12:353–359.
15. Andreassen TT, Melsen F, Oxlund H. The influence of growth hormone on cancellous and cortical bone of the vertebral body in aged rats. J Bone Miner Res 1996;11: 1094–1102.
16. Wüster CHR, Blum WF, Schlemilch S, Ranke MB, Ziegler R. Decreased serum levels of insulin like growth factors 1 and 2 and IGF binding protein-3 in patients with osteoporosis. J Intern Med 1993;234:249–255.
17. Wüster C, Köppler D, Müller C, Seibel MJ, Schmidt-Gayk, Blum HW et al. Normal GH-, PICP- and ICTP- and decreased PTH-24 hour-secretion in osteoporosis. Osteoporos Int 1996;6(Suppl 1):102.
18. Mosekilde L, Danielsen C, Gasser JA. The effect on vertebral bone mass and strength of long term treatment with antiresorptive agents (estrogen and calcitonin), human parathyroid hormone (1–38), and combination treatment, assessed in aged ovariectomized rats. Endocrinology 1994;134:2126–2134.
19. Lane NE, Kimmel DB, Nilsson MH, Cohen FE, Newton S, Nissenson RA, et al. Bone-selective analogs of human PTH(1–34) increase bone formation in an ovariectomized rat model. J Bone Miner Res. 1996;11:614–625.

20. Lane NE; Thompson JM; Strewler GJ; Kinney JH. Intermittent treatment with human parathyroid hormone (hPTH[1-34]) increased trabecular bone volume but not connectivity in osteopenic rats. J Bone Miner Res 1995;10:1470–1477.
21. Reeve J, Meunier PJ, Parsons JA, Bernat M, Bijvoet OL, Courpron P, et al. Anabolic effect of human parathyroid hormone fragment on trabecular bone in involutional osteoporosis: a multicentre trial. BMJ 1980;280:1340–1344.
22. Yuan ZZ, Jee WS, Ma YF, Wei W, Ijiri K. Parathyroid hormone therapy accelerates recovery from immobilization-induced osteopenia. Bone 1995;17(Suppl 4):219S–223S.
23. Andreassen TT, Jorgensen PH, Flyvbjerg A, Orskov H, Oxlund H. Growth hormone stimulates bone formation and strength of cortical bone in aged rats. J Bone Miner Res. 1995;10:1057–1067.
24. Ørtoft G, Brüel A, Andreassen, Oxlund H. Growth hormone is not able to counteract osteopenia of rat cortical bone induced by glucocorticoid with protracted effect. Bone 1995;17:543–548.
25. Sandstedt J, Tornell J, Norjavaara E, Isaksson OG, Ohlsson C. Elevated levels of growth hormone increase bone mineral content in normal young mice, but not in ovariectomized mice. Endocrinology. 1996;137:3368–3374.
26. Denis I, Zerath E, Pointillart A. Effects of exogenous growth hormone on bone mineralization and remodeling and on plasma calcitriol in intact pigs. Bone 1994;15:419–424.
27. Brixen K, Nielsen Hk, Mosekilde L, Flyvbjerg A. A short course of recombinant human growth hormone treatment stimulates osteoblasts and activates bone remodeling in normal human volunteers. J Bone Miner Res 1990;5:609–618.
28. Marcus R, Butterfield G, Holloway L, Gilliland L, Baylink Dj, Hintz Rl, et al. Effects of short term administration of recombinant human growth hormone to elderly people. J Clin Endocrinol Metab 1990;70:519–527.
29. Rudman D, Feller AG, Nagraj HS, Gergnas GA, Laltha PY, Goldberg AF, et al. Effects of growth hormone in men over 60 years old. N Engl J Med 1990;323:1–6.
30. Holloway L, Butterfield G, Hintz Rl, Gesundheit N, Marcus R. Effects of recombinant human growth hormone on metabolic indices, body composition, and bone turnover in healthy elderly women. J Endocrinol Metab 1994;79:470–479.
31. Kruse HP, Kuhlencordt F. On an attempt to treat primary and secondary osteoporosis with human growth hormone. Horm Metab Res 7:488–91 (1975).
32. Aloia JF, Zanzi I, Ellis K, Jowsey J, Roginski M, Wallach S, et al. Effects of growth hormone in osteoporosis. J Clin Endocr Metab 1976;43:922–999.
33. Aloia JF, Vaswani A, Kapoor A, Yeh JK, Cohn SH. Treatment of osteoporosis with calcitonin with and without growth hormone. Metabolism 1985;34:124–131.
34. Aloia JF, Vaswani A, Meunier PJ, Edourd CM, Arlot ME, Yeh JK, et al. Coherence treatment of postmenopausal osteoporosis with growth hormone and calcitonin. Calcif Tissue Int 1987;40:253–259.
35. Dambacher MA, Lauffenberger T, Haas HG. Vergelich verschiedener medikamentöser Therapieformen bei Osteoporose (NaF, NaF + Vitamin D, 1,25$(OH)_2D_3$ und menschliches Wachstumshormon) Kurz- und Langzeituntersuchungen. Akt Rheumatol 1982;7:249–252.
36. Johannson AG, Lindh E, Blum WF, Kollerup G, Sorensen OH, Ljunghall S. Effects of growth hormone and insulin-like growth factor I in men with idiopathic osteoporosis J Clin Endocrinol Metab 1996;81:44–48.
37. Erdtsieck RJ, Pols HAP, Valk NK, van Ouwerkerk BM, Lamberts SWJ, Birkenhäger JC. Treatment of postmenopausal osteoporosis with a combination of growth hormone and pamidronate: a placebo-controlled trial. Clin Endocrinol 1995;43:557–565.
38. Harms HM, König S, Wüstermann PR, von zur Mühlen A, Hesch RD. Knochenstoffwechselparameter bei Patienten mit Osteoporose unter Therapie mit humanem Parathormon-(1–38)(hPTH1–38) und rekombinantem Wachstumshoromon (rhGH). In: Wüster C, Raue R, Ziegler R, editors. Osteologie`92. Heidelberg: Merges, 1992:29.
39. Gonelli S, Cepollaro C, Montomoli M, Gennari L, Montagnani A, Plamieri R. Treatment

of postmenopausal osteoporosis with recombinant human growth hormone and salmon calcitonin: a placebo-controlled study. Clin Endocrinol 1997;46:55–61.
40. Ebeling PR, Jones JD, O`Fallon WM, Janes CH, Riggs BL. Short term effects of recombinant IGF-I on bone turnover in normal women. J Clin Endocrinol Metab 1990;70:1292–1298.
41. Johannson AG, Lindh E, Ljunghall S. IGF-I stimulates bone turnover in osteoporosis. Lancet 1992;339:1619.
42. Miyauchi A, Notoya K, Taketomi S, Takagi Y, Fujii Y, Jinnai K, et al. Novel ipriflavone receptors coupled to calcium influx regulate osteoclast differentiation and function. Endocrinology 1996;137:3544–3550.
43. Giossi M, Caruso P, Civelli M, Bongrani S. Inhibition of parathyroid hormone-stimulated resorption in cultured fetal rat long bones by the main metabolites of ipriflavone. Calcif Tissue Int 1996; 58:419–422.
44. Cecchini MG, Fleisch H, Mühlbauer RC. Ipriflavone inhibits bone resorption in intact and ovariectomized rats. Calcif Tissue Int 1997;61(Suppl 1):S9–11.
45. Ghezzo C, Civitelli R, Cadel S, Borelli G, Maiorino M, Bufalino L, et al. Ipriflavone does not alter bone apatite crystal structure in adult male rats. Calcif Tissue Int 1996;59:496–499.
46. Agnusdei D, Bufalino L. Efficacy of ipriflavone in established osteoporosis and long-term safety. Calcif Tissue Int 1997;61(Suppl 1):S23–S27.
47. Szanto F. Experience with ipriflavone therapy in postmenopausal osteoporosis. F Orv Hetil 1997;138:2801–2803.
48. Gennari C, Adami S, Agnusdei D, Bufalino L, Cervetti R, Crepaldi G, et al. Effect of chronic treatment with ipriflavone in postmenopausal women with low bone mass. Calcif Tissue Int 1997;61(Suppl 1): S19–S22.
49. De Aloysio D, Gambacciani M, Altieri P, Ciaponi M, Ventura V, Mura M, et al. Bone density changes in postmenopausal women with the administration of ipriflavone alone or in association with low-dose ERT. Gynecol Endocrinol 1997;11:289–293.
50. Reginster JY, Bufalino L, Christiansen C, Devogelaer JP, Gennari C, Riis BJ, et al. Design for an ipriflavone multicenter European fracture study. Calcif Tissue Int 1997;61(Suppl 1):S28–S32.
51. Rosen CJ, Donahue LR, Hunter SJ. Insulin-like growth factors and bone: the osteoporosis connection. Proc Soc Exp Biol Med 1994;206:83–102.
52. Johansson A, Lindh E, Ljunghall S. Growth hormone, insulin-like growth factor I, and bone: a clinical review. J Intern Med 1993:234:553–560.
53. Slootweg MC. Growth hormone and bone. Horm Metab Res 1993;25:335–343.
54. Inzucchi SE, Robbins RJ. Clinical review 61: effects of growth hormone on human bone biology. J Clin Endocrinol Metab 1994;79:691–694.
55. Parfitt AM. Growth hormone and adult bone remodelling. Clin Endocrinool 1991;35: 467–470.
56. Eriksen EF, Kassem M, Langdahl B. Growth hormone, insulin-like growth factors and bone remodelling. Eur J Clin Invest 1996;26:525–534.
57. Ohlsson C, Bengtsson BÅ, Isaksson OG, Andreassen TT, Slootweg MC. Growth hormone and bone. Endocr Rev 1998;19:55–79.
58. Bouillon R, editor. GH and bone. London: OCC, 1998.
59. Wüster C, Slenczka E, Ziegler R. Erhöhte Prävalenz von Osteoporose und Arteriosklerose bei konventionell substituierter Hypophysenvorderlappeninsuffizienz: Bedarf einer zusätzlichen Wachstumshormonsubstitution? Klin Wochenschr 1991;69: 769–773.
60. Wüster C, et al. Benefits of growth hormone treatment on bone metabolism, bone density and bone strength in growth hormone deficiency. Growth Horm IGF Res 1998;8(Suppl A):87–94.

Part VI

Identification and Management of Secondary or Localized Bone Loss

36 Osteoporosis in Rheumatoid Arthritis

J. Dequeker, R. Westhovens, I. Ravelingien

Is Osteoporosis an Extra-articular Manifestation of Rheumatoid Arthritis?

Bone loss has been recognized as a complication of the rheumatoid process for more than a century. Barwel was the first to apply the term "osteoporosis" to the bone disease in rheumatoid arthritis (RA) [1]. Osteoporosis, as recognized by Soila [2], McConkey et al. [3], Saville and Kharmosh [4] and Kennedy and Lindsay [5], may be localized, occurring close to the site of inflamed joints, or generalized, involving the whole skeleton.

There have been a number of controversial reports regarding the systemic effect of RA on bone metabolism. Parathyroid overactivity and hypercalcemia, as well as osteomalacia, have been proposed as part of the rheumatoid process. RA affects more women (pre- and postmenopausal) than men and leads to chronic immobility in some but not others. It is accompanied by serum protein alterations and requires a variety of drug treatment regimens. These different factors all influence bone remodelling indices, so that evaluation of the effect of RA is complicated and very difficult [6]. For these reasons, we [7] prospectively studied bone metabolism indices in a homogeneous group of postmenopausal women with RA who were hospitalized because of exacerbation of their disease activity. Patients with RA who never had steroid treatment differed from the control population as they had significantly higher serum phosphorus concentrations, alkaline phosphatase activity, and osteocalcin concentrations. Calcitropic hormone concentrations (parathyroid hormone, 25-hydroxy- and 1,25-dihydroxyvitamin D concentrations) were normal. Serum calcium concentrations were also normal when corrected for serum albumin. Excretion of urinary hydroxyproline and glycosaminoglycan was significantly increased [8–10]. These results have been confirmed with newer bone turnover markers [11–14]. Oelzner et al. [13] found a decreased 1,25-vitamin D level in RA and this was correlated with disease activity. These data, in particular the 1,25-vitamin D decrease, should be corrected for changes in vitamin D protein levels.

In two population-based studies, one from Finland [15] and one from the United States [16], a lower axial bone density in RA patients who never used corticosteroids was found. In the Finnish study, the decrease at the spine of 5.5% was not significant, but the decrease of 8.7% at the hip was highly significant. In the United

States study, elderly patients taking part in a population study, with self-reported RA (confirmed by a hand radiograph) and who never had taken corticosteroids, had a significantly lower lumbar bone mineral density (BMD) (−8.4%) than controls, while those currently on steroids ($n = 13$) had a BMD that was not significantly lower. These findings are in contrast with the other studies mentioned above. Because the RA patients in this study had mean disease duration of ± 24 years, and a mean age of 74 years, probably other factors such as selection or concomitant diseases are involved.

Recent studies using dual-energy X-ray absorptiometry (DXA) of the spine and proximal femur demonstrated a reduction in BMD at the hip, but not the spine, in postmenopausal women and men with RA [11,17–21]. The hip–spine discrepancy remains unexplained, but it would appear that the hip is a more vulnerable site than the spine for osteopenia in RA. The reduction in BMD at the hip is related to disability and knee/foot arthritis, and therefore cannot be considered as a parameter for a systemic effect of RA on bone. Although the data suggest a higher metabolic bone activity in RA, no increased bone loss in the vertebral column was detected. Massive osteolysis in RA occurs rarely and is usually associated with concomitant diseases [22]. Compston et al. [23], using computed tomography, found no difference in spinal bone content between female RA patients age > 50 years and controls. Two longitudinal studies of axial bone loss in RA revealed either no or only a moderate difference between patients (most of them were on low-dose corticosteroids) and controls in the rate of loss at the spine, but a tendency toward more rapid femoral bone loss in the RA patients was noted [24].

Periarticular Osteoporosis Reflects Disease Activity in Early Arthritis

Juxta-articular bone loss, or osteopenia, affecting the hands and feet, is one of the earliest radiological changes in RA. Juxta-articular bone loss precedes the development of erosions and probably results from the release of bone-resorbing cytokines, such as interleukins 1 and 6 and tumor necrosis factor, from the diseased synovium [25]. However, osteopenia does not become apparent radiologically until a considerable proportion of the bone mineral has been lost. Quantification of juxta-articular bone loss could be a sensitive index of joint damage.

Juxta-articular bone mass has been found to be decreased in RA using metacarpal indices [26] and by measurement of the distal radius using either single photon absorptiometry (SPA) [27] or quantitative computed tomography (QCT) [28]. Sambrook et al. [28] demonstrated that bone loss from the distal radius was more rapid in patients with early RA than in normal controls, while there was no between-group difference in the rates of loss from the lumbar spine or mid-radius. Precise quantification of bone loss from the site of the earliest radiological changes in RA, namely the hand, may predict joint destruction [11,29].

The development of DXA has enabled the precise and accurate measurement of BMC and BMD of the entire skeleton or of selected regions of interest.

Peel et al. [30] used DXA measurements to determine hand BMD in a series of postmenopausal RA patients and examined the relationship between hand BMD, disease activity and disability in patients with relatively early disease. Hand BMD correlated negatively with disease activity as assessed by erythrocyte sedimentation rate (ESR) ($r = 0.81$), and with disability ($r = 0.49$) as estimated by grip strength. In a longitudinal study Gough et al. [24]found a significant bone loss at the lumbar spine related to disease activity (CRP) in patients with early RA, but they did not separate corticosteroid-treated and non-corticosteroid-treated cases.

The same group reported recently longitudinal data on biochemical markers of bone turnover in RA [12]. They found that mean urinary pyridinoline and deoxypyridinoline levels correlated strongly with BMD changes at all sites, were increased in patients with active disease ($p < 0.005$), and correlated closely with mean C-reactive protein (CRP) ($p < 0.005$, $r \geqslant 0.41$ for both).

Pathophysiology of Bone Loss in RA

There is much evidence to suggest that interleukin-1 (IL-1) plays a crucial role in the pathophysiology of periarticular bone loss in RA, in addition to disuse bone loss. The plasma levels of IL-1 beta are significantly higher in RA patients than in controls and correlate positively with clinical disease activity, (Ritchie index, pain score and ESR) and negatively with hemoglobin concentration [25].

Many activities of IL-1 are relevant to RA [31]. IL-1 increases the release from synovial cells of vasoactive agents and mediators of tissue damage (e.g., prostaglandins, proteinolytic enzymes and reactive oxygen molecules) and is a powerful stimulus of bone and cartilage resorption. It also induces the acute-phase response and fever and may potentiate chronic inflammation by induction of lymphocyte growth factors such as interleukin 2 and its receptor.

Local factors such as tumor necrosis factor (TNF), and systemic hormones such as parathyroid hormones and 1,25-dihydroxyvitamin D_3, promote the development of osteoclasts through their ability to stimulate the production of cytokines such as IL-6 and IL-1.

The recognition that changes in the number of bone cells, rather than changes in the activity of individual cells, form the pathogenetic basis of osteoporosis is a major advance in understanding the mechanisms of this disease [32]. Because cytokines are produced by activated leukocytes, they may be instrumental in inducing the local osteolysis commonly observed in bone adjacent to inflammatory sites. However, it is difficult to discern a clear adaptive role for local osteolysis in inflammation and this may not be their primary role. TNFα appears to be an agent of the systemic response to inflammatory and injurious agents and enhanced bone resorption by effecting a shift in skeletal homeostasis towards catabolism [33]. Local inflammatory osteolysis may be explicable as a perturbation of normal physiological mechanisms through immigration into bone of inflammatory cells that produce TNF for other purposes.

Symptomatic Fractures in RA and Ankylosing Spondylitis

In contrast to the abundant information on bone density measurements in RA, data on symptomatic fracture incidence in RA are scarce [34]. The available data suggest an increased relative risk for hip fracture: 1.51 (95% confidence intervals (CI) 1.01, 2.17) [35] and 2.1 (95% CI 1.0, 4.7) [36]. After excluding patients with corticosteroid use, the odds ratio is still increased, but not statistically significant: 1.9 (95% CI 0.9, 4.3) [36].

With the focus on patients with severe functional impairment – that is, Steinbrocker scores 3 and 4 – the hip fracture risk is markedly increased: relative risk 4.2 (95% CI 1.8, 8.3) [35] and 4.4 (95% CI 2.4, 8.4) respectively [36].

In a cross-sectional study [37], 12.1% of patients with RA had vertebral fractures, compared with 6.2% of the age- and sex-matched controls (odds ratio 2.1; 95% CI 1.2, 3.7). These data suggest a doubling of the rate of vertebral and hip fractures in patients with severe RA, because of disability or because of RA itself.

In a large RA population follow-up study of 6.7 years in 395 cases, multivariate analysis identified use of corticosteroids in women and prior to diagnosis of osteoporosis as an important risk for fracture. Among patients taking 5 mg or more of prednisone, female sex strongly predicted fractures: the 5-year probability of having a fracture was 34% [38].

Vertebral fractures are a recognized complication of advanced ankylosing spondylitis (AS) and are generally thought to result from chronic inflammation of the axial skeleton and from enhanced biomechanical fragility of an ankylosed spine. Cooper et al. [39], in a population-based cohort study of 2398 person-years of observation, found that there was no increase in the risk of limb fractures but a pronounced increase in the risk of thoracolumbar compression fractures (standardized morbidity ratio = 7.6; 95% CI 4.3, 12.6) among those with ankylosing spondylitis.

Cervical Spine Instability in RA: Treatment Challenges

RA may affect the cervical spine and in particular the C1–2 region, without much pain. Tenosynovitis of the transverse ligament of C1, which stabilizes the odontoid process (dens) of C2, may produce significant C1–2 instability allowing myelopathy due to pressure on the cord. Careful neurological examination is mandatory because, for example, positive Hoffman–Trömer sign of the fingers, sensation of electricity in the fingers and general power loss in the limbs are alarming signs of myelopathy. A lateral spinal radiograph of the cervical spine in flexion will show subluxation of the C1–2 region (Fig. 36.1) and a through-the-mouth view will show the erosions of the odontoid and eventually instability of the apophyseal joint (Fig. 36.2) [40].

Preoperatively, more accurate staging of a neurological compression using magnetic resonance imaging (MRI) is indicated. MRI is for this situation a better imaging procedure than computed tomography (CT) (Fig. 36.3). It is recommended that the MRI examinations also be done in the cervical spine in flexion.

The prevalence of cervical subluxation in RA has been reported to be 43–86%, the magnitude being related to the severity of the systemic disease process [41]. Atlanto-axial subluxation is the most common type and can be anterior (30–70%), posterior (2%), vertical (14–27%) or lateral (14%) [41–44]. Most surgeons will intervene in a patient with myelopathy or intractable cervical pain. However, on the question of prophylactic surgery for a patient with an abnormal atlanto-dens interval and no neurological signs, there is less unanimity. The divergence of opinion as to when surgery is appropriate arises from the unpredictability of radiological progression and the poor correlation between an increasing atlanto-dens interval and the development of neurological signs (only 7–34%) [41]. Damage to the spinal cord is believed to be mechanical in origin. Repeated minor trauma from the spinal cord causes incremental damage.

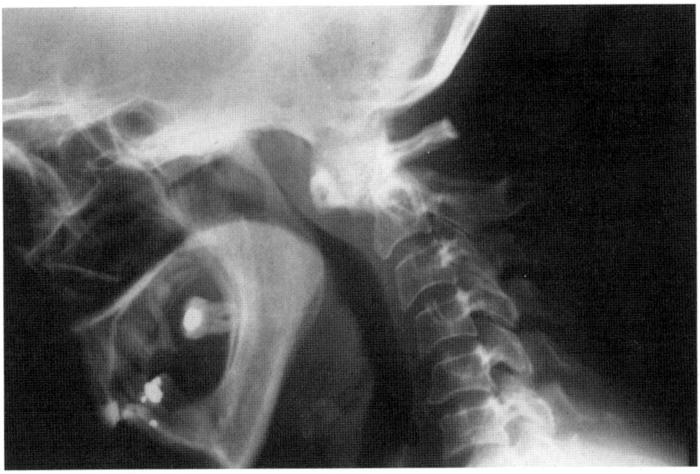

Figure 36.1. Lateral radiograph of the cervical spine in flexion.

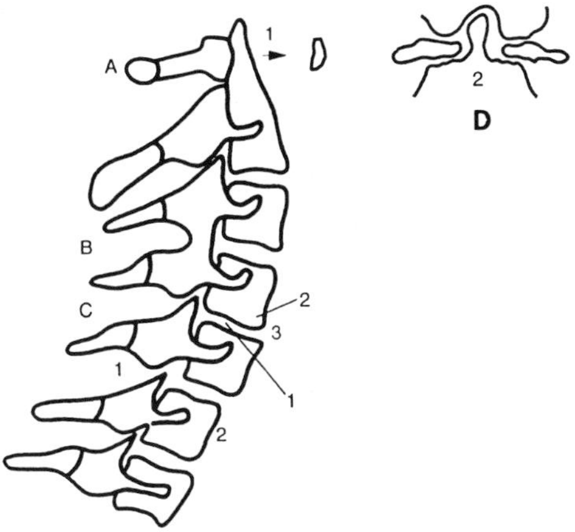

Figure 36.2. The radiographic alterations in the cervical spine in RA. *A* Subluxation of C1–2 *(1)*. The atlas (C2) is more than 3 mm separated from the anterior face of the odontoid (C1) on a lateral radiograph of the cervical spine in flexion. There is erosion of the odontoid *(2)*. *B* Fusion of the apophyseal joint C3–4. *C* Rheumatoid spondylodiscitis. Note the disc narrowing *(1)*, erosion of the vertebral endplates *(2)* and moderate osteophyte formation *(3)*. *D* Destruction of the apophyseal joint C5–6 *(1)* with anterolisthesis of C5–6 *(2)*. From [40], by permission of Marcel Dekker.

Recently [45], early operative treatment for any evidence of neurological dysfunction that is caused by subluxation of the cervical spine due to RA has been advocated by many authors because of the risk of myelopathy that can be irreversible. Conservative treatment (a soft collar) often delays surgery to a stage at which the operation is more extensive and hazardous, and may have little to offer. In a recent study [42], patients with Ranawat classification IIIa (ambulatory, paresis and long tract signs) and IIIb (quadriparesis, not ambulatory) were compared. The crucial

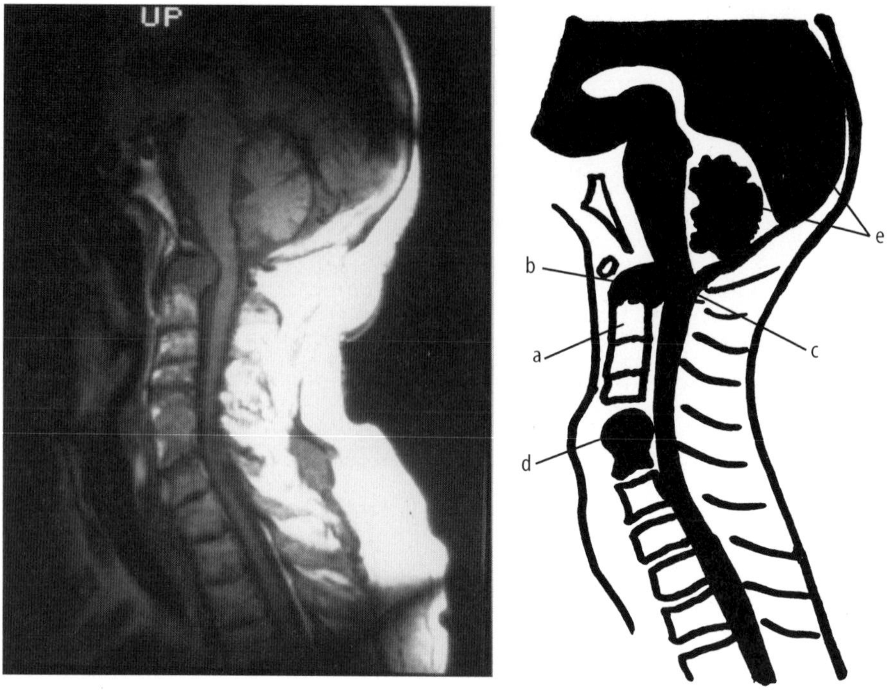

Figure 36.3. Sagittal T1-weighted MR spin-echo image of the cervical spine: *(a)* corpus of C2, *(b)* pannus tissue, *(c)* replaced upper cervical, *(d)* cerebellum, *(e)* rheumatoid discitis C5–6.

point is that surgery on these class IIIb patients has a much higher morbidity and mortality than in class IIIa, with poorer neurological and functional recovery.

The primary goal of arthrodesis is to prevent irreversible neurological complaints. Some authors [41] recommend operative stabilization of the rheumatoid cervical spine, in the presence or absence of a neurological deficit, for patients who have atlanto-axial subluxation and a posterior atlanto-odontoid interval of 14 mm or less, patients who have atlanto-axial subluxation and at least 5 mm of basilar invagination, and patients who have subaxial subluxation and a sagittal diameter of the spinal canal of 14 mm or less. The anterior atlanto-odontoid interval has traditionally been reported as the determinant of atlanto-axial instability, but in recent studies [41] the posterior atlanto-odontoid interval was a more reliable predictor of the development and severity of paralysis.

The surgery involved in RA is often demanding: poor bone quality, impaired wound healing, susceptibility to infection and joint disability may limit postoperative rehabilitation. Factors that influence the extent and type of surgery are listed in Tables 36.1 and 36.2.

There is much discussion regarding the preferred technique. There is no simple answer. One of the most difficult questions in terms of the choice of surgical procedure is assessment of bone quality. Manifestly osteoporotic bone will not "take" any form of screw fixation. By spreading the load over more segments than one would normally immobilize, the construct/bone interface may survive. In such a situation the lamina may be the strongest part of the segment and a cable construct

Table 36.1. Management strategies for cervical instability in RA

	Advantages	Disadvantages
Collar	Feels good	No effect
Traction	Reduction (sometimes)	Complications of recumbency
Halo	Immobilization (reduction sometimes)	Very difficult for patient
Laminectomy	Decompression	Kyphos formation Further compression
Anterior plates	Anterior tension band	Screw "pull-out" in poor bone
Vertebrectomy	Decompression	Kyphos; needs halo or posterior surgery
Posterior implant	Posterior tension band; good fixation	May need anterior decompression as well
Transoral	Decompression	Difficult surgery needs posterior fixation as well
Lateral mass screws	Good fixation	Needs good bone
Occipitocervical fixation	Good fixation	Stiff neck; occasional subaxial subluxation
Bone graft	Fusion	High nonfusion rate; donor site infection

Stainless steel implants should be avoided to allow postoperative magnetic resonance studies
From [43].

Table 36.2. Various surgical strategies for cervical instability in RA

	Good bone quality	Poor bone quality
Halo	4+	2+
Anterior plate alone	2+	–
Vertebrectomy	+	–
Post-fixation alone	4+	–
Anterior and posterior surgery	4+	3+
Transoral decompression	4+	4+
Transoral fixation	–	–
Lateral mass screws	4+	–
Bone graft alone	–	–
Bone graft with implant	4+	–
Occipitocervical fixation	4+	3+
Screws	4+	–
Sublaminar cables	4+	3+
Interspinous cables/wires	–	–
Laminectomy	–	–

From [43].

The advisability varies from expected good results (4+) to potential disaster (–).
++++ = 4+; +++ = 3+; ++ = 2+; + = 1; – = minus.

may be preferable to a screw construct. But even with the most aggressive surgery and the application of a halo body jacket there may still be up to a 20% nonunion in the end-stage disease [43].

In summary, though cervical surgery in RA patients is difficult, there is growing evidence that perhaps it should be considered earlier before irreversible damage is done.

Corticosteroid Osteoporosis: Is There a Threshold Dose?

The deleterious effects of corticosteroids on bone mass and the fracture rate are well known. A number of older as well as more recent studies [46–49] using modern technology to estimate bone mass, have clearly shown that even relatively low doses of corticosteroids have a negative effect on bone and that ultimately the cumulative dose of corticosteroids is the cause for concern rather than the actual dosage of corticosteroids. However, a temporary use of corticosteroids in very active inflammatory disease states could prevent severe bone loss due to immobilization and/or disease activity.

Multivariate analysis of the BMD data obtained by Dykman et al. [50], using SPA at the radius and previous corticosteroid therapy, demonstrated clearly that the cumulative dose of prednisone is the most important factor determining corticosteroid osteopenia. Patients who had taken a cumulative dose of > 30 g of prednisone had the highest incidence of fracture (53%) and osteopenia (78%).

It is evident that a daily dose of 5 mg will take 16 years to reach the 30 g cumulative dose but a daily dose of 30 mg will reach this point in 2.7 years. Therefore, cross-sectional and longitudinal studies looking only at actual daily doses may be misleading.

Few longitudinal studies on the effect of corticosteroids on bone have been reported, and some of those were done in patients receiving corticosteroid treatment for some time [26,38,51]. In addition, some studies showed no increased rates of bone loss as this occurs early in the course of corticosteroid therapy [52,53].

Laan et al. [48] studied the effect of short course of low-dose corticosteroids (10 mg/day initially) on bone mass in 40 cases with RA, using dual-energy computed tomography (DEQCT). The study design was carefully elaborated, using a method which could evaluate trabecular bone changes better than the usual integral cortical–trabecular DXA method, by selectively looking at trabecular bone. The authors found an impressive bone loss of −8.2% within 6 months compared with placebo-treated patients, and a recovery of 5.3% after stopping corticosteroid treatment compared with no changes in the placebo group. In their cross-sectional study also using DEQCT they found, after correction for confounding variables, that the lumbar BMD was highly significantly influenced by low-dose prednisone therapy (< 10 mg) in postmenopausal patients: −31.2% on trabecular BMD and −37.2% on cortical BMD [47].

These impressive results of marked bone loss under corticosteroids and recovery after withdrawal deserve some comment [54]. Although the authors correctly used DEQCT, the interpretation of the data requires thoughtful consideration. One of the major problems of QCT is the influence of fat replacement on the density measurements. The loss of "bone density" measured by QCT in conditions of bone loss due to estrogens, corticosteroids and immobilization necessitates correct interpretation. In these conditions of bone loss, adipose tissue will fill the resulting space and this can introduce errors in the technique of measurement. Even though DEQCT has only about half the fat error of single energy QCT (SEQCT), the error remains large. For CT scanners operating at 140 kVp this amounts to 15 mg/cm^3 for each 100 mg/cm^3 of fat with SEQCT and ±7 mg/cm^3 for DEQCT. A change of 100 mg/cm^3 can occur rapidly with corticosteroids, leading to an apparent decrease in bone density [55].

In addition, the extent of bone loss and the reversibility of corticosteroid-induced osteoporosis should be reconsidered. This study demonstrates clearly that corticosteroid-induced bone loss occurs at a lower rate than previously reported. How much of the corticosteroid-induced osteoporosis is really reversible is questionable, despite the fact that also in Cushing's disease a reversal of BMD has been observed [56].

It is of interest to compare total corticosteroid bone loss with what is lost early in RA. Gough et al. [24] published results of an early arthritis clinic in Birmingham.

At 1 year, loss was greater in patients than in controls and reached statistical significance for women with early RA, in particular at the proximal femur measurement site (−2 vs −1% in the spine). The greatest loss was associated with the use of intermediate doses of corticosteroids (1–5 mg/day). Persistent elevation of C-reactive protein was a consistent predictor of BMD loss at all sites. These results are in line with data reported earlier by Hall et al. [17] in a larger group of postmenopausal patients with RA compared with 597 postmenopausal control subjects. Compared with controls, the never users had no difference in BMD at the lumbar spine but a 6.9% reduction at the femur. In current users (mean daily prednisone dosage 6.9 mg), BMD was reduced by 6.5% at the spine and by 7.4% at the hip, compared with never users after adjustment for age, weight, duration of menopause and functional disability. Also in men with RA, BMD is significantly reduced at the femoral neck in steroid and nonsteroid-treated group and at the spine in the steroid-treated group [18].

The effect of low-dose corticosteroids on bone density in the absence of several independent factors was studied longitudinally in polymyalgia rheumatica cases and found to be deleterious, involving trabecular and cortical bone [57,58].

Intra-articular administration of corticosteroids has no net effects on bone resorption and only a transient systemic effect on bone formation [59].

In conclusion, most studied agreed that osteoporosis in postmenopausal women and men with RA is more evident in the hip than the spine, and the most important determinants of bone loss are disability and cumulative corticosteroid dose. Low-dose steroids should not be used with complacency. Recovery after discontinuation is doubtful and unproven. Patients taking steroids probably have vertebral fractures and femoral neck fractures at higher thresholds of spine and hip density than nonusers, but by no means all patients taking steroids develop fractures. The wide variation may reflect genetic differences in susceptibility to corticosteroids or variability in the pharmacokinetics or bone quality changes among individuals.

Pathophysiology of Corticosteroid-Induced Osteoporosis

The strategy for prevention and treatment of corticosteroid-induced osteoporosis has to be based on solid scientific evidence. Fig. 36.4 shows the pathophysiology of corticosteroid-induced osteoporosis [60]. Corticosteroid excess causes bone loss by two mechanisms: suppression of osteoblast function and increased osteoclastic resorption. The suppression of osteoblast function results in the reduced synthesis of bone matrix and therefore in reduced bone formation. As shown by serum osteocalcin concentrations, osteoblast function decreases within a week after the initiation of treatment and remains depressed for as long as treatment continues [61]. Increased bone resorption may be caused by secondary hyperparathyroidism, the stimulus for which is a corticosteroid-induced decrease in intestinal absorption. In addition, chronic corticosteroid therapy inhibits gonadotropin secretion in women and in men [62]. Because of this feedback inhibition of adrenocorticotropic hormone secretion, androgen production in the adrenals and ovaries is reduced and thus the main source of estrogens after menopause, i.e., aromatization of androstenedione to estrone, is eliminated.

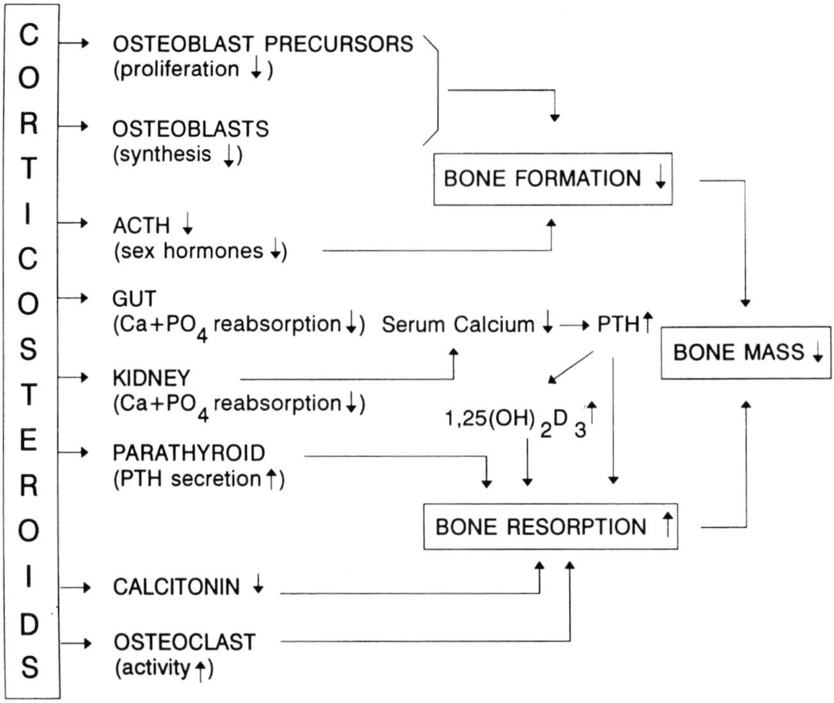

Figure 36.4. Pathophysiology of corticosteroid-induced osteoporosis.

Assessment of Patients at Risk for Corticosteroid-Induced Osteoporosis and Treatment of Osteoporosis

The first strategic step in corticosteroid-induced osteoporosis is prophylaxis [54]. It is easier to maintain bone than to restore it. In our unit we found the following general guidelines useful for prevention at the start of long-term corticosteroid therapy (Table 36.3). The principle of "look before you leap" is of particular relevance for rheumatologists. We all know the miraculous results corticosteroids can produce in early inflammatory disease. Our experience has taught us that miracles may turn into disasters. To avoid disasters, clinicians should first consider alternatives to corticosteroids. If corticosteroids do prove necessary, then it is wise to "go low, go slow". If available, deflazacort, an oxazoline derivative with reduced effects on bone and calcium metabolism [63] should be preferred. Although the bio-equivalents of deflazacort and prednisone in inflammatory conditions are said to be 1.2, no significant differences at the lumbar spine have been found in 2 mg/day deflazacort compared with 10 mg/day prednisone [64]. Try to encourage change of adverse lifestyles such as smoking, inactivity and alcohol abuse. Of particular importance is regulating calcium consumption. A calcium supplement is given at bedtime because it is now well known that there is a circadian rhythm of bone loss that starts after midnight when there is no calcium available in the gut. Evening calcium supplementation suppresses the circadian rhythm of bone resorption as measured

Table 36.3. Prophylaxis of corticosteroid osteoporosis

1. *Look before you leap* Are corticosteroids necessary ? Is there an alternative ? Go low, go slow
2. *General lifestyle advice* Remain active and fit Eliminate risk factors: smoking, excess alcohol Add calcium at bedtime (milk or tablet: 600–1,000 mg) Assure adequate vitamin D (400–800 U/day)
3. *Estimate risk for osteoporosis* Age, weight, height Expected cumulative dose CS Determine bone turnover: low–high Urine: fasting Ca/Cr (normal < 0.15) Hypro/Cr (normal < 0.05) (D-pyr) 24 h calciuria Serum calcium, phosphorus, alkaline phosphatase, osteocalcin
4. *Consider preventive therapy in high risk patients according to clinical, laboratory findings and bone mass reserves* Hypercalciuria: thiazides Hypocalciuria: vitamin D High turnover: antiresorbtive drugs: sex hormones, anabolic steroids (elderly), bisphosphonates, "perimenopausal pill", vitamin D, and metabolites 1-alpha vitamin D/1,25-vitamin D
5. *Follow testosterone levels in men and augment if necessary*

by deoxypyridinolinium crosslink excretion in the urine; morning calcium supplementation had no significant effect [65]. Therefore, a supplement of calcium, preferentially as a milk product (600–1000 mg), should be given at bedtime [66]. Controlled studies in steroid-treated cases have shown positive effects of calcium supplementation at night on bone [67,68].

A further step in the prophylaxis is to determine the risk of osteoporosis on the basis of clinical and laboratory variables. Risk of osteoporosis depends on sex, age, weight, height, expected cumulative dose of corticosteroids and on the bone mass capital at the cortical and trabecular sites, as measured by the newer techniques such as DXA and QCT.

Apart from scientific interest, information on the bone turnover status (low or high) at the start of therapy is useful in deciding on the most effective drug regimen (Fig. 36.5). Simple urinary fasting calcium/creatinine ratio, hydroxyproline/creatinine, deoxypyridinolinium crosslinks if available, 24 h calcium and serum levels of calcium, phosphorus, alkaline phosphatase and osteocalcin can give important information on the bone turnover status of the patient. According to the clinical and laboratory findings, a rational therapy can be proposed: for example, when there is hypercalciuria, thiazides to reduce calcium excretion are a good choice [69]; for hypocalciuria, vitamin D; with high turnover rates antiresorbtive drugs such as sex hormones, tibolone, calcitonin and bisphosphonates are indicated; in low turnover states fluoride, anabolic steroids, 1-alpha vitamin D (1,25-vitamin D) should be given; in cases of low testosterone levels in men testosterone should be substituted.

Recently, a number of studies have been published showing that pamidronate [70], etidronate [71,72] and alendronate [73] can prevent bone loss in corticosteroid-treated patients.

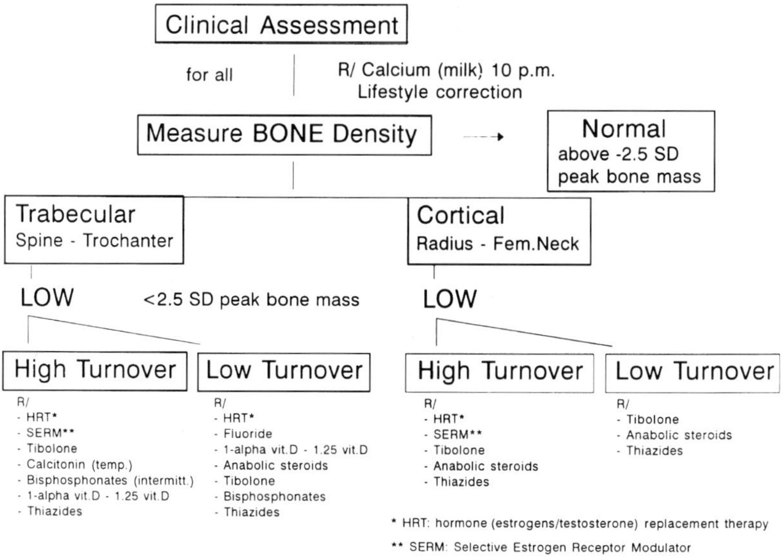

Figure 36.5. Decision tree for determining treatment choice.

Are Stress (Fatigue–Insufficiency) Fractures Rare in RA?

Periarticular osteoporosis, as well as a slight increase in the relative risk for hip fracture (RR 1.5–2.1) [74,36], are well recognized in non-steroid-treated RA. However, in a number of case reports [75–81] attention has been drawn to stress fractures occurring at the pelvis, the upper and lower tibia, and the hindfoot. The patients experienced a gradual onset of pain, walking difficulties and swelling in one lower extremity, suggestive of either cellulitis, thrombophlebitis or osteomyelitis. In the early phase, radiographs are misleading and may show an irregular sclerotic line, but bone scintigraphy will show increased uptake of the radiotracer at the fracture site as early as 48 h after its occurrence. CT has been reported to be very useful for the diagnosis of pelvic insufficiency fracture in elderly women with normal or inconclusive findings on radiographs [79]. The presence of knee deformity has been reported to be a risk factor for the occurrence of proximal, but not distal, tibial fracture in patients with RA. Other predisposing factors are aging, corticosteroid treatment, unaccustomed exercises after reconstructive surgery, frailness and metabolic bone diseases such as osteomalacia [75,77,82].

Stress, fatigue and insufficiency fractures are probably not rare in RA but are underdiagnosed or misdiagnosed as an exacerbation of synovitis. We have seen several patients who experienced stress fractures while receiving methotrexate therapy [83]. Whether chronic low-dose methotrexate is an additional predisposing factor for the development of osteoporosis is as yet unknown.

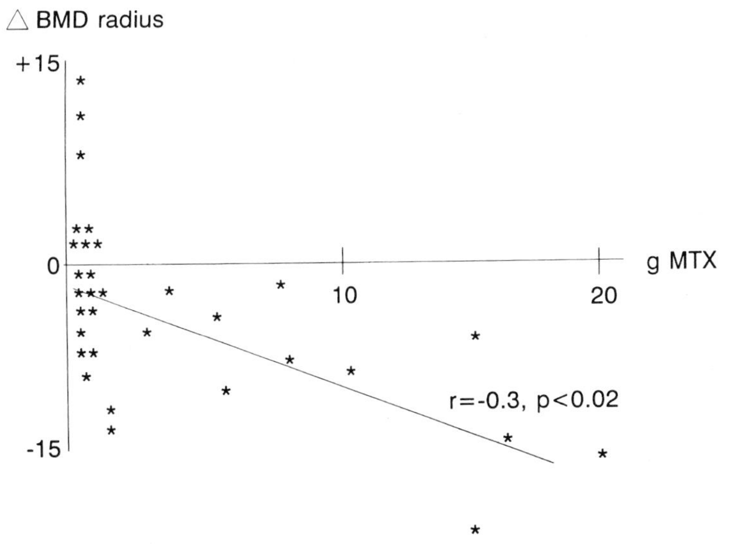

Figure 36.6. Effect of methotrexate (MTX) on bone loss ((BMD: change in bone mineral density) rheumatoid arthritis (J. Verwilghen, unpublished data).

Is Methotrexate Toxic for Bone?

Methotrexate osteopathy is a well-known entity in pediatric oncology, the initial reports being published as early as 1971 by Ragab et al. [84]. In some children with acute lymphatic leukemia, high-dose oral maintenance therapy with methotrexate caused localized osteoporosis, severe lower extremity pain and spontaneous fractures. Preston et al. [85] recognized a similar pattern in two RA patients treated with low-dose methotrexate. Similar problems were noticed in our unit [86] as well as by others [86].

The pathophysiological effects of methotrexate on bone are not known, and a direct antifolate action has been proposed to contribute to the negative effect of methotrexate on bone metabolism. The drug is present at high concentrations in trabecular bone as well as in cortical bone [87]. Animal models suggest that methotrexate inhibits osteoblastic activity [88,89] and, in addition, stimulates osteoclast recruitment, resulting in increased bone resorption [89].

No large studies on the role of methotrexate on bone in humans have been published. One small study examined the relationship between the effects of low-dose methotrexate in RA patients and the BMD. The authors did not find a difference between the methotrexate-treated patients and the control RA patients [90].

In a retrospective study our group found a cumulative dose-dependent cortical bone loss at the radius in RA patients treated with low-dose methotrexate when compared with RA controls not treated with methotrexate (Fig.36. 6) (J. Verwilghen, unpublished data). The methotrexate dose used in childhood leukemia far exceeds that currently used for the rheumatic population. Large prospective studies are needed to assess whether the doses used in RA patients predispose them yet further to the development of osteoporosis.

In recent years there have been reports suggesting that low-dose prednisone (7.5 mg daily), given for 2 years in early active RA in addition to other treatments, substantially reduces the rate of radiologically detected progression of disease [91,92].

Can Subchondral Bone Be Improved and Does It Matter?

Theoretically, drugs with anti-bone-resorbing activity could have a beneficial effect on rheumatoid bone erosions. If bone erosions can be prevented, then the long-term progression of RA could be substantially delayed. We investigated in a controlled study the effects of intranasal calcitonin, a strong inhibitor of osteoclast activity, on erosion progression and bone loss in RA. The age-related bone loss at the lumbar spine was temporarily stopped, but no effect on bone erosion (evaluated using the Larsen score) was seen [93]. Studies of the effect of bisphosphonates on radiological progression of RA also failed to show an effect [94–96]. The absence of effect could be because focal erosive disease may have progressed as a result of a non-osteoclast-related mechanism, probably cytokines.

There are almost no controlled prospective reports in the literature that have examined the relationship between subchondral bone quantity/quality and the outcome of joint replacement at the hip and knee. Obrant and his group have studied hip prosthetic loosening in early phase RA, using roentgen stereophotogrammetric techniques, comparing RA cases with osteoarthritis cases. Their results suggest that, unlike the acetabular socket, the cemented Charnley femoral component is equally secure in osteoarthritis and in RA, and that its initial fixation is not influenced by the quality of the local cancellous bone [97]. Further studies on micromotion of the acetabular component and periarticular bone morphology revealed that micromotions as long as 24 months after surgery were related to the periarticular cancellous bone quality as assessed by histomorphometric methods from samples taken during surgery. Acetabular components migrated more in hips with RA than in those with osteoarthritis. Hips with RA had approximately 4 times more non-mineralized bone (osteoid volume) than hips with osteoarthritis [98,99]. The DXA measurements at the hip showed that RA patients had 20% lower bone mineral content in the proximal femur compared with the osteoarthritis patients. The decreased BMD in the periarticular region in RA might be an additional reason for the socket anchorage to fail under load.

In a recent study of 1600 consecutive RA patients, seen during a period of observation that extended 23 years, who underwent a total joint arthroplasty (TJA), overall failure was low [100]. Six percent of knees and 4% of hips will have failed sufficiently to require a second TJA at 10 years of follow-up, and 12% of knees and 13% of hips will have required either a revision TJA or TJA-AP (arthroplasty-associated procedures) within the same 10-year period. These results provide confirmatory quantitative data on the tolerability of the surgery, even among those receiving second-line drugs and steroids.

In this series life table estimates indicated that 25% of RA patients will undergo TJA. In a multivariate predictor study, using time-varying covariates, the ESR, white blood count, hemoglobin level, HAQ disability scale score, global severity score, erosion and smoking (current or past) remained significant in a multivariate Cox regression, controlling for age and disease duration.

The most important lesson for the surgeon from these studies is that a patient with RA should be treated or have been treated appropriately by rheumatologists with extensive experience in the management of RA so that disease activity and disability are controlled early and consistently with disease-modifying drugs and the aid of a multidisciplinary team. This multidisciplinary team includes, besides the rheumatologist, nurses, a physiotherapist, an occupational therapist, a social worker and a psychologist, who are concerned about selfcare and education programs for the patients.

In conclusion, osteoporosis is not a common systemic extra-articular manifestation of RA for the following reasons. In postmenopausal women and in men with RA, osteoporosis is more evident at the hip and radius than at the spine. In addition, the most important determinants of bone loss in RA are disability, local disease activity and the cumulative corticosteroid dose. However, in exceptional cases of RA sustained massive osteolysis may be seen which is in excess of local disability due to excess cytokine production [22].

Periarticular osteoporosis reflects disease activity in early arthritis but not in chronic arthritis. Due to periarticular erosions and osteoporosis, cervical disability especially at the C1–2 level, is of particular importance and might be life-threatening.

In patients with severe RA, the rate of vertebral and hip fracture is doubled. Use of corticosteroids is a more important risk factor for fracture than disability.

The cumulative dose of corticosteroids is more important for osteoporosis and fragility fractures, and therefore there is no threshold dose. There is no evidence at present that anti-bone-resorbing drugs can prevent the progression of RA, except maybe for low-dose corticosteroids in early arthritis. Stress fractures are underdiagnosed in RA. There is a strong possibility that methotrexate is toxic for bone and may induce lower leg stress fractures.

References

1. Barwel H. Disease of the joints. London: Hardwick, 1865.
2. Soila P. Roentgen manifestations of adult rheumatoid arthritis. Acta Rheumatol Scand 1985;Suppl 1.
3. McConckey B, Frazer G, Eligh A. Transparent skin and osteoporosis. A study in patients with rheumatoid disease. Ann Rheum Dis 1965;24:219–223.
4. Saville PD, Kharmosh P. Osteoporosis of rheumatoid arthritis: influence of age, sex and corticosteroids. Arthritis Rheum 1967;10:423–430.
5. Kennedy AC, Lindsay R. Bone involvement in rheumatoid arthritis. Clin Rheum Dis 1977;3:403–420.
6. Bijlsma JWJ. Bone metabolism in patients with rheumatoid arthritis. Clin Rheumatol 1988;7:16–23.
7. Dequeker J, Geusens P. Osteoporosis and arthritis. Ann Rheum Dis 1990;49:276–280.
8. Mbuyi JM, Dequeker J, Teblick M, Merlevede M. Relevance of urinary excretion of alcian blue glycosaminoglycan complexes and hydroxyproline to disease activity in rheumatoid arthritis. J Rheumatol 1982;9:579–583.
9. Gevers G, Devos P, De Roo M, Dequeker J. Increased levels of osteocalcin (serum bone gla protein) in rheumatoid arthritis. Br J Rheumatol 1986;25:260–262.
10. Verstraeten A, Dequeker J. Mineral metabolism in postmenopausal women with active rheumatoid arthritis. J Rheumatol 1986;13:43–46.
11. Gough AKS, Peel NFA, Eastell R, Holder RL, Lilley J, Emery P. Excretion of pyridinium crosslinks correlates with disease activity and appendicular bone loss in early rheumatoid arthritis. Ann Rheum Dis 1994;53:14–17.

12. Gough A, Sambrook P, Devlin J, Huissoon A, Njeh C, Robbins S, et al. Osteoclastic activation is the principal mechanism leading to secondary osteoporosis in rheumatoid arthritis. J Rheumatol 1998;25:1282–1289.
13. Oelzner P, Müller A, Deschner F, Hüller M, Abendroth K, Hein G, et al. Relationship between disease activity and serum levels of vitamin D metabolites and PTH in rheumatoid arthritis. Calcif Tissue Int 1998;62:193–198.
14. Westhovens R, Nijs J, Taelman V, Dequeker J. Body composition in rheumatoid arthritis. Br J Rheumatol 1997;36:444–448.
15. Kröger H, Honkanen R, Saarikoski S, Alhava E. Decreased axial bone mineral density in perimenopausal women with rheumatoid arthritis: a population based study. Ann Rheum Dis 1994;53:18–23.
16. Lane NE, Pressman AR, Star VL, Cummings SR, Nevitt MC, and the Study of Osteoporotic Fractures Research Group. Rheumatoid arthritis and bone mineral density in elderly women. J Bone Miner Res 1995;10:257–263.
17. Hall GM, Spector TD, Griffin AJ, Jawad ASM, Hall ML, Doyle DV. The effect of rheumatoid arthritis and steroid therapy on bone density in postmenopausal women. Arthritis Rheum 1993;36:1510–1516.
18. Garton MJ, Reid DM. Bone mineral density of the hip and of the anteroposterior and lateral dimensions of the spine in men with rheumatoid arthritis. Arthritis Rheum 1993;36:222–228.
19. Towheed TE, Brouillard D, Yendt E, Anastassiades T. Osteoporosis in rheumatoid arthritis: findings in the metacarpals, spine and hip and a study of the determinants of both localized and generalized osteoporosis. J Rheumatol 1995;22:440–443.
20. Hansen M, Florescu A, Stoltenberg M, Podenphant J, Pedersen-Zbinden B, Horslev-Petersen K, et al. Bone loss in rheumatoid arthritis. Scand J Rheumatol 1996;25:367–376.
21. Martin JC, Munro R, Campbell MK, Reid DM. Effects of disease and corticosteroids on appendicular bone mass in postmenopausal women with rheumatoid arthritis: comparison with axial measurements. Br J Rheumatol 1997;36:43–49.
22. Mbuyi-Muamba JM, Dequeker J, Burssens A. Massive osteolysis in a case of rheumatoid arthritis: clinical, histologic and biochemical findings. Metab Bone Dis Rel Res 1983;5:101–106.
23. Compston JE, Crawley EO, Evans C, O'Sullivan MM. Spinal trabecular bone mineral content in patients with non-steroid treated rheumatoid arthritis. Ann Rheum Dis 1988;47:660–664.
24. Gough AKS, Lilley J, Eyre S, Holder RL, Emery P. Generalised bone loss in patients with early rheumatoid arthritis. Lancet 1994;344:23–27.
25. Eastgate JA, Wood NC, Di Giovine FS, Symons JA, Grinlinton FM, Duff GW. Correlation of plasma interleukin 1 levels with disease activity in rheumatoid arthritis. Lancet 1988;II:706–709.
26. Dequeker J, Wielandts L, Koentges D, Nijs J. The assessment of bone loss in rheumatoid arthritis. In: Feltkamp TEW, van der Korst JK, editors. Disease evaluation and assessment in rheumatoid arthritis. Alphen aan den Rijn/Brussels: Stafleu's Scientific Publishing Company, 1979:54–63.
27. Verstraeten A, Dequeker J. Vertebral and peripheral bone mineral content and fracture incidence in postmenopausal patients with rheumatoid arthritis: effect of low dose corticosteroids. Ann Rheum Dis 1986;45:852–857.
28. Sambrook PN, Ansell BM, Foster S, Gumpel JM, Hesp R, Reeve J. Bone turnover in early rheumatoid arthritis. 2. Longitudinal bone density studies. Ann Rheum Dis 1985;44:580–584.
29. Chan E, Pandith V, Towheed TE, Brouillard D, Zee B, Anastassiades TP. Comparison of the combined cortical thickness of the second metacarpal with Sharp's method for scoring hand microradiographs in rheumatoid arthritis. J Rheumatol 1998;25:1290–1294.
30. Peel NFA, Spittlehouse AJ, Bas DE, Eastell R. Bone mineral density of the hand in rheumatoid arthritis. Arthritis Rheum 1994;37:983–991.

31. Duff GW. Immune diseases: many roles for interleukin 1. Nature 1985;313:352–353.
32. Manolagas SC, Jilka RL. Bone marrow, cytokines and bone remodeling. N Engl J Med 1995;332:305–311.
33. Thomson BM, Mundy GR, Chambers TJ. Tumor necrosis factors α and β induce osteoblastic cells to stimulate osteoclastic bone resorption. J Immunol 1987;138: 775–779.
34. Lems WF, Dijkmans BAC. Should we look for osteoporosis in patients with rheumatoid arthritis? Ann Rheum Dis 1998;57:325–327.
35. Hooyman JR, Melton LJ, Nelson AM, O'Fallon WM, Riggs BL. Fractures after rheumatoid arthritis. Arthritis Rheum 1984;27:1353–1361.
36. Cooper C, Coupland C, Mitchell M. Rheumatoid arthritis, corticosteroid-therapy and hip fracture. Ann Rheum Dis 1995;54:49–52.
37. Spector TD, Hall GM, McCloskey EV, Kanis JA. Risk of vertebral fracture in women with rheumatoid arthritis. BMJ 1993;306:58.
38. Michel BA, Bloch DA, Fries JF. Predictors of fractures in early rheumatoid arthritis. J Rheumatol 1991;18:804–808.
39. Cooper C, Carbone L, Michet CJ, Atkinson EJ, O'Fallon WM, Melton LJ III. Fracture risk in patients with ankylosing spondylitis: a population based study. J Rheumatol 1994;21:1877–1882.
40. Dequeker J, Panayi G, Pincus T, Grahame R. Polyarthritis: rheumatoid arthritis and related conditions. In: Dequeker J, Panayi G, Pincus T, Grahame R, editors. Medical management of rheumatic musculoskeletal and connective tissue diseases. New York: Marcel Dekker, 1997:101–152.
41. Boden SD, Dodge LD, Bohlman HH, Rechtine GR. Rheumatoid arthritis of the cervical spine. J Bone Joint Surg Am 1993;75:1282–1297.
42. Casey ATH, Crockard HA, Bland JM, Stevens J, Moskovich R, Ransford AO. Surgery on the rheumatoid cervical spine for the non-ambulant myelopathic patient: too much, too late ? Lancet 1996;347:1004–1007.
43. Crockard HA. Surgical management of cervical rheumatoid problems. Spine 1995;20: 2584–2590.
44. Lesoin F, Duquesnoy B, Destee A, Leys D, Rousseaux M, Carini S, et al. Cervical neurological complications of rheumatoid arthritis. Surgical treatment techniques and indications. Acta Neurochir 1985;78:91–97.
45. Santavirta S, Slätis P, Kankaanpää U, Sandelin J, Laasonen E. Treatment of the cervical spine in rheumatoid arthritis. J Bone Joint Surg Am 1988;70:658–667.
46. Buckley LM, Leib ES, Cartularo KS, Vacek PM, Cooper SM. The effects of low dose corticosteroids on the bone mineral density of patients with rheumatoid arthritis. J Rheumatol 1995;22:1055–1059.
47. Laan RFJM, Van Riel PLCM, Erning LITHO, Lemmens JAM, Ruijs SHJ, Van de Putte LBA. Vertebral osteoporosis in rheumatoid arthritis patients: effect of low dose prednisone therapy. Br J Rheumatol 1992;31:91–96.
48. Laan RFJM, Van Riel PLCM, Van de Putte LBA, Van Erning LITHO, Van 't Hof MA, Lemmens JAM. Low-dose prednisone induces rapid reversible axial bone loss in patients with rheumatoid arthritis. Ann Intern Med 1993;119:963–968.
49. Nagant de Deuxchaisnes C, Devogelaer JP, Huaux JP. Influence of the menopausal state and the effect of low-dose glucocorticoids on bone mass in rheumatoid arthritis patients. Arthritis Rheum 1986;29:693–694.
50. Dykman TR, Gluck OS, Murphy WA, Hahn TJ, Hahn BH. Evaluation of factors associated with glucocorticoid-induced osteopenia in patients with rheumatic diseases. Arthritis Rheum 1985;28:361–368.
51. Nagant de Deuxchaisnes C, Devogelaer JP, Esselinckx W, Bouchez B, Depresseux G, Rombouts-Lindemans C, et al. The effect of low dosage glucocorticoids on bone mass in rheumatoid arthritis: a cross-sectional and a longitudinal study using single photon absorptiometry. Adv Exp Med Biol 1984;171:209–239.
52. Sambrook PN, Cohen ML, Eisman JA, Pocock NA, Champion GD, Yeates MG. Effects

of low dose corticosteroids on bone mass in rheumatoid arthritis: a longitudinal study. Ann Rheum Dis 1989;48:535–538.
53. Reid DM, Kennedy NSJ, Smith MA, Nicoll J, Brown N, Tothill P, et al. Bone loss in rheumatoid arthritis and primary generalized osteoarthrosis: effects of corticosteroids, suppressive antirheumatic drugs and calcium supplements. Br J Rheumatol 1986;25: 253–259.
54. Dequeker J, Westhovens R. Low dose corticosteroid associated osteoporosis in rheumatoid arthritis and its prophylaxis and treatment: bones of contention. J Rheumatol 1995;22:1013–1019.
55. Karantanas AH, Kalef-Ezra J, Glaros D. Limitations of quantitative CT in corticosteroid induced osteopenia. Acta Radiol 1991;32:339–341.
56. Manning P, Evans MC, Reid IR. Axial bone density following cure of Cushing's syndrome: Evidence for reversibility of steroid osteoporosis. In: Christiansen C, Overgaard K, editors. Osteoporosis. Copenhagen: Osteopress, 1990:1585–1586.
57. Pearce G, Ryan PFJ, Delmas PD, Tabensky DA, Seeman E. The deleterious effects of low-dose corticosteroids on bone density in patients with polymyalgia rheumatica. Br J Rheumatol 1998;37:292–299.
58. Saito JK, Davis JW, Wasnich RD, Ross PD. Users of low-dose glucocorticoids have increased bone loss rates: a longitudinal study. Calcif Tissue Int 1995;57:115–119.
59. Emkey RD, Lindsay R, Lyssy J, Weisberg JS, Dempster DW, Shen V. The systemic effect of intraarticular administration of corticosteroid on markers of bone formation and bone resorption in patients with rheumatoid arthritis. Arthritis Rheum 1996;39:277–282.
60. Geusens P, Dequeker J. Locomotor side-effects of corticosteroids. Baillieres Clin Rheumatol 1991;5:99–118.
61. Dequeker J. Kortikoide, Knochenmasse und Frakturen bei rheumatischen Erkrankungen. Akt Rheumatol 1993;18:14–18.
62. MacAdams MR, White RH, Chipps BE. Reduction of serum testosterone levels during chronic glucocorticoid therapy. Ann Intern Med 1986;104:648–651.
63. Olgaard K, Storm T, van Wowern N, Daugaard H, Egfjord M, Lewin E, et al. Glucocorticoid-induced osteoporosis in the lumbar spine, forearm, and mandible of nephrotic patients: a double-blind study on the high-dose long-term effects of prednisone versus deflazacort. Calcif Tissue Int 1992;50:490–497.
64. Messina OD, Barreira JC, Zanchetta JR, Maldonado-Cocco JA, Boagado CE, Sebastian ON, et al. Effect of low doses of deflazacort vs prednisone on bone mineral content in premenopausal rheumatoid arthritis. J Rheumatol 1992;19:1520–1526.
65. Blumsohn A, Herrington K, Hannon RA, Shao P, Eyre DR, Eastell R. The effect of calcium supplementation on the circadian rhythm of bone resorption. J Clin Endocrinol Metab 1994;79:730–735.
66. van de Voorde M, Dequeker J, Geusens P. Effect of one late evening dose of calcium on bone resorption in postmenopausal women. In: Christiansen C, Overgaard K, editors. Osteoporosis. Copenhagen: Osteopress, 1990:1192–1193.
67. Reid IR, Ibbertson HK. Calcium supplements in the prevention of steroid-induced osteoporosis. Am J Clin Nutr 1986;44:287–290.
68. Bijlsma JWJ, Raymakers JA, Mosch C, Hoekstra A, Derksen RH, Baart de la Faille H, et al. Effect of oral calcium and vitamin D on glucocorticoid-induced osteopenia. Clin Exp Rheumatol 1988;6:113–119.
69. Adams JS, Wahl TO, Luker BP. Effects of hydrochlorothiazide and dietary sodium restriction on calcium metabolism in corticosteroid treated patients. Metabolism 1981;30:217–221.
70. Boutsen Y, Jamart J, Esselinckx W, Stoffel M, Devogelaer JP. Primary prevention of glucocorticoid-induced osteoporosis with intermittent intravenous pamidronate: a randomized trial. Calcif Tissue Int 1997;61:266–271.
71. Adachi JD, Bensen WG, Brown J, Hanley T, Hodsman A, Josse R, et al. Intermittent etidronate therapy to prevent corticosteroid-induced osteoporosis. N Engl J Med 1997;337:382–387.

72. Roux C, Oriente P, Laan R, Hughes RA, Ittner J, Goemaere S, et al. Randomized trial of effect of cyclical etidronate in the prevention of corticosteroid-induced bone loss. J Clin Endocrinol Metab 1998;83:1128–1133.
73. Saag KG, Emkey R, Schnitzer TJ, Brown JP, Hawkins F, Goemaere S, et al. Alendronate for the prevention and treatment of glucocorticoid-induced osteoporosis. N Engl J Med 1998;339:292–299.
74. Hooyman JR, Melton LJ III, Nelson AM, O'Fallon WM, Riggs BL. Fractures after rheumatoid arthritis. A population-based study. Arthritis Rheum 1991;34:912–915.
75. Dequeker J, Heylen H, Burssens A. Spontaneous fractures of pelvis in rheumatoid arthritis. BMJ 1972;I:29:314.
76. Schneider R, Kaye JJ. Insufficiency and stress fractures of the long bones occurring in patients with rheumatoid arthritis. Radiology 1975;116:595–599.
77. Young A, Kinsella P, Boland P. Stress fractures of the lower limb in patients with rheumatoid arthritis. J Bone Joint Surg Br 1981;63:239–243.
78. Reynolds MT. Stress fractures of the tibia in the elderly associated with knee deformity. Proc R Soc Med 1972;65:377–380.
79. Straaton KV, Lopez-Mendez A, Alarcon GS. Insufficiency fractures of the distal tibia misdiagnosed as cellulitis in three patients with rheumatoid arthritis. Arthritis Rheum 1991;34:912–915.
80. Semba CP, Mitchell MJ, Sartoris DJ, Resnick D. Multiple stress fractures in the hindfoot in rheumatoid arthritis. J Rheumatol 1989;16:671–676.
81. Kahanpal S, McLeod RA, Luthra HS. Insufficiency-type stress fractures in rheumatoid arthritis: report of an interesting case and review of the literature. Clin Exp Rheumatol 1986;4:151–154.
82. Wordsworth BP, Vipond S, Woods CG, Mowat AG. Metabolic bone disease among inpatients with rheumatoid arthritis. Br J Rheumatol 1984;23:251–257.
83. Maenaut K, Westhovens R, Dequeker J. Methotrexate osteopathy: does it exist? J Rheumatol 1996;23:2156–2159.
84. Ragab AH, Fresh RS, Vietti TJ. Osteoporotic fractures secondary to methotrexate therapy of acute leukemia in remission. Cancer 1970;25:580–585.
85. Preston SJ, Diamon T, Scott A, Laurent MR. Methotrexate osteopathy in rheumatic disease. Ann Rheum Dis 1993;52:582–585.
86. Ansell G, Evans S, Jackson CT, Lewis-Jones S. Cytotoxic drugs for non-neoplastic disease. BMJ 1983;287:762.
87. Bologna C, Edno L, Anaya J, Canovas F, Vanden Berghe M, Jorgensen C, et al. Methotrexate concentrations in synovial membrane and trabecular and cortical bone in rheumatoid arthritis patients. Arthritis Rheum 1994;37:1770–1773.
88. Friedlaender GE, Tross RB, Doganis AC, Kirkwood JM, Baron R. Effects of chemotherapeutic agents on bone. J Bone Joint Surg 1984;66:602–607.
89. May KP, West SG, McDermott MT, Huffer WE. The effect of low-dose methotrexate on bone metabolism and histomorphometry in rats. Arthritis Rheum 1994;37:201–206.
90. Katz JN, Leboff MS, Wade JP, Brown EM, Liang MH. Effect of methotrexate on bone density and calcium homeostasis in rheumatoid arthritis. Clin Res 1989;37:509A.
91. Kirwan JR. The effect of glucocorticoids on joint destruction in rheumatoid arthritis. The Arthritis and Rheumatism Council low-dose glucocorticoid study group. N Engl J Med 1995;333:142–146.
92. Boers M, Verhoeven AC, Markusse HM, van de Laar MAFJ, Westhovens R, van Denderen JC, et al. Randomised comparison of combined step down prednisolone methotrexate and sulphasalazine versus sulphasalazine alone in early rheumatoid arthritis. Lancet 1997;350:309–318.
93. Sileghem A, Geusens P, Dequeker J. Intranasal calcitonin for the prevention of bone erosion and bone loss in rheumatoid arthritis. Ann Rheum Dis 1992;51:761–764.
94. Ralston SH, Hacking L, Willocks L, Bruce F, Pitkeathly DA. Clinical, biochemical and radiographic effects of aminohydropropylidene bisphosphonate treatment in rheumatoid arthritis. Ann Rheum Dis 1989;48:396–399.

95. Bird HA, Hill J, Sitton NG, Dixon JS, Wright V. A clinical and biochemical assessment of etidronate disodium in patients with active rheumatoid arthritis. Clin Rheumatol 1988;7:18–23.
96. Maccagno A, Di Giorgio E, Roldan EJA, Caballero LE, Perez Lloret A. Double blind radiological assessment of continuous oral pamidronic acid in patients with rheumatoid arthritis. Scand J Rheumatol 1994;23:211–214.
97. Önsten I, Åkesson K, Besjakov J, Obrant KJ. Migration of the charnley stem in rheumatoid arthritis and osteoarthritis.J Bone Joint Surg Br 1995;77:18–22.
98. Önsten I, Åkesson K, Obrant KJ. Micromotion of the acetabular component and periacetabular bone morphology. Clin Orthop 1995;310:103–110.
99. Åkesson K, Önsten I, Obrant KJ. Periarticular bone in rheumatoid arthritis versus arthrosis. Acta Orthop Scand 1994;65:135–138.
100. Wolfe F, Zwillich SH. The long-term outcomes of rheumatoid arthritis. Arthritis Rheum 1998;41:1072–1082.

37 Regional Demineralization and Osteoporosis

M. Chigira

Introduction

There is vast confusion about regional loss of bone mass. It has been difficult to demonstrate the pathogenesis of several disorders including transitory demineralization, migratory osteoporosis, Sudeck´s bone atrophy and idiopathic femoral head necrosis. However, recent advances in magnetic resonance imaging (MRI) have revealed the pathogenesis of these disorders, and these disorders should be classified as "circulatory disturbances" rather than "osteoporosis". Therefore, it is important to differentiate regional demineralization from systemic osteoporosis and to demonstrate the pathophysiology of bone mineral loss in osteoporosis.

Transitory Demineralization of the Femoral Head

In 1959, Curtis and Kincaid [1] reported 3 cases of transitory loss of calcium content of the femoral head during pregnancy. In all 3 patients the pain began during the last trimester. In this condition, the pain in the hip joint rapidly subsides within several months after delivery [2,3]. Claudication is usually obvious. The range of motion of the hip joint is limited and severe pain on motion is observed. Joint cartilage is well preserved after remineralization in the patients without pathological fracture of the femoral head. No clear demineralization can be demonstrated at other sites of the skeleton. A few reports have suggested a loss of bone mineral at the ipsilateral lower extremity, but multiple lesions may, of course, be secondary due to disuse after immobilization [4]. Systemic osteoporosis cannot be demonstrated. Complete recovery of bone mineral is usually observed within a year after delivery. Laboratory findings reveal no evidence of infection or inflammatory processes including tuberculosis. Transitory demineralization of the hip has also been reported in middle-aged men, though differentiation between transitory demineralization and avascular necrosis of the hip is difficult. Only the relationship with pregnancy may be clear evidence on which to differentiate transitory demineralization from avascular necrosis.

On the basis of the close relationship with pregnancy, mechanical compression of the obturator nerve was proposed to be a cause of transitory demineralization [1]. Hunder and Kelly [2] also suggested a neurogenic process in the etiology of demineralization. However, motor palsy of the obturator nerve has not been reported. Experimentally, artificial compression of the nerve using a metal clip did not result in any demineralization of the hip [3]. In addition, bilateral and earlier onset of the disorder do not support the theory of direct compression of the obturator nerve by the fetus [4]. There is thus no evidence of a neurogenic pathogenesis of the transitory demineralization of the femoral head as shown in reflex sympathetic dystrophy (Sudeck´s atrophy). Abnormal metabolism of hydroxyproline has also been suggested as a cause of this disorder [3] but this has not been supported by further investigations.

Rosen [5] showed accumulation of erythrocytes in bone marrow and suggested that obstruction of venous return during pregnancy was an etiology of this disorder. Histological findings of bone marrow suggest that transitory edema plays an important role in the pathogenesis of transitory osteoporosis and that there is no increase of fatty bone marrow due to loss of trabeculae [5]. The intertrabecular space is filled with blood cells in transitory demineralization of the femoral head. MRI reveals three stages of the disorder: a diffuse stage, a focal stage, and a residual stage with increased water content and "bone edema" [6]. It has widely been accepted that transitory demineralization of the hip is caused by "marrow edema" as demonstrated by MRI findings [7,8]. MRI findings are generally compatible with the histological characteristics in transitory demineralization.

In general, in transitory demineralization there is need for protective immobilization of the hip joint until complete recovery from the demineralization in order to prevent pathological fracture of the femoral neck. Core decompression as suggested by Hofmann et al. [7] may be a useful procedure to relieve symptoms by lowering marrow pressure. However, it is not clear whether mechanical decompression is necessary in the treatment of this disorder. Finally, transitory demineralization cannot be differentiated from avascular necrosis on the basis of the radiological and MRI findings, since bone marrow edema is common to the two disorders.

Avascular Necrosis of the Femoral Head

Avascular necrosis of the femoral head is a well-known disorder of middle-aged men. Circulatory disturbance of the femoral head has been believed to be an important pathogenetic factor. Liver dysfunction, smoking, steroid administration and Caisson disease cause this disorder, since a decrease in blood flow in these conditions plays an important role in the appearance of necrosis. Recently, venous stasis caused by intra-medullary bleeding has been suggested to be a cause of this disorder. Bone marrow edema, demonstrated by MRI, is an initial finding of avascular necrosis [9]. In the last stage, necrotic change within the femoral head due to loss of blood flow is demonstrated. These MRI findings have been supported by histological examinations.

It is noteworthy that spontaneous recovery from demineralization has been reported in some cases of avascular necrosis in the early phase. However, most patients do not recover. In these cases, avascular necrosis cannot be differentiated from transitory demineralization, since the results of radiological and MRI examinations are similar in avascular necrosis in its initial phase and transitory demineralization.

Regional Migratory Osteoporosis

Regional migratory osteoporosis, first described by Duncan et al. [10], is a rare syndrome characterized by arthralgia, severe intercurrent focal osteoporosis and gradual spontaneous recovery [11]. Swelling with a rapid onset of osteoporosis is observed in the painful areas. Severe periarticular osteoporosis with preservation of the cartilage space is occasionally accompanied by periosteal new bone formation. Although acetabular preservation, as seen in transitory demineralization of the hip, has not been demonstrated in migratory osteoporosis, these two disorders are occasionally confused. Spontaneous involvement of multiple regions may occur concomitantly or sequentially. The symptoms last 6–9 months, followed by remineralization that may take as long as 2 years. From the variety of clinical findings, it is speculated that migratory osteoporosis is a nontraumatic variety of Sudeck´s atrophy, since the signs of reflex sympathetic dystrophy, including swelling and skin changes, are commonly observed in this disorder [11].

With the exception of bone scintigraphy, laboratory findings do not indicate any abnormalities. A distinctive pattern of radiotracer uptake in the delayed phase of a triphasic bone scan indicates increased blood flow to the bone [12]. The scintigraphic abnormalities may even precede the development of clinical symptoms of reflex sympathetic dystrophy [12]. MRI supports the scintigrapic findings that blood flow to the bone increases in migratory osteoporosis. Venous stasis and bone marrow edema cannot be demonstrated in migratory osteoporosis as is seen in transitory demineralization and avascular necrosis of the hip [13]. There is increased blood flow in this disease, in contrast to the decrease of blood flow in transitory demineralization of the hip and in avascular necrosis. From the viewpoint of circulation to the bone, migratory osteoporosis is thus different from bone marrow edema as seen in transitory demineralization.

Blocking the sympathetic nerve seems to be an effective treatment for migratory osteoporosis [12]. Such treatment may normalize the increased bone blood flow since it is likely that the pathological vasomotor functions in this disease are involved in bone decalcification. The effectiveness of the relief of symptoms of such sympathetic nerve blocking, supports the contention that abnormalities of the sympathetic nerve may cause migratory osteoporosis. Furthermore, it has not been reported that blocking the sympathetic nerve improves the bone marrow edema found in transitory demineralization and avascular necrosis of the hip. Core decompression used in the treatment of transitory demineralization has not been reported in migratory osteoporosis. Immobilization as used in the treatment of transitory demineralization of the hip is not effective for treatment of migratory osteoporosis. On the contrary, it is believed that such immobilization of the extremity worsens the abnormalities of the sympathetic nerve. A neural or neurovascular mechanism is thus suggested in the pathogenesis of migratory osteoporosis. From the viewpoint of pathophysiology and response to treatment there seems thus to be an overlap between migratory osteoporosis and reflex sympathetic dystrophy. Furthermore, the bone marrow edema associated with transitory demineralization and avascular necrosis of the hip does not accompany migratory osteoporosis. Therefore, migratory osteoporosis should be differentiated from transitory demineralization of the hip.

Regional Demineralization

Circulatory disturbances cause loss of bone mineral, as seen in several disorders described above. "Regional osteoporosis" is a misnomer, since there is no histological evidence of osteoporosis within the regional bone. MRI and scintigraphical evidence do not support the assumption that regional osteoporosis is present. Therefore, regional demineralization as an entity should phenomenologically be used to describe several disorders, including transitory demineralization, the initial phase of avascular necrosis, and migratory osteoporosis. In these disorders, circulatory disturbances play important roles in the pathogenesis. However, the relationship between changes in blood flow and loss of bone mineral is not clear. MRI indicates both an increase and a decrease in blood flow with regional loss of bone minerals.

It may be reasonable that an increase in blood flow can accelerate bone remodelling. However, spontaneous recovery of bone structure cannot be explained. If an increase in blood flow enhances bone remodelling, bone structure cannot completely recover. It is noteworthy that transitory demineralization is not accompanied by the remodelling seen in systemic osteoporosis. It is suspected that bone matrix is preserved after demineralization. On the other hand, the loss of bone mineral observed in systemic osteoporosis is usually accompanied by increased remodelling and loss of bone matrix.

Complete remineralization of bone matrix in transitory demineralization indicates secondary suppression of the mineralization process. Systemic osteoporosis must be different from transitory demineralization, since the capability of mineralization is well preserved in the latter.

The exact cause of bone marrow edema has not been identified, although several mechanisms, including marrow haemorrhage and embolism, have been investigated in avascular necrosis. On the other hand, the natural course of transitory demineralization has not been demonstrated, because of its rarity. No clear evidence has been demonstrated, albeit recent reports suggest that a larger area of the femoral head suffers change in transitory demineralization than in avascular necrosis. Bone marrow edema has been demonstrated in the limited, small area of the femoral head in avascular necrosis [9]. Therefore, it is reasonable to suppose that the anatomical structure of the venous system may play an important role in stasis. Recent advances in MRI technology will reveal the differences between transitory demineralization and avascular necrosis.

A direct mechanism of demineralization due to bone marrow edema has not been indicated. From the histological findings of transitory demineralization, it is suggested that chemical mediators secreted from blood cells play a role in demineralization. Venous stasis results in their increase in inflammatory lesions. Osteoclasts may be activated by these agents.

Regional Demineralization and Systemic Osteoporosis

Regional demineralization due to circulatory disturbances is frequently observed in the disorders described above. It is questionable whether regional demineralization is related to systemic osteoporosis or not. A common mechanism underlying systemic osteoporosis and transitory demineralization has not been demonstrated.

Bone marrow edema, as seen in transitory demineralization and avascular necrosis of the hip, has not been demonstrated in postmenopausal and senile osteoporosis by MRI or histological examination. In systemic osteoporosis, the bone marrow is filled with fibrous and fatty tissue. Cellularity in the marrow is generally decreased in osteoporosis compared with that in normal marrow. Mature erythrocytes are generally rare in osteoporotic marrow. On the other hand, many blood cells are demonstrated in bone marrow edema described above. Furthermore, the increased blood flow in bone marrow as seen in migratory osteoporosis and Sudeck's bone atrophy is not observed in systemic osteoporosis. Neurological abnormalities suggested as a cause of Sudeck's atrophy have not been demonstrated in systemic osteoporosis. There is no evidence that circulatory disturbances play an important role in the pathogenesis of systemic osteoporosis.

Morphologically, the trabecular pattern of bone marrow is well preserved in regional demineralization. Furthermore, expansion of the cortex has not been demonstrated in regional demineralization. On the other hand, in senile osteoporosis the expansion of the cortex is a major pathological finding, and the trabecular pattern of bone marrow is also lost [14]. These findings suggest that regional demineralization is not a "degenerative" disorder, and that it is different from aging processes such as systemic osteoporosis. Altered bone remodelling does not seem to play an important role in the pathogenesis of regional demineralization, although senile osteoporosis may be caused by such bone remodelling [14].

References

1. Curtiss PH, Kincaid WE. Transitory demineralization of the hip in pregnancy. J Bone Joint Surg 1959;41:1327–1333.
2. Hunder GG, Kelly PJ. Roentgenologic transient osteoporosis of the hip. A clinical syndrome? Ann Intern Med 1968;68:539–552.
3. Longstreth PL, Malinak LR, Facoq, Stratton Hill C Jr. Transient osteoporosis of the hip in pregnancy. Obstet Gynecol 1973;41:563–569.
4. Chigira M, Watanabe H, Udagawa E. Transient osteoporosis of the hip in the first trimester of pregnancy. A case report and review of Japanese literature. Arch Orthop Trauma Surg 1988;107:178–180.
5. Rosen RA. Transitory demineralization of the femoral head. Radiology 1970;94:509–512.
6. Grimm J, Higer HP, Benning R, Meairs S. MRI of transient osteoporosis of the hip. Arch Orthop Trauma Surg 1991;110:98–102.
7. Hofmann S, Engel A, Neuhold A, Leder K, Kramer J, Plenk H Jr. Bone-marrow edema syndrome and transient osteoporosis of the hip. J Bone Joint Surg Br 1993;75:210–216.
8. Hauzeur J-P, Hanquinet S, Gevenois PA, Appelboom T, Bentin J, Perlmutter N. Study of magnetic resonance imaging in transient osteoporosis of the hip. J Rheumatol 1991;18:1211–1217.
9. Takatori Y, Kokubo T, Ninomiya S, Nakamura S, Morimoto S, Kusaba I. Avascular necrosis of the femoral head. Natural history and magnetic resonance imaging. J Bone Joint Surg Br 1993;75:217–221.
10. Duncan H, Frame B, Frost H, Arnstein R. Migratory osteolysis of the lower extremities. Ann Intern Med 1967;66:1165–1173.
11. Banas MP, Kaplan FS, Fallon MD, Haddad JG. Regional migratory osteoporosis. A case report and review of the literature. Clin Orthop 1990;250:303–309.
12. Mailis A, Inman R, Pham D. Transitory migratory osteoporosis: A variant of reflex sympathetic dystrophy? Report of 3 cases and literature review. J Rheumatol 1992;19: 758–764.

13. Schweitzer ME, Karasick D. MRI of the ankle and hindfoot. Semin Ultrasound CT MR 1994;15:410–422.
14. Chigira M. Mechanical optimization of bone. Med Hypoth 1996;46:327–330.

38 Immobilization and Post-traumatic Osteopenia

C. Trevisan and S. Ortolani

Introduction

Over 300 years ago Galileo and Vesalius suspected skeletal architecture might depend on mechanical usage [1] and more than 100 years ago Julius Wolff stated the relationship between bone function and its architecture [2]. Therefore, the effects of reduced mechanical usage on bone have been known for a long time. In 1924, J.W. Dowden wrote: "the musculature of a limb is reflected in the bones, so that it is easy to distinguish the long bone of a strong man, by its solidity and powerful ridges for muscular attachment, from the bone of a disuse limb, by the lightness and smoothness of the latter. The results of disuse are rapidly seen, even in the X-ray photographs" [3]. In 1941, Albright and colleagues reported the case of a young boy who developed hypercalcemia as a consequence of the immobilization for a fracture. During the 1940s and 1950s, alterations in calcium and phosphorus metabolism were described by Whendon and colleagues in poliomyelitic patients and immobilized volunteers and an elevated rate of bone turnover after fracture was described by Bauer [4] and confirmed by others [5,6].

Since then, immobilization and post-traumatic osteopenia have been extensively studied in experimental animals, in patients and human volunteers from the metabolic and endocrinological point of view and by histomorphometry, radiomorphometry and bone densitometry.

While immobilization osteopenia is due to muscular inactivity and reduction in weightbearing which lead to the decrease in bone mechanical loading, in post-traumatic osteopenia there is the adjunctive effect of the trauma itself and of the possible related surgical procedures. These two conditions partially share a common pathogenesis but they usually depict two different clinical situations: the patient with a chronic illness and the patient who has sustained an acute injury. They will thus be treated separately and for the same reason the studies on immobilization induced by surgical methods will not be discussed in the section on immobilization osteopenia.

Immobilization Osteopenia

Influence of Load and Strain on Bone Modelling and Remodelling

The skeleton's bone tissue is controlled by three mechanisms: longitudinal growth, which adds new supplies of primary spongiosa and new length to cortices, bone modelling which shapes bones according to functional demands; and lastly bone remodelling which controls bone turnover and replacement [1,7]. While bone growth is genetically determined and terminated, modelling and remodelling continue throughout life and are mainly controlled by nongenetic factors [8].

Bone modelling moves bone surfaces around in tissue space by means of the "formation drifts" in which osteoblasts can add bone to periosteal, cortical-endosteal and trabecular surfaces, and "resorption drifts" in which osteoclasts can resorb bone. In this way they move tissue from one surface to another, shaping bones. Modelling is mechanically controlled and responds to some time-averaged history of repeated loads: large loads probably receive significantly more weight in governing bone modelling than smaller ones [9–11]. When bone surface local strains reach or exceed a threshold range (perhaps near 1000 microstrains in adults and near 2000 microstrains in growing subjects) modelling is activated until the changes operating on bone structure reduce the local strains below that threshold [12,13]. In disuse, strains stay below the modelling threshold strain range and bone modelling simply turns off. Its results may be seen in the case of limbs that were paralyzed well before skeletal maturity whose bone shape – reduced length, slim diaphysis, narrow cortices and medullary cavity and smaller epiphysis – reveals the absence of functional adaptation to load provided by modelling (Fig. 38.1).

Remodelling has the primary task of renewing bone. Bone tissue is particularly prone to fatigue: at 1000 microstrains, the normal lamellar bone's fatigue life exceeds 60 years, but under 4000 microstrains (about 16% of the fracture strain) its fatigue life could be less than 2 months (20 000 cycles or less) [1,14]. Only a periodically renewed material can safely withstand an infinite number of loading cycles.

Remodelling activity is performed by functionally coupled osteoclasts and osteoblasts that form the basic multicellular units for remodelling (BMUs). A stimulus can make resting cells on or near a bone surface create or activate a new BMU that first removes and then replaces a small packet of bone. Activation frequency and the number of active BMUs determine how much bone is turned over annually. Averaged over the whole skeleton, in adults the balance between resorption and formation in completed packets is slightly negative and may be the cause of the annual loss of around 0.75% of the skeleton bone [15]. This balance is different in different skeletal envelopes: positive in the periosteal envelope, near equilibrium in the haversian envelope and negative in the cortical-endosteal and trabecular envelope [1,16,17]. This means that in the long term remodelling determines periosteal mineral deposition and endosteal mineral resorption with enlargement of bone diameter, and a substantial impoverishment of the trabecular network.

Remodelling responds to some time-averaged loading history too. In healthy adults, when typical peak bone strains are below 50–100 or so microstrains, BMU creations are stimulated; in the window of adapted mechanical usage between about 50 and 1000 microstrains BMU creations are normal; and when typical bone strains rise above about 1000 microstrains, BMU creations are depressed [1]. Therefore, acute disuse of normally used bone can increase BMU creations to over 5 times the

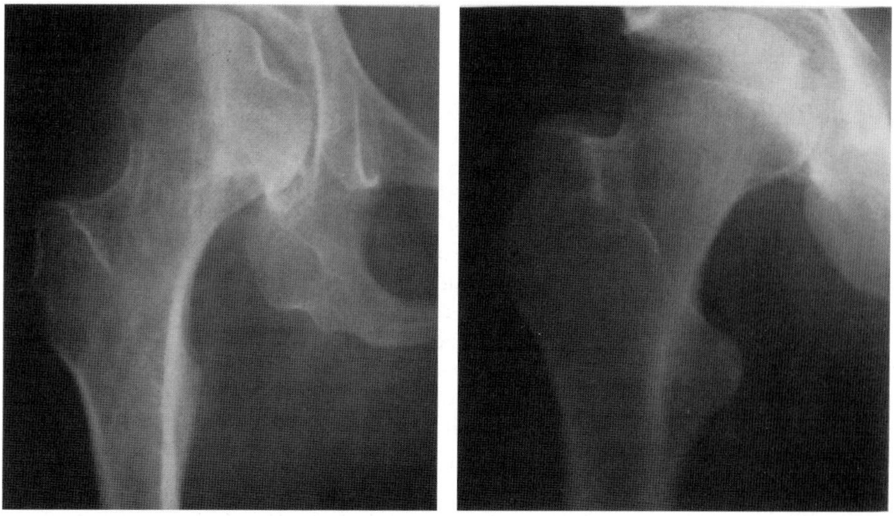

Figure 38.1. Comparison of the proximal femur in a poliomyelitic patient (*left*) and in an healthy subject (*right*). In the paralyzed limb of the poliomyelitic patient, the longstanding disuse and reduced muscle activity has resulted in a very low level of modelling activation with smaller bones with abnormal shape, narrow cortices and medullary cavity and decreased bone mass.

normal level. Acute disuse may also slightly increase the amount of bone completed BMUs resorb. Next to marrow, BMU bone formation is decreased or even blocked or delayed for months. The net result is a decrease in bone mass that in turn drives back local bone strains (per surface unit) toward the threshold range of normal mechanical usage, in a feedback loop that reduces the activation of new BMUs. When the new steady state is reached at a lower bone mass, remodelling returns toward normal and bone loss stops [1].

Calcium Metabolism

The experimental and clinical data on immobilization osteopenia fit well in this model of skeletal physiology. The earliest experimental studies on inactivity evaluated the derangement on calcium metabolism. In 1948, Dietrick et al. [18] studied 4 healthy men who were placed in a body plaster cast for 6–7 weeks and found a marked increase in urinary calcium, nitrogen and phosphorus with corresponding negative calcium balance. A negative calcium balance with increased urinary and/or fecal calcium excretion, suggesting an increased remodelling activity with bone resorption exceeding formation, has been reported in several other investigations. Issekutz et al. [19] confirmed the rise in urinary calcium as an effect of prolonged bed rest and its decrease with quiet standing and Rose [20] found hypercalciuria despite a decrease in calcium absorption in 139 patients confined to bed for fractured legs or prolapsed discs. In the longest study on inactivity, Donaldson et al. [21] reported a negative calcium balance of around 200 mg/day (representing a loss of whole-body mineral of about 0.5% each month) and increased urinary and fecal calcium excretion for all the 7 months of bed rest in healthy adult volunteers.

Weightless spaceflights are another model of disuse osteopenia. The increase in urinary calcium excretion during the Vostok 2 and 3 flights was the first suggestion of undesirable changes in bone metabolism during space missions [22]. A negative calcium balance consequent to the removal of the constant pull of gravity in spaceflight was confirmed by increased urinary calcium on the 18 day flight of Soyuz 9 [23], by high urinary and fecal calcium losses in the lunar flight of Apollo 17 [24] and in the three Skylab flights in 1973–74 [25,26]. During space flight, the reduced mechanical stimulus on bones leads to an increased bone turnover with a rise in urinary hydroxyproline and plasma calcium. In its turn, the latter induces a fall in serum parathyroid hormone which accounts for both the rise in urinary calcium excretion and the lesser stimulation of the 1-hydroxylation of 25-hydroxycholecalciferol with increased fecal calcium loss [27]. Suppression of the parathyroid–vitamin D axis due to primary loss of mineral from bone was also found in a group of patients with recent spinal cord injury [28] and may be considered the standard hormonal and metabolic pattern after immobilization.

Histology

Histological characteristics and histomorphometric analysis of immobilization-induced bone tissue changes have also been investigated in humans and in animal models. In the iliac crest bone biopsies of paralytic patients with spinal cord trauma, Minaire et al. [29] found a rapid initial trabecular bone loss with increased resorption activity and a reduced bone formation. Similar findings were observed by Vico et al. [30] in healthy volunteers after 120 days of bed rest, in whom an increased osteoclastic activity and a reduced mineralization rate were found.

Experimental animal models provided additional information: increased resorption activity, sustained by an increased number and perimeter of active osteoclasts, prevails at the endosteal envelope, whereas osteoblastic activity is reduced mainly in the endosteal and trabecular envelopes [31–33]. Cancellous bone responds faster to immobilization with decreased bone volume, trabecular thinning and increased trabecular spacing [34,35]; its mechanical properties appear to decline accordingly [36]. Cortical bone has a slower response and the induced porosity is highly nonuniform, prevailing in the plane of application of prevalent stresses during normal activity [32,34]. A steady state appears to occur at about 24 weeks of immobilization, both in human [29] and in animal models [37].

Noninvasive Quantitative Assessment of Bone Mass

Quantitative assessment of bone mass is useful to substantiate the extent and the site of immobilization osteopenia and its possible recovery. The amount of bone loss observed in different reports depends on the technique used in measuring bone mass, the site of measurement and the time of immobilization and may also vary between a few percentage points to over 50%.

In a few days of spaceflight, weightlessness induced a decrease in the heel density of the Cosmos 110 dogs by around 10% and the two-man crews of Gemini IV, V and VIII, whose missions lasted 4, 8 and 14 days respectively, showed a calcaneus bone loss by radiographic densitometry ranging from 2.9% to 15.1%. A more precise assessment of bone mass by single photon absorptiometry confirmed a detectable bone loss in the heel but not in the radius or ulna of the Apollo, Skylab and Soyuz crews [27].

In nonambulant elderly women, calcaneal density by Compton scattering was lower than that of ambulant controls [38], and in chronic continuing care patients with restricted mobility, a reduction of the calcaneal density more than 1 standard error below the predicted density was found in 57% of patients [39].

When activity is more restricted or the immobilization period is longer, bone loss may become considerable. At the end of a bed rest period averaging 27 days (range 11–61 days) for low back pain due to protrusion of a lumbar intervertebral disc, Krølner and Toft [40] found in their 34 patients a 3.6% decrease in L2–4 bone mineral density. In teenage girls during 2–6 weeks of bed rest after corrective surgery for scoliosis, Hansson et al. [41] found a 6.1% decrease in spinal bone density in those patients allowed to mobilize after 2 weeks and a 10.7% decrease in those patients allowed to mobilize after 4 weeks. Prolonged bed rest in healthy volunteers (5–36 weeks) caused a 25–40% depletion of calcaneal mineral but maintenance of forearm bone density [42,43]. In another study on the bone changes after 17 weeks of continuous bed rest in healthy volunteers, Leblanc et al. [44] found a reduction in bone mineral density at the total body, lumbar spine, femoral neck, trochanter, tibia and calcaneus of 1.4%, 3.9%, 3.6%, 4.6%, 2.2% and 10.4%, respectively. In experimental animal models, prolonged and complete immobilization by means of noninvasive methods may results in bone density reduction in the immobilized limb of between 15% and 50% depending on the measured site [35–37,45].

The rate of bone loss following immobilization ranges from 4% to 8% per month [40–43], which is a huge depletion compared with the 0.75–1% per year of involutional bone loss.

Skeletal sites appeared to respond differently: in weightlessness, weightbearing bones had a greater bone loss than non-weightbearing bones which probably are more sensitive to stress induced by muscle activity [27,42,43,46], and the sites with prevalent trabecular content showed an earlier and greater response than cortical sites, as already observed histologically [34,36,44,46–49]. Cortical bone is generally lost with prolonged immobilization [47,50,51]. In immobilized limbs, a proximal–distal gradient of bone loss is likely to occur [37,49] as well as a selective osteopenia below the level of neurological impairment in paraplegic patients [52].

Reversibility

The potential for recovery of morphological and mechanical properties following a period of immobilization is controversial. Young individuals have a greater potential for bone recovery. Jaworski and Uhthoff [51] studied the reversibility of nontraumatic disuse osteoporosis in young and old beagle dogs: young dogs recovered 70% of immobilization-induced bone loss whereas older dogs recovered only 40%. A better restoration of bone tissue in younger rats has been observed by Tuukkanen et al. [53] and also in humans affected by post-traumatic osteopenia; growing subjects have demonstrated a complete recovery which is unattainable in older subjects [54,55].

The period of remobilization necessary for the highest possible recovery is longer than the period of immobilization and the cancellous bone recovers earlier than cortical bone [34,40,44,47]. In young adult dogs, after 16 weeks of immobilization, cortical and cancellous bone mechanical properties returned to control values only after 32 weeks of remobilization [36]. Normal activity results in poor compensation of the immobilization-induced osteopenia and greater than normal activity is necessary to restore bone mass [45,56,57].

It may be questionable whether the incomplete recovery of immobilization-induced osteopenia observed in many studies should be ascribed to the short period of follow-up or to insufficient mechanical loading, but it may be reasonable to conclude that in adult individuals, even for experimental animal models, complete recovery is indeed impossible. The observation of a long-lasting osteopenia in the calcaneus of the Skylab astronauts 5 years after their flights [27] and the necessity of an indefinitely increased level of activity to preserve bone mass at its original value in experimental animals with immobilization osteopenia [57] supports this opinion.

Clinical Consequences

From the clinical point of view immobilization osteopenia is associated with paralytic medical conditions (spinal cord injury or stroke) or with a variety of nonparalytic conditions (prolonged bed rest for severe illness, for prolapsed spinal disc, for scoliosis correction) that differ from the former in their limited duration in time. In both cases osteopenia may lead to severe consequences. In patients with spinal cord injury nontraumatic fractures of the lower limb (typically of the distal femur) are relatively common (6% of the patients) and may not be recognized at the time, due to the absence of pain sensation. If untreated or healed without proper management these fractures may result in deformity and loss of function. With the current advances in early medical treatment and rehabilitation of spinal cord injuries and stroke many of these patients may retain or regain substantial motor function. This makes immobilization osteopenia even more clinically relevant and its prevention worthwhile, as the occurrence of pathological fractures may severely interfere with the continuation of rehabilitation programs and impair functional recovery. In nonparalytic conditions many patients will suffer a permanent residual bone loss, despite the limited duration of immobilization, because complete recovery after remobilization is seldom achieved.

Prevention

The importance of the prevention as well as the active treatment of immobilization-induced osteopenia is evident given the high rate of bone loss and the sequelae seen in this condition. Kannus et al. [56] clearly illustrated the main steps in the management of immobilization osteopenia: avoidance of full immobility, limitation of immobilization time, effective muscular training during and after immobilization, and early weightbearing.

Avoidance of full immobility is definitely beneficial. In healthy subjects prescribed bed rest, 4 h of daily ambulation corrected negative calcium balance [58] and standing, with simple periodic shifts in position, appears to limit mineral depletion [19]. Conversely, not all exercise regimens are equally effective. Exercise on bicycle ergometers had no effect on bone loss of bed-rested men and neither static compression harnesses nor a harness system to generate cyclic compression equivalent to walking reduced bone loss in bed rest volunteers [19,21]. There is a dose–response relationship between physical loading and mechanical competence of bone, and adaptive bone modelling and remodelling are sensitive to unusual strain distribution, high strain and high strain rates, which seem to be particularly osteogenic [59,60]. Therefore, exercise protocols that load bone with high peak forces and high strain rates, create versatile strain distributions throughout the bone structure, consist of relatively short repetition and training sessions but are long term and progressive by nature should be the most effective to increase bone mass [61,62].

Many pharmacological regimens have been proposed for the treatment of immobilization osteopenia. Indeed, immobilization osteopenia is one of the few available experimental models to induce osteoporosis in animals and is therefore widely used to test candidate molecules for the treatment of osteoporosis. Bisphosphonates effectively prevent or reduce immobilization-induced osteopenia in different rat models [63–65], in healthy bed rest volunteers [66,67] and in paraplegic patients [68,69]. Calcitonin reduced bone loss in neurectomized rats but not in cast-immobilized rats [70] and was ineffective in immobilized sheep [71]. Anti-inflammatory drugs have also been shown to produce some effect: acetylsalicylic acid had a 13% bone sparing effect in casted hind limb of the dog [72] and ketoprofen inhibited bone loss in a nontraumatic immobilization model in the rat [73]. A preventive effect has also been demonstrated for tamoxifen in immobilized growing dogs [74] and for parathyroid hormone in rats with one hindlimb immobilized by bandage [75].

Unfortunately, the majority of the available data have been obtained in animals and only a few in small series of humans. Adequate controlled clinical studies demonstrating the efficacy of any pharmacological treatment in patients are still lacking. Nevertheless, as increased bone resorption is the more dramatic change in bone metabolism seen during the active early phase of immobilization osteopenia, there is a rationale for the use of antiresorptive agents to prevent its development. The efficacy of these agents may be much less in the late inactive phase, when bone turnover returns toward normal. Bisphosphonates are the most potent antiresorptive drugs available and should therefore be considered a valid option for the early prevention of immobilization osteopenia. Vitamin D and calcium supplements should be used very carefully and only when a deficit is present, as plasma and urinary calcium spontaneously rise in this condition, increasing the risk of urinary lithiasis.

Physical therapy may also be useful: electrical muscle stimulation and pulsed electromagnetic fields can induce bone formation and prevent bone and cartilage deterioration in cast-immobilized experimental animals and in humans [76,77].

Post-traumatic Osteopenia

Regional Acceleratory Phenomenon

In a recent experimental study on the high turnover osteopenia of inflammatory arthritis, Bogoch et al. [78] found that arthritis and not immobilization plays the major role in the related bone loss. In another very common orthopaedic problem, the aseptic loosening of joint implants, the macrophage activation promoted by inflammatory cytokines has been considered responsible for the observed periprosthetic osteoclast-mediated bone resorption [79]. In many other events, such as fractures, crushing injuries, contusions, surgical operations, burns, infections and inflammations, all the ongoing regional processes – blood flow, cell metabolism and turnover, capillarization and reparative cellular activities – are greatly accelerated.

First postulated by Frost in 1983, this mechanism has been called the regional acceleratory phenomenon (RAP) and it may also increase any growth, modelling or remodelling of bone [1,5,80]. The activation of RAP in post-traumatic conditions is the main difference between immobilization and post-traumatic osteopenia. The biochemical and cellular constituents of the RAP as an operational entity have recently been delineated in several investigations on the complex interrelationships between the cellular components of inflammatory reactions, bone cells, cytokines, prostaglandins and growth factors. According to the latest knowledge, cells of the mononuclear-phagocyte lineage form the precursor cells of osteoclasts and it has recently been shown that monocytes and macrophages, as a result of activation, can change to osteoclast-like cells capable of extensive bone resorption [81].

Cytokines (IL1, IL3, IL6, IL11, MCSF1) and growth factors (TNF[αβ]) activate macrophages, induce their production of neutral proteases which are responsible for the digestion of nonmineralized osteoid, and promote the recruitment, differentiation or activation of osteoclasts. The degradation products of osteoid act as chemotactic stimuli for osteoclasts [79]. Finally, inflammatory cytokines also have a pronounced effect on the proliferation of osteoblasts [82].

It is now clear that post-traumatic osteopenia is an event driven not only by functional impairment and consequent disuse but also by RAP. As a consequence, bone resorption may sometimes occur at a faster rate and to a greater extent than in immobilization osteopenia, as already observed in surgically induced experimental disuse models [47]. Histomorphological changes in bones affected by post-traumatic osteopenia confirm the presence of a high-turnover condition with an increased number of both osteoclasts and osteoblasts and an increased osteoid volume and surface [83,84].

Soft Tissue Injury

The occurrence of osteopenia was reported principally as a consequence of fractures but soft tissue injuries may cause bone loss too. In 1969 Nilsson and Westlin [85], measuring bone content by single photon absorptiometry in the distal aspect of the femur of 54 patients time after a meniscectomy, found a residual 9% decrease with respect to the contralateral side. An average 10% bone loss in the proximal aspect of the tibia was found by Andersson and Nilsson [86] in patients with partial rupture of a knee ligament, whereas in patients with a complete rupture the average acute bone loss was 18%. Kannus et al. [87] investigated bone mass in the proximal and distal femur, proximal tibia, patella and calcaneus of 42 patients with acute knee ligament injury surgically treated 10–11 years earlier: no difference between sides was found in patients with moderate injury (isolated rupture of the collateral medial ligament), whereas in patients with severe injury (cruciate ligament rupture) the reduction in bone density of the affected side was 6% at the distal femur, 9% at the patella and 3.3% at the proximal tibia. Neither the proximal femur nor the calcaneus showed any difference. Using dual photon absorptiometry, Petersen et al. [88] found that 12 years after surgery the reduction of bone density at the proximal tibia was 2.8% in patients with total meniscectomy and 1.3% in patients with partial medial meniscectomy. Also at the shoulder, soft tissue inflammatory conditions lead to bone loss. Lundberg and Nilsson [89] reported considerable bone loss in the proximal humerus of patients affected by the so-called frozen-shoulder syndrome. Kannus et al. [90] examined by dual-energy X-ray absorptiometry 34 men who had been managed operatively 9 years earlier for a rupture of the rotator cuff of the dominant shoulder. The reduction in bone density at the operated side was 3.5% at the proximal humerus, 2.6% at the humeral shaft, 0.4% at the radial shaft and 0.2% at the distal forearm. Marchetti et al. [91] calculated the proximal humerus bone mass before surgery and at 3, 6 and 12 weeks after surgery in 22 patients immobilized 6 weeks for soft tissue shoulder surgery. At 6 weeks the reduction in bone density was 13.9% at the lateral region of the humeral head, 11.8% at the medial region of the humeral head, 6% at the humeral neck and 2.3% at the diaphysis. A slight reversal of bone density losses occurred in the humeral head and neck after 6 weeks of remobilization, but in the same period a further slight decrease in bone density was recorded at the diaphyseal level [91]. Finally, Houde et al. [92] recorded a significant bone loss at the distal forearm after wrist or hand surgical procedure and immobilization. The bone loss persisted even after 4.7 weeks of remobilization in all the regions considered, with final values between 5.1% and 7.8%.

Fracture

Changes in bone density were investigated after femoral fracture, tibial shaft fractures, ankle fracture and distal radius fractures. In the different studies, the amount of post-traumatic osteopenia after bone fracture ranged from 9% to 25% for the upper limb and from 4% to 50% for the lower limb depending on the site measured, the technique used, the time elapsed from fracture and other variables (Fig. 38.2) [93]. The bone loss is typically greater when measured closer to the site of fracture and at the metaphyseal or epiphyseal bone regions, which have a prevalent trabecular composition. In 25 patients operated on because of a displaced femoral neck fracture, Neander et al. [94] found that, after 6 months, the bone density reduction was 2% at the cortical location of the middle diaphysis, and 11% and 19% at the more trabecular regions of the distal femur and proximal tibia. In a series of patients with surgically treated femoral shaft fracture, Kannus et al. [95] found that 10 years after the fracture the residual bone loss was 6.8% at the distal femur, 5.4% at the patella, 4.7% at the proximal tibia and 2.2% at the calcaneus. The mainly cortical femoral neck region did not show any reduction of bone density. The same group investigated the long-term effects of tibial fracture on bone density on the same skeletal regions and found, 9 years after the fracture, greater bone loss at the mainly trabecular sites of distal femur, patella and proximal tibia. Moreover, the patients with primarily nonunited fractures showed bone loss greater than patients with primarily united fractures [96]. Bone changes after tibial shaft fracture were also investigated by Finsen and Haave [97]: after 16–68 months, they found an average 7–8% bone loss at the metaphysis of the distal femur and of the proximal and distal tibia while the bone loss at the femoral and tibial diaphysis was 3%. In a similar study on ankle fractures, Finsen and Benum [98] found a bone loss at the metaphysis of the distal femur and proximal tibia of 5% and 9% respectively after 2 years, while the corresponding values at the femoral and tibial diaphysis were 3.5% and 6%. At 1 year after unstable fractures of the leg, Van der Wiel et al. [99] found a greater bone loss in the mainly trabecular trochanteric region than in the mainly cortical neck region of the proximal femur (9% vs 5%).

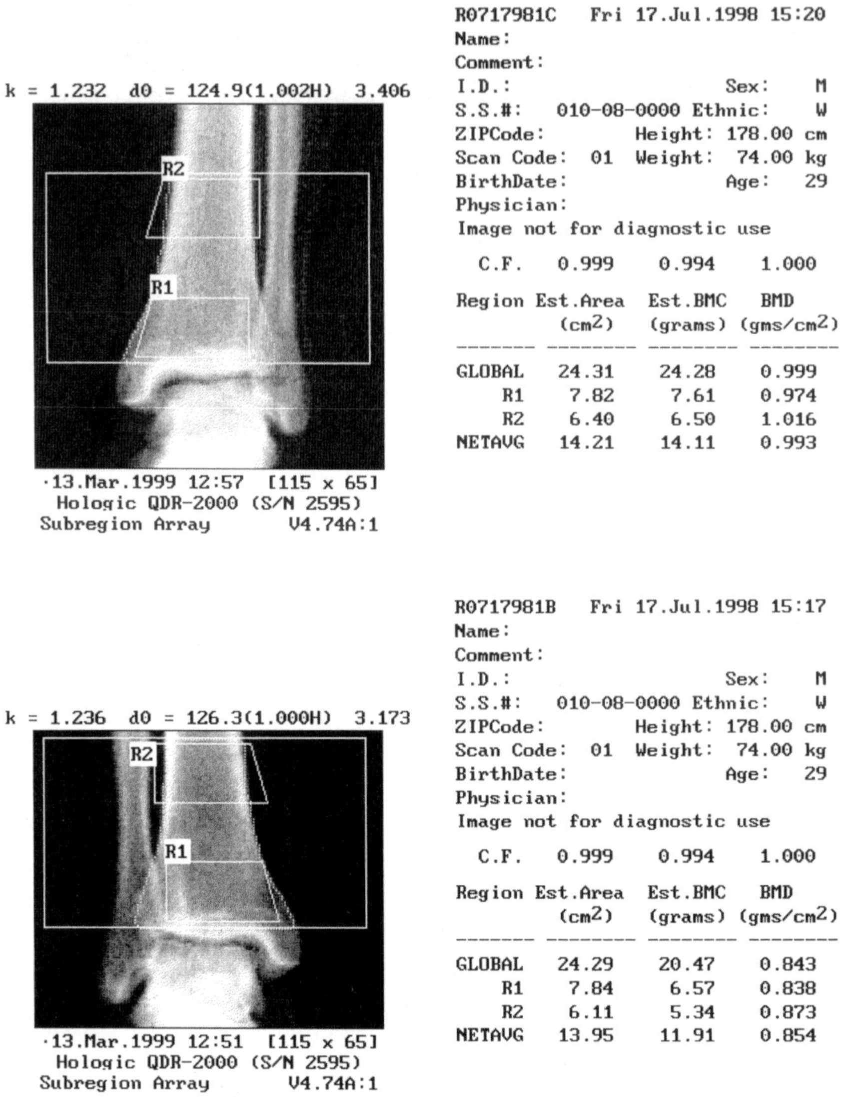

R0717981C Fri 17.Jul.1998 15:20
Name:
Comment:
I.D.: Sex: M
S.S.#: 010-08-0000 Ethnic: W
ZIPCode: Height: 178.00 cm
Scan Code: 01 Weight: 74.00 kg
BirthDate: Age: 29
Physician:
Image not for diagnostic use
k = 1.232 d0 = 124.9(1.002H) 3.406
R2
R1
C.F. 0.999 0.994 1.000
Region Est.Area (cm2) Est.BMC (grams) BMD (gms/cm2)
GLOBAL 24.31 24.28 0.999
R1 7.82 7.61 0.974
R2 6.40 6.50 1.016
NETAVG 14.21 14.11 0.993
·13.Mar.1999 12:57 [115 x 65]
Hologic QDR-2000 (S/N 2595)
Subregion Array V4.74A:1
R0717981B Fri 17.Jul.1998 15:17
Name:
Comment:
I.D.: Sex: M
S.S.#: 010-08-0000 Ethnic: W
ZIPCode: Height: 178.00 cm
Scan Code: 01 Weight: 74.00 kg
BirthDate: Age: 29
Physician:
Image not for diagnostic use
k = 1.236 d0 = 126.3(1.000H) 3.173
R2
R1
C.F. 0.999 0.994 1.000
Region Est.Area (cm2) Est.BMC (grams) BMD (gms/cm2)
GLOBAL 24.29 20.47 0.843
R1 7.84 6.57 0.838
R2 6.11 5.34 0.873
NETAVG 13.95 11.91 0.854
·13.Mar.1999 12:51 [115 x 65]
Hologic QDR-2000 (S/N 2595)
Subregion Array V4.74A:1

Figure 38.2. Dual-energy X-ray absorptiometry bone densitometry of the distal legs of a young adult man 2 years after a traumatic fracture of the proximal right tibia. Bone mineral density in the fractured tibia is 14% lower than in the contralateral healthy leg, indicating a relevant residual post-traumatic bone loss.

Longitudinal studies have also reported a substantial agreement on the chronological succession of the repair events: the lowest values of bone mass are reached from 4 to 12 months after injury [55,94,98–102]. Trabecular bone responds faster to injury and immobilization but also to remobilization, while cortical bone has a greater latency [92,94].

When the repair processes are complete, the bone mineral density at the site of the fracture is higher than at the contralateral healthy site: this increase was found after diaphyseal radial fractures by Nilsson and Westlin [103], after Colles' fractures by Finsen and Benum (+39%) [104], after tibial fractures by Finsen and Haave (+28%) [97] and by Eyers and Kanis (+72% in adults, +30% in children) [55].

Severity and Recovery

Time for recovery is much greater than the time elapsed for the development of osteopenia. In the study of Nilsson and Westlin [105] on bone loss in 74 women who had sustained a Colles' fracture from 1 month to 12 years earlier, there was a significant trend for post-traumatic osteopenia to decrease with time with a long-term pattern. Four months after a tibial shaft fracture, Andersson and Nilsson found an average bone loss of 40% which was reduced to 25% after 1 year [100] and further reduced in a subgroup of patients 15 years later [106]. The amount of bone loss within the first months after a tibial fracture in the trabecular site of the proximal or distal tibia ranges between 43% and 50% in different studies [98,100,102,107], but in long-term follow-up the residual osteopenia ranged from 1.5% to 29% [55,96,97]. A full recovery from post-traumatic osteopenia is not possible in adults but may be expected in children. Nilsson and Westlin [54], studying 14 young adults who had sustained a tibial shaft fracture approximately 11 years earlier, found a complete restoration of bone mass in children who were younger than 10 years old at the time of the fracture. In their 10 patients studied 5–10 years after a tibial fracture occurred when they were children, Eyers and Kanis [55] showed a complete recovery of bone mass. A complete recovery in children after a tibial fracture was also found by Henderson et al. [108], but only in those who had been immobilized for less than 4 weeks [108].

The degree of post-traumatic osteopenia was correlated with the severity of the fracture but not with early weightbearing in the study of ankle fracture by Ahl et al. [109], with duration of unloading but not with age, basal value of bone mass or body weight and body mass index in the study of Van der Wiel et al. [99], with disability and duration of plaster fixation in one of the first studies by Nilsson [110] and with muscle strength in the study by Henderson et al. [108].

Kannus et al. [87,90,95,96] performed four studies on post-traumatic osteopenia after knee ligament injuries, tibial fractures, femur fractures and rotator cuff ruptures. In these studies, bone mass in the affected limb was primarily correlated with some parameters of function: with knee functional scores in the case of ligament injuries and femur fractures, with knee functional scores, muscle strength, short immobilization time and low pain assessment in the case of tibial fracture, and with objective assessment of shoulder function in the case of rotator cuff ruptures. Other parameters such as patient's age, type of surgery and fracture type or location did not show any significant correlation with the bone mass status.

It may be argued that the degree of post-traumatic osteopenia and its potential restoration are not strictly tied to a time limit beyond which the bone loss become irreversible, as suggested by some authors [111,112]. It seems more probable that a more severe injury induces a greater bone loss and that the pattern of bone mass recovery is linked to the pattern of functional recovery.

Clinical Considerations

Some epidemiological data enlighten the meaning of post-traumatic osteopenia: the enduring lower limb reduction of bone density after certain type of fractures is linked to a higher probability of subsequent ipsilateral fractures at a different level [114,115] and raise concern for the effects on the risk of fragility fractures in osteopenic and osteoporotic elderly people [93].

The cornerstones of the management of post-traumatic osteopenia are those already described for the immobilization-induced osteopenia: limitation of immobilization time, effective muscular training during and after immobilization, early functional rehabilitation. Data concerning pharmacological treatment of post-traumatic osteopenia are scarce, the efficacy still unproven and additional rigorous clinical studies are needed [116,117]. Theoretically, there may be a place also for treatments able to interfere with RAP.

References

1. Frost HM. Introduction to a new skeletal physiology. Vol. I: Bone and bones. Pueblo, CO: Pajaro Group, 1995.
2. Wolff J. Concerning the interrelationship between form and function of the individual parts of the organism. Clin Orthop 1988;228:2–12.
3. Dowden JW. The principle of early active movement in treating fractures of the upper extremity. Clin Orthop 1980;146:4–8.
4. Bauer GCH. Rate of bone salt formation in healing fractures determined in rats by means of radiocalcium. Acta Orthop Scand 1954;23:169–191.
5. Frost HM. The biology of fracture healing: an overview for clinicians, part. 1. Clin Orthop 1989;248:283–293.
6. Wendeberg B. Mineral metabolism of fractures of the tibia in man studied with external counting of Sr85. Acta Orthop Scand 1961;Suppl 52:130.
7. Frost HM. The mechanostat: a proposed pathogenic mechanism of osteoporoses and the bone mass effects of mechanical and nonmechanical agents. Bone Miner 1987;2: 73–85.
8. Frost HM. Perspectives: on artificial joint design. J Long Term Eff Med Impl 1992;2: 9–35.
9. Epker BN, Frost HM. Correlation of patterns of bone resorption and formation with physical behaviour of loaded bone. J Dent Res 1965;44:33–42.
10. Epker BN, O'Ryan F. Determinant of Class II dentofacial morphology. I. A biomechanical theory. In: McNamara JA, Carlson DS and Ribbens KA, editors. Effects of surgical intervention on craniofacial growth. Ann Arbor: University of Michigan, 1982:169–205.
11. Frost HM. Orthopaedics biomechanics. Springfield: Thomas, 1973.
12. Lanyon LE. Functional strain as a determinant for bone remodelling. Calcif Tissue Int 1984;36 (Suppl):s56–s61.
13. Turner CH. Homeostatic control of bone structure: an application of feedback theory. Bone 1991;12:203–217.
14. Pattin CA, Carter DR. Bone mechanical energy dissipation during cycling loading. Trans Orthop Res Soc 37th annual meeting, 1991:129.
15. Melton LJ, Kan SH, Wahner HW, Riggs BL. Lifetime fracture risk: an approach to hip fracture risk assessment based on bone mineral density and age. J Clin Epidemiol 1988;10:985–994.
16. Sedlin ED. Uses of bone as a model system in the study of ageing. In: HM Frost, editor. Bone biodynamics Boston: Little Brown, 1964:655–666.

17. Frost HM. Perspectives: the role of changes in mechanical usage setpoints in the pathogenesis of osteoporosis. J Bone Miner Res 1992;7:253–261.
18. Dietrick JE, Whedon GD, Shorr E. Effects of immobilization upon various metabolic and physiologic functions of normal men. Am J Med 1948;4:3–36.
19. Issekutz B Jr, Blizzard JJ, Birkhead NC, Rodahl K. Effects of prolonged bed rest on urinary calcium output. J Appl Physiol 1966;21:1013–1020.
20. Rose GA. Immobilization osteoporosis: study of extent, severity and treatment with bendrofluazide. Br J Surg 1966;53:769–774.
21. Donaldson CL, Hulley SB, Vogel JM, Hattner RS, Boyers JH, MacMillan DE. Effects of prolonged bed rest on bone mineral. Metabolism 1970;19:1071–1084.
22. Davids H. Russians discuss space radiation in conference. Missiles and Rockets 1963 (Oct 21):34.
23. Birykov N, Krasnykh IG. Changes in optical density of bone tissue and calcium metabolism in cosmonauts, Nikolayev AG, Sevastyanov VI. Kosmicheskaya Biologiya i Meditsina 1970;4:42–45.
24. Rambaud PC, Leach CS, Johnson PC. Calcium and phosphorus changes of the Apollo 17 crewmembers. Nutr Metab 1975;182:62–69.
25. Rambaud PC, Leach CS, Whedon GD. A study of metabolic balance in crewmembers of Skylab IV. Acta Astronautica 1979;6:1113–1122.
26. Rambaud PC, Johnson PC. Prolonged weightlessness and calcium loss in man. Acta Astronautica 1979;6:1313–1322.
27. Rambaud PC, Goode AW. Skeletal changes during space flight. Lancet 1985;I:1050–1052.
28. Steward AF, Adler M, Byers CM, Segre GV, Broadus AE. Calcium homeostasis in immobilization: an example of resorptive hypercalciuria. N Engl J Med 1982;306:1136–1140.
29. Minaire P, Meunier P, Edouard C, Bernard J, Courpron P, Bourret J. Quantitative histological data on disuse osteoporosis: comparison with biological data. Calcif Tissue Res 1974;17:57–73.
30. Vico L, Chappard D, Alexandre C, Palle S, Minaire P, Riffat G, et al. Effects of 120 day period of bed-rest on bone mass and bone cell activities in man: attempts at countermeasure. Bone Miner 1987;2:383–394.
31. Weinreb M, Rodan GA, Thompson DD. Depression of osteoblastic activity in immobilized limbs of suckling rats. J Bone Miner Res 1991;6:725–731.
32. Gross TS, Rubin CT. Uniformity of resorptive bone loss induced by disuse. J Orthop Res 1995;13:708–714.
33. Wronski TJ, Morey ER. Inhibition of cortical and trabecular bone formation in the long bones of immobilized monkeys. Clin Orthop 1983;181:269–276.
34. Lane NE, Kaneps AJ, Stover SM, Modin G, Kimmel DB. Bone mineral density and turnover following forelimb immobilization and recovery in young adult dogs. Calcif Tissue Int 1996;59:401–406.
35. Thomas T, Vico L, Skerry TM, Caulin F, Lanyon LE, Alexandre C, et al. Architectural modifications and cellular response during disuse-related bone loss in calcaneus of the sheep. J Appl Physiol, 1996;80:198–202.
36. Kaneps AJ, Stover SM, Lane NE. Changes in canine cortical and cancellous bone mechanical properties following immobilization and remobilization with exercise. Bone 1997;21:419–423.
37. Uhthoff HK, Jaworski ZFG. Bone loss in response to long-term immobilization. J Bone Joint Surg Br 60:1978;420–429.
38. Roberts JG, Ditomasso E, Weber CE. Photon scattering measurements of calcaneal bone density: results of in vivo cross-sectional studies. Invest Radiol 1982;17:20–28.
39. Gross M, Roberts JG, Foster J, Shankardass K, Weber CE. Calcaneal bone density reduction in patients with restricted mobility. Arch Phys Med Rehabil 1987;68: 158–161.
40. Krølner B, Toft B. Vertebral bone loss: unheeded side effect of therapeutic bed rest. Clin Sci 1983;64:537–540.

41. Hansson TH, Roos BO, Nachemson A. Development of osteopenia in fourth lumbar vertebra during prolonged bed rest after operation for scoliosis. Acta Orthop Scand 1975;46:621–630.
42. Hulley SB, Vogel JM, Donaldson CL, Bayers JH, Friedman RJ, Rosen SN. Effects of supplemental oral phosphate on the bone mineral changes during prolonged bed rest. J Clin Invest 1971;50:2506–2518.
43. Schneider VS, McDonald. Skeletal calcium homeostasis and countermeasures to prevent disuse osteoporosis. Calcif Tissue Int 1984;36(Suppl1):s151–s154.
44. Leblanc AD, Schneider VS, Evans HJ, Engelbretson DA, Krebs JM. Bone mineral loss and recovery after 17 weeks of bed rest. J Bone Miner Res 1990;5:843–850.
45. Skerry TM, Lanyon LE. Interruption of disuse by short duration walking exercise does not prevent bone loss in the sheep calcaneus. Bone 1995;16:269–274.
46. Cann CE, Genant HK, Young DR. Comparison of vertebral and peripheral mineral losses in disuse osteoporosis in monkeys. Radiology 1980;134:525–529.
47. Maeda H, Kimmel DB, Raab DM, Lane NE. Musculoskeletal recovery following hindlimb immobilization in adult female rats. Bone 1993;14:153–159.
48. Young DR, Niklowitz WJ, Brown RJ, Jee WSS. Immobilization-associated osteoporosis in primates. Bone 1986;7:109–117.
49. Uhthoff HK, Sekaly G, Jaworski ZFG. Effect of long-term immobilization on metaphyseal spongiosa in young adult and old beagle dogs. Clin Orthop 1985;192:278–283.
50. Jaworski ZFG, Liskova-Kiar M, Uhthoff HK. Effect of long-term immobilization on the pattern of bone loss in older dogs. J Bone Joint Surg Br 1980;62:104–110.
51. Jaworski ZFG, Uhthoff HK. Reversibility of nontraumatic disuse osteoporosis during its active phase. Bone 1986;7:431–439.
52. Griffith JH, D'Orsi CJ, Zimmerman RE. Use of 125I photon scanning in evaluation of bone density in group of patients with spinal cord injury. Invest Radiol 1972;7: 107–111.
53. Tuukkanen J, Peng Z, Väänänen HK. The effect of training on the recovery from immobilization-induced bone loss in rats. Acta Physiol Scand 1992;145:407–411.
54. Nilsson BE, Westlin NE. Restoration of bone mass after fracture of the lower limb in children. Acta Orthop Scand 1971;42:78–81.
55. Eyres KS, Kanis JA. Bone loss after tibial fracture: evaluated by dual-energy X-ray absorptiometry. J Bone Joint Surg Br 1995;77:473–478.
56. Kannus P, Sievänen H, Järvinen TLN, Järvinen M, Kvist M, Oja P, et al. Effects of free mobilization and low- to high-intensity treadmill running on the immobilization-induced bone loss in rats. J Bone Miner Res 1994;10:1613–1619.
57. Kannus P, Järvinen TLN, Sievänen H, Kvist M, Rauhaniemi J, Maunu V-M, et al. Effects of immobilization, three forms of remobilization, and subsequent deconditioning on bone mineral content and density in rat femora. J Bone Miner Res 1996;11:1339–1346.
58. Anderson SA, Cohn SH. Bone demineralization during space flight. Physiologist 1985; 28:212–217.
59. Smith EL, Gilligan C. Dose–response relationship between physical loading and mechanical competence of bone. Bone 1996;18(Suppl):45S–50S.
60. Lanyon LE. Using functional loading to influence bone mass and architecture: objectives, mechanisms, and relationship with estrogen of the mechanically adaptive process in bone. Bone 1996;18(Suppl):37S–43S.
61. Kannus P, Sievänen H, Vuori I. Physical loading, exercise and bone. Bone 1996; 18(Suppl):1S–3S.
62. Skerry TM. Mechanical loading and bone: what sort of exercise is beneficial to the skeleton? Bone 1997;20:179–181.
63. Thompson DD, Seedor JG, Weinreb M, Rosini S, Rodan GA. Aminohydroxybutane bisphosphonate inhibits bone loss due to immobilization in rats. J Bone Miner Res 1990;5:279–286.
64. Lepola V, Jalovaara P, Vaananen K. The influence of clodronate on the torsional strength of the growing rat tibia in immobilization osteoporosis. Bone 1994;15:367–371.

65. Morukov BV, Saichik VE, Ivanov VM, Orlov OI. The use of bisphosphonates for correcting changes of calcium turnover and mineral state of bone tissue during 60-day rat hypokinesia. Patol Fiziol Eksp Ter 1987;2:75–77.
66. Grigoriev AI, Morukov BV, Oganov VS, Rakhmanov AS, Buravkova LB. Effect of exercise and bisphosphonate on mineral balance and bone density during 360 day antiorthostatic hypokinesia. J Bone Miner Res 1992;7(Suppl 2):S449–S455.
67. Chappart D, Alexandre C, Palle S, Vico L, Morukov BV, Rodionova SS, et al. Effect of a bisphosphonate (1-hydroxy ethyldene-1,1 biphosphonic acid) on osteoclast number during prolonged bed rest in healthy humans. Metabolism 1989;38:822–825.
68. Minaire P, Depassio J, Berard E, Meunier PJ, Edouard C, Pilonchery G, et al. Effects of clodronate on immobilization bone loss. Bone 1987;8 (suppl.1):S63–S68.
69. Chappart D, Minaire P, Privat C, Berard E, Mendoza-Sarmiento J, Tournebise H, et al. Effects of tiludronate on bone loss in paraplegic patients. J Bone Miner Res 1995;10:112–118.
70. Tuukkanen J, Jalovaara P, Väänänen HK. Calcitonin treatment of immobilization osteoporosis in rats. Acta Physiol Scand 1991;141:119–124.
71. Thomas T, Skerry TM, Vivo L, Caulin F, Lanyon LE, Alexandre C. Ineffectiveness of calcitonin on a local-disuse osteoporosis in the sheep: a histomorphometric study. Calcif Tissue Int 1995;57:224–228.
72. Waters DJ, Caywood DD, Trachte GJ, Turner RT, Hodgson SF. Immobilization increases bone prostaglandin E. Effect of acetylsalicylic acid on disuse osteoporosis studied in dogs. Acta Orthop Scand 1991;62:238–243.
73. Fiorentino S, Melillo G, Fedele G, Clavenna G, D'Agostino C, Mainetti E, et al. Ketoprofen lysine salt inhibits disuse-induced osteopenia in a new non-traumatic immobilization model in the rat. Pharmacol Res 1996;33:277–281.
74. Waters DJ, Caywood DD, Turner RT. Effect of tamoxifen citrate on canine immobilization (disuse) osteoporosis. Vet Surg 1991;20:392–396.
75. Ma YF, Jee WS, Ke HZ, Lin BY, Liang XG, Li M, Yamamoto N. Human parathyroid hormone-(1–38) restores cancellous bone to the immobilized, osteopenic proximal tibial metaphysis in rats. J Bone Miner Res 1995;10:496–505.
76. Burr DB, Frederickson RG, Pavlinch S, Sickles M, Burkhard S. Intracast muscle stimulation prevents bone and cartilage deterioration in cast-immobilized rabbits. Clin Orthop 1984;189:264–278.
77. Rubin CT, McLeod KJ, Lanyon LE. Prevention of osteoporosis by pulsed electromagnetic fields. J Bone Joint Surg Am 1989;71:411–417.
78. Bogoch ER, Moran E, Crowe S, Fornasier V. Arthritis not immobilization causes bone loss in the carrageenan injection model of inflammatory arthritis. J Orthop Res 1995;13:777–782.
79. Lassus J, Salo J, Jiranek WA, Santavirta S, Nevalainen J, Matucci-Cerinic M, et al. Macrophage activation results in bone resorption. Clin Orthop 1998;352:7–15.
80. Frost HM. The regional acceleratory phenomenon: a review. Henry Ford Hosp Med J 1983;31:3–9.
81. Quinn JM, Sabokbar A, Athanasou NA. Cells of the mononuclear phagocyte series differentiate into osteoclastic lacunar bone resorbing cells. J Pathol 1996;179:106–111.
82. Frost A, Jonsson KB, Nilsson O, Ljunggren O. Inflammatory cytokines regulate proliferation of cultured human osteoblasts. Acta Orthop Scand 1997;68:91–96.
83. Obrant KJ. Trabecular bone changes in the greater trochanter after fracture of the femoral neck. Acta Orthop Scand 1984;55:78–82.
84. Obrant KJ, Nilsson BE . Histomorphologic changes in the tibial epiphysis after diaphyseal fracture. Clin Orthop 1984;185:271–275.
85. Nilsson BE, Westlin NE. Osteoporosis following injury to the semilunar cartilage. Calcif Tissue Res 1969;4:185–187.
86. Andersson SM, Nilsson BE. Changes in bone mineral content following ligamentous knee injuries. Med Sci Sports 1979;11:351–354.

87. Kannus P, Sievänen H, Järvinen M, Heinonen A, Oja P, Vuori I. A cruciate ligament injury produces considerable, permanent osteoporosis in the affected knee. J Bone Miner Res 1992;7:1429–1434.
88. Petersen MM, Olsen C. Lauritzen JB, Lund B, Hede A. Late changes in bone mineral density of the proximal tibia following total or partial medial meniscectomy. J Orthop Res 1996;14:16–21.
89. Lundberg BJ, Nilsson BE. Osteopenia in the frozen shoulder. Clin Orthop 1965; 60:187–191.
90. Kannus P, Leppälä J, Lehto M, Sievänen H, Heinonen A, Järvinen M. A rotator cuff rupture produces permanent osteoporosis in the affected extremity, but not in those whom shoulder function has returned to normal. J Bone Miner Res 1995;10:1263–1271.
91. Marchetti ME, Houde JP, Steinberg GG, Crane GK, Goss TP, Baran DT. Humeral bone density losses after shoulder surgery and immobilization. J Shoulder Elbow Surg 1996;5:471–475.
92. Houde JP, Schulz LA, Morgan WJ, Breen T, Warhold L, Crane GK, Baran D. Bone mineral changes in the forearm after immobilization. Clin Orthop 1995;317:199–205.
93. Järvinen M, Kannus P. Injury of an extremity as a risk factor for the development of osteoporosis. J Bone Joint Surg Am 1997;79:263–276.
94. Neander G, Adolphson P, Hedström, von Siver K, Dahlborn M, Dalén N. Decrease in bone mineral density and muscle mass after femoral neck fracture. A quantitative computed tomography study in 25 patients. Acta Orthop Scand 1997;68:451–455.
95. Kannus P, Järvinen M, Sievänen H, Järvinen TAH, Oja P, Vuori I. Reduced bone mineral density in men with a previous femur fracture. J Bone Miner Res 1994;11:1729–1736.
96. Kannus P, Järvinen M, Sievänen H, Oja P, Vuori I. Osteoporosis in men with a history of tibial fracture. J Bone Miner Res 1994;9:423–429.
97. Finsen V, Haave O. Changes in bone-mass after tibial shaft fracture. Acta Orthop Scand 1987;58:369–371.
98. Finsen V, Benum P. Osteopenia after ankle fractures: the influence of early weight bearing and muscle activity. Clin Orthop 1989;245:261–268.
99. Van der Wiel HE, Lips P, Nauta J, Patka P, Haarman HJThM, Teule GJJ. Loss of bone in the proximal part of the femur following unstable fractures of the leg. J Bone Joint Surg Am 1994;76:230–236.
100. Andersson SM, Nilsson BE. Changes in bone mineral content following tibial shaft fractures. Clin Orthop 1979;144:226–229.
101. Ulivieri FM, Bossi E, Azzoni R, Ronzani C, Trevisan C, Montesano A, et al. Quantification by dual photon absorptiometry of local bone loss after fracture. Clin Orthop 1990;250:291–296.
102. Westlin NE. Loss of bone mineral after Colles' fracture. Clin Orthop 1974;102:194–199.
103. Nilsson BE, Westlin NE. Bone mineral content in the forearm after fracture of the upper limb. Calcif Tissue Res 1977;22:329–331.
104. Finsen V, Benum P. Refracture rate after removal of fixation device from healed hip fractures. Acta Orthop Scand 1986;57:434–435.
105. Nilsson BE, Westlin NE. Long-term observations on the loss of bone mineral following Colles' fracture. Acta Orthop Scand 1975;46:61–66.
106. Karlsson MK, Nilsson BE, Obrant KJ. Bone mineral loss after lower extremity trauma. 62 cases followed for 15–38 years. Acta Orthop Scand 1993;64:362–364.
107. Andersson SM, Nilsson BE. Post-traumatic bone mineral loss in tibial shaft fractures treated with a weight-bearing brace. Acta Orthop Scand 1979;50:689–691.
108. Henderson RC, Kemp GJ, Campion ER. Residual bone mineral density and muscle strength after fractures of the tibia or femur in children. J Bone Joint Surg Am 1992;74:211–218.
109. Ahl T, Sjoberg H, Dalen N. Bone mineral content in the calcaneus after ankle fracture. Acta Orthop Scand 1988;59:173–175.

110. Nilsson BE. Post-traumatic osteopenia: a quantitative study of the bone mineral mass in the femur following fracture of the tibia in man using Americium-241 as a photon source. Acta Orthop Scand 1966;37(Suppl 91).
111. Minaire P. Immobilization osteoporosis: a review. Clin Rheumatol 1989;8(Suppl): 95–103.
112. Mazess RB, Whedon GD. Immobilization and bone. Calcif Tissue Int 1983;35:265–267.
113. Finsen V, Haave O, Benum P. Fracture interaction in the extremities: the possible relevance of post-traumatic osteopenia. Clin Orthop 1989;240:244–249.
114. Karlsson MK, Hasserius R, Obrant KJ. The ankle fracture as an index for future fracture risk. A 25–40 years follow-up of 1063 cases. Acta Orthop Scand 1993;64:482–484.
115. Mallet E, Lefort J, Caulin F. Prevention of trabecular bone loss in children's femoral fracture: effects of treatment with calcitonin. Clin Sci 1986;70 (Suppl 13):82.
116. Crespo R, Revilla M, Crespo E, Villa LF, Rico H. Complementary medical treatment for Colles' fracture: a comparative, randomized, longitudinal study. Calcif Tissue Int 1997;60:567–570.
117. Petersen MM, Lauritzen JB, Schwarz P, Lund B. Effect of nasal calcitonin on post-traumatic osteopenia following ankle fracture. A randomized double-blind placebo-controlled study in 24 patients. Acta Orthop Scand 1998;69:347–350.

39 Reflex Sympathetic Dystrophy

J. H. B. Geertzen and P. U. Dijkstra

Introduction

Reflex sympathetic dystrophy (RSD) is a complex regional pain syndrome that was probably first described by Ambroise Paré in the sixteenth century [1]. Paré treated King Charles IX of France for severe pain after a phlebotomy. The pain disappeared within several months. In the centuries between Paré and Sudeck (1900), only two papers are known in which RSD or a related syndrome (causalgia) is described: Denmark in 1813 and Mitchell et al. in 1864 [2,3]. Sudeck reported in 1900 for the first time the atrophy of the bones seen on radiography [4]. "Sudeck atrophy" is the name frequently used for this pain syndrome. Over the centuries the supposed pathogenesis of RSD has changed many times, and probably as a consequence of that the names and definitions and the therapies of RSD have changed [5,6]. Many names have been given to RSD. For instance, more than 30 different names can be found in the French literature, more than 80 different names in the Anglo-Saxon literature, and more than 50 in the German literature [7–10]. In Dutch literature a mere 15 names for this syndrome can be found [7]. The names are related either to a supposed pathogenesis (e.g., reflex sympathetic dystrophy, paralyse de ordre reflexe), to the clinical signs (e.g., swollen atrophic hand, Stauungsatrophie), to the diagnostic findings in radiographs (e.g., Sudecksche Knochenatrophie, osteotrophie traumatique) or to the inciting event (e.g., rhumatisme neurotrophique, post-traumatic dystrophy) [10,11].

The diagnosis of RSD is usually made on the basis of clinical signs and symptoms; however, no uniformly defined criteria exist [5,6,8,12–17]. To make the diagnosis of RSD on the basis of internationally acknowledged criteria is very complex because (1) its etiology is poorly understood; (2) the natural causes are quite diverse; (3) many definitions (and related criteria) concerning RSD are proposed; and (4) many therapies have been described [6,12,13,16–18].

There is dissatisfaction with the most frequently used terms "reflex sympathetic dystrophy" and "causalgia". The term RSD does not cover the complete picture of the syndrome it describes; moreover, the role of the sympathetic system in RSD is controversial [15]. Additionally the dystrophic component is not always present in every patient. Recently both terms, RSD and causalgia, were renamed by the International Association for the Study of Pain (IASP) and the terms "complex regional pain syndrome (CRPS)", type I and type II, respectively, were introduced

[5,6,15,19–21]. The definition of CRPS type I, according to the IASP, is as follows: "CRPS type I is a syndrome that usually develops after a noxious event, is not limited to the distribution of a single nerve, and is apparently disproportionate to the inciting event. It is associated at some point with evidence of edema, changes in skin blood flow, abnormal sudomotor activity in the region of pain, or allodynia or hyperalgesia." The criteria for CRPS type I are the following:

1. The presence of an initiating noxious event, or a cause of immobilization.
2. Continuing pain, allodynia, or hyperalgesia with which the pain is disproportionate to any inciting event.
3. Evidence at some time of edema, changes in skin blood flow or abnormal sudomotor activity in the region of the pain.
4. The diagnosis is excluded by the existence of conditions that would otherwise account for the degree of pain and dysfunction.
5. Criteria 2, 3 and 4 must be satisfied.

All the definitions used have their limitations in daily practice [4–8,12–17,22–24]. The fifth criterion is rather strange; there are five criteria and only criteria 2, 3 and 4 must be satisfied. Why not define three mandatory criteria? The suggested symptoms are difficult to handle in daily clinical practice. The suggested criteria can change over time and are not consistently manifest. There is a need for more manageable criteria. A suggestion for criteria to define RSD for clinical daily practice, which are easy to handle, is as follows: RSD is a complex of symptoms that may develop after trauma, disease or "spontaneously" and has obligatory pain and at least three of the four following symptoms:

1. Difference in skin color relative to the other limb.
2. Diffuse edema.
3. Difference in skin temperature relative to the other limb
4. Limited active range of motion.

The definition of CRPS type II, according to the IASP, is as follows: "CRPS type II is a burning pain syndrome with allodynia, and hyperpathia usually in the hand or foot after partial injury of a nerve or one of its major branches [5]". The only criterion according to which it can be distinguished from CRPS type I is the nerve lesion.

Etiology

The inciting event for RSD may vary considerably from minor strain, contusion, fracture, frostbite to myocardial infarction and cancer; in short it can arise from almost anything [7,22,25]. Sometimes RSD may arise spontaneously or seemingly spontaneously because the inciting event was too small for the patient to remember. The incidence described in the literature varies widely, probably due to the different definitions and criteria used for RSD. For instance, after fractures of the wrist the incidence in the literature varies from 0.03% to 37% [26,27].

Women between 40 and 70 years of age are more at risk than others [7,23]. Other risk factors for RSD are coexisting diseases (endocrine and neurological disorders) such as hyperlipidemia, diabetes mellitus, hemiplegia or alcoholism [7,9]. However,

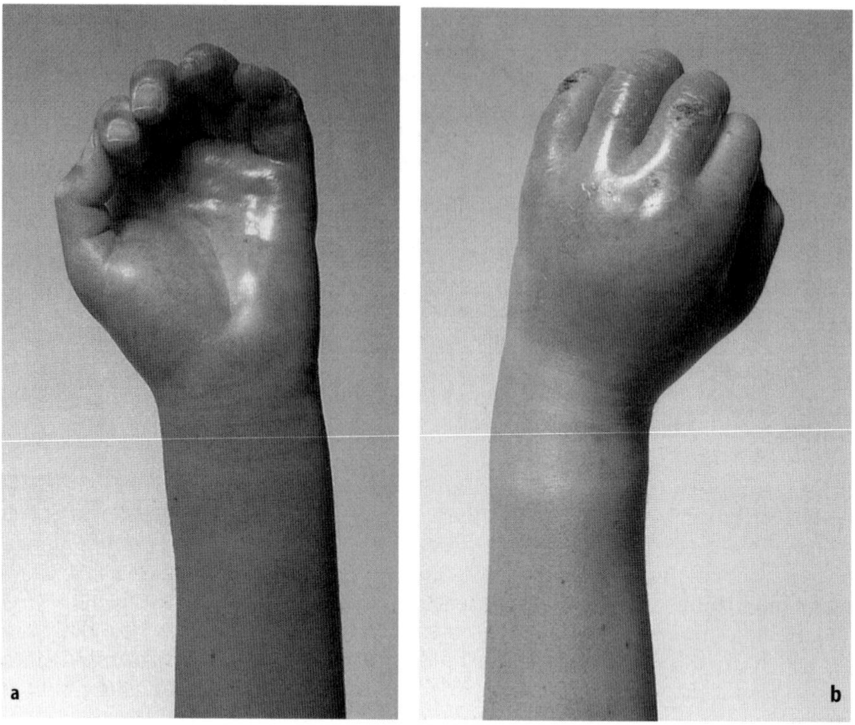

Figure 39.1. **a** Volar aspect of a RSD hand. **b** Dorsal aspect of a RSD hand.

these so-called risk factors have only been described in case studies with a very small number of patients.

It has been suggested that the disproportionate relation between the inciting event and the extensive pain might be regarded as an exaggerated pain response. The pain suggested by the patients seems to have more impact clinically than the pain suggested by multitrauma patients or amputees. This disproportionate relation, in for example CRPS type II, was very well described in 1864 by Weir Mitchell et al. and by Sunderland and Kelly in 1948 [3,24]. These descriptions suggest a behavioral or psychological component. Since then, many authors have expressed ideas about the involvement of psychological or psychosocial aspects in the development of RSD, whereas others have thought that the psychological or psychosocial effects are the result of RSD [13,28–41]. Social life events (SLE) play a role in the pathogenesis of RSD but there is no direct causal relation between psychological disorders or the experience of SLE and the onset of RSD [13].

Symptoms

RSD has many clinical symptoms, which can vary over time, such as pain, edema, discoloration and hyperhidrosis [8]. The intensity of the pain is often disproportionate in relation to the inciting event. In a study by Veldman et al. [8] of the 829 RSD patients, 93% had pain, 91% had discoloration of the skin and 93% had altered skin temperature. Edema was present in 96% of patients and 88% had limitation in the active range of motion of the affected limb. They divided the symptoms into inflammatory signs (e.g., pain, edema, limited range of motion), neurological signs (e.g., hyperpathy, tremor, paresis), atrophy (e.g., atrophy of skin, nails, bone, muscle) and sympathetic signs (hyperhidrosis, changed growth of hairs and nails) [8]. The different symptoms are variable in their intensity and their combinations (Fig. 39.1).

In a study by Jonker [42] in which 183 publications were reviewed, 15 different symptoms (or criteria) were used to describe RSD. Unfortunately the syndrome does not always develop in a typical way with typical symptoms. Due to this problem the syndrome is not always diagnosed early and is sometimes missed altogether.

In short, RSD can have a wide variety of symptoms of different intensities and combinations that change over time. A definition is therefore difficult to establish internationally.

Pathogenesis

In the pathogenesis of RSD two main theories exist: involvement of the sympathetic nervous system or an abnormal inflammatory tissue reaction [6,18,21,28]. The involvement of the sympathetic system is assumed to be sympathetic overactivity in the affected limb [19]. This assumption is based on the observation that in some patients, skin blood flow and consequently the temperature are reduced in the affected limb, and that blocking of the sympathetic efferent pathway to the affected limb relieves these symptoms [19,43]. Others have hypothesized that peripheral interactions between efferent sympathetic and afferent nociceptive pathways are responsible for maintaining a central vicious circle accounting for vascular, sensory and motor disturbances [20].

The theory regarding the abnormal inflammatory tissue reaction was described in 1982 by Fantone et al. [44]. According to that theory, hydroxyl radicals play an important role in the inflammatory processes. The hydroxyl radicals are produced by activated phagocytes or by ischemia. Excessive production of the radicals leads to destruction of healthy tissue which may lead to RSD. Positive results of treatment with scavengers substantiate this theory [8,18,44].

Diagnosis

Many physicians believe that the diagnosis RSD can be made only with additional laboratory investigations such as a nuclear scan, thermography, testing of the sympathetic system or radiography [45–47]. Evidence for this belief is lacking however. In the literature there is consensus about the description of the radiographs in RSD patients. Sudeck described the radiographs of RSD patients as "a patchy osteoporosis" [4].

In 1981, Kozin [16] wrote: "the plain radiograph may show a patchy osteopenia in about half of all patients with RSD, and this may be observed as early as 2 to 3 weeks after the onset of symptoms; however, the patchy osteopenia cannot be differentiated from disuse osteopenia". The rapid bone loss is generally thought to be exclusively due to increased osteoclastic activity following, for example, local tissue acidosis, that explains the peculiar patchy bone loss (Fig. 39.2). Osteopenia may not be considered a reliable diagnostic criterion. Scintigraphy (nuclear bone scan)

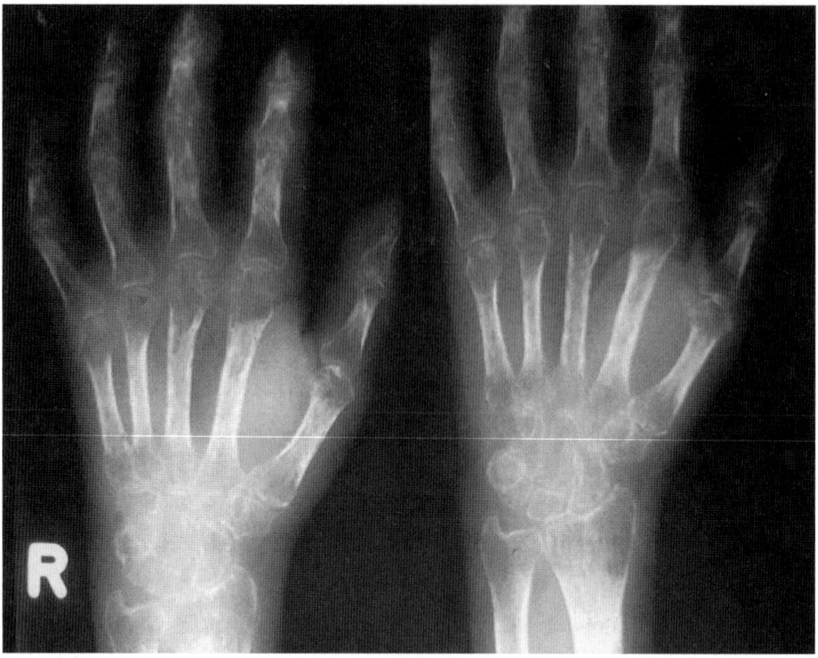

Figure 39.2. Radiograph of a RSD hand after distal radius fracture.

or a three-phase bone scan are more specific but no more sensitive than radiography [16]. In a review by Veldman [7] 11 studies are compared concerning the sensitivity and specificity of bone scans. Sensitivity varied from 29% to 96% and specificity from 77% to 98%. Bone scans are not positive in the so-called late stage of RSD. Magnetic resonance imaging (MRI) appears to be insensitive and nonspecific for the diagnosis RSD [48]. Probably the osteopenia is rather a secondary effect of the immobilization resulting from RSD than a direct effect of RSD itself. A detailed history of the present illness and a conscientious physical examination are usually enough to diagnose RSD.

Differential Diagnosis

Perhaps the most difficult and challenging patients are those with a diversity of clinical symptoms with RSD. Some may have nerve entrapment syndrome (e.g., carpal tunnel syndrome), a myofascial pain syndrome, an undiscovered fracture, an occupational overuse syndrome, tennis elbow, bursitis or fibromyalgia [15]. Pain, tenderness, swelling, warmth and a limitation in range of motion may also occur in patients with arthritis or thrombosis.

Acute compartment syndrome, arterial insufficiency, rheumatological disorders, Raynaud's phenomenon or neurological symptoms such as polyneuropathy may also be present in an atypical way, making the differential diagnosis with RSD difficult [7,15].

As mentioned in the section on diagnosis, a careful interview and physical examination can in many cases solve the differential diagnostic dilemma, though additional laboratory measurements are sometimes necessary: for example, radiographs are necessary to exclude a missed fracture, electromyography to exclude, for example, carpal tunnel syndrome, and blood tests to exclude arthritis.

Treatment

More than 50 types of treatment are described in literature for RSD patients [11]. These treatments can be divided into a few subgroups: physical therapy, occupational therapy, immobilization with a cast or brace, drugs applied to the skin (DMSO), drugs administered regionally (guanethidine), drugs administered systemically (corticosteroids), drugs administered at the level of the spinal cord (opiates), nerve blocks with local anesthetics, surgical procedures such as paravertebral ganglionectomy or periarterial sympathectomy, neurosurgical procedures (thalamotomy), electrical neurostimulation, and others such as radiation therapy or acupuncture [11]. Most authors claim success rates of about 60–70% [16,43,49–51]. These claims are in contrast to the clinical finding that many patients frequently go from doctor to doctor (medical shopping). Some patients undergo, over the years, many types of treatment, including sympathectomy, and long or permanent physical therapy, occupational therapy and/or pharmacotherapy.

With respect to the osteopenia, treatments with intramuscular injections with calcitonin (anti-osteoclastic properties; therapeutic effect in osteoporosis) are proposed. Calcitonin is a hormone and has been the treatment most frequently used for RSD in France [39]. Besides its anti-osteoclastic action it diminishes pain and edema, probably due partly to its analgesic and vascular side-effects. Results of nasal administration were disappointing [39]. If given sufficiently early in the course of RSD, bisphosphonate (inhibits osteoclastic resorption) treatment only arrests bone loss and does not replace lost bone [39].

RSD seldom leads to chronic invalidism or amputation of the affected limb [7,21]. Jänig and Stanton-Hicks [20] concluded that there is a lack of knowledge regarding the efficacy of treatment, time-dependent symptoms of RSD and psychological and psychosomatic aspects of RSD.

In 1994 we published the results of a randomized clinical trial concerning the treatment of of 26 patients who had RSD of the hand. The treatment was initiated within 3 months of the diagnosis RSD [13]. Thirteen patients were treated with regional intravenous ismelin blocks and 13 with a hydroxyl radical scavenger, dimethylsulfoxide (DMSO). After 9 weeks there was a statistically significant better result, as well as a clinically significant better result (e.g., increasing range of motion and reduction of pain and edema), in the group treated with DMSO. The patients applied the DMSO themselves and the costs of the DMSO treatment were less than the treatment with ismelin [13].

Prognosis

In order to inform RSD patients well about their prognosis, extensive knowledge concerning the long-term outcome of RSD is necessary. The World Health Organization suggests a sequence involving disease–impairment–disability–handicap [52]. This sequence is the foundation upon which rehabilitation medicine is built. The activities in rehabilitation medicine regarding diagnosis and prognosis involve not only the examination of impairments but also the determination of disabilities and handicaps. Clinically, each of the factors can be assessed in the course of a rehabilitation process. The rehabilitation team can intervene at each level. It is thus necessary to have knowledge about the sequence disease–impairment–disability–handicap and their relationship. Does an impairment always lead to a disability? To treat or prevent a handicap, should one focus on treatment of the impairments or disabilities? Until recently, only a few studies [14,26,28,53–55] described the long-term outcomes; in only one study [53] were the instruments for measuring the impairments described. Consequently, quantification of the extent of the impairments in RSD in other studies is almost impossible. Disabilities and handicap are mentioned anecdotally [14,28]. To quantify the extent of impairments, disabilities and handicaps in RSD, we performed a long-term follow-up study [56]. The study group consisted of 65 patients with RSD of the upper extremity. RSD appeared after fractures of the wrist or hand in 29 patients (45%) or after a carpal tunnel release in 9 patients (14%). The mean follow-up period was 5.5 years. The main outcome measurements were the impairments measured by standard physical examination. According to the American Medical Association guidelines the impairments found in our study should not result in disabilities. Pain was the most disabling factor.

Another objective of our long-term follow-up study was to identify the general health status, long-term vocational outcome and psychosocial aspects such as social life events (SLE) at the time or shortly after the inciting event of RSD, and to identify the psychological history of the same 65 patients [32]. SLEs, (life change unit (≥ 35), were present in 32 patients (49%). A psychological (or psychiatric) history was present in 22 patients (34%). In total, 60% of the patients had a SLE or/and a psychological history. In total 17 patients (26%) had to change profession due to RSD. Nearly 30% of the patients had to stop working for more than 1 year. These results show a high coincidence between RSD and interacting psychosocial disorders. This co-incidence may play a role in intensifying and prolonging the symptomatology of RSD.

The results of our study also showed that after RSD of the upper extremity, 62% of the RSD patients were limited in the activities of daily life (ADL) and/or instrumental activities of daily life (IADL) to some extent [57]. Pain and restriction in forward flexion of the shoulder, thumb opposition and grip strength were the most important impairments limiting ADL and IADL. Pain was the most important factor contributing to handicap. We found a weak to moderate relationship between impairments and disability and between disability and handicap in RSD patients. It was concluded that pain is the most important factor leading to disability and handicap [57]. As a consequence of the described longstanding impairments after RSD, the (early) treatment for RSD patients should also focus on pain treatment and strength training programs of the affected limb.

Conclusion

RSD is classified as a complex regional pain syndrome, type I. It can develop after a variety of incidents. Because the pathogenesis is unknown, the therapy cannot be causal. RSD can become a chronic pain syndrome and is associated with psychosocial disorders. Pain is the most disabling complaint of RSD.

Acknowledgments. The authors thank J. W. Groothoff, MSc, PhD, of the Northern Centre for Health Care Research, for his positive and critical comments on the manuscript.

References

1. Rogge CWL. De betekenis van A. Paré (1510–1590); mens, leermeester en chirurg. Thesis, University of Groningen, the Netherlands, 1973.
2. Denmark A. An example of symptoms resembling tic doloreux produced by a wound in the radial nerve. Med Chir Trans 1813;4:48–52.
3. Mitchell SW, Morehouse GR, Keen WW. Gunshot wounds and other injuries of nerves. Philadelphia: Lippincot, 1864.
4. Sudeck P. Uber die akute entzündliche Knochenatrophie. Arch Klin Chir 1900;62: 147–156.
5. Merskey H, Bogduk N,editors. Classification of chronic pain: descriptions of chronic pain syndromes and definition of terms, 2nd ed. Seattle: IASP press, 1994.
6. Stanton-Hicks M, Jänig W, Hassenbuch S, et al. Reflex sympathetic dystrophy: changing concepts and taxonomy. Pain 1995;63:127–133.
7. Veldman PHJM. Clinical aspects of reflex sympathetic dystrophy. Thesis, University of Nijmegen, the Netherlands, 1995.
8. Veldman PHJM, Reynen HM, Arntz IE, Goris RJA. Signs and symptoms of reflex sympathetic dystrophy: prospective study of 829 patients. Lancet 1993;342:1012–1016.
9. Vries de J. Schouderpijn bij de hemiplegische patiënt. Thesis, University of Groningen, the Netherlands, 1978.
10. Wagner W. Das Sudeck-Syndrom. Vienna: Wilhelm Maudrich Verlag, 1960.
11. Kurvers HAJM. Reflex sympathetic dystrophy: a clinical and experimental study. Thesis, University of Maastricht, the Netherlands, 1997.
12. Amadio PC, Mackinnon S, Merrit WH, Brody GS, Terzis JK. Reflex sympathetic dystrophy syndrome: Consensus report of an ad hoc committee of the American Association for Hand Surgery on the definition of reflex sympathetic dystrophy syndrome. Plast Reconstr Surg 1991;87:371–375.
13. Geertzen JHB, de Bruijn H, de Bruijn-Kofman AT, Arendzen JH. Reflex sympathetic dystrophy: early treatment and psychological aspects. Arch Phys Med Rehabil 1994;75:442–446.
14. Gibbons JJ, Wilson PR. RSD score: criteria for the diagnosis of reflex sympathetic dystrophy and causalgia. Clin J Pain 1992;8:260–263.
15. Jänig W. The puzzle of "reflex sympathetic dystrophy": mechanisms, hypotheses, open questions. In: Jänig W, Stanton-Hicks M, editors. Reflex sympathetic dystrophy: a reappraisal. Seattle: IASP Press, 1996:1–24.
16. Kozin F, Ryan LM, Carrera GF, Soin JS, Wortman RL. The reflex sympathetic dystrophy syndrome (RSDS). III. Scintigraphic studies, further evidence for the therapeutic efficacy of systemic corticosteroid, and proposed diagnostic criteria. Am J Med 1981;70: 23–30.
17. Lankford LL. Reflex sympathetic dystrophy. In: Omer GF, Spinner M, editors. Management of peripheral nerve problems. Philadelphia: Saunders, 1980:216–244.

18. Goris RJA. Treatment of reflex sympathetic dystrophy with hydroxyl radical scavengers. Unfallchirurgie 1985;88:330–332.
19. Bonica JJ. Causalgia and other reflex sympathetic dystrophies. In: Bonica JJ, Liebeskind JC, Albe-Fessard DG, editors. Advances in pain research and therapy, vol 3. New York: Raven Press, 1990:220–243.
20. Jänig W, Stanton-Hicks M. Future perspectives: experimental neurobiological research in reflex sympathetic dystrophy and its interaction with clinical research. In: Stanton-Hicks M, Jänig W, Boas RA, editors. Reflex sympathetic dystrophy. Dordrecht: Kluwer Academic, 1990:201–205.
21. Jänig W, Stanton-Hicks M. Epilogue. In: Jänig W, Stanton-Hicks M, editors. Reflex sympathetic dystrophy: a reappraisal. Seattle: IASP Press, 1996:239–241.
22. Steinbrocker O. The shoulder-hand syndrome: present perspective. Arch Phys Med Rehabil 1968;49:388–395.
23. Subbarao J, Stillwell GK. Reflex sympathetic dystrophy syndrome of the upper extremity: analysis of total outcome of management of 125 cases. Arch Phys Med Rehabil 1981;62:549–554.
24. Sunderland S, Kelly M. The painful sequelae of injuries to peripheral nerves. Aust N Z J Surg 1948;18:75–118.
25. Johnson AC. Disabling changing in the hands resembling sclerodactylea following myocardial infarctions. Ann Intern Med 1943;19:433–456.
26. Atkins R, Duckworth T, Kanis JA. Features of algodystrophy after Colles' fracture. J Bone Joint Surg Br 1990;72:105–110.
27. Böhler L. Ist das Sudeck-Syndrom nach geschlossenen Verletzungen eine unabwendbare Unfallfolge oder eine vermeidbare Behandlungfolge? Langenbecks Arch Klin Chir 1956;284:43–53.
28. Bruehl S, Carlson CR. Predisposing psychological factors in the development of reflex sympathetic dystrophy: a review of the empirical evidence. Clin J Pain 1992;8: 287–299.
29. Bruehl S, Husfeldt B, Lubenow TR, Nath H, et al. Psychological differences between reflex sympathetic dystrophy and non-RSD chronic pain patients. Pain 1996;67: 107–114.
30. Covington EC. Psychological issues in reflex sympathetic dystrophy. In: vasomotor function, hypotheses, open questions. In: Jänig W, Stanton-Hicks M, editors. Reflex sympathetic dystrophy: a reappraisal. Seattle: IASP Press 1996:191–215.
31. Egle UT, Hoffmann SO. Psychosomatische Zusammenhange bei sympathischer reflex dystrophie (Morbus Sudeck). Psychother Med Psychol 1990;40:123–135.
32. Geertzen JHB, Dijkstra PU, Groothoff JW, Duis HJ ten, Eisma WH. Reflex sympathetic dystrophy of the upper extremity. A 5.5.-year follow up. II. Social life events, general health and changes in occupation. Acta Orthop Scand (Suppl 279) 1998;69:19–23.
33. Haddox JD. Psychological aspects of reflex sympathetic dystrophy. In: Stanton-Hicks M editor. Pain and the sympathetic nervous system. Boston: Kluwer Academic, 1990:207–224.
34. Haddox JD, Abram SE, Hopwood MH. Comparison of psychometric data in RSD and radiculopathy. Reg Anaesth 1988;12(1S):27.
35. Hardy MA, Merritt WH. Psychological evaluation and pain assessment in patients with reflex sympathetic dystrophy. J Hand Ther 1988;155–164.
36. Houdenhove van B. Neuro-algodystrophy: a psychiatrist's view. Clin Rheum 1986;3: 399–406.
37. Houdenhove van B, Vasquez G, Onghena P, et al. Etiopathogenesis of reflex sympathetic dystrophy: a review and biopsychosocial hypothesis. Clin J Pain 1992;8: 300–306.
38. Lynch ME. Psychological aspects of reflex sympathetic dystrophy: a review of the adult and paediatric literature. Pain 1992;49:337–347.
39. Pollack HJ, Neumann R, Pollack EM. Sudeck und Psyche. Beitrag Orthop Traumatol 1990;27:H8.

40. Spaendonck van KPM, Heusden van HA, The R et al. Post-traumatische dystrophie en persoonlijkheidstype. In: Goris RJA, editor. Post-traumatische dystrofie. Nijmegen: Post-Academisch Onderwijs Geneeskunde Katholieke Universiteit Nijmegen, 1992:39–43.
41. Zucchini M, Alberti G, Moretti MP. Algodystrophy and related psychological features. Funct Neurol 1989;4:153–156.
42. Jonker D. Post-traumatische Dystrofie. Feiten en fabels over de behandeling. Wetenschapswinkel Geneesmiddelen Utrecht, Universiteit Utrecht, 1995.
43. Hannington-Kiff JG. Relief of Südeck's atrophy by regional intravenous guanethidine. Lancet 1977;I:1132–1133.
44. Fantone JC, Ward PA. Role of oxygen derived free radicals and metabolites in leukocyte-dependent inflammatory reactions. Am J Pathol 1982;107:397.
45. Davidof G, Werner R, Cremer S, Jackson MD, Ventocilla C, Wolf L. Predictive value of the three-phase technetium bone scan in diagnosis of reflex sympathetic dystrophy syndrome. Arch Phys Med Rehabil 1989;70:135–137.
46. Kozin F, Soin JS, Ryan LM, Carrera GF, Wortman RL. Bone scintigraphy in the reflex sympathetic dystrophy syndrome. Radiology 1981:138:437–443.
47. Schwartzman RJ, McLellan TL. Reflex sympathetic dystrophy. A review. Arch Neurol 1987;44:555–561.
48. Koch E, Hofer HO, Sialer G, et al. Failure of MR imaging to detect reflex sympathetic dystrophy of the extremities. AJR 1991;156:113–115
49. Glick EN. Reflex dystrophy (algoneurodystrophy): results of treatment by corticosteroids. Rheum Rehab 1973;88:84–88.
50. Langendijk PNJ, Zuurmond WWA, Apeldoorn van HAC, Loenen van AC, Lange de JJ. Goede resultaten van behandeling van acute reflectoire sympatische dystrofie met een 50%-dimethylsulfoxide-creme. Ned Tijdschr Geneesk 1993;137:500–503.
51. Wang JK, Johnson KA, Ilstrup DM. Sympathetic blocks for reflex sympathetic dystrophy. Pain 1985;23:13–17.
52. WHO. International classification of impairments, disabilities and handicaps: a manual of classification relating the consequences of disease. Geneva: WHO, 1980.
53. Bickerstaff DR, Kanis JA. Algodystrophy: an underrecognized complication of minor trauma. Br J Rheumatol 1994;33:240–248.
54. Field J, Warwick D, Bannister C. Features of algodystrophy ten years after Colles' fracture. J Hand Surg [Br] 1992;17:318–320.
55. Inhofe PD, Garcia-Moral CA. Reflex sympathetic dystrophy; a review of the literature and a long-term outcome study. Orthop Rev 1994;23:655–661.
56. Geertzen JHB, Dijkstra PU, Groothoff JW, Duis HJ ten, Eisma WH. Reflex sympathetic dystrophy of the upper extremity. A 5.5-year follow-up. Part I. Impairments and perceived disability. Acta Orthop Scand (Suppl 279) 1998;69:12–18.
57. Geertzen JHB, Dijkstra PU, Sonderen FLP van, Groothoff JW, Duis HJ ten, Eisma WH. Relationship between impairments, disability and handicap in reflex sympathetic dystrophy patients: a long-term follow-up study. Clin Rehabil 1998;12:412–422.
58. Renier JC, Masson C. In: Ficat CCJ, editor.Reflex sympathetic dystrophy. Baillieres Clin Orthop 1996;1:315–326.

40 Localized Osteolysis after Joint Replacement Surgery

A. S. Shanbhag and H. E. Rubash

Introduction

Osteolysis is currently the most common cause of failure of total joint replacements [1–4]. Numerous in vitro and in vivo studies have investigated and elucidated the cellular mechanisms involved in periprosthetic osteolysis, and particulate wear debris from materials used in the prostheses is believed to be the causative agent [2,5–9]. Among the types of wear debris, ultrahigh-molecular-weight polyethylene (UHMWPE) from the acetabular liner is particularly implicated, since billions of submicrometer-sized UHMWPE particles are released into the joint cavity each year [3,6,10]. While macrophages are able to clear modest amounts of wear debris via the lymphatic system, large amounts of debris overwhelm the clearance capacity, resulting in a local accumulation of the debris [11]. Macrophages are then stimulated to release lysosomal enzymes and inflammatory mediators such as prostaglandin E_2 (PGE_2), interleukin (IL)-1, tumor necrosis factor (TNF) and IL-6 [8, 12–16] which stimulate osteoclasts to resorb the surrounding bone, causing loosening of the prosthesis, which in turn necessitates revision surgery to replace the components (Fig. 40.1).

In the United States, it is estimated that approximately 38,000 joint replacements are revised each year due to osteolysis and aseptic loosening alone. Revision surgeries are more expensive not only in their initial cost, but also because they have a significantly higher rate of local and systemic complications, and length of hospital stay. Revision surgeries also have less favorable outcomes than primary joint replacement, translating into more frequent surgeries in progressively less optimal bone. Thus the impact of osteolysis on the lifestyle of the arthritis patient cannot be overemphasized.

Solutions for Osteolysis

Through the decades there have been several successful attempts at improving the quality of the primary arthroplasty and thereby reducing the incidence of osteolysis and aseptic loosening. Several modifications to the cementing technique have been instituted, including vacuum mixing, using cement guns to pressurize the cement, medullary plugs to enhance the penetration of cement into the bony

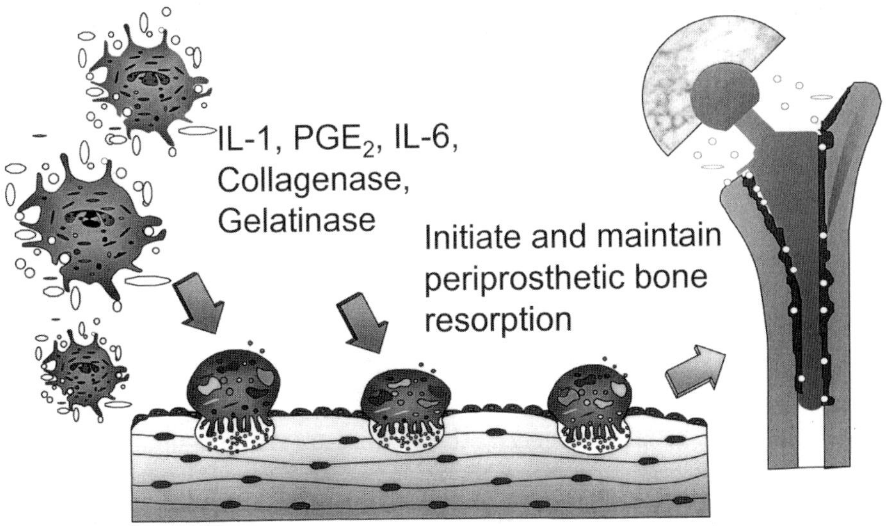

Figure 40.1. Schematic of osteolysis. Wear debris generated at the articulating surfaces migrates to the bone-implant interface. Macrophages phagocytoze the wear debris and are stimulated to release inflammatory mediators such as TNF, IL–1, PGE_2 and IL–6. These cytokines and mediators initiate and perpetuate osteoclastic bone resorption. Periprosthetic bone resorption results in loss of fixation and a painfully loose implant.

interstices, and precoating the implant surface to enhance bonding to the bone cement [17–20]. Numerous implant modifications have also been advanced to decrease the wear debris burden. Femoral head size was reduced to lower volumetric wear rates and slow the generation of wear debris. In addition, better metaphyseal filling and circumferentially porous coated implants with hardened and polished surfaces have been designed to reduce abrasive wear and limit access of debris to the bone–implant interface, by improving biologic tissue ingrowth. Bone ingrowth into implant porosities could also be enhanced by coating the bulk implant and the porous coatings with hydroxyapatite [21–23] or growth factors such as transforming growth factors β (TGF-β) [24] and bone morphogenic protein-2 (BMP-2) [25]. While these modifications have improved the outcomes of total joint replacements, periprosthetic osteolysis remains a relentless impediment to their long-term success.

A significant effort is directed at reducing the amount of UHMWPE debris generated. In this regard, alternative bearing materials such as metal-on-metal and ceramic-on-ceramic components are being used. The wear resistance of UHMWPE has been improved by modifying the sterilization protocols to prevent oxidation-induced damage and cross-linking [26,27]. Re-designs of the metal backing of the UHMWPE shell, improved locking mechanisms, and thicker UHMWPE liners are also incorporated in the currently used implant systems. For alternative approaches, investigators have looked to modifying the host response to the materials by using non-steroidal anti-inflammatory drugs (such as naproxen) to inactivate the inflammatory mediators [28,29], and gene transfer techniques to neutralize the pro-inflammatory mediators (IL-1β, TNF-β) released in the periprosthetic tissues [30]. Despite implementation of several of these modifications, osteolysis and aseptic loosening persist. Their resistance to technical and design innovations underscores the need for a better understanding of their pathophysiology and the investigation of alternative targeted therapeutic modalities.

In surveying pharmaceutical agents, we have considered systemic diseases such as osteoporosis and Paget's disease, which are also characterized by significant bone loss, and in which bisphosphonates have been successfully used to inhibit the osteoclasts and treat these pathologies [31–34]. It was thus logical to consider bisphosphonates to prevent or treat wear debris-mediated osteolysis in total joint replacements, wherein the end effector cell is also the osteoclast. Here we briefly summarize the studies investigating the potential of bisphosphonates to protect the bone from breakdown in response to wear debris-mediated inflammatory processes. Using bisphosphonates is not without its drawbacks and we have attempted to highlight the causes for concern as well.

Inhibiting Wear Debris Mediated Osteolysis

The authors studied the efficacy of oral bisphosphonate therapy to inhibit wear debris-mediated bone resorption in a canine total hip replacement (THR) model [35]. Adult dogs were randomized to three groups ($n = 8$ each) and a right uncemented THR was performed on all animals. The femoral and acetabular components were porous coated titanium-alloy (TiAlV) with a UHMWPE liner similar to those used clinically (Zimmer, Warsaw, IN). Group I (control) dogs received no particulate debris. In groups II and III, a mixture of fine UHMWPE, TiAlV and cobalt chrome-alloy (Co-Cr) particles was introduced intraoperatively into the proximal femoral gap. Group III dogs additionally received oral drug therapy (5 mg once a day, alendronate sodium, Fosamax, Merck, Rahway, NJ) which was begun on postoperative day 7 and continued until the dogs were killed. Postoperatively, all dogs were allowed 24 weeks of full ambulation before euthanasia. Radiographs obtained preoperatively, postoperatively, and at the time the dogs were killed were studied for bone apposition, remodelling and periprosthetic osteolysis. One dog receiving debris (group II) suffered a periprosthetic fracture and was omitted from the study. Radiographically, 1 of 8 control dogs developed periprosthetic radiolucencies with endosteal scalloping. The characteristics of the wear debris and their challenge dose was very effective and 6 of 7 group II dogs developed periprosthetic osteolysis (Fig. 40.2). In contrast, of 8 group III animals which received the massive debris challenge and were additionally treated with oral alendronate, only 1 developed periprosthetic radiolucencies (Fig. 40.2) [35].

In this study, while bisphosphonate treatment was very effective in preventing radiographic evidence of osteolysis in the face of massive debris challenge, it did not affect the macrophage-mediated inflammatory response [35]. Histologically, periprosthetic tissues harvested when the dogs were sacrificed had significant macrophage and foreign body giant cell infiltration. Biochemically, levels of PGE_2 and IL-1 released by periprosthetic tissues were significantly elevated in both experimental groups compared with controls. Thus it appears that although bisphosphonate therapy suppresses bone resorption, it does not influence the underlying wear debris-induced inflammation [35]. This is consistent with the literature indicating that bisphosphonates act as specific inhibitors of osteoclast-mediated bone resorption with no known anti-inflammatory effects [34,36].

Since bone remodelling is achieved by a combination of osteoclastic bone resorp-

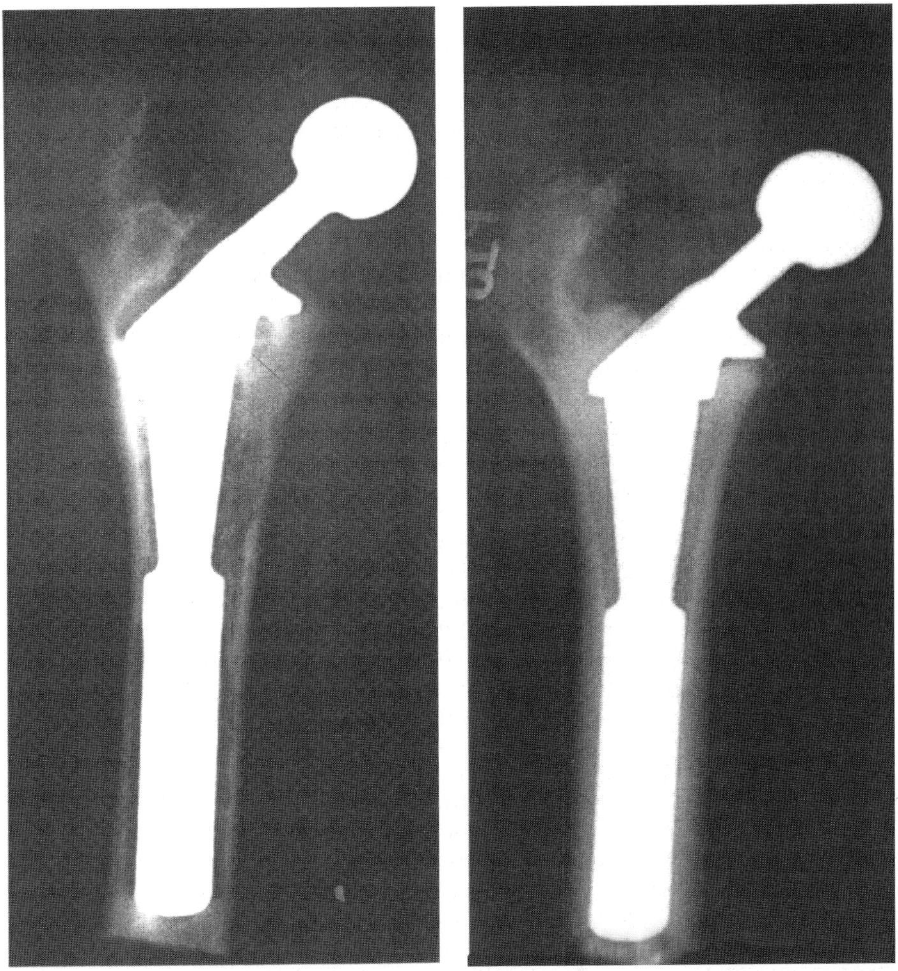

Figure 40.2. Radiographs of femoral components in dogs at 24 weeks postoperatively. *Left*: dogs with wear debris introduced intraoperatively at the bone-implant interface. The periprosthetic bone loss is discernible. *Right*: dogs with wear debris introduced intraoperatively and additionally treated with oral alendronate for 23 weeks which prevented periprosthetic bone loss. Reproduced with permission from Shanbhag et al. [35] and Shanbhag and Rubash [4].

tion and osteoblastic bone formation, it can be argued that continuous alendronate treatment may block the normal bone remodeling process by inhibiting osteoclastic bone resorption. If this is indeed the case, the bone microstructure and mechanical properties of alendronate-treated animals would be different and weaker, respectively, from that of control animals. This aspect takes on added importance if bisphosphonates are to be considered for human clinical use in relatively younger, healthy individuals with joint replacements for long-term use. To address this issue, contralateral femurs were harvested from the above study and the biomechanical properties of bisphosphonate-treated bones were studied [37]. The 23 week bisphosphonate treatment did not reduce the mechanical properties such as fracture toughness, elastic modulus, tensile strength and microhardness of bone. The weight fraction of the mineral and organic phases was also similar and micrographs of bone cross-sections did not show any differences in microstructure between the two groups [37]. These still represent short-term studies and the long-term effects of bisphosphonate treatment are yet to be investigated.

Inhibiting Bone Loss

At the 1998 Orthopaedic Research Society (ORS) Meeting in New Orleans, LA, Goodship et al. [38] hypothesized that bisphosphonates may be effective in preventing stress-shielding related bone loss as well. In an ovine femoral hemi-arthroplasty model, local stress shielding in the region of the calcar and medial cortex resulted in significant bone loss at 16 weeks postoperatively. Intravenous infusion of 10 μg of zoledronate 1 month preoperatively, during surgery and monthly thereafter, was able to reduce calcar bone resorption as assessed by radiography and bone mineral densitometry [38]. Lyons et al. [39] studied the beneficial effects of bisphosphonates in patients with THR. Patients who had undergone a primary THR and received alendronate (10 mg/day) demonstrated increases in bone mineral density compared with controls given a placebo. However, patients who either had a well-functioning THR or demonstrated aseptic loosening and were awaiting revision surgery, did not demonstrate any advantages of the therapy [39].

It is also clear that bisphosphonates are not a panacea for all bone resorption. Astrand and Aspenberg [40] reported the ineffectiveness of bisphosphonates in inhibiting instability-induced bone resorption. In a rat motion model, while treatment with alendronate from 2 to 6 weeks resulted in a dramatic increase in unremodelled bone, it was ineffective in preventing bone resorption around the moving component [40]. The ash weights of bone samples were significantly increased in animals with alendronate treatment, confirming the systemic inhibition of osteoclasts. The findings in this model can be reconciled with known mechanisms of bisphosphonates, if the bone loss observed around the moving plate is a consequence of decreased osteoblastic bone formation with only a minor role, if any, for osteoclasts.

These recent in vivo studies using bisphosphonates around implants, highlight the potential application and benefits of using pyrophosphate analogs to treat a variety of osteoclast-mediated pathologies.

Macrophage-Mediated Responses

Horowitz et al. [36,41] explored the effect of bisphosphonates on macrophage-mediated bone resorption in a murine calvarial model. Macrophages cultured with particulate wear debris released appreciable amounts of PGE_2 and TNF-α in the culture conditioned medium. The ability of this conditioned medium to elicit ^{45}Ca release was inhibited by the addition of pamidronate to the calvarial organ culture, which protected the bone from osteoclastic resorption [36,41].

Ritchie et al. [42] reported that in addition to inhibiting osteoclastic bone resorption, alendronate cultured with macrophages and particles inhibited TNF-α release, suggesting that bisphosphonate may affect macrophages as well. This study was complicated by the finding that significant cell death had also occurred in the macrophage population at the end of the culture period. Bisphosphonate-induced cell death is consistent with the findings of other investigators who reported that alendronate, clodronate, ibandronate and risedronate caused DNA fragmentation and changes in nuclear morphology (apoptosis) of J774 macrophages [43,44].

Mechanism of Bone Resorptive Activity of Bisphosphonates

Bisphosphonates are synthetic analogs of pyrophosphate that contain a carbon atom [P–C–P] instead of an oxygen atom [P–O–P] as found in-situ. Bisphosphonates bind avidly to hydroxyapatite crystals and thus have a strong affinity for bone mineral. Bisphosphonates retard the dissolution of hydroxyapatite crystals in vitro and also inhibit bone resorption in vivo [45,46]. It is because of this ability that bisphosphonates are well established as effective therapeutic agents in clinical pathologies such as Paget's disease, hypercalcemia of malignancy and osteoporosis, which are characterized by increased bone loss [31,32,47].

Bisphosphonates when present in the surrounding fluid, bind to hydroxyapatite wherever the bone mineral is exposed. Bound bisphosphonates can easily be released from the bone particles on acidification of the medium [48]. In newly formed bone, alendronate deposits preferentially under the osteoclasts, where the bone is being actively resorbed [34,49], and on new bone formation surfaces lined by osteoid and osteoblasts [48,50]. Normal bone is formed on top of the bisphosphonate already incorporated within the hydroxyapatite, indicating that bisphosphonate does not impair osteoblastic bone formation [34,48]. While the mechanism of action of bisphosphonates is still being elucidated, it is now widely accepted that bisphosphonates have an important effect on the osteoclast, the primary bone resorbing cell.

In organ culture, bisphosphonates decrease the destruction of bone in embryonic long bones and in neonatal calvaria [48,49,51,52]. In vitro mineralized substrata such as dentine, ivory and bone slices, or bone particles when preincubated with bisphosphonates will inhibit the formation of pits by isolated osteoclasts.

While the mechanisms by which bisphosphonates inhibit the osteoclast are still under study, in vitro and in vivo studies demonstrate that the primary effect is via the acidification processes at the cell–mineral interface [49,53]. Bisphosphonates appear to have a minimal effect on the formation, recruitment and maturation of osteoclasts [47,54,55]. Osteoclasts attach normally to the bisphosphonate-containing bone forming the ruffled border and the underlying clear zone in preparation for bone resorption. The ensuing acidification process underneath the osteoclasts liberates the bisphosphonates within the clear zones. The localized high concentration of bisphosphonates increases the membrane permeability to calcium and other ions and causes an influx of bisphosphonates in the cytoplasm [56]. These activities disrupt the actin attachment sites on the bone surfaces [54] and interfere with the ruffled border function and the acidification process, which in turn paralyzes the bone resorption process [34,48,54]. This appears to be a self-contained process and as the clear zone returns to a neutral pH, re-adsorption of the bisphosphonates to the hydroxyapatite causes a drop in the free bisphosphonate at the interface [48]. The bisphosphonate therefore remains conserved in the bone mineral and can thus be conceptualized as an enzyme catalyzing the inhibition of osteoclasts.

Recent Study on Enhancing Bone Ingrowth

In our canine study discussed earlier, we had noticed from radiographic analysis that in bisphosphonate-treated animals the bone had filled in the gap and ingrown well into the fiber mesh – so much so that, in trying to remove the implant after the femur was split, we had to tear apart the metal fibers. This was an interesting observation and difficult to understand, since the only action of the bisphosphonates was reportedly in inhibiting osteoclasts. To explore this finding further, and since we still had the acetabular components, we investigated whether bisphosphonate enhances net bone ingrowth into porous implants [57]. After analyzing and quantifying the acetabular components, we concluded that alendronate therapy enhances net bone ingrowth in implant porosities by 115% in bone contacting areas. However, granulomas were still detected behind the acetabular shell and were associated with migrated wear debris. We believe that since bisphosphonates do not affect the osteoblasts, normal bone formation continues, at least temporarily, resulting in the net positive bone mass. This finding, in concert with their ability to inhibit osteolysis, makes bisphosphonates invaluable in extending the useful life of implants.

Update on Clinical Trials for Periprosthetic Osteolysis

Alendronate is currently approved by the Food and Drug Administration (FDA, USA) for the treatment of Paget´s disease and postmenopausal osteoporosis. This situation, combined with the striking findings in our canine study, permitted its expedient investigation in a clinical trial. The aims of the clinical study are to evaluate two doses of alendronate, 10 mg and 35 mg, in a placebo-controlled, double-masked, prospective randomized multicenter trial. The radiographic progression of the disease will be studied, comparing a daily oral dose approved for Paget´s disease (35 mg), the osteoporosis dose (10 mg) and a placebo. Not only the prevention or the progression of osteolysis but also the changes that may occur once bisphosphonate therapy has been discontinued will be assessed. Currently 11 centers are involved and patient enrollment has already begun. The expected enrollment period is approximately 6 months and the actual study will take approximately 18 months per patient enrolled.

Summary

The studies reviewed here indicate that an oral bisphosphonate can effectively prevent the periprosthetic bone loss associated with osteolysis and aseptic loosening in a canine model. It is currently not known whether the drug is effective if it is administered after osteolysis is detected, or whether osteolysis recurs once the drug is discontinued. There is also the distinct possibility that bisphosphonates have the added benefit of enhancing bone ingrowth into the implant porosities. The issues of bone fragility and interference with bone remodelling also require serious consideration if the drug needs to be administered during the entire duration of the arthroplasty. The inflammatory response to particulate debris continues unabated with alendronate treatment and has the potential for late complications.

We plan to address these questions with further animal studies so that patients can benefit with more durable joint replacements. The FDA approval of bisphosphonates for human clinical use in the United States for the treatment of Paget´s disease and osteoporosis has facilitated a multicenter prospective, randomized trial which is under way to study the effects of alendronate on patients with established progressive femoral osteolysis. Another bisphosphonate, risedronate, was recently approved by the FDA for the treatment of Paget´s disease. With the reported potency of this drug being at least 5 times that of alendronate, creative therapeutic regimens can be explored that can take advantage of the antiresorptive activity and simultaneously further reduce bone fragility in younger patients. Bisphosphonates are thus appropriate candidates in a growing arsenal of materials development, implant designs, and pharmaceutical agents to combat periprosthetic osteolysis.

References

1. National Institutes of Health. Total hip replacement. NIH Consensus Statement, Bethesda, MD, Sept 12–14 1994; 12(5):1–31.
2. Friedman RJ, Black J, Galante JO, Jacobs JJ, Skinner HB. Current concepts in orthopaedic biomaterials and implant fixation. J Bone Joint Surg Am 1993;75: 1086–1109.
3. Wright TM, Goodman SB. Implant wear: the future of total joint replacement. Rosemont, IL: American Academy of Orthopaedic Surgeons, 1996.
4. Shanbhag AS, Rubash HE. Bisphosphonate therapy for the prevention of osteolysis in total joint replacements. Curr Opin Orthop 1998;9:81–87.
5. Galante JO, Lemmons J, Spector M, Wilson PD Jr, Wright TM. The biologic effects of implant materials. J Orthop Res 1991;9:760–775.
6. Shanbhag AS, Rubash HE. Wear: the basis of particle disease in total hip arthroplasty. Tech Orthop 1994;8:269–274.
7. Dowd JE, Schwendeman LJ, Macaulay W, Doyle JS, Shanbhag AS, Wilson S, et al. Aseptic loosening in uncemented total hip arthroplasty in a canine model. Clin Orthop 1995;319:106–121.
8. Chiba J, Rubash HE, Kim KJ, Iwaki Y. The characterization of cytokines in the interface tisssue obtained from failed cementless total hip arthroplasty with and without femoral osteolysis. Clin Orthop 1994;300:304–312.
9. Howie DW, Vernon-Roberts B, Oakeshott R, Manthey B. A rat model of resorption of bone at the cement-bone interface in the presence of polyethylene wear particles. J Bone Joint Surg Am 1988;70:257–263.
10. Shanbhag AS, Jacobs JJ, Glant TT, Gilbert JL, Black J, Galante JO. Composition and morphology of wear debris in failed uncemented total hip replacement arthroplasty. J Bone Joint Surg Br 1994;76:60–67.
11. Willert HG, Semlitsch M. Reactions of the articular capsule to wear products of artificial joint prostheses. J Biomed Mater Res 1977;11:157–164.
12. Goldring SR, Schiller AL, Roelke M, Rourke CM, O'Neill DA, Harris WH. The synovial-like membrane at the bone-cement interface in loose total hip replacements and its proposed role in bone lysis . J Bone Joint Surg Am 1983;65:575–584.
13. Kim KJ, Rubash HE, Wilson SC, D'Antonio JA, McClain EJ. A histological and biochemical comparison of the interface tissues in cementless and cemented hip prosthesis. Clin Orthop 1993; 287:142–152.
14. Dorr LD, Bloebaum R, Emmanual J, Meldrum R. Histologic, biochemical and ion analysis of tissue and fluids retrieved during total hip arthroplasty. Clin Orthop 1990;261:82–95.
15. Goodman SB, Knoblich G, O'Connor M, Song Y, Huie P, Sibley R. Heterogeneity in

cellular and cytokine profiles from multiple samples of tissue surrounding revised hip prostheses. J Biomed Mater Res 1996;31:421–428.
16. Shanbhag AS, Jacobs JJ, Black J, Galante JO, Glant TT. Cellular mediators secreted by interfacial membranes obtained at revision total hip arthroplasties. J Arthroplasty 1995;10:498–506.
17. Berger RA, Steel MJ, Schleiden M, Rubash HE. Preventing distal voids during cementation of the femoral component in total hip arthroplasty. J Arthroplasty 1993;8: 323–329.
18. Harris WH, Davies JP. Modern use of modern cement for total hip replacement. Orthop Clin North Am 1988;19:581–589.
19. Mulroy WF, Estok DM, Harris WH. Total hip arthroplasty with use of so-called second-generation cementing techniques. J Bone Joint Surg Am 1995;77:1845–1852.
20. Mulroy RD Jr, Harris WH. The effect of improved cementing techniques on component loosening in total hip replacement. J Bone Joint Surg Br 1990;72:757–760.
21. D'Antonio JA, Capello WN, Manley MT. Remodeling of bone around hydroxyapatite-coated femoral stems. J Bone Joint Surg 1996;78:1226–1234.
22. Jaffe WL, Scott DF: Total hip arthroplasty with hydroxyapatite-coated prostheses. J Bone Joint Surg Am 1996;78:1918–1934.
23. Dean JC, Tisdel CL, Goldberg VM, Parr J, Davy D, Stevenson S. Effects of hydroxyapatite tricalcium phosphate coating and intracancellous placement on bone ingrowth in titanium fibermetal implants. J Arthroplasty 1995;10:830–838.
24. Sumner DR, Turner TM, Purchio AF, Gombotz WR, Urban RM, Galante JO. Enhancement of bone ingrowth by transforming growth factor-β. J Bone Joint Surg 1995:77:1135–1147.
25. Riley EH, Lane JM, Urist MR, Lyons KM, Lieberman JR: Bone morphogenetic protein-2: biology and applications. Clin Orthop 1996;324:39–46.
26. Bragdon CR, O'Connor DO, Muratoglu OK, Jasty M, Ramamurti BS, Merrill E, et al. A new polyethylene with undetectable wear at 12 million cycles. Trans Soc Biomater 1998;21:2–2.
27. Shen F-W, McKellop HA, Salovey R: Improving the resistance to wear and oxidation of acetabular cups of UHMWPE by gamma radiation crosslinking and remelting. Trans Soc Biomater 1998;21:3–3.
28. Spector M, Shortkroff S, Hsu H-P, Lane N, Sledge CB, Thornhill TS. Tissue changes around loose prostheses. A canine model to investigate the effects of an antiinflammatory agent. Clin Orthop 1990;261:140–152.
29. Goodman SB, Chin RC, Chiou SS, Lee JS: Suppression of prostaglandin E_2 synthesis in the membrane surrounding particulate polymethylmethacrylate in the rabbit tibia. Clin Orthop 1991;271:300–304.
30. Wooley PH, Sud S, Robbins PD, Whalen JD, Evans CH. Contrasting effects of gene therapy to inhibit interleukin-1β or tumor necrosis factor alpha in the murine inflammatory response to wear particles. Trans Orthop Res Soc 1998;23:122–122.
31. Liberman UA, Weiss SR, Broll J, Minne HW, Quan H, Bell NH, et al. Effect of oral alendronate on bone mineral density and the incidence of fractures in postmenopausal osteoporosis. N Engl J Med 1995;333:1437–1443.
32. Black DM, Cummings SR, Karpf DB, Cauley JA, Thompson DE, Nevitt MC, et al. Randomised trial of effect of alendronate on risk of fracture in women with existing vertebral fractures. Lancet 1996;348:1535–1541.
33. Garnero P, Shih WJ, Gineyts E, Karpf DB, Delmas PD. Comparison of new biochemical markers of bone turnover in late postmenopausal osteoporotic women in response to alendronate treatment. J Clin Endocrinol Metab 1994;79:1693–1700.
34. Rodan GA, Fleisch HA: Bisphosphonates: mechanisms of action. J Clin Invest 1996;97:2692–2696.
35. Shanbhag AS, Hasselman CT, Rubash HE. Inhibition of wear debris-mediated osteolysis in a canine total hip arthroplasty (THA) model. Clin Orthop 1997;344:33–43.

36. Horowitz SM, Algan SA, Purdon MA. Pharmacologic inhibition of particulate-induced bone resorption. J Biomed Mater Res 1996;31:91–96.
37. Wang X, Shanbhag AS, Rubash HE, Agrawal CM. Short-term effects of bisphosphonates on the biomechanical properties of canine bone. J Biomed Mater Res 1999; 44:456–460.
38. Goodship AE, Lawes TJ, Green J, Eldridge JD, Kenwright J. The use of bisphosphonates to inhibit mechanically related bone loss in aseptic loosening of hip prostheses. Trans Orthop Res Soc 1998;23:2.
39. Lyons AR, Owen JE, Freedholm DA, Miller CG, Fasano G, Pye D, et al. Effect of alendronate on periprosthetic bone mass. Trans 10th Combined Mtg Orthop. Assoc. of the English Speaking World, Feb 1–6, Auckland, New Zealand; 1998;209.
40. Astrand J, Aspenberg P. Alendronate does not inhibit instability-induced bone resorption. Trans Orthop Res Soc 1998;23:28.
41. Horowitz SM, Gonzales JB. Effects of polyethylene on macrophages. J Biomed Mater Res 1997;15:50–56.
42. Ritchie CK, Patel MA, Stamos BD, Horowitz SM. Alendronate reduces particle-induced cytokine production in macrophages. Trans Orthop Res Soc 1998;23:357.
43. Luckman SP, Hughes DE, Coxon FP, Russell RGG, Rogers MJ. Nitrogen-containing bisphosphonates inhibit the mevalonate pathway and prevent post-translational prenylation of GTP-binding proteins, including Ras. J Bone Miner Res 1998;13:581–589.
44. Frith JC, Monkkonen J, Blackburn GM, Russel RGG, Rogers MJ. Clodronate and liposome-encapsulated clodronate are metabolized to a toxic ATP analog, adenosine 5′-(β,gamma-dichloromethylene)triphosphate, by mammalian cells in vitro. J Bone Miner Res 1997;12:1358–1367.
45. Fleisch H, Russel RGG, Francis MD. Diphosphonates inhibit hydroxyapatite dissolution in vitro and bone resorption in tissue culture and in vivo. Science 1969; 10:1262–1264.
46. Russel RGG, Kislig A-M, Casey PA, Fleisch H, Thornton J, Schenk R, et al. Effect of diphosphonates and calcitonin on the chemistry and quantitative histology of rat bone. Calcif Tissue Res 1973; 11:179–195.
47. Flanagan AM, Chambers TJ. Inhibition of bone resorption by bisphosphonates: Interactions between bisphosphonates, osteoclasts and bone. Calcif Tissue Int 1991;49: 407–415.
48. Sato M, Grasser W, Endo N, Akins R, Simmons H: Bisphosphonate action: alendronate localization in rat bone and effects on osteoclast ultrastructure. J Clin Invest 1991; 88:2095–2105.
49. Fleisch H. Bisphosphonates in bone disease, 2nd ed. New York: Parthenon, 1995.
50. Azuma Y, Sato H, Oue Y, Okabe K, Ohta T, Tsuchimoto M, tet al. Alendronate distributed on bone surfaces inhibits osteoclastic bone resorption in vitro and in experimental hypercalcemia models . Bone 1995;16:235–245.
51. Sato M, Grasser W. Effects of bisphosphonates on isolated rat osteoclasts as examined by reflected light microscopy. J Bone Miner Res 1990;5:31–39.
52. Reynolds JJ, Minkin C, Morgan DB, Spycher D, Fleisch H. The effect of two diphosphonates on the resorption of mouse calvaria in vitro. Calcif Tissue Res 1972;10: 302–313.
53. Zimolo Z, Wesolowski G, Rodan GA. Acid extrusion is induced by osteoclast attachment to bone. J Clin. Invest 1995;96:2277–2283.
54. Murakami H, Takahashi N, Sasaki T, Udagawa N, Tanaka S, Nakamura I, et al. A possible mechanism of the specific action of bisphosphonates on osteoclasts: tiludronate preferentially affects polarized osteoclasts having ruffled borders. Bone 1995;17:137–144.
55. Tanzi MC, Sket I, Gatti AM, Monari E. Physical characterization of acrylic bone cement cured with new accelerator systems. Clin Mater 1991;8:131–136.
56. Felix R, Guenther HL, Fleisch H. The subcellular distribution of [^{14}C]dichlorometh-

ylene bisphosphonate and [^{14}C]1-hydroxyethylidene-1,1-bisphosphonate in cultured calvaria cells. Calcif Tissue Int 1984;36:108–113.

57. Shanbhag AS, May D, Cha CC, Hasselman CT, Rubash HE. Oral bisphosphonate therapy enhances net bone formation in implant porosities. Trans Soc Biomater 1999;22:66.

Part VII

Concluding Remarks

41 A Personal Algorithm for the Prevention of Fractures in Orthopaedic Practice

K. Obrant

Introduction

No other medical doctor sees so many elderly patients with osteoporosis as does the orthopaedic specialist. Since there are now proven effective prevention and treatment modalities for osteoporosis it is therefore the responsibility of the orthopaedic surgeon to arrange for these patients to be properly advised and/or investigated for osteoporosis. Each and every orthopaedic surgeon should be aware of the different treatment modalities that exist and give professional advice to the patient. This is not, however, to say that the investigation and treatment of osteoporosis is a matter for the orthopaedic surgeon, but the referral of the patient to the right doctor interested in such an investigation and treatment should be done by the orthopaedic surgeon. There are now pharmacological and non-pharmacological resources which reduce the incidence of osteoporotic fractures, including hip fracture, by 50% or even more. A bone mass measurement has a better predictive ability for future fractures than a blood pressure measurement has for future stroke. The medical community has never resisted treating a large number of individuals with antihypertensive drugs but there is a resistance among orthopaedic surgeons to treat patients with fractures with anti-osteoporotic drugs. The reason for this discrepancy is probably the different accessibility to the measuring devices of bone mass and of blood pressure, the second of course being so much easier. I am convinced that the accessibility to devices for the measurement of bone mass will increase, thus making such a measurement a more natural part of the medical care of individuals who have already had osteoporotic fractures. Today, the cost of a bone mass measurement with the DXA technique has been estimated to be on average US$ 65 and, as a minimum, US$ 40, depending on the technical equipment and on the extent to which it is used [1].

Which Equipment Should Be Used for Bone Mass Measurement?

It is well known that the accuracy is poor for all existing in vivo bone mass measurement techniques – seldom better than 10%. This is, however, of limited clinical significance. Of much more importance is the precision error of the different techniques. This is true especially when longitudinal bone mass measurements are performed to assess the effects of treatment, for instance. Mathematical statistical calculations show that, for instance, with an instrumental precision of 1%, the difference between two measurements in a single patient must be 2.8% if this difference can be judged as not being due to technical variation. If, on the other hand, the precision error of the apparatus is worse, say 5%, the observed difference must be as high as 14% between two measurements in order to be able to rule out random variation. If, for instance, an individual loses 3% of bone mass per year, which is not an unusual situation shortly after menopause, or if another individual gains 3% per year after treatment with a certain drug, which is also not an unusual situation, it would take a year to detect this bone loss or bone gain using equipment with a 1% precision error and almost 5 years if the precision error of the equipment is 5%.

Theoretically today four different types of equipment can be used to measure bone mass noninvasively:

Dual-energy X-ray absorptiometry (DXA) should be regarded as the gold standard for two main reasons: the very low precision error (0.5–1.5%) and the availability of measuring deep-seated skeletal sites such as the hip and the lumbar spine.

Single energy X-ray absorptiometry has the clear disadvantage of not being able to define the skeletal location in the spine and the hip but only in peripheral skeletal sites.

Ultrasound is also limited to peripheral skeletal sites. One advantage of the equipment is that it exists in a portable version and that it is also less expensive and, further, that X-ray radiation is avoided. So far, the precision of this technique is not comparable to that of DXA and, therefore, the existing equipment is, at least to date, not really suited for follow-up examinations.

Quantitative computed tomography (QCT) is the only technique with which a true volumetric density of the bone mineral mass can be identified. For clinical reasons, however, this has proven not to be of significant value so far. Evident disadvantages of this technique are the very expensive equipment and the amount of radiation the patient receives at each examination, as well as an inferior precision compared with DXA.

Where Should the Equipment Be Located?

So far osteoporosis research has not been a major field for orthopaedic surgeons – sadly, I should like to add. Mostly doctors in other specialities such as rheumatology, endocrinology, radiology, pathology, clinical chemistry and others have been engaged in this area of research. I am convinced that this will change in the future, the reason being that orthopaedic surgeons come into daily contact with patients with osteoporosis and have daily evidence of the sometimes devastating fractures resulting in patients with severe osteoporosis. To me it seems obvious that the bone mass measurement equipment should be located where the patients are, i.e., at the Department of Orthopaedics or at the Department of Diagnostic Radiology.

In Orthopaedic Practice, Who Should Be Considered for a Bone Mass Measurement?

It has been proven that a previously sustained fragility fracture is one of the most important predictors for future fragility fractures [2]. For instance, of all patients with hip fracture, 12% have already sustained such a fracture earlier in life [3]. It is, therefore, my firm belief that for the benefit of our patients and in order to avoid repeated fragility fractures, all patients presenting with a fragility fracture should be offered a bone mass measurement – provided they have a positive attitude toward preventive treatment for further fractures. It may be a matter of opinion whether the biologically oldest individuals should also be offered bone mass measurement. In this age group factors other than bone mass seem to be of more importance for repeated fractures, among these are impaired vision, balance and confusion. Also, in these very old persons we lack data to substantiate evidence of the protective effect of modern pharmacological drugs. There is strong evidence based on data, however, that reasonably high doses of calcium and vitamin D may give protection from fractures, even hip fractures, in this age group [4]. Therefore, the very oldest and most frail individuals may benefit from calcium and vitamin D supplementation, and bone mass measurement may not always be necessary for this decision to be made.

Judging Risk Factors in Orthopaedic Practice

In the literature there are numerous risk factors associated with the propensity to fall and sustain a fracture as well as risk factors closely correlated with osteoporosis per se. Apart from advanced age and female gender, a history of falls and a history of fragility fractures are the most important. The orthopaedic fracture patient meets most of these criteria and the orthopaedic doctor has to arrange for a strategy of how to handle this group of patients with clinical evidence of osteoporosis and thus risk of future fracture. A decision has to be made for each and every case as to whether a bone mass measurement should be performed or not and also whether basic biochemical tests should be performed.

Biochemistry Tests to Identify Metabolic Bone Disease and to Monitor Treatment.

Numerous different biochemical tests have been suggested for individuals with osteoporosis. In orthopaedic practice I am of the opinion that, for the sake of feasibility, these analyses should be kept to a minimum. The following suggestion, I admit, is controversial but sedimentation rate, hemoglobin, serum calcium, serum alkaline phosphatase and serum creatinine should be sufficient as screening tests in orthopaedic practice in order to exclude metabolic bone disease other than osteoporosis. It is true that several other analyses have been suggested to be carried out more or less routinely in patients with osteoporosis, such as serum thyroid stimulating hormone, serum albumin, serum phosphate, serum glutamine transferase and, in men, serum testosterone. It is my opinion that these analyses should be done only in special cases when there is a clinical suspicion of related disease.

Biochemical markers of bone turnover are, in the individual patient from a clinical point of view, of limited or no value. The problem with these analyses is their low specificity and sensitivity. I myself use these markers, and especially the resorption markers, in very few cases and, if so, as a means to encourage the patient to comply with the instruction to take the drug continuously. To explain this further I once again make the comparison with the treatment for hypertonia, where the patient can very soon note a positive result, namely decreased blood pressure, as early as a few weeks after treatment is started. By contrast, in osteoporosis such a prompt treatment result is not possible by re-measuring bone mass. As mentioned earlier this takes at least 1–2 years. Therefore, some patients who are doubtful about continuing their anti-osteoporosis medication may be helped in a positive way if a marker for decreased bone resorption can give evidence that the drug is working on their skeleton already after a few months.

A Critical Review of Papers on Nonpharmacological Prevention of Osteoporotic Fractures

Physical Activity

From a theoretical point of view it is quite feasible to believe that increased physical activity will result in increased bone and muscle mass and thus in a decreased risk of fracture. There is no doubt, as evidenced by several studies, that an increased muscle mass and bone mass after increased physical activity are a reality. There is no convincing evidence, however, that this leads to a decreased risk of fracture.

From numerous cross-sectional studies it is evident that physically active individuals have a higher bone mass than normally sedentary controls. This seems to be true for both sexes at all ages. The type of activity required for a positive effect on bone mass is high-impact, short-term and weightbearing activities. There is no clear evidence that, for instance, swimming is positive from the point of view of increasing bone mass [5–8]. Endurance training such as long distance running may even be negative in terms of bone mass. It is difficult to judge the above studies as regards what is the chicken and what is the egg. However, evidence that players of racket sports have considerably higher bone mass in the dominant arm than in the non-dominant arm [9] can be taken as evidence that increased physical activity leads to increased bone mass.

Better than judging bone mass from the results of cross-sectional studies is evidence from prospective studies. Also, from prospective studies it seems evident that bone mass increases, on a yearly basis by a few percent. This is true also in women and after menopause [10–13]. The limitations of these prospective studies cited are numerous. Mostly the individuals included are very few and the time-span studied is only 1 year. It is, of course, difficult, if not impossible, to carry out proper randomized studies of large groups of individuals over a long period of time and to avoid drop-outs from either of the two groups when they, ideally, come from the same catchment area and know that they are part of an investigation on physical activity. Nevertheless, there seems to be enough evidence in the literature that physical activity increases bone mass.

On the other hand, there is no evidence whatsoever from prospective studies that increased physical activity leads to a decreased risk of fracture. Theoretically, this would be plausible, not only because of the increased bone mass but also the increased muscle mass and thus possible improved balance. On the other hand the increased physical activity in itself may lead to tumbles and falls and thus fractures.

We do recommend our patients to try to increase their physical activity and we feel that this would probably be advantageous not only from the point of view of the risk of sustaining fracture but also for many other biological functions. However, we must bear in mind that to date we lack clear evidence that the number of fractures will decrease in individuals who start to increase their physical activity.

Nutrition

Although there is good evidence that calcium and vitamin D supplementation can reduce the risk of sustaining hip fracture in an elderly, institutionalized population [4] we still lack evidence that any other nutritional compound has the same effect. Nevertheless there is evidence that increased protein intake can reduce the hospital stay in elderly individuals who have already suffered a fracture [14]. We also know that seriously decreased food intake, such as in anorexia, leads to decreased bone mass and thus, probably, an increased risk of fracture. It is also well known that hip fracture patients are considerably leaner than age-matched individuals without fracture [15]. It is therefore feasible that increased intake of nutrition, not only calcium and vitamin D but also proteins, may to some extent protect from future fractures. However, unequivocal evidence for this is still lacking.

Hip Protectors

Ever since the introduction of hip protectors by Lauritzen et al. [16] there has been considerable interest in studies trying to avoid hip fracture. Not many publications have been produced, however. I am aware of only one other sufficiently large randomized study [17] in which the same protective effect as Lauritzen found was reached. From a scientific point of view and with a deliberately critical analysis of the two studies mentioned, it is noteworthy that, although prospective and randomized, both studies ran for 11 months and the results of both were barely significant in terms of proving a protective effect on hip fracture of hip protectors. We must also bear in mind the difficulties involved in designing and judging randomized studies on hip protectors. The randomization in the two studies cited was of residents in wards, not individual patients, and therefore one can suspect that the entire environment in the designated wards where the hip protector probands were staying was in many ways protective against falls. In fact, in the study by Ekman et al. [17] if the number of fractures per fall instead of per individual is calculated, the significant protective effect of the protectors disappears. It is also noteworthy that not only were the number of fractures in the hip protector group fewer than expected, but also the number of fractures in the control group was higher than expected in the study by Lauritzen et al. [16].

This is not to say that hip protectors are not effective, only that there is room for scientific caution. I believe that hip protectors are effective in the prevention of hip fracture in the very elderly and most frail individuals in nursing homes. In less frail individuals or even in free-living individuals compliance is a serious problem and in these two studies, undertaken in nursing homes, the compliance was 24% and 44%, respectively.

A Critical Review of Papers on Pharmacological Preventive Measures of Osteoporotic Fractures

Prospective and randomized and sometimes even masked studies on prevention of fracture with pharmacological treatment must be judged on the basis of the statistics used. As pointed out by Windeler and Lange [18], "counting events instead of patients, although having been used in papers published in journals of high scientific reputation, is suitable merely for a chapter in Methodological Errors in Medical Research." This is to say that in many recent publications the number of fractures has been calculated instead of the number of individuals with fractures. From a basic statistical point of view this is not sound. It is understandable, however, that this statistical technique has been used when the numbers of probands in the treated and the placebo groups are too small to reach significant effects otherwise. It is, of course, not appropriate to calculate, for instance, 8 vertebral fractures in one patient since these fractures are not independent observations. Therefore, in the following I will try to adhere to the appropriate way of comparing data, i.e., the number of individuals with a new fracture. I will also, almost entirely, report results from prospective, randomized and often masked studies. The number of individuals with a fracture in the treated and the control groups in the studies referred to will be given below, but since the treatment and the control groups were not always of equal size, I have extrapolated the number of individuals in the control group to the same number as in the treatment group. The figures for most studies are also given in Table 41.1.

Calcium or/and Vitamin D

Calcium

To my knowledge there are three prospective, randomized and masked studies on the prevention of fracture with calcium alone. The number of individuals included in each study, the selection criteria, the age of the probands, the time span studied and the specific fractures studied, are given in Table 41.1. All these studies were performed in the 1990s [19–21]. None was sufficiently large to prove any fracture-preventive effect of calcium alone. The time span studied varied between 1.5 years and 4.3 years.

It is noticeable that although there was no effect on prevention of fracture for the whole group in the largest of the studies cited above, the title of the paper indicates an effect: "Correcting calcium nutritional deficiency prevents spine fractures in elderly women" [21]. However, this conclusion was reached by performing subgroup analyses of only those women with a previous fracture for whom a significant protective effect of calcium was found. From a critical point of view it can thus be argued that, since there was no effect for the whole group of women studied, there must be an increased risk of fracture after calcium supplementation in women without previous fracture. Indeed the proportion of women treated with calcium without previous fracture, who sustained a new fracture, was higher than for the controls although statistical significance was not reached.

Personal conclusion: My conclusion from these three studies is that calcium alone may have a protective effect against future fractures since there is the same tendency in all three studies, but that this has not been proven with certainty.

Vitamin D

There is one very large study from Amsterdam [22] in which elderly individuals, both institutionalized and free-living, were given, by a randomized, masked selection, 400 IU of vitamin D or placebo daily for more than 3 years. The number of individuals with new fractures did not differ in the two groups after this time period. The two groups were of the same size and actually there were slightly more individuals (certainly not statistically significant) with hip fractures and with other fractures in the group treated with Vitamin D.

Personal conclusion: My conclusion from the above study is that it is doubtful whether vitamin D alone is protective against fracture, especially in free-living individuals and at the age studied here. If higher doses were given, and in the case of elderly people, particularly those in nursing homes lacking daily exposure to sunshine, an effect may have been found.

Calcium and Vitamin D

There are two studies in which a combination of calcium and vitamin D was given in a prospective, randomized and masked placebo-controlled procedure. In a French study by Chapuy et al. [4] high doses of calcium and vitamin D, namely, 1.2 g calcium + 800 IU of vitamin D were given daily for 18 months to nursing home residents of advanced age. The oldest individual was 106 years old. This was a well-designed study including a sufficiently large number of probands. There was a 30% reduction of hip fracture cases among the individuals receiving medication. Also, a significant positive effect was found for other, nonvertebral fractures.

In a more recent but somewhat smaller American study [23] lower doses of calcium and vitamin D (500 mg calcium + 700 IU of vitamin D) were given for 3 years. Also in this study a positive protective effect was found when all clinical fractures were taken into account.

Personal conclusion: My conclusion from these two studies is clear. Calcium and vitamin D given together and in sufficiently large doses seem to provide protection against hip fracture and other clinical fractures, especially in elderly individuals living in nursing homes who may lack sufficient exposure to sunshine and nutrients.

Estrogen

There are numerous retrospective studies revealing a positive effect of estrogen on osteoporosis and fractures. There are serious difficulties, however, to judge from these studies, as to what is the chicken and what is the egg. Women who take estrogen in their postmenopausal period tend to be healthier than women who do

Table 41.1. Prospective randomized placebo controlled masked studies on prevention of osteoporotic fracture with drugs.

Drug	Author, publication year and reference	Selection criteria	Age (years)	Total no. of individuals in trial	Time span studied (years)	Fractures studied	No. of individuals with fracture in treatment group	No. of individuals with fracture in placebo group[a]
Calcium	Chevalley et al. 1994 [19]	Healthy women and men	62–87	93	1.5	Vertebral fractures	6	9 (4)
	Reid et al. 1995 [20]	Healthy women	Post-menopausal	78	4	All	2	7
	Recker et al. 1996 [21]	Women living independently	62–87	197	4.3	Vertebral fractures	27	32 (34)
Vitamin D	Chapuy et al. 1992 [4]	Women in nursing homes	69–106	3 270	1.5	All non vertebral fractures Hip fractures	160 80	215 110
	Lips et al. 1996 [22]	"Reasonably" healthy women and men	⩾ 70	2 578	3.5 (median)	Hip fractures Other peripheral fractures	58 77	48 74
	Dawson-Hughes et al. 1997 [23]	Women and men living independently	> 65	389	3	Nonvertebral fractures	11	26
Etidronate	Storm et al. 1990 [30]	Women with 1–4 vertebral fractures	56–75	66	3	All	5	6
	Watts et al. 1990 [31]	Postmenopausal women with 1–4 vertebral fractures	< 75	429	2	Vertebral fractures Nonvertebral fractures	8 34	18 (17) 30 (28)
	Harris et al. 1993 [32]	Postmenopausal women with 1–4 vertebral fractures		< 75	423	2 + 1 Nonvertebral fractures	Vertebral fractures 40	28 34 (32) 34 (32)
Alendronate	Liberman et al. 1995 [34]	Women with BMD <−2.5 SD	45–80	994	3	Vertebral fractures Nonvertebral fractures	17 45	33 (22) 57 (38)
	Black et al. 1996 [35]	Women with BMD <−2.1 SD + vertebral fracture	55–81	2 027	2.9	Hip fractures Wrist fractures 1 new vertebral fracture Multiple new vertebral fractures Other clinical fractures	11 22 78 5 44	22 41 145 47 28 (14)

Table 41.1. (*continued*)

	Hosking et al. 1998 [36]	Postmenopausal women, mainly non-osteoporotic	45–59	1499	2	Nonvertebral fractures	44	28 (14)
	Cummings et al. 1998 [37]	Postmenopausal women with BMD<–1.6 SD	54–81	4272	4	Vertebral fractures Clinical fractures	43 272	75 312
Risedronate	Harris et al. 1999 [38]	Postmenopausal women with vertebral fracture	< 85	1628	3	Vertebral fractures Nonvertebral fractures	61 33	93 52
Estrogen	Lufkin et al. 1992 [25]	Postmenopausal women with vertebral fracture	47–75	75	1	Vertebral fractures	7	12
	Hulley et al. 1998 [26]	Postmenopausal women with coronary heart disease	< 80	2763	4, 1	Hip fracture Other fractures	12 119	11 129
Raloxifene	Ettinger et al. 1999 [39]	Postmenopausal women	31–80	6828	3	Vertebral fractures Other clinical fractures	272 437	457 (231) 475 [240]
Calcitonin	Overgaard et al. 1992 [44]	Women with low bone mass	68–72	208	2	All	7	27 (9)
Fluoride	Riggs et al. 1990 [38]	Postmenopausal women with prevalent vertebral fractures	50–75	202	4	Nonvertebral fractures	31	28 (22)
	Kleerekoper et al. 1991 [39]	Postmenopausal women with prevalent vertebral fractures	45–75	84	4	Vertebral fractures	31	28 (22)
	Meunier et al. 1998 [41]	Postmenopausal women with prevalent vertebral fractures	47–76	354	2	Vertebral fractures Other fractures	74 29	55 (39) 24 (17)
	Reginster et al. 1998 [42]	Postmenopausal women with T-score <–2.5 for BMD of the spine	63 (mean)	200	4	Vertebral fractures Peripheral fractures	2 3	12 11
	Ringe et al. 1998 [43]	Men with osteoporosis	33–68	64	3	Vertebral fractures Non-vertebral fractures	3 3	12 11

[a]Figures within brackets denote actual figures while figures without brackets are corrected for by me as though the treatment and placebo groups were of equal size.

not and when a postmenopausal woman taking estrogen becomes ill for some reason it is plausible to believe that she also tends to stop taking estrogen at that time. Because of this it is difficult to determine with certainty, from retrospective studies, whether estrogen in itself is protective against fracture or not.

A more satisfactory method is a prospective study. There a numerous (more than 20) studies on estrogen and its effect on bone mass. Data have been collected from prospective, randomized, masked studies [24]. It appears that 1 year of estrogen treatment results, on average, in a 3% higher bone mass compared with controls. Once again, however, bone mass is only a secondary outcome variable; it is the fracture event in itself that estrogen should be seen to provide protection against. Also, nearly all these prospective, randomized, masked studies have been performed in the early postmenopausal period when the risk of osteoporotic fracture has not yet increased very much. Nearly all studies are also limited in the time span studied, to 2 years or even less.

There is only one prospective, randomized, masked study in which the number of individuals suffering fractures has been investigated and this has also been done at a somewhat older age [25]. In 47- to 75-year-old women and with a 1-year follow-up, no significant difference was found in the number of women sustaining a new vertebral fracture between the estrogen-treated group and the placebo-treated group. The number of women included in this study was clearly too low ($n = 75$), however, to be powered for such an outcome variable as fracture (Table 41.1). In a recent, much larger prospective, randomized, placebo, controlled study, aimed at studying secondary prevention of coronary heart disease, the fractures sustained were also studied. No preventive effect of estrogen was found [26].

It is evident that there are difficulties in performing large, prospective, randomized studies on estrogen and fracture outcome, not only from a commercial point of view but also because it is difficult to keep the study masked with the well-known side-effects of estrogen such as menstruation. From large, prospective, cohort studies on estrogen and fracture, including many thousands of women [27–29], it appears that estrogen, while currently being taken, has a certain protective effect on all types of fractures, including hip fractures. Already a few years after cessation of estrogen administration this protective effect seems to disappear.

Personal conclusion: It is my conclusion that estrogen, provided it is given in sufficient amount, i.e., orally either 0.625 mg of conjungated estrogen or 2 mg of estradiol or as a dermal application 50 μg of estradiol, is to some extent protective against all types of fractures while being taken. Since administration of estrogen is difficult because of side-effects in older women, usually over 70 years, this protective effect is not very pronounced for hip fractures.

Bisphosphonates

Although there are newer bisphosphonates emerging on the market, to date three specific compounds dominate the international arena: etidronate, sometimes also called didronate, alendronate with the commercial name Fosamax and risedronate (Optinate). These three compounds differ in their potency and as to their risk of causing osteomalacia as a side-effect. Didronate, therefore, has to be given intermittently with 2 weeks on and 11 weeks off, while alendronate and risedronate should be given every day. With these dosage regimens there have been no reports of the development of osteomalacia for either of the three compounds.

Also, it is important to be aware of the poor gastrointestinal absorption of bisphosphonates, namely that only a few percent or even less than 1% is absorbed. This absorption decreases even further if the drug is taken together with other nutrients such as orange juice, coffee, milk or even other drugs, especially calcium. Therefore, it is vital for efficacy that the drugs are taken on an empty stomach. It is also vital that they are taken together with appreciable water in order to avoid a local irritative side-effect on the esophagal mucosa that, in some cases, may lead to erosive esophagitis. To avoid this the patients should, after having taken the drug, refrain from lying down for a while.

Etidronate

There are a few prospective, randomized and masked studies on the effect of didronate on fracture prevention (Table 41.1). The first study, performed in 1990 by Storm et al. [30], showed an increase in bone mass, but the number of probands was too small to reveal any fracture preventive effect. However, in the same year Watts et al. [31] found that in postmenopausal women under age 75 years, who were followed for 2 years, there was a protective effect on vertebral fractures in the treated group compared with the placebo group also when the number of individuals and not only the number of fractures were counted. In a 1-year, continuous masked extension of the above study by Watts et al. [31], Harris et al. [32] proved, however, that this preventive effect on fractures disappeared when the number of individuals with a fracture was counted. There was no effect on either vertebral fractures or nonvertebral fractures after 3 years with etidronate. In another, recent, further extension of the Watts and Harris studies, Miller et al. [33] found that after 7 years of didronate treatment, of which 2 years had been open-labelled, there was a significant difference between those who had, for the 7 year study, been on 7 years or 2 years of didronate.

Personal conclusion: It is evident from several studies that didronate increases bone mass. It is less evident that it also decreases the risk of sustaining fracture. Data on this matter are rather inconsistent. I find no reason to believe, however, that the number of fractures sustained should not be reduced also after didronate therapy, albeit to a lesser extent than after therapy with alendronate or risedronate.

Alendronate

Fosamax has been investigated in considerably larger studies including more patients than has didronate. In 1995 Liberman et al. [34] concluded, from studying in a prospective, randomized, masked study almost 1000 postmenopausal women between 45 and 80 years of age for 3 years, that Fosamax decreased the risk of vertebral fractures by almost 50%. This reduction was in number of women and not number of fractures. In line with this and continuously in another, even larger study Black et al. [35] found a reduction of vertebral fractures almost identical to that Liberman had found, i.e., 50%. There was an astonishing 90% reduction in individuals who sustained multiple vertebral fracture and a reduction was also found for wrist fracture and for hip fracture. The hip fracture data, however, are in my view not very convincing. Firstly, they are just barely significant – one patient more in the treated group or one fewer in the control group and the significance would have disappeared. This I could accept if the intended 3 year trial had been allowed to continue for 3 years, but for some reason (efficacy as stated by the investigators) the otherwise exemplarily designed study was discontinued after 2.9 years instead of the intended 3 years.

Alendronate seems also to be effective in terms of increasing bone mass in recently postmenopausal women without osteoporosis. There is no evidence, however, that this increased bone mass is paralleled by a decreased fracture rate [36,37].

Personal conclusion: In individuals with osteoporosis there is no doubt that Fosamax is sufficient in terms of preventing future fractures, especially those involving the trabecular bone, such as vertebral fractures and distal radius fracture. It is also possible that this preventive effect is valid for hip fractures too, although such data are considerably weaker.

Risedronate

Just recently Risedronate (Optinate) has also been approved in many countries for treatment of osteoporosis. The basis for this approval is a study by Harris et al. [38] including initially 2458 postmenopausal women. Subjects were randomly assigned to receive oral treatment of Risedronate (2,5 or 5 mg daily) or placebo for three years. Due to negative results from other studies the 2,5 mg arm was discontinued already after a year. In Table 1 the figures of the 5 mg and the placebo groups are given. 5 mg Risedronate/day seems to prevent from not only vertebral factures but also from nonvertebral fractures.

Personal conclusion: In high risk postmenopausal women, that is women with prevalent vertebral fractures with low bone mass, Risedronate does prevent from further fractures. It has not been proven so far that the efficacy of Risedronate outshines that of Alendronate. Rather it is reasonable to believe the two drugs to be comparable.

Selective Estrogen Receptor Modulators (SERMs)

The SERMs have been developed recently and, so far, one of them, raloxifene (Evista), has been approved for clinical practice [39].

SERMs are targeted at estrogen receptors in specific organs: the skeleton, for instance. Therefore, this drug acts as an agonist in some ways with estrogen and as antagonist in other ways. Preclinical and clinical data reveal a positive effect of the drug on the skeleton. An increase in bone mass is achieved after treatment with this drug, as is fracture prevention, at least as found in radiomorphometric evaluation of vertebral bodies in a large, randomized, placebo, controlled study involving several thousand women [39]. Preliminary data suggest also that the drug is not only without the negative effects of estrogen for the evolution of breast cancer but that SERMs may even be positive in this respect, thus leading to a reduced number of breast cancers compared with the number in women who are not taking this drug. This is also in line with one of the earlier drugs of this family – tamoxifen – which has for a long time has been used as an anti-estrogen for treatment of women with breast cancer.

Personal conclusion: SERMs are very interesting new drugs not only for the treatment of osteoporosis but for possible prevention of future fractures, potential positive effects on the cardiovascular system and as inhibitors for the development of breast cancer. It is, however, still too early to decide with certainty what clinical role this drug will have in the future treatment of osteoporosis. There are reports of a high incidence of side-effects such as thromboembolism, which may limit their usefulness.

Other Drugs

Fluoride

There are numerous, randomized, double-masked studies on fluoride treatment and fracture [40–45]. The outcome of fracture prevention in these studies is conflicting, as increased, unaltered and decreased fracture rates have all been found. In some of the studies also significant side-effects were found after such treatment. The therapeutic window for fluoride treatment seems to be narrow. Fluoride is still, however, of great interest as the most efficient anabolic drug in terms of increasing bone mass.

Personal conclusion: Significant side-effects and conflicting results of studies are at present the reason why fluoride treatment can be disregarded in clinical practice. For continuing research purposes and possibly in combination with other drugs, fluoride is still interesting.

Calcitonin

There is only one prospective, randomized, masked study on the prevention of fracture with calcitonin [46]. Although the drug has a protective effect on bone loss after fracture [47] there are no convincing data to prove that calcitonin can decrease the risk of sustaining fracture (Table 41.1).

Parathyroid Hormone Peptides

There are two recent, small studies showing that parathyroid hormone (PTH) given cyclically is more effective in increasing bone mass than PTH given cyclically with sequential calcitonin [48]. Also, PTH with estrogen seem to be more efficient for increasing bone mass than estrogen alone [49]. This latter study was done in only 34 women and therefore there are no evident fracture data.

Personal conclusion: PTH-related peptides given in small and intermittent doses are promising compounds in terms of an anabolic effect on bone mass and thus a possible fracture preventive effect. To date there are no published data on the effect on fracture prevention of PTH.

Other Medicines

There are trials in progress using several other drugs intended to increase bone mass and/or decrease fracture risk. Such drugs may work primarily through anabolic stimulation of bone formation or by reducing bone resorption and thus creating a net positive effect on bone mass. To date there are no data to suggest that anabolic steroids, growth factors, prostaglandins or any other drug can prevent future fractures. Currently, the pharmaceutical industry is showing great interest in developing this type of drug and more than 20 different drugs are being tested in phase II and phase III studies [50].

Conclusion and Suggestion for an Algorithm for Investigating and Treating Osteoporosis in Orthopaedic Clinical Practice

Based on the available published data it is my conclusion that future osteoporotic fractures can to varying degrees be prevented by different nonpharmacological and pharmacological treatments.

Fracture Prevention

Physical activity:	Probably
Hip protectors:	Yes
Calcium alone:	Perhaps
Vitamin D alone:	Perhaps
Vitamin D and calcium:	Yes
Estrogen:	Yes
Etidronate:	Probably
Alendronate:	Yes
Risedronate	Yes
Raloxifen	Yes
Others	?

In orthopaedic practice almost everyone presenting with a fragility fracture is at a high risk of sustaining a new fragility fracture. As stated before, I therefore strongly advocate that all patients with such a fracture, sustained by low-energy trauma, and provided they have a positive attitude towards treatment, should be investigated by measuring their bone mass and possibly be treated for osteoporosis. Since the strict medical indications for such a bone mass measurement may vary in different age groups and depending on sex and since, furthermore, the specific treatment implemented is not uniform for all ages and for both sexes, I here conclude by providing a suggestion for how to handle these patients in orthopaedic practice. This algorithm is given in Fig. 41.1.

Patients Presenting with Low Energy Fracture

Calcium + vitamin D has been proven to be efficient for the prevention of future fractures in the very elderly and in individuals in nursing homes. In this age group there are no data on the prevention of future fractures by any other drug. Calcium + vitamin D is cheap and has few side-effects. Most of the very old, especially those in nursing homes, can be expected to lack calcium and vitamin D. Therefore there is no need for bone mass measurement in this age group. Treatment for such elderly and frail patients with calcium and vitamin D can be started without performing a bone mass measurement.

Those still living independently, excluding the biologically very oldest, should have a bone mass measurement performed, provided they are positive towards treatment. This measurement should include the hip region and possibly also the lumbar spine, the latter only if there is no coexisting and already known degenerative

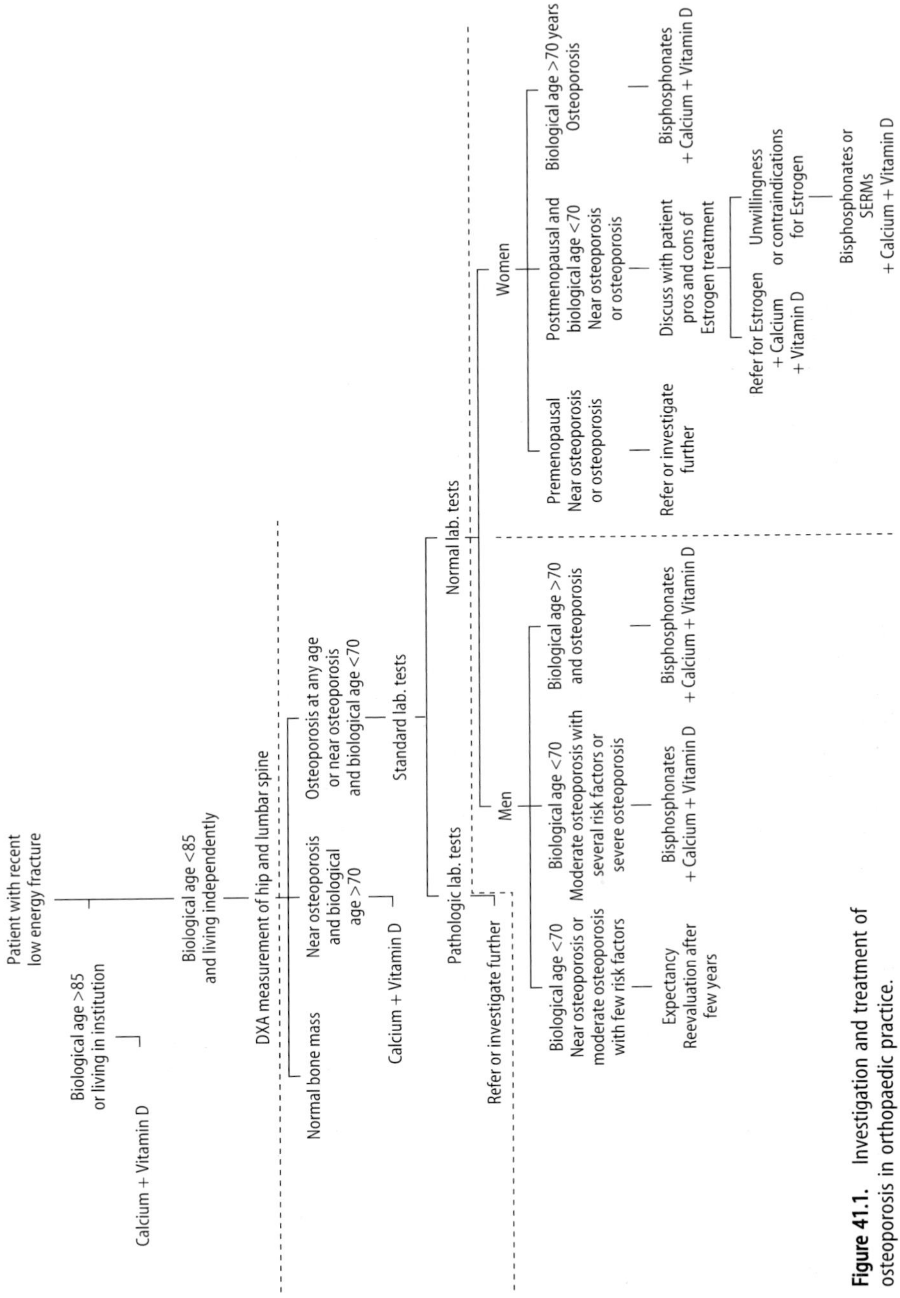

Figure 41.1. Investigation and treatment of osteoporosis in orthopaedic practice.

spine disease which may result in falsely high values for the lumbar spine. It must also be remembered that lumbar vertebrae with existing fractures will also give falsely high BMD values for the lumbar spine. Therefore, a measurement of the lumbar spine does not always give accurate results. Individuals with near-osteoporosis, i.e. a *T*-score usually between −2.0 and −2.5 and of a certain age, should benefit from prophylactic calcium and vitamin D treatment. On younger individuals with near-osteoporosis or osteoporosis, standard laboratory tests should be performed. If these tests reveal pathological results other metabolic bone disease must be suspected, such as myeloma, cancer metastasis, parathyroid hormone disease or other general and serious disease. The patient should therefore usually be referred from orthopaedic practice to the appropriate speciality. On the other hand, if the laboratory test results are normal, treatment for osteoporosis can start. Such treatment differs, of course, for the two sexes.

In men, I suggest three different treatment tracks. In fairly young individuals below biological age about 70 years and with near-osteoporosis or a moderate osteoporosis combined with few risk factors, I suggest no pharmacological treatment and re-evaluation after a few years. The reason for this is that the diagnosis of osteoporosis in men is not clearly defined and a *T*-score of −2.5 represents more absolute bone mass than in a woman and thus, at least theoretically, a lower risk of fragility fracture. Furthermore, there are no data on fracture prevention with pharmacological drugs in men, although we have no reason to expect that, for instance, the bisphosphonates should not be as effective in men as in women.

If, on the other hand, the man is still fairly young but has osteoporosis with several risk factors, I suggest treatment with bisphosphonates + calcium and vitamin D for the reason just mentioned.

For the same reason elderly men with osteoporosis should be treated with bisphosphonates + calcium and vitamin D. The indication for such treatment increases, of course, with an increased number of risk factors.

In women, I suggest three different treatment tracks. Premenopausal women with osteoporosis or near-osteoporosis should be suspected of having a metabolic bone disease and thus referred for investigation. Postmenopausal women, on the other hand, and below a biological age of about 70 years and with near-osteoporosis or osteoporosis, should be considered for estrogen treatment and this should be discussed with the patient. If the patient has a positive attitude and there are no contraindications, she should be given estrogen + calcium and vitamin D. If, on the other hand, there is an unwillingness or contraindications, bisphosphonates or SERMs should be given together with calcium and vitamin D.

In women with a biological age of or over 70 years and certified osteoporosis, I would suggest bisphosphonates + calcium and vitamin D to be given. The reason why I do not suggest the administration of SERMs at this age is the limited data and clinical experience, so far, with this new type of drug. There is no contraindication to giving estrogen instead of bisphosphonates at this age but clinical experience reveals a low compliance with estrogen at this age because of its side-effects and difficulties in coping with these.

References

1. The Swedish Council on Technology Assessment in Health Care. Mätning av bentäthet. [Bone density measurement.] SBU report no.127, 1995. In Swedish.

2. Cummings SR, Nevitt MC, Browner WS et al. Risk factors for hip fracture in white women. N Engl J Med 1995;332:767–773.
3. Johnell O, Sernbo I. Health and social status in patients with hip fractures and controls. Age Ageing 1986;15:285–291.
4. Chapuy MC, Arlot ME, Duboeuf F, et al. Vitamin D3 and calcium to prevent hip fractures in the elderly women. N Engl J Med 1992;327:1637–1642.
5. Risser WL, Lee EJ, LeBlanc A, et al. Bone density in eumenorrheic female collage athletes. Med Sci Sports Exerc 1990;22:570–574.
6. Fehling PC, Alekel L, Clasey J, Rector A, Stillman RJ. A comparison of bone mineral densities among female athletes in impact loading and active loading sports. Bone 1995;17:205–210.
7. Taaffe DR, Snow-Harter C, Connolly DA, Robinson TL, Brown MD, Marcus R. Differential effects of swimming versus weight-bearing activity on bone mineral status of eumenorrheic athletes. J Bone Miner Res 1995;10:586–593.
8. Orwoll ES, Ferar J, Oviatt SK, McClung MR, Huntington K. The relationship of swimming exercise to bone mass in men and women. Arch Intern Med 1989;149:197–200.
9. Kannus P, Haapasalo H, Sankelo M, et al. Effect of starting age of physical activity on bone mass in the dominant arm of tennis and squash players. Ann Intern Med 1995;123:27–31.
10. Krölner B, Toft B, Nielsen S, Töndevold E. Physical exercise as prophylaxis against involutional vertebral bone loss: a controlled trial. Clin Sci 1983;64:541–546.
11. Chow R, Harrison J, Notarius C. Effect of two randomized exercise programs on bone mass of healthy postmenopausal women. BMJ 1987;295:1441–1444.
12. Dalsky G, Stocke K, Ehsani A, Slatopolsy E, Lee W, Birge S. Weight-bearing exercise training and lumbar bone mineral content in postmenopausal women. Ann Intern Med 1988;108:824–828.
13. Krall E, Dawson-Hughes B. Heritable and life-style determinants of bone mineral densiy. J Bone Miner Res 1993;8:1–9.
14. Tkatch L, Rapin CH, Rizzoli R, et al. Benefits of oral protein supplementation in elderly patients with fracture of the proximal femur. J Am Coll Nutr 1992;11:519–525.
15. Karlsson KM, Johnell O, Nilsson BE, Sernbo I, Obrant KJ. Bone mineral mass in hip fracture patients. Bone 1993;14:161–165.
16. Lauritzen JB, Petersen MM, Lund B. Effect of external hip protectors on hip fractures. Lancet 1993;341:11–13.
17. Ekman A, Mallmin H, Michaelsson K, Ljunghall S. External hip protectors to prevent osteoporotic hip fractures. Lancet 1997;350:563–564.
18. Windeler J, Lange S. Events per person year: dubious concept. BMJ 1995;310:454–456.
19. Chevalley T, Rizzoli R, Nydegger V, et al. Effects of calcium supplements on femoral bone mineral density and vertebral fracture rate in vitamin-D-replete elderly patients. Osteoporos Int 1994;4:245–252.
20. Reid IR, Ames RW, Evans MC, Gamble GD, Sharpe SJ. Long-term effects of calcium supplementation on bone loss and fractures in postmenopausal women: a randomized controlled trial. Am J Med 1995;98:331–335.
21. Recker RR, Hinders S, Davies KM, et al. Correcting calcium nutritional deficiency prevents spine fractures in elderly women. J Bone Miner Res 1996;11:1961–1966.
22. Lips P, Graafmans WC, Ooms ME, Bezemer PD, Bouter LM. Vitamin D supplementation and fracture incidence in elderly persons. Ann Intern Med 1996;124:400–406.
23. Dawson-Hughes B, Harris SS, Krall EA, Dallal GE. Effect of calcium and vitamin D supplementation on bone density in men and women 65 years of age or older. N Engl J Med 1997;337:670–676.
24. Johnell O. Prevention of fractures in the elderly. A review. Acta Orthop Scand 1995;66:90–98.
25. Lufkin EG, Wahner HW, O´Fallon WM, et al. Treatment of postmenopausal osteoporosis with transdermal estrogen. Ann Intern Med 1992;117:1–9.

26. Hulley S, Grady D, Bush T, et al. Randomized trial of estrogen plus progestin for secondary prevention of coronary heart disease in postmenopausal women. Heart and estrogen/progestin replacement study (HERS) research group. JAMA 1998;280:605–613.
27. Naessen T, Persson I, Adami HO, Bergström R, Bergkvist L. Hormone replacement therapy and the risk for first hip fracture. A prospective, population-based cohort study. Ann Intern Med 1990;113:95–103.
28. Paganini-Hill A, Chao A, Ross RK, Henderson BE. Exercise and other factors in the prevention of hip fracture: the Leisure World study. Epidemiology 1991;2:16–25.
29. Cauley JA, Seeley DG, Ensrud K, Ettinger B, Black D, Cummings SR. Estrogen replacement therapy and fractures in older women. Study of Osteoporotic Fractures Research Group. Ann Intern Med 1995;122:9–16.
30. Storm T, Thamsborg G, Steiniche T, Genant HK, Sörensen OH. Effect of intermittent cyclical etidronate therapy on bone mass and fracture rate in women with postmenopausal osteoporosis. N Engl J Med 1990;322:1265–1271.
31. Watts NB, Harris ST, Genant HK, et al. Intermittent cyclical etidronate treatment of postmenopausal osteoporosis. N Engl J Med 1990;323:73–79.
32. Harris ST, Watts NB, Jackson RD, et al. Four-year study of intermittent cyclic etidronate treatment of postmenopausal osteoporosis: three years of blinded therapy followed by one year of open therapy. Am J Med 1993;95:557–567.
33. Miller PD, Watts NB, Licata AA, et al. Cyclical etidronate in the treatment of postmenopausal osteoporosis: efficacy and safety after seven years of treatment. Am J Med 1997;103:468–476.
34. Liberman UA, Weiss SR, Broll J, Minne HW, Quan H, Bell NH. Effect of oral alendronate on bone mineral density and the incidence of fractures in postmenopausal osteoporosis. The alendronate phase III osteoporosis treatment study group. N Engl J Med 1995;222:1437–1443.
35. Black DM, Cummings SR, Karpf DB, et al. Randomised trial of effect of alendronate on risk of fracture in women with existing vertebral fractures. Lancet 1996;348:1535–1541.
36. Hosking D, Chilvers CED, Christiansen C, et al. Prevention of bone loss with alendronate in postmenopausal women under 60 years of age. N Engl J Med 1998;338: 485–492.
37. Cummings SR, Black DM, Thompson DE, et al. Effect of alendronate on risk of fracture in women with low bone density but without vertebral fractures. JAMA 1998;280:2077–2082.
38. Harris ST, Watts NB, Genant HK, et al. Effects of risedronate treatment on vertebral and non vertebral fractures in women with postmenopausal osteoporosis. JAMA 1999;282:1344–1352.
39. Ettinger B, Black DM, Mitlak BH, et al. Reduction of vertebral fracture risk in postmenopausal women with osteoporosis treated with raloxifene. JAMA 1999;282:637–645.
40. Riggs BL, Hodgson SF, O´Fallon WM, et al. Effect of fluoride treatment on the fracture rate in postmenopausal women with osteoporosis. N Engl J Med 1990;322:802–809.
41. Kleerekoper M, Peterson EL, Nelson DA, et al. A randomized trial of sodium fluoride as a treatment for postmenopausal osteoporosis. Osteoporos Int 1991;1:155–161.
42. Pak CY, Sakhaee K, Piziak V, et al. Slow-release sodium fluoride in the management of postmenopausal osteoporosis. A randomized controlled trial. Ann Intern Med 1994;120:625–632.
43. Meunier PJ, Sebert JL, Reginster JY, et al. Fluoride salts are no better at preventing new vertebral fractures than calcium–vitamin D in postmenopausal osteoporosis: the FAVO Study. Osteoporos Int 1998;8:4–12.
44. Reginster JY, Meurmans L, Zegels B, et al. The effect of sodium monofluorophosphate plus calcium on vertebral fracture rate in postmenopausal women with moderate osteoporosis. A randomized, controlled trial. Ann Intern Med 1998;12:1–8.
45. Ringe JD, Dorst A, Kipshoven C, Rovati LC, Setnikar I. Avoidance of vertebral fractures in men with idiopathic osteoporosis by a three year therapy with calcium and low-dose intermittent monofluorophosphate. Osteoporos Int 1998;8:47–52.

46. Overgaard K, Hansen MA, Jensen SB, Christiansen C. Effect of salcatonin given intranasally on bone mass and fracture rates in established osteoporosis: a dose response study. BMJ 1992;305:556–561.
47. Ljunghall S, Gärdsell P, Johnell O, et al. Synthetic human calcitonin in postmenopausal osteoporosis: a placebo-controled, double-blind study. Calcif Tissue Int 1991;49:17–19.
48. Hodsman AB, Fraher LJ, Watson PH, et al. A randomized controlled trial to compare the efficacy of cyclical parathyroid hormone versus cyclical parathyroid hormone and sequential calcitonin to improve bone mass in postmenopausal women with osteoporosis. J Clin Endocrinol Metab 1997;82:620–628.
49. Lindsay R, Nieves J, Formica C, et al. Randomised controlled study of effect of parathyroid hormone on vertebral-bone mass and fracture incidence among postmenopausal women on oestrogen with osteoporosis. Lancet 1997;350:550–555.
50. Holmer AF. Pharmaceutical companies tackle diseases of aging with 178 new medicines in testing. In: New medicines in development for older Americans. PhRMA 8, 1997

Index